CYTOKINES IN THE GENESIS AND TREATMENT OF CANCER

CANCER DRUG DISCOVERY AND DEVELOPMENT

BEVERLY A. TEICHER, SERIES EDITOR

CYTOKINES IN THE GENESIS AND TREATMENT OF CANCER

Edited by

MICHAEL A. CALIGIURI, MD

*The Ohio State University Comprehensive Cancer Center
Columbus, OH*

MICHAEL T. LOTZE, MD

*University of Pittsburgh Cancer Center
Pittsburgh, PA*

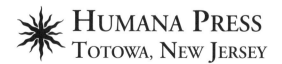

HUMANA PRESS
TOTOWA, NEW JERSEY

© 2007 Humana Press Inc.
999 Riverview Drive, Suite 208
Totowa, New Jersey 07512

www.humanapress.com

Due diligence has been taken by the publishers, editors, and authors of this book to assure the accuracy of the information published and to describe generally accepted practices. The contributors herein have carefully checked to ensure that the drug selections and dosages set forth in this text are accurate and in accord with the standards accepted at the time of publication. Notwithstanding, as new research, changes in government regulations, and knowledge from clinical experience relating to drug therapy and drug reactions constantly occurs, the reader is advised to check the product information provided by the manufacturer of each drug for any change in dosages or for additional warnings and contraindications. This is of utmost importance when the recommended drug herein is a new or infrequently used drug. It is the responsibility of the treating physician to determine dosages and treatment strategies for individual patients. Further it is the responsibility of the health care provider to ascertain the Food and Drug Administration status of each drug or device used in their clinical practice. The publisher, editors, and authors are not responsible for errors or omissions or for any consequences from the application of the information presented in this book and make no warranty, express or implied, with respect to the contents in this publication.

Cover design by Donna Niethe

Cover illustrations: B16–F10 melanoma cell-derived tumors generated in IL-5 transgenic mice display increased eosinophil accumulation in the necrotic and capsule regions with evidence of extensive eosinophil degranulation. Immunohistochemistry with the rabbit polyclonal anti-mouse MBP antisera demonstrated a dramatic eosinophilia in tumors from hypereosinophilic IL-5 transgenic mice, which replicated the spatial distribution observed in tumors from wild type mice (i.e., eosinophils accumulated only in the necrotic and capsule regions of the tumors). Higher magnification views of tumor sections revealed evidence of extensive eosinophil degranulation within the necrotic areas (i.e., diffuse reddish-purple extracellular matrix staining). Photographs were taken by Anna Taranova, Nancy Lee, and Jamie Lee (Mayo Clinic Arizona).

This publication is printed on acid-free paper. ∞

ANSI Z39.48-1984 (American National Standards Institute) Permanence of Paper for Printed Library Materials
For additional copies, pricing for bulk purchases, and/or information about other Humana titles, contact Humana at the above address or at any of the following numbers: Tel.:973-256-1699; Fax: 973-256-8341; Email: humanapr.com; or visit our Website: http://humanapress.com

Printed in the United States of America.   10 9 8 7 6 5 4 3 2 1

eISBN: 1-59745-455-9

Library of Congress Cataloging-in-Publication Data

Cytokines in the genesis and treatment of cancer / edited by Michael A. Caligiuri, Michael T. Lotze.
   p. ; cm. -- (Cancer drug discovery and development)
 Includes bibliographical references and index.
 ISBN 978-0-89603-820-2 (alk. paper)
 1. Cytokines--Therapeutic use. 2. Cancer--Chemotherapy. 3. Carcinogenesis. I. Caligiuri, Michael
A. II. Lotze, Michael T. III. Series.
 [DNLM: 1. Cytokines--therapeutic use. 2. Neoplasms--therapy. 3. Cytokines--immunology. 4.
Neoplasms--genetics. QZ 266 C997 2007]
 RC271.C95C982 2007
 616.99'406--dc22
                                                                           2007005215

For our families and those who have loved us, helped us,
and supported us along the way

FOREWORD

Cancer initiation and progression reflect the combined effects of tumor cell-autonomous genetic alterations and the complex interplay of tumor cells with nontransformed host elements. Whereas intense effort has been directed towards elucidating the mechanisms by which mutations in oncogenes and tumor suppressors give rise to the hallmarks of cancer, increasing attention is being devoted to clarifying the role of host reactions in tumor pathogenesis. Hal Dvorak's concept of cancer as a "wound that does not heal" has stimulated detailed investigations of the molecular pathways by which tumor cells subvert host factors released in response to tissue injury. While chronic inflammatory reactions usually fail to effectuate tissue repair, they may result in the persistent production of cytokines that, perhaps unintentionally, promote tumor cell growth, attenuate apoptosis, and facilitate angiogenesis, invasion, and metastasis. The delineation of these pathways and the recognition that they contribute to multiple stages of disease progression support the crafting of therapeutic strategies aimed at antagonizing these responses.

In contrast to the diverse ways in which tumor cells may exploit host reactions, other compelling data indicate that the immune system sometimes may impede tumor development. Indeed, mice rendered immune deficient by gene targeting techniques display increased tumor susceptibility, and studies in immunocompetent animals illustrate that host responses profoundly shape the immunogenicity of nascent tumors. Despite these provocative findings, however, the formation of clinically evident tumors implies a failure of protective host reactions. Some of the mechanisms underlying this immune escape have been unraveled; these include inefficient tumor antigen presentation and negative immune regulatory circuits that normally function to maintain tolerance to self-antigens. These insights have provided a strong framework for devising new approaches to enhance antitumor immunity. Early-stage clinical testing of dendritic cell-based vaccines, defined immune adjuvants, antibodies that block regulatory pathways, adoptive transfer of antigen-specific T cells, and cytokine therapies have shown considerable promise.

In *Cytokines in the Genesis and Treatment of Cancer*, Drs. Caligiuri and Lotze bring together an impressive array of internationally distinguished investigators who are devoted to the study of cytokines and cancer. Collectively, these reviews provide a comprehensive picture of the dual role of host responses in promoting and inhibiting tumor progression. The emerging intersection of cancer biology and cancer immunology is creating synergies that should accelerate the design of efficacious therapies; this volume represents an important contribution to that effort.

Glenn Dranoff, MD
Dana-Farber Cancer Institute
and Harvard Medical School
Boston, MA

Selected Reading

Dvorak, H F. Tumors: wounds that do not heal. Similarities between tumor stroma generation and wound healing. N Engl J Med 315, 1650-9 (1986).

Hanahan, D and Weinberg, RA. The hallmarks of cancer. Cell 100, 57-70. (2000).

Coussens, L and Werb, Z. Inflammation and cancer. Nature 420, 860-867 (2002).

Dranoff, G. Cytokines in cancer pathogenesis and cancer therapy. Nat Rev Cancer 4, 11-22 (2004).

Dunn, GP, Old, LJ, and Schreiber, RD. The immunobiology of cancer immunosurveillance and immunoediting. Immunity 21, 137-48 (2004).

PREFACE

A flea and a fly in a flue,
Were imprisoned, so what could they do?
Said the fly "Let us flee!"
"Let us fly!" said the flea,
And they flew through a flaw in the flue.

1. INTRODUCTION

For over two decades it has been clear that cancer is a disease of the genes, associated with stepwise acquisition of mutations or molecular flaws arising in oncogenes and tumor suppressor genes that lead to abnormal cell death and unscheduled, reparative, cellular growth. More recently, it has also become clear that cancer in adults arises most often in the setting of chronic inflammation and that critical cytokines, the hormones that regulate cell growth, cell death, and cell function, also contribute to the pathogenesis of these cancers and can be commandeered to either prevent or treat patients with cancer. This volume collects the most exciting components of this evolving story so as to further cross-fertilize the worlds of immunology and oncology, enabling conception of novel interventions for the prevention and treatment of patients with cancer. In addition, we provide an up-to-date summary and assessment of the use of cytokines in harnessing components of the body's immune and hematopoietic systems for the direct and supportive treatment of patients with cancer.

2. CYTOKINE BIOLOGY

The components of the immune system, including cytokines and the cells they act on, sit between inflammation and the genesis of cancer. Cytokines are largely released by immune cells in response to tissue inflammation caused by danger, damage, or injury secondary to either infection (providing so-called pathogen-associated molecular patterns or PAMPs, cueing inflammatory cells) or chemical/physical induced cellular damage-associated molecular patterns or DAMPs (similarly driving recruitment and activation of myeloid cells). If such insults cannot be resolved quickly, chronic cytokine deregulation can contribute to the initiation and progression of cancer through a variety of mechanisms detailed in the ensuing chapters. The dizzying array of malignancies most commonly associated with chronic inflammation as the result of infection or chemical injury include bladder cancer from infection with schistosomiasis or analine dye exposure, lung cancer from smoking or asbestos exposure, colon cancer subsequent to inflammatory bowel disease and excessive red meat consumption, gastric cancer from *Helicobacter pylori* infection, cervical cancer arising in the setting of human papilloma virus, skin cancer from ultraviolet irradiation or chronic ulceration, esophageal cancer from gastric acid reflux, esophageal and head and neck cancer from excessive alcohol and/or tobacco consumption, hepatocellular carcinoma from hepatitis B or hepatitis C viral infections, lymphoma from Epstein-Barr virus infection, and lymphoma or Kaposi's sarcoma from human herpes virus 8 infection. In some instances, the chronic use of anti-inflammatory agents has been associated with a lower incidence of cancer, lending further support to the role of chronic inflammation in the etiology of cancer.

3. MOLECULAR MECHANISMS OF CYTOKINE ASSOCIATED CARCINOGENESIS

The molecular mechanisms used by cytokines to initiate or promote carcinogenesis are fascinating yet varied and incompletely understood. Several insights derived from in vitro systems and mouse models are covered in the first two parts of this text. The cytokine macrophage-migration inhibitory factor, an active component of both local and systemic inflammation, is capable of functionally inactivating the tumor suppressor p53 as well as the Rb-E2F pathway (1,2), whereas dysregulation of IL-15 is associated with acute leukemia and a genome-wide, nonrandom methylation in the 5' regulatory regions of select genes that results in their silencing (3). The interleukin-1 [IL-1] gene is polymorphic, some variants of which strongly associate with altered secretion and the subsequent development of gastric cancer (4), appearing to be important for both tumor invasion and angiogenesis (5). TNF inhibits skeletal muscle differentiation by suppressing MyoD mRNA at the post-transcriptional level and inducing NFκB (6). These changes are associated with comorbid conditions including cancer-associated muscle wasting or cachexia, described in detail in Chapter 16.

The chapters contained within the first half of this book detail the diverse ways that individual host cytokines contribute to cancer initiation and cancer progression. Thus neutralization or disruption of their effect on host tissues should presumably prevent cancer, slow its progression, or favorably alter the threshold for apoptosis in the context of cytotoxic anticancer therapy. Most recent studies are consistent with the notion that life in the tumor microenvironment is indeed disordered, associated with hypoxia, mitotic catastrophe, autophagy, and frank necrosis and apoptosis—all means of death driven by genomic instability and chronic inflammation. In experimental animal models, elimination or neutralization of individual cytokines can adversely impact the genesis of cancer, often arising in the setting of chronic inflammation. For example, although TGF-β likely promotes the late stages of colon carcinogenesis, its absence in Rag2 deficient mice renders them more susceptible to the spontaneous development of colon cancer only when these mice are not maintained under pathogen-free conditions (ref. 7 and Chapter 5). It is more likely that a balanced symphony of cytokines is required to finely regulate tissue homeostasis, responding to tissue damage in some instances, and in others promoting neoplastic progression and reparative expansion of neoplastic clones. Elimination of any one cytokine may go unnoticed because of redundancy or may advance local environmental dysfunction in a way that exacerbates inflammation because of unexpected pleiotropy or unopposed action of other mutually antagonistic cytokines. A multitude of such scenarios is considered throughout this treatise and the results are carefully interpreted in the context of these experimental systems.

The first three chapters focus on the interface of cytokines with three infectious agents, H. pylori, HTLV-1, and human herpes viruses associated with the genesis of cancer. In each instance, only a small fraction of individuals infected with these agents eventually develop cancer. Gastric infection with H. pylori induces a persistent proinflammatory cytokine response, resulting in malignant transformation depending on the host's immune response genes along with the individual pathogen's virulence factors. Although infection with HTLV-1 is endemic in many regions of the world, the molecular mechanisms used by the virus to establish persistent infection while simultaneously circumventing immune surveillance is only partially understood. The role of cytokines and chemokines in both the transformation of infected lymphocytes to adult T-cell leukemia/lymphoma and their spread into tissues, as occurs in a small fraction of those infected with HTLV-1, is complex and carefully detailed in Chapter 2. Both human herpesvirus-4 (the Epstein-Barr virus or EBV) and human herpesvirus-8 are associated with the activation of numerous cellular cytokines and the induction of their own viral homologues of cellular cytokines. Chapter 3 reviews both viral and cellular encoded cytokines and explores their roles in malignant transformation as well as in modulating the host's immune, angiogenic, and stromagenic response.

Chapters 4–10 focus on specific cytokines and their complex roles in the initiation and promotion of cancer, providing insights in cancer prevention and treatment. Several of the factors have seemingly paradoxical functions in these processes. For example, TNF plays a role in the processes of tumor angiogenesis, metastasis, promotion, and growth, but is also applied successfully as an anticancer agent in treating patients with melanomas or sarcomas restricted to the limb in the setting of isolated limb perfusion and in combination with alkylating agents, now approved for clinical use in Europe but not yet in the United States. A review of the most recent biology of this pleiotropic molecule and its receptors here provides some clarification to help understand these seemingly contradictory observations. Likewise, TGF-β is a fascinating cytokine with a complex signaling network that alters malignant transformation by at least two distinct processes. Early in cancer initiation, TGF-β acts as a tumor suppressor inducing both cell cycle arrest and programmed cell death. However, during cancer progression, genetic mutations at the level of the receptor or in the SMAD signaling pathway can alter the tumor's response to TGF-β resulting in its paradoxical promotion of tumor invasion, metastasis, and angiogenesis. This can occur through additional signaling molecules including MAPK, JNK, ERK, PI3K, and others as discussed in Chapter 5. IL-6 is another example of a pleiotropic cytokine, this time with a pivotal role in the systemic clinical manifestations of multicentric Castleman disease and in the pathogenesis and prognosis of multiple myeloma, both detailed in Chapters 6 and 10. In addition, several other cytokines and growth factors are important in multiple myeloma and include many of those mentioned above (e.g., vascular endothelial growth factor, IL-1, and a variety of TNF family members). All of these are carefully discussed in the context of this complex and lethal disease in Chapter 10.

Several type 2 cytokines are considered in the context of oncogenesis as well as experimental therapeutics. IL-4 and IL-13 are considered collectively in Chapter 7 as their cognate receptors share at least two subunits with each other. IL-13 is implicated as an autocrine growth factor for Reed-Sternberg cells in classical Hodgkin's lymphoma. More recent experimental therapeutic interventions with a soluble IL-13 decoy receptor inhibited growth of Hodgkin's lymphoma in vitro and in vivo (8). In addition, such therapy may favorably alter the type 1/type 2 cytokine balance for enhancement of immune surveillance and tumor immunity, such as has been observed with neutralization of TGF-β (9). In addition to these neutralization approaches, this chapter reviews recently completed phase I investigations of a genetically altered IL-4 molecule linked to a toxin, exploiting the high number of IL-4 receptors expressed on the surface of certain solid tumors such as glioblastoma. Although IL-10 is primarily known as a cytokine that dampens the immune responsiveness of antigen presenting cells, it also has an immune enhancing antitumor effect for NK cells and CD8(+) T-cells. This dichotomous cytokine is carefully considered in the context of initiating the local response surrounding tumor cells as well as its role in regulating systemic responses in Chapter 9.

5. COMPLEX INTERACTIONS BETWEEN CYTOKINES AND ONCOGENESIS

Following the review of selected individual cytokines in the genesis of cancer and their uses in experimental treatment of cancer, we review more complex interactions between cytokines and cancer. Chapters 11 and 12 examine selected murine models of both cytokine-induced cancer as well as cytokine-induced prevention of cancer. Chapters 13 and 14 examine some of the early work now emerging from the study of cytokines within the tumor stroma. This is followed by a review of the network of chemokines and chemokine-receptor expression in the context of both the tumor microenvironment and tumor progression. Chapter 16 deals with the complex and poorly understood process of cancer-induced cachexia or muscle wasting, with a special focus on the role of TNF-α in this condition that so often limits the successful treatment of certain solid tumors.

6. APPLICATION OF CYTOKINE-BASED THERAPEUTICS

Although cytokine networks are complex, there has been notable progress, both in animal models of cancer and in humans with cancer or cancer susceptibility, in demonstrating the use of cytokine or anticytokine therapies for the prevention and treatment of cancer. In the second half of the book, we focus on cytokines that have either been FDA approved for the treatment of patients with cancer or are now in clinical development. The first cytokine commercially approved for the treatment of patients with cancer was IL-2. The history of its development, as well as the data supporting the two cancers for which IL-2 is approved (renal cell carcinoma and melanoma), and a multitude of experimental avenues currently being investigated are all reviewed in Chapter 17. Although IL-12 is not commercially approved for the treatment of patients with cancer, this fascinating cytokine has a strong preclinical track record supporting its use as an anticancer agent. Chapter 18 reviews IL-12 biology, preclinical and clinical development in a variety of solid and hematologic malignancies, as well as its use in combination with antibodies and chemotherapy. The application of IL-18, another interferon-γ inducing cytokine recently introduced in the treatment of patients with cancer in phase I and II studies, is considered in the chapter on the IL-1 family members, which now number ten. Perhaps the best-studied cytokines are the type I interferons, approved for the treatment of patients with chronic myeloid leukemia, melanoma, and renal cell carcinoma. The successes and limitations with interferon therapy are carefully reviewed in Chapter 19 along with an excellent summary of its cellular and molecular effects as well as our understanding of its role in the immune response. Chapter 20 reviews preclinical rationale and clinical development of cytokine combinations for the treatment of patients with cancer. Virtually every combination that is reviewed in this chapter contains cytokines as individual agents previously presented in this book. This is next followed by a chapter reviewing the history and current preclinical and clinical status of tumor reactive antibodies chemically linked to immune activating cytokines for the experimental treatment of patients with cancer, with an emphasis on pediatric solid tumors in the setting of minimal residual disease. Given that most cytokines regulate immunity at a local or regional level, Chapter 22 reviews the limitations to date in systemic delivery of cytokines to enhance vaccination with tumor-associated antigens, as well as the history and future application of loco-regional delivery of cytokines in the form of gene therapy as a more promising means to boost such vaccination.

Insights in cytokine biology enabling the successful treatment of patients with cancer are summarized here. Chapter 23 reviews the experimental use of tumor necrosis factor-α (TNF-α)-neutralization to enhance tolerance and sensitivity to cancer chemotherapy, whereas Chapter 24 reviews the highly successful application of cytokines including GM- and G-CSF in the reduction of serious infection encountered by cancer patients undergoing intensive myelosuppressive chemotherapy with curative intent.

7. SUMMARY

To be sure, we are only at the beginning of understanding what is now appreciated as a very complex relationship between the immune cells, the extended family of cytokines, chemokines, and defensins, and the genesis and treatment of patients with cancer. As this book is being assembled there are hundreds of articles being published that cannot be included but serve as the basis for updates and the next edition. Clearly, a deep understanding of the Darwinian nature of cancer/cytokine biology is in its infancy. The interventions to come from genetically altered mouse models as well as preclinical and clinical trials will provide enormous advances in our understanding of how immune cells and the cytokines that they respond to and secrete influence cancer progression. As we begin to dissect this relationship and target individual components of the cytokine milieu for the prevention and treatment of patients with cancer, we will begin to make real progress. It is with this in the forefront of our minds that we provide this first edition on the subject. It is our hope that this stimulates provocative approaches that both promote protective antitumor host responses and inhibit those that appear to contribute to the genesis of cancer.

Michael A. Caligiuri, MD
Michael T. Lotze, MD

REFERENCES

1. Hudson JD, Shoaibi MA, Maestro R, Carnero A, Hannon GJ, Beach DH. A proinflammatory cytokine inhibits p53 tumor suppressor activity. J Exp Med 1999; 190:1375-1382.
2. Petrenko O, Moll UM. Macrophage migration inhibitory factor MIF interferes with the Rb-E2F pathway. Mol Cell 2005; 17:225-236.
3. Kukita T, Arima N, Matsushita K, et al. Autocrine and/or paracrine growth of adult T-cell leukaemia tumour cells by interleukin 15. Br J Haematol 2002; 119:467-474.
4. El-Omar EM, Carrington M, Chow WH, et al. The role of interleukin-1 polymorphisms in the pathogenesis of gastric cancer. Nature 2001; 412:99.
5. Voronov E, Shouval DS, Krelin Y, et al. IL-1 is required for tumor invasiveness and angiogenesis. Proc Natl Acad Sci USA 2003; 100:2645-2650.
6. Langen RC, Van Der Velden JL, Schols AM, Kelders MC, Wouters EF, Janssen-Heininger YM. Tumor necrosis factor-alpha inhibits myogenic differentiation through MyoD protein destabilization. FASEB J 2004; 18:227-237.
7. Engle SJ, Ormsby I, Pawlowski S, et al. Elimination of colon cancer in germ-free transforming growth factor beta 1-deficient mice. Cancer Res 2002; 62:6362-6366.
8. Trieu Y, Wen XY, Skinnider BF, et al. Soluble interleukin-13Rα2 decoy receptor inhibits Hodgkin's lymphoma growth in vitro and in vivo. Cancer Res 2004; 64:3271-3275.
9. Dierksheide JE, Baiocchi RA, Ferketich AK, et al. IFN-γ gene polymorphisms associate with development of EBV+ lymphoproliferative disease in hu PBL-SCID mice. Blood 2005; 105:1558-1565.

CONTENTS

CONTRIBUTORS

MARK R. ALBERTINI, MD • *Associate Professor, Section of Hematology and Medical Oncology, Department of Medicine, University of Wisconsin Medical School, Madison, WI*

PAOLA ALLAVENA, MD • *Department of Immunology and Cell Biology, Istituto Mario Negri, Milano, Italy*

G. MARK ANDERSON, PHD • *Assistant Director, Oncology Research, Centocor, Inc., Malvern, PA*

KENNETH C. ANDERSON, MD • *The Jerome Lipper Multiple Myeloma Center, Department of Medical Oncology, Dana Farber Cancer Institute, Harvard Medical School, Boston, MA*

TIMOTHY E. BAEL, MD • *Biologic Therapy Program, Division of Hematology and Oncology, Duke University Medical Center, Durham, NC*

ALYSSA R. BONINE-SUMMERS • *Vanderbilt-Ingram Comprehensive Cancer Center, Department of Cancer Biology, Vanderbilt University Medical Center, Nashville, TN*

CHARLES K. BROWN, MD, PHD • *Assistant Professor of Surgery, Division of Surgical Oncology, University of Pittsburgh School of Medicine, Pittsburgh, PA*

MICHAEL A. CALIGIURI, MD • *The Ohio State University Comprehensive Cancer Center, Columbus, OH*

WILLIAM E. CARSON, III, MD • *Departments of Medical Microbiology, Virology, and Immunology and of Surgery, The Comprehensive Cancer Center, The Ohio State University College of Medicine, Columbus, OH*

DHARMINDER CHAUHAN, JD, PHD • *The Jerome Lipper Multiple Myeloma Center, Department of Medical Oncology, Dana Farber Cancer Institute, Harvard Medical School, Boston, MA*

JOSEPH CLARK, MD • *Departments of Medicine and Hematology/Oncology, Cardinal Bernardin Cancer Center, Loyola University Health System, Maywood, IL*

SETH M. COHEN, MD • *Division of Hematology/Oncology, Continuum Cancer Center, St. Luke's–Roosevelt Hospital Center, New York, NY*

MEGAN A. COOPER, MD, PHD • *The Jerome Lipper Multiple Myeloma Center, Department of Medical Oncology, Dana Farber Cancer Institute, Harvard Medical School, Boston, MA*

ERIKA CRETNEY • *Cancer Immunology Program, Peter MacCallum Cancer Centre, Melbourne, Victoria, Australia*

MARK DEWITTE, DVM • *Director, Clinical Hematology/Oncology Research, Centocor Inc., Malvern, PA*

TODD A. FEHNIGER, MD, PHD • *Division of Hematology and Oncology, Department of Internal Medicine, Washington University School of Medicine, St. Louis, MO*

SHIN-ICHIRO FUJII, MD, PHD • *Unit for Cellular Immunotherapy, RIKEN Research Center for Allergy and Immunology (RCAI), Laboratory for Cellular Immunotherapy, Yokohama, Japan*

STEPHEN D. GILLIES, PHD • *EMD-Lexigen Research Center, Billerica, MA*

JOHN A. GLASPY, MD • *Professor of Medicine, Sanders Endowed Chair in Cancer Research, Division of Hematology-Oncology, Department of Medicine, UCLA School of Medicine, Jonsson Comprehensive Cancer Center, Los Angeles, CA*

JARED A. GOLLOB, MD • *Director, Biologic Therapy Program, Associate Professor of Medicine and Immunology, Duke University Medical Center, Durham, NC*

DENIS C. GUTTRIDGE, PHD • *Human Cancer Genetics Program, Department of Molecular Virology, Immunology, and Medical Genetics, The Ohio State University College of Medicine, Columbus, OH*

JACKIE A. HANK, PHD • *University of Wisconsin Paul P. Carbone Comprehensive Cancer Center, Madison, WI*

YOSHIHIRO HAYAKAWA, PHD • *Cancer Immunology Program, Peter MacCallum Cancer Centre, Melbourne, Victoria, Australia*

HEATHER R. HENSLER, BS • *Department of Infectious Diseases and Microbiology, University of Pittsburgh School of Medicine, Pittsburgh, PA*

TERU HIDESHIMA, PHD • *The Jerome Lipper Multiple Myeloma Center, Department of Medical Oncology, Dana Farber Cancer Institute, Harvard Medical School, Boston, MA*

FRANK J. JENKINS, PHD • *Departments of Pathology and of Infectious Diseases and Microbiology, University of Pittsburgh School of Medicine, Pittsburgh, PA*

HOWARD L. KAUFMAN, MD, FACS • *Chief, Division of Surgical Oncology, Columbia University College of Physicians and Surgeons, New York, NY*

KOJI KAWAKAMI, MD, PHD • *NCI, Division of Cellular and Gene Therapies, CBER-FDA, Bethesda, MD*

JOHN M. KIRKWOOD, MD • *Division of Hematology and Oncology, Department of Medicine, University of Pittsburgh Cancer Institute, Pittsburgh, PA*

MICHAEL D. LAIRMORE, DVM, PHD • *Professor and Chair, Department of Veterinary Biosciences, The Ohio State University, Columbus, OH*

BRIAN K. LAW, PHD • *Department of Pharmacology and Therapeutics, University of Florida College of Medicine, Gainesville, FL*

GREGORY B. LESINSKI, PHD • *Department of Medical Microbiology, Virology, and Immunology, The Comprehensive Cancer Center, The Ohio State University College of Medicine, Columbus, OH*

MICHAEL T. LOTZE, MD • *Director, Translational Research, Molecular Medicine Institute, University of Pittsburgh School of Medicine, Pittsburgh, PA*

ALBERTO MANTOVANI, MD • *Department of Immunology and Cell Biology, Mario Negri Institute; Centro IDET, Institute of General Pathology, University of Milan, Milan, Italy*

FEDERICA MARCHESI • *Department of Immunology and Cell Biology, Mario Negri Institute, Milan, Italy*

KIM MARGOLIN, MD • *City of Hope National Medical Center, Duarte, CA*

STERGIOS J. MOSCHOS, MD • *Department of Medicine, University of Pittsburgh Cancer Institute, Pittsburgh, PA*

HAROLD L. MOSES, MD • *Vanderbilt-Ingram Comprehensive Cancer Center, Department of Cancer Biology, Vanderbilt University Medical Center, Nashville, TN*

MARIAN T. NAKADA, PHD • *Senior Director, Oncology Research, Centocor Inc., Malvern, PA*

NORIHIRO NISHIMOTO, MD, PHD • *Professor, Laboratory of Immune Regulation, Graduate School of Frontier Biosciences, Osaka University, Osaka, Japan*

HIDEHO OKADA MD, PHD • *Assistant Professor of Neurosurgery and Surgery, University of Pittsburgh Medical Center/Cancer Institute, Research Pavilion at the Hillman Cancer Center, Pittsburgh, PA*

MICHAEL C. OSTROWSKI, PHD • *Professor and Chair, Department of Molecular and Cellular Biochemistry, The Ohio State University Comprehensive Cancer Center, Columbus, OH*

RICHARD M. PEEK, JR., MD • *Director, Division of Gastroenterology, Vanderbilt University School of Medicine, Nashville, TN*

RAJ K. PURI, MD, PHD • *NCI, Division of Cellular and Gene Therapies, CBER-FDA, Bethesda, MD*

LEE RATNER, MD, PHD • *Department of Medicine, Pathology, and Molecular Microbiology, Washington University School of Medicine, St. Louis, MO*

SHARMILA ROY-CHOWDHURY, MD • *Assistant Professor of Surgery, Loma Linda University School of Medicine, Loma Linda, CA*

DAVID J. SHEALY, PHD • *Associate Director, Immunobiology Research, Centocor Inc., Malvern, PA*

MARK J. SMYTH • *Cancer Immunology Program, Peter MacCallum Cancer Centre, Melbourne, Victoria, Australia*

PAUL M. SONDEL, MD, PHD • *Professor, Departments of Pediatrics and Human Oncology, University of Wisconsin Medical School; University of Wisconsin Paul P. Carbone Comprehensive Cancer Center, Madison WI*

SHAYNA E. A. STREET, PHD • *Cancer Immunology Program, Peter MacCallum Cancer Centre, Melbourne, Victoria, Australia*

MIGUEL A. VILLALONA-CALERO, MD, FACP • *Division of Hematology–Oncology, Department of Internal Medicine, The Ohio State University College of Medicine, Columbus, OH*

I

INFECTIOUS AGENTS, CYTOKINES, AND CANCER

1

Helicobacter pylori and Cytokines in the Genesis of Gastric Cancer

Richard M. Peek, Jr.

CONTENTS

1. INTRODUCTION

Rudolph Virchow pioneered the hypothesis that inflammation exerts a profound influence on the development and biological behavior of cancer nearly 150 years ago, and since that time it has become increasingly apparent that microbial pathogens contribute to the genesis of a substantial number of malignancies worldwide *(1)*. Conservative estimates indicate that nearly 15% of all cancer cases are attributable to infectious agents, translating to a malignant burden of 1.2 million cases per year *(1)*. One mechanism that contributes to carcinogenesis induced by chronic pathogens is the concomitant inflammatory response that leads to the production of mutagenic substances, such as nitric oxide *(2)*. Nitric oxide, in turn, can be converted to reactive nitrogen species, which nitrosylate a variety of cellular targets including DNA and proteins, and similarly, superoxide anion radicals generated by polymorphonuclear cells induce DNA damage through the formation of DNA adducts. Viral agents can directly transform host cells by integrating active oncogenes into the host genome *(1)*. Thus, there is precedence and support for the concept that infectious agents can initiate or promote pathways that eventuate in neoplasia.

Gastric adenocarcinoma is the second leading cause of cancer-related death in the world *(3)*, and two histologically distinct variants have been described. Diffuse-type

From: *Cancer Drug Discovery and Development,*
Cytokines in the Genesis and Treatment of Cancer
Edited by: M. A. Caligiuri and M. T. Lotze © Humana Press Inc., Totowa, NJ

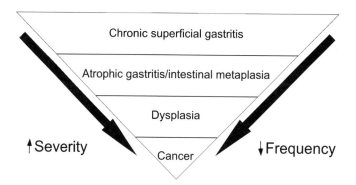

Fig. 1. Complications of *Helicobacter pylori* colonization.

gastric cancer most commonly affects younger persons and consists of individually infiltrating neoplastic cells that do not form glandular structures *(4)*. In contrast, intestinaltype adenocarcinoma occurs at a later age and progresses through a well-defined series of histologic steps initiated by the transition from normal mucosa to chronic superficial gastritis, which then leads to atrophic gastritis and intestinal metaplasia, and finally to dysplasia and adenocarcinoma (Fig. 1) *(3,4)*. *Helicobacter pylori* is a Gram-negative bacterial species that selectively colonizes gastric mucosa, and virtually all persons who are colonized by this organism develop coexisting gastritis, a signature feature of which is the capacity to persist for decades. This is in marked contrast to inflammatory reactions induced by other Gram-negative enteric pathogens, such as *Salmonella*, that either resolve within days to weeks or progress to eliminate the host. However, there is a biological cost incurred by long-term relationships between *H. pylori* and humans in that chronic inflammation confers a significantly increased risk of serious disease, including gastric adenocarcinoma (Fig. 1; refs. *5–20*).

Epidemiological studies in humans and experimental infections in rodents have clearly demonstrated that interactions between *H. pylori* and its host significantly increase the risk for atrophic gastritis, intestinal metaplasia, and distal gastric adenocarcinoma *(2,3)*. Based on these data, the World Health Organization has classified *H. pylori* as a class I carcinogen for gastric cancer, and because virtually all infected persons have superficial gastritis, it is likely that the organism plays a causative role early in this progression (Fig. 1). Although persistent *H. pylori* infection is the strongest identified risk factor for malignancies that arise within the stomach, only a small percentage of colonized persons ever develop neoplasia, raising the hypothesis that enhanced cancer risk involves specific and well-choreographed interactions between pathogen and host, which, in turn, are dependent on strain-specific bacterial factors and inflammatory responses governed by host genetic diversity. The inflammatory infiltrate that develops in response to *H. pylori* is orchestrated by cytokines, which facilitate chemoattraction of hematopoietic populations, recruit downstream effector cells, and determine the natural history of an inflammatory response. Thus, a clear understanding of how *H. pylori* initiates gastric cancer necessitates understanding how *H. pylori* induces gastritis and this chapter will therefore focus on specific mechanisms by which *H. pylori* colonization leads to gastric inflammation and injury via manipulation of the host cytokine response.

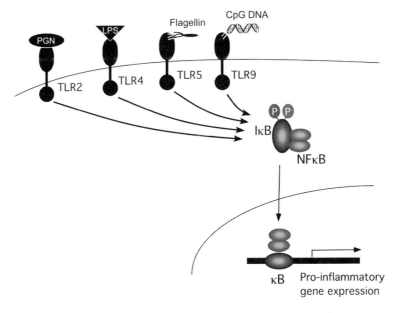

Fig. 2. Toll-like receptors (TLRs) that recognize microbe-associated molecular patterns. PGN, peptidoglycan; LPS, lipopolysaccharide; CpG, cytidine-phosphate-guanosine.

2. *H. PYLORI*-INDUCED GASTRIC INFLAMMATION

If a bacterial species is to persistently colonize a mammalian host, its most formidable challenge is to evade immune clearance. One mechanism through which *H. pylori* may persist is by limiting the bactericidal effects of pro-inflammatory molecules, such as nitric oxide *(21)*. Another level of host defense that may be circumvented by *H. pylori* is innate immunity. Toll-like receptors (TLRs) are an evolutionarily conserved family of eukaryotic receptors that function in innate immunity via recognition of invariant regions in bacterial molecules termed pathogen- or microbe-associated molecular patterns *(22–24)*. Although the bacterial ligands for TLRs are distinct, signaling pathways used by these receptors all appear to eventuate in NF-κB activation and pro-inflammatory gene expression (Fig. 2). It is becoming increasingly clear, however, that *H. pylori* has evolved strategies to avoid activation of this system. For example, TLR4 recognizes bacterial lipopolysaccharide (LPS), yet *H. pylori* LPS is relatively anergic compared with that of other enteric bacteria, primarily because of lipid A core modifications *(25–27)*. In contrast to flagellins expressed by Gram-negative mucosal pathogens that activate TLR5-mediated pro-inflammatory responses, *H. pylori* flagellin is noninflammatory *(28,29)*. *H. pylori* can also facilitate persistence by varying the antigenic repertoire of surface-exposed proteins *(30)* and by actively suppressing the host adaptive immune response *(31–34)*. However, despite these strategies for evading clearance, substantial immune activation still occurs during colonization as manifested by epithelial cytokine release, infiltration of the gastric mucosa by inflammatory cells, and cellular and humoral recognition of *H. pylori* antigens *(27)*.

The gastric inflammatory response induced by *H. pylori* consists of neutrophils, lymphocytes (T and B-cells), plasma cells, and macrophages, along with varying degrees of epithelial cell degeneration and injury *(35)*. Invasion of the gastric mucosa is rarely if at all identified in vivo, and therefore other potential mechanisms for induction of inflammation must be postulated. One possibility is that *H. pylori* secrete substances that stimulate mucosal inflammation from afar. For example, urease has been detected within the lamina propria and the urease complex of *H. pylori* stimulates chemotaxis by both monocytes and neutrophils and activates mononuclear cells as well *(35)*. Similarly, *H. pylori* porins and low-molecular-weight molecules possess chemotactic properties *(36)*. *H. pylori* water extracts promote neutrophil-endothelial cell interactions in vitro and increase leukocyte adherence via CD11a/CD18 and CD11b/CD18 interactions with intercellular adhesion molecule type-1 (ICAM-1) *(38,39)*.

2.1. H. pylori *Contact-Mediated Cytokine Release and the Development of Acute Inflammation*

The presence of acute inflammatory components within *H. pylori*-infected mucosa suggests that soluble mediators capable of attracting polymorphonuclear cells (PMNs) are key regulators in disease development. Therefore, another mechanism through which *H. pylori* may induce inflammation is via direct contact with gastric epithelial cells and stimulation of cytokine release. Gastric epithelium from infected persons contains increased levels of interleukin-1β (IL-1β), IL-2, IL-6, IL-8, and TNF-α *(40–44)*, and within this group, IL-8 has been studied most intensively as a mediator of *H. pylori*-induced gastritis. IL-8 is a potent neutrophil-activating chemokine that is secreted by gastrointestinal epithelial cells in response to infection with pathogenic bacteria *(45)*, and IL-8 produced by activated enterocytes binds to the extracellular matrix and establishes a haptotactic gradient that directs inflammatory cell migration towards the epithelial cell surface *(46–49)*. Consistent with these observations for infected intestinal epithelial cells, expression of IL-8 is increased within *H. pylori*-colonized gastric mucosa *(43,50)* where it localizes to gastric epithelial cells *(50)*, and levels of IL-8 are directly related to the severity of gastritis *(43)*. In vitro, *H. pylori* stimulates IL-8 expression and release from gastric epithelial cells and these events are dependent on an active interplay between viable bacteria and epithelial cells *(51–53)*. Thus, a paradigm for the acute component of *H. pylori*-induced gastric inflammation is that contact between bacteria and epithelial cells stimulates IL-8 secretion, which then regulates neutrophilic infiltration into the gastric mucosa.

2.1.1. MOLECULAR REGULATION OF *H. PYLORI*-INDUCED IL-8 GENE EXPRESSION

Pro-inflammatory cytokine expression is often regulated at the mRNA level by soluble transcription factors and the human IL-8 gene contains several motifs within its promoter region including binding sites for NF-κB, NF-IL6, AP-1 (which is composed of the binding elements c-*fos* and c-*jun*), and a recently identified novel element that is homologous to an interferon-stimulated responsive element (ISRE) (Fig. 3) *(54–57)*. NF-κB constitutes a family of transcription factors sequestered in the cytoplasm, whose activation is tightly controlled by a class of inhibitory proteins termed IκBs *(58)*. Multiple signals, including microbial contact, stimulate phosphorylation of IκB by IκB kinase β (IKKβ), which leads to proteasome-mediated degradation of phospho-IκB, thereby liberating NF-κB to enter the nucleus where it regulates transcription of a variety of genes, including immune response genes (Fig. 3) *(59)*. Stimulation and activation of NF-κB does not require protein synthesis, thereby allowing efficient activation of target genes, such as IL-8. This system is particularly used in immune and inflammatory

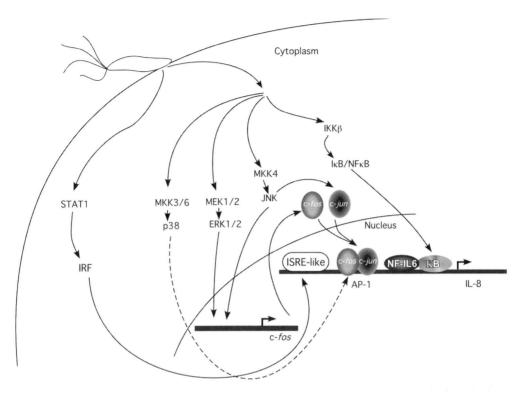

Fig. 3. *Helicobacter pylori* activates multiple signaling pathways in gastric epithelial cells. IKK, IκB kinase; MKK, MAP kinase kinase; JNK, c-Jun amino-terminal kinase; MEK, mitogen-activated protein kinase kinase; ERK, extracellular signal-regulated protein kinase; IRF, interferon-regulatory factor; STAT, signal transducer and activator of transcription; ISRE, interferon-stimulatory response element; κB, Kappa B; NF, nuclear factor; AP-1, activation protein-1.

responses where rapid activation of defense genes following exposure to pathogens such as bacteria is critical for survival of an organism. Several studies have demonstrated that contact between *H. pylori* and gastric epithelial cells results in brisk activation of NF-κB, which is followed by increased IL-8 expression (Fig. 3) *(54,57,60–62)*. The ability of *H. pylori* to activate NF-κB in vitro has also been corroborated in vivo as activated NF-κB is present within gastric epithelial cells of infected, but not uninfected patients *(60)*, which mirror the topography of increased IL-8 protein within colonized mucosa.

Mitogen-activated protein kinases (MAPK) also mediate *H. pylori*-dependent IL-8 expression. MAPK are signal transduction networks that target transcription factors such as AP-1 and participate in a diverse array of cellular functions, including cytokine expression *(63–65)*. MAPK cascades are organized in three-kinase tiers consisting of a MAPK, an MAPK kinase (MKK), and an MKK kinase (MKKK), and transmission of signals occurs by sequential phosphorylation and activation of components specific to a respective cascade (Fig. 3). In mammalian systems, at least five MAPK modules have been identified and characterized to date; these include extracellular signal-regulated kinase 1 and 2 (ERK 1/2), p38, and c-Jun N-terminal kinase (JNK) *(63–65)*. Our laboratory and others have demonstrated that *H. pylori* activates p38, ERK 1/2, and JNK in gastric epithelial cells in vitro *(66–68)* (Fig. 3), and that activation of ERK1/2 is dependent on transactivation of the EGF receptor, a receptor tyrosine kinase *(69)*. An important question raised by these studies is whether *H. pylori*-induced IL-8 production is dependent on NF-κB, MAPK, or both.

Cell culture studies have revealed that *H. pylori*-induced IL-8 expression is dependent on both NF-κB and MAPK activation of AP-1 *(54)*, and such cross-talk between NF-κB and MAPK pathways has been demonstrated previously. For example, MEKK1, a hierarchical MAPK kinase, can directly activate the IκB kinase signal *(59,70)*. However, inhibition of ERK 1/2 attenuates *H. pylori*-induced IL-8 secretion without affecting NF-κB *(66)*, raising the possibility that synergistic interactions between AP-1 and NF-κB occur within the IL-8 promoter. Consistent with these data, *H. pylori* activation of ERK 1/2 results in enhanced c-*fos* transcription *(67,68)*, indicating that ERK 1/2 may exert regulatory effects on IL-8 production that are primarily dependent on AP-1 (Fig. 3). An additional layer of complexity is added when one considers the recent finding that maximal *H. pylori*-induced IL-8 gene transcription requires the presence of NF-κB, AP-1, and ISRE elements (Fig. 3) *(57)*. Collectively, these data indicate that the mucosal inflammatory reaction that develops in response to *H. pylori* involves multiple intracellular pathways converging on the IL-8 promoter and that *H. pylori*-mediated host signaling is of central importance for understanding the inflammatory response to this pathogen, which if left untreated over decades, may progress to gastric cancer.

2.2. Humoral Responses to **H. pylori**

Although *H. pylori* colonization induces an exuberant systemic and mucosal humoral response directed at multiple antigens *(71–76)*, antibody production does not result in eradication even though this organism is susceptible in vitro to antibody-dependent complement-mediated phagocytosis and killing *(77,78)*. The ineffective humoral response generated against *H. pylori* and its components have led some investigators to speculate that this may actually contribute to pathogenesis. Monoclonal antibodies directed against *H. pylori* cross-react with gastric epithelium of both mice and humans and delivery of these antibodies alone to mice can induce gastritis *(79)*. In colonized human patients, *H. pylori* induces the formation of antibodies that recognize the H^+–K^+ ATPase epitope on the luminal surface of acid-secreting parietal cells *(79,80)*. IgM antibodies generated by immortalized B-cells obtained from *H. pylori*-colonized gastric mucosa also recognize gastric epithelium *(81)*. These findings indicate that the humoral response to *H. pylori* may contribute to the development of distinct histologic lesions. For example, an autoimmune reaction against parietal cells may lead to gastric atrophy with a concomitant reduction in gastric acidity; conversely, immunoglobulin-mediated destruction of epithelial cells may initiate or maintain mucosal inflammation and epithelial cell injury.

2.3. Cell-Mediated Adaptive Immune Responses to **H. pylori**

The ability of the gastrointestinal tract to discern pathogenic bacteria from commensals is regulated through T-cell-dependent responses. CD4$^+$ T-cells can be broadly divided into two functional subsets, type 1 (Th1) and type 2 (Th2) T-helper cells, each of which are defined by distinct patterns of cytokine secretion. Th1 cells produce IL-2 and IFN-γ and promote cell-mediated immune responses whereas Th2 cells secrete IL-4, IL-5, IL-6, and IL-10 and induce B-cell activation and differentiation *(82)*. The type of immune response to a particular microbial agent is governed by preferential expansion of one T-helper cell subset accompanied by a corresponding and relative down-regulation of the other *(82)*. In general, most intracellular bacteria induce Th1 responses, whereas extracellular pathogens stimulate Th2 type responses. The importance of CD4$^+$ T-cells in *H. pylori*-induced inflammation is evidenced by studies using genetic models of immunodeficiency. Compared to wild-type mice, severe combined immunodeficiency (SCID) and T-cell deficient mice infected with *Helicobacter* develop less severe mucosal injury despite similar levels of bacterial density, whereas infected B-cell deficient mice are no different than wild-type littermates in the progression to gastric atrophy or metaplasia *(83–85)*.

Although the acquired immune response to *H. pylori* is composed of both Th1- and Th2-type cells, cytokine profiles indicate a Th1 predominance, as the majority of *H. pylori* antigen-specific T-cell clones isolated from infected gastric mucosa produce higher levels of IFN-γ than IL-4 *(86)*. Consistent with these observations, *H. pylori* stimulates the production of IL-12 in vitro, a cytokine that promotes Th1 differentiation *(87)*. This is somewhat counterintuitive based on the fact that *H. pylori* is noninvasive and that infection is accompanied by an exuberant humoral response, but studies now suggest that this Th1-biased response may actually play an important role in pathogenesis. *H. pylori* infection of IFN-γ deficient mice (that fail to mount an appropriate Th1 response) leads to decreased levels of gastric inflammation and atrophy compared to wild-type mice *(88–90)*. In vivo neutralization of IFN-γ in mice infected with a related *Helicobacter* species (*H. felis*) similarly reduces the severity of gastritis *(91)*, whereas gastric inflammation and atrophy can be correspondingly induced by delivering infusions of IFN-γ, even in the absence of *Helicobacter (92)*. Certain strains of mice (C57/BL6) infected with *H. felis* that mount a polarized Th1-type response develop extensive gastric inflammation, whereas genetically distinct strains (BALB/c) that respond to infection with a Th2-like response develop only minimal gastritis *(93)*. Adoptive transfer of Th1-type cells from *Helicobacter*-infected donor mice into infected recipients increases the severity of gastritis, whereas transfer of Th2-primed lymphocytes reduces colonization density *(94)*. Finally, antecedent challenge with a helminth *(Heligmosomoides polygyrus)* that induces a Th2-type mucosal reaction significantly attenuates the development of Th1-mediated gastritis and atrophy in response to *H. felis (95)*. These data are consistent with a model in which an inappropriate host T-cell response towards *H. pylori* facilitates the development of gastric inflammation and injury.

3. ADDITIONAL EFFECTORS OF INFLAMMATION THAT MAY BE RELATED TO *H. PYLORI*-INDUCED GASTRIC CARCINOGENESIS

In addition to stimulating the production of cytokines, *H. pylori* also activates proinflammatory cyclooxygenase (COX) enzymes. Cyclooxygenases catalyze key steps in the conversion of arachidonic acid to endoperoxide (PGH$_2$), a substrate for a variety of prostaglandin synthases that, in turn, catalyze the formation of prostaglandins and other eicosanoids (Fig. 4) *(96)*. Prostaglandins regulate a diverse array of physiologic processes including immunity, maintenance of vascular tone and integrity, nerve development, and bone metabolism *(96)*. Three isoforms of cyclooxygenase have been identified to date, each possessing similar activities, but differing in expression characteristics and inhibition profiles by nonsteroidal anti-inflammatory drus (NSAIDs). COX-1 was purified in 1976 and is expressed constitutively in many cells and tissues *(97,98)*. A second COX enzyme, COX-2, was later identified *(99,100)*, and in contrast to COX-1, COX-2 expression is inducible in cells transformed with the oncogene *v-src* or treated with phorbol esters

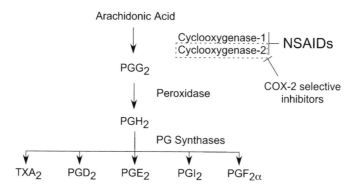

Fig. 4. Prostaglandin (PG) synthesis in despendent on cyclooxygenases. PG, prostaglandin; TXA, thromboxane; NSAIDs, nonsteroidal antiinflammatory drugs.

(100,101). Subsequent studies have now shown that COX-2 can be induced by a variety of growth factors and pro-inflammatory cytokines such as TNF-α, IFN-γ, and IL-1 in a number of pathophysiologic conditions *(98).* COX-2 expression is increased in gastric epithelial cells co-cultured with *H. pylori (102,103)* and within gastric mucosa of *H. pylori*-infected individuals *(104,105).* COX-2 expression is further increased within *H. pylori*-induced premalignant (atrophic gastritis and intestinal metaplasia) and malignant (adenocarcinoma) lesions *(106,107)* and COX-inhibitors such as aspirin and other NSAIDs have been shown to decrease the risk for distal gastric cancer *(108,109).* *H. pylori* also activates phospholipase A$_2$, an enzyme that catalyzes the formation of the prostaglandin precursor arachidonic acid, in vitro and in vivo *(110,111).*

The inflammatory response induced by *H. pylori* leads to the production of mutagenic substances, such as metabolites of inducible nitric oxide synthase (iNOS), which promote oncogenesis *(105,112).* iNOS-generated nitric oxide can be converted to reactive nitrogen species, which nitrosylate a variety of cellular targets including DNA and proteins. Superoxide anion radicals generated by PMNs also induce DNA damage through the formation of DNA adducts *(113).* Serum levels of vitamin C, a scavenger of reactive oxygen species and nitrates, are inversely proportional to the prevalence of gastric cancer *(114).* Eradication of *H. pylori* has been reported to raise gastric intraluminal ascorbic acid levels *(115),* so the presence of *H. pylori* also affects gastric mucosal antioxidant defenses.

In summary, the chronic and persistent inflammatory response induced by *H. pylori* can lower the threshold for malignancy through the production of a variety of effector molecules. The capacity of cytokines, COX-2 generated products, and reactive nitrogen and oxygen species to promote neoplasia is well-described and specific mechanisms used by these molecules include stimulation of proliferation and inhibition of apoptosis (which leads to a heightened retention of mutagenized cells), promotion of cellular adhesion, stimulation of angiogenesis, and cellular transformation. Based on the available data, it appears that the types and levels of mediators present (i.e., Th1 cytokines vs prostaglandins) may differentially alter the risk for gastric carcinogenesis *(2).*

4. *H. PYLORI* STRAIN VARIATION AND CARCINOGENESIS

Colonization of humans by *H. pylori* is relatively common, but the development of cancer follows in only a fraction of infected persons. Consideration must be given to

Table 1. *H. pylori* Virulence Determinants and Gastric Carcinogenesis

Genetic locus	Conservation between strains	Function	Genotype associated with gastric cancer
cag pathogenicity island	60–70% Western strains 95–100% Eastern strains	CagA injected into host epithelial cells; induction of pro-inflammatory cytokine release	*cagA*[+]
VacA	Always present, alleles vary	Apoptosis; increase paracellular permeability; decreases T-cell function	*vacA* s1ml
babA2	~85%	Adhesion	*babA2*[+]
oipA	Always present, promoter framestatus varies	Induction of IL-8	*oipA* "on"
iceA	Always present, alleles vary	?	*iceAl*

strain-specific differences that exist among *H. pylori* isolates, as well as the functions associated with such differences. *H. pylori* strains from different individuals are extremely diverse because of point mutations, gene insertions, or deletions *(116–119)*, and our group has previously demonstrated that genetically unique derivatives of a single strain are present simultaneously within an individual human host, and that isolates can modify their genetic composition over time *(120)*. Although this extraordinary diversity has hindered characterization of bacterial factors associated with various disease outcomes, five different genetic loci have been identified (*cag* island, *vacA*, *babA*, *oipA*, and *iceA*) for which persons harboring particular alleles have different risks of disease (Table 1). These markers are not completely independent of each other and importantly, are not absolutes, but instead reflect degrees of risk.

4.1. The cag *Pathogenicity Island*

The most well-characterized *H. pylori* virulence determinant is the *cag* pathogenicity island, a 31-gene locus that is present in approx 60% of US strains *(116,117, 121,122)*. Although all *H. pylori* strains induce gastritis, *cag*[+] strains significantly augment the risk for severe gastritis, atrophic gastritis, and distal gastric cancer compared to that incurred by *cag*[-] strains *(43,74,75,123–132)*. Several *cag* genes encode products that bear homology to components of a type IV bacterial secretion system, which functions as a molecular syringe to export proteins, and the product of the terminal gene in the island (CagA) is translocated into host epithelial cells after bacterial attachment. Following its injection into epithelial cells by the *cag* secretion system, CagA undergoes tyrosine phosphorylation by members of the Src family of kinases, which have been implicated in many human malignancies *(133–142)*. Phospho-CagA subsequently activates a eukaryotic phosphatase (SHP-2) as well as ERK, a member of the MAPK

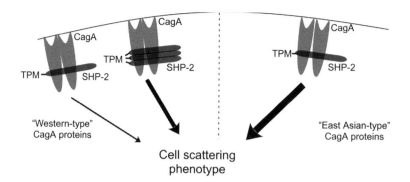

Fig. 5. CagA biological activity is determined by variation in the number and sequence of tyrosine phosphorylation motifs (TPMs). CagA, cytotoxin-associated gene A; TPM, tyrosine phosphorylation motif; SHP-2, Src homology 2 domain.

family, leading to morphological changes (e.g., cell scattering) that are reminiscent of unrestrained stimulation by growth factors. It is likely no coincidence that manipulation of the IL-6 family coreceptor gp130 leading to altered SHP-2 signaling similarly culminates in the development of intestinal-type gastric adenocarcinoma in genetically engineered mice *(143,144)*. *H. pylori cag*⁺ strains also selectively induce transactivation of the EGF receptor via activation of HB-EGF in vitro and *H. pylori*-induced EGF receptor transactivation is required for Ras-mediated activation of ERK1/2 *(69)*.

Recent studies have sought to define differences in the biological activity of CagA proteins that are present in different *H. pylori* strains. Higashi et al. demonstrated that the number of tyrosine phosphorylation motifs (TPMs) within CagA proteins isolated from persons residing in Western countries can vary substantially and that SHP-2 binding affinity and induction of cell scattering are potentiated by an increasing number of such motifs (Fig. 5) *(141)*. In contrast, TPMs within CagA proteins from East Asian *H. pylori* strains are unique and the sequences flanking East Asian-type TPMs perfectly match the consensus binding site for SHP-2 *(141)*. As expected, binding of SHP-2 and cell scattering are induced more potently by CagA proteins containing East Asian-type TPMs compared with Western-type TPMs (Fig. 5), which may explain, in part, the strikingly different rates of gastric cancer in these regions.

In addition to the effects of phospho-CagA on signaling pathways that alter cellular morphology, CagA phosphorylation also results in activation of C-terminal Src kinase, which inhibits the activity of Src, leading to a reciprocal decrease in the level of phosphorylated CagA *(142,145)*. Although this negative feedback loop likely contributes to the long-term equilibrium between *H. pylori* and its host, emerging data indicate that unphosphorylated CagA can also exert effects within the cell that contribute to pathogenesis. For example, unmodified CagA binds to growth factor receptor bound 2 (Grb2), which results in activation of the Ras/MEK/ERK MAPK pathway *(146)*. Translocation, but not phosphorylation, of CagA leads to disruption of apical-junctional complexes in polarized epithelial cells and a loss of cellular polarity, alterations that also play a role in carcinogenesis *(147)*.

A CagA-independent consequence of *cag*-mediated epithelial contact is secretion of IL-8. Clinical observations that the *cag* island represented a disease-associated locus led to subsequent molecular investigations and, not surprisingly, the first *H. pylori* strain-specific constituent identified as being required for IL-8 production was a component of the *cag* island, *cagE (148)*. Inactivation of *cagE* not only attenuates IL-8 expression but also decreases activation of NF-κB and MAPK in vitro. Numerous *cag* island genes (*cagG, cagH, cagI, cagL,* and *cagM*) have now been demonstrated to be required for NF-κB and MAPK-mediated IL-8 production *(66–68,149–151)*, and clinical *cag*[+] strains are more potent in stimulating IL-8 production than *cag*[−] strains *(51–53)*. Consistent with these findings, *H. pylori cag*[+] strains induce an enhanced IL-8 and inflammatory response in human tissue *(43,44)*, and inactivation of *cagE* and/or the entire *cag* locus attenuates the development of gastritis and atrophy in a rodent model of *H. pylori*-induced gastric adenocarcinoma, Mongolian gerbils *(152,153)*. Collectively, these data indicate that *cag*[+] strains are disproportionately represented among hosts who develop serious sequelae of *H. pylori* infection, including gastric cancer, and that genes within the *cag* island are necessary for induction of pathogenic epithelial responses, which may heighten the risk for transformation, particularly over prolonged periods of colonization.

4.2. H. pylori *vacA and Carcinogenesis*

The aforementioned studies have contributed to the genesis of a molecular portrait through which CagA and the *cag* island commandeer host signaling pathways that regulate cellular responses and cytokine production. However, most persons colonized by *cag*[+] strains remain completely asymptomatic. This paradox has fostered the need for studies to identify other microbial factors that may influence disease.

An independent *H. pylori* locus linked with pathologic outcomes such as ulcer disease and gastric cancer is *vacA*, which encodes a secreted bacterial toxin (VacA) *(154–159)*. When added to epithelial cells in vitro, VacA induces multiple structural and functional alterations in cells, the most prominent of which is the formation of large intracellular vacuoles *(160)*. There is a strong correlation between vacuolating cytotoxin activity and the presence of *cagA*. However, *vacA* and *cagA* map to two distinct loci on the *H. pylori* chromosome, and mutation of *cagA* does not affect toxin production, indicating that expression of the two proteins is independent *(161)*.

Unlike the *cag* island, *vacA* is present in virtually all *H. pylori* strains examined (Table 1) *(155,162)*; however, strains vary considerably in cytotoxic activity, and this variation is primarily owing to variations in *vacA* gene structure. The regions of greatest diversity are localized near the 5′ end of *vacA* (allele types s1a, s1b, s1c, or s2) and in the midregion of *vacA* (allele types m1 or m2) *(162–164)*. Most type s1 VacA toxins possess detectable cytotoxic activity in vitro, whereas type s2 VacA proteins possess little if any cytotoxic activity *(162)*. This is attributable to the presence of a 12-amino-acid hydrophilic segment at the N-terminus of type s2 toxins, which abolishes cytotoxic activity *(165,166)*. The mid-region of VacA contains a cell-binding site; m1-type toxins exhibit higher binding affinities than do m2-type toxins.

In addition to vacuolation, inoculation of mice with either purified VacA or VacA-containing filtrates leads to epithelial injury, and in vitro, VacA induces gastric epithelial cell apoptosis *(167–171)*. VacA also functions as transmembrane pore, permeabilizing host epithelial cells to urea, which, in turn, may allow *H. pylori* to manipulate the pH of its environment by generating ammonia. When added to polarized epithelial cell monolayers, acid-activated VacA increases paracellular permeability to organic molecules, iron, and nickel. VacA has also recently been shown to actively suppress T-cell proliferation and activation in vitro *(31–33)*, which may contribute to the longevity of *H. pylori* colonization. Collectively, these data indicate that VacA can induce multiple physiologic consequences that may contribute to pathogenesis.

H. pylori strains that possess a type s1/m1 *vacA* allele are associated with an increased risk of gastric cancer *(172–175)* and enhanced gastric epithelial cell injury *(176,177)* compared to *vacA* s2/m2 strains. The relationship between s1/m1 alleles and gastric cancer is consistent with the distribution of *vacA* genotypes throughout the world. In regions where the prevalence rate of distal gastric cancer is high, such as Colombia and Japan, most *H. pylori* strains contain type s1/m1 alleles *(164)*, whereas the converse is true in regions of the world with low rates of noncardia adenocarcinoma, underscoring the importance of *vacA* as a bacterial locus related to high-grade host responses within the gastric niche.

4.3. H. pylori *BabA*

Sequence analysis of the genomes from the completely sequenced *H. pylori* prototype strains 26695 and J99 has revealed that an unusually high proportion (1%) of identified open reading frames are predicted to encode outer membrane proteins (OMPs) *(116,117)*. Consequently, recent attention has been directed toward a possible role of these OMPs in *H. pylori* pathogenesis *(116,117,178,179)*. BabA, a member of a family of highly conserved outer membrane proteins, and encoded by the strain-specific gene *babA2*, binds the Lewis[b] histo-blood-group antigen on gastric epithelial cells *(172,180)*. *H. pylori* strains possessing *babA2* are associated with increased risk for gastric adenocarcinoma *(172)*. The presence of *babA2* is associated with *cagA* and *vacA* s1 and strains that possess all three of these genes incur the highest risk for gastric cancer *(172)*. Recently, another *H. pylori* adhesin, SabA, has been shown to bind the sialyl-Lewis a antigen, an established tumor antigen and marker of gastric dysplasia that is up-regulated by chronic gastric inflammation *(181)*, further emphasizing the pivotal role of *H. pylori* adherence in the induction of gastric inflammation and injury.

4.4. H. pylori *oipA, Mucosal Inflammation, and Gastric Carcinogenesis*

Another *H. pylori* outer membrane protein that may influence disease development is a 34-kD proinflammatory protein encoded by *oipA (182)*. Yamaoka et al. were the first to demonstrate that the vast majority of *cag*[+] strains isolated from patients in East Asia have an in-frame copy of *oipA* and when cocultured with gastric epithelial cells in vitro, these strains were found to induce high levels of IL-8. Inactivation of *oipA* decreased IL-8 levels by approx 40%, whereas inactivation of both *oipA* and *cagE* in the same strain completely abolished IL-8 production *(182)*. A recent analysis of IL-8 promoter activation in gastric epithelial cells revealed that maximal *H. pylori*-induced IL-8 transcription requires the presence of NF-κB, AP-1, and the ISRE-like binding sites, and that *oipA* selectively induced STAT1 phosphorylation, which functions as an upstream mediator of ISRE activation (Fig. 3) *(57)*.

H. pylori strains that contain an in-frame or functional copy of *oipA* are linked with more severe gastric inflammation, higher bacterial colonization density, and enhanced mucosal levels of IL-8 *(183)*. In a mouse model of *H. pylori*-induced gastritis, infection with an isogenic *oipA* mutant led to a significant decrease in the severity of gastritis as well as a reduction in chemokine production compared to levels induced by the parental wild-type *H. pylori* strain *(184)*, indicating a potential role of OipA in *H. pylori* pathogenesis.

4.5. H. pylori iceA *and Disease*

An independent strain-specific *H. pylori* locus associated with disease is *iceA*, a gene whose transcription is up-regulated following adherence to gastric epithelial cells *(185)*. Although *iceA* exists in two major allelic sequence variants, *iceA1* and *iceA2*, only *iceA1* is induced following contact with epithelial cells. The deduced *H. pylori iceA1* product demonstrates strong homology to a restriction endonuclease, *Nla*III in *Neisseria lactamica (186)* however, mutations including insertions and deletions found in the majority of *iceA1* sequences preclude translation of a full-length homolog. In contrast, *iceA2* has no homology to known proteins.

H. pylori iceA1 strains are significantly associated with the presence of peptic ulceration and distal gastric adenocarcinoma in certain populations *(185,187,188)*, and levels of *iceA1* expression within colonized human gastric mucosa are directly related to the severity of acute inflammation and IL-8 expression (Table 1) *(189)*. *iceA1* is associated with the presence of *cagA* and the *vacA* s1 allele, but is only found in 25% of US *H. pylori* isolates, which approximates the percentage of infected persons who progress to peptic ulceration or gastric cancer *(185)*. The association of *iceA1* with increased tissue damage and disease, its allelic distribution in a minority of clinical strains, its linkage disequilibrium with *cagA* and *vacA* s1 alleles, and its induction by physiologic events that induce pathologic responses (adherence), collectively suggest that *iceA1* may be a marker for strains that induce more severe gastric inflammation and injury.

5. HUMAN GENETIC POLYMORPHISMS THAT INFLUENCE THE PROPENSITY TOWARDS GASTRIC CANCER DEVELOPMENT

Although *H. pylori* strain-specific constituents clearly influence disease outcome, these factors are not absolute determinants of virulence. Most persons colonized with disease-associated *H. pylori* strains remain asymptomatic and *H. pylori cag*[+] toxigenic strains are related to both duodenal ulcer disease and distal gastric cancer, two mutually exclusive disease outcomes *(190)*. The inability of bacterial virulence components to completely account for pathologic outcomes has highlighted the need to explore host factors that may influence diseases, particularly gastric cancer.

The critical components that regulate the *H. pylori*-induced cascade to carcinogenesis are (1) the presence of the bacterium, (2) the concomitant inflammatory response, and (3) a reduction in acid secretion, because inflammation that involves the acid-secreting gastric corpus increases the risk of developing gastric adenocarcinoma by inducing hypochlorhydria and atrophic gastritis *(191)*. A host effector molecule that interacts with all three of these parameters, therefore, would represent an ideal candidate to investigate. The Th1 cytokine IL-1β, a pleiotropic pro-inflammatory molecule that is increased within the gastric mucosa of *H. pylori*[+] persons, robustly satisfies these criteria (Fig. 6) *(192)*. IL-1β both amplifies the host inflammatory response and potently inhibits gastric acid secretion by parietal cells *(193)*. Further, the *IL-1β* gene cluster, consisting of *IL-1β* and *IL-1RN* (encoding the naturally occurring IL-1β receptor antagonist), contains a number of functionally relevant polymorphisms that are associated with either increased or decreased IL-1β production and this has facilitated case-control studies to be performed that relate host genotypes and disease. The seminal report in this series was published by El-Omar and colleagues who demonstrated that *H. pylori*-colonized persons

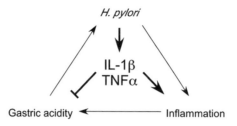

Fig. 6. Immune response genes and *H. pylori*-induced carcinogenesis. IL, interleukin; TNF, tumor necrosis factor.

with "high-expression" *IL-1β* promoter region polymorphisms have a significantly increased risk for hypochlorhydria, gastric atrophy, and distal gastric adenocarcinoma than persons with genotypes that limit *IL-1β* expression *(194)*. An increase in disease risk was only present among *H. pylori*-colonized persons and not uninfected individuals, emphasizing the importance of host–environment interactions and inflammation in the progression to gastric cancer, and these results have now been replicated by investigators in geographically distinct regions of the world *(195,196)*. The associations between genotypes and disease also mirror alterations in mucosal IL-1β production induced by *H. pylori* as gastric tissue levels of this cytokine are significantly higher in colonized patients possessing high- vs low-expression *IL-1β* polymorphisms, and increased IL-1β levels are significantly related to the intensity of gastric inflammation and atrophy *(197)*.

Rodent models also support this paradigm; in *H. pylori*-infected Mongolian gerbils and hypergastrinemic INS-GAS mice, gastric mucosal IL-1β levels increase 6–12 weeks postchallenge, and for gerbils, this is accompanied by a reciprocal decrease in gastric acid output *(198,199)*. That administration of recombinant IL-1 receptor antagonist to *H. pylori*-infected gerbils normalizes acid outputs *(198)*, implicates IL-1β as a pivotal modulator of acid secretion within inflamed mucosa. Because IL-1β is the most powerful known inhibitor of acid secretion, is profoundly pro-inflammatory, is induced by *H. pylori*, and is regulated by a promoter with informative polymorphisms, this molecule is likely to be of substantial importance in regulating the development of gastric cancer (Fig. 6).

Although IL-1β appears to be the ideal host candidate, other molecules are legitimate targets. For example, TNF-α is a pro-inflammatory acid-suppressive cytokine that is increased within *H. pylori*-colonized mucosa (Fig. 6) *(40)*. *TNF-α* polymorphisms that increase *TNF-α* expression have now been associated with an increased risk of gastric cancer and its precursors *(200)*. Smith and colleagues recently reported that polymorphisms within the *IL-8* promoter that increase *IL-8* expression also augment the risk for atrophic gastritis among *H. pylori*-infected subjects *(201)*. Conversely, polymorphisms that reduce the production of anti-inflammatory cytokines may similarly increase the risk for gastric cancer and indeed El-Omar et al. demonstrated that "low-expression" polymorphisms within the locus controlling expression of the anti-inflammatory cytokine IL-10 are associated with an enhanced risk for distal gastric cancer *(200)*. This group also examined the combinatorial effect of polymorphisms within immune response genes on cancer risk and found that the relative risk for noncardia gastric cancer increased progressively with an increasing number of pro-inflammatory polymorphisms to the point that three polymorphisms increased the risk of cancer 27-fold over baseline *(200)*.

6. MICROBIAL AND HOST INFLAMMATORY GENOTYPES AND GASTRIC CANCER RISK

An important question raised by these studies focused on immune response gene polymorphisms is whether *H. pylori* strain characteristics can further augment cancer risk exerted by host genotypes. To directly address this, Figueiredo et al. stratified *H. pylori*-infected subjects on the basis of both high-expression *IL-1β* polymorphisms and virulence genotype of their infecting *H. pylori* strains *(202)*. Odds ratios for distal gastric cancer were greatest in those persons with high-risk host and bacterial genotypes, and in persons with high-expression *IL-1β* alleles that were colonized by *H. pylori vacA* s1-type strains, the relative risk for gastric cancer was 87-fold over baseline *(202)*, indicating that interactions between specific host and microbial characteristics are biologically significant for the development of gastric cancer.

On the basis of these case-control studies in human populations, it is apparent that *H. pylori* are able to send and receive signals from their hosts, allowing host and bacteria to become linked in a dynamic equilibrium *(2,203)*. The equilibrium is different for each colonized individual, as determined by both host and bacterial characteristics and may explain why certain *H. pylori* strains augment the risk for carcinogenesis. For example, *H. pylori cag⁺* strains induce an intense inflammatory response that involves production of IL-8. This leads to increased production of IL-8, IL-1β, and TNF-α that can not only amplify the mucosal inflammatory response, but may also inhibit acid production, especially in hosts with polymorphisms that permit high expression levels of these molecules. *H. pylori* has also been shown recently to increase gastric mucosal levels of macrophage migratory inhibitory factor (MIF), a cytokine that may link inflammation to carcinogenesis *(204)*. Although the host genotype remains stable over time, *H. pylori cag⁺* and *cag⁻* strains can coexist and recombine within the same host, and thus the percentage of *cag⁺* strains is likely to vary over time, which will affect the amplitude of this equilibrium. An augmented inflammatory response induced by *cag⁺* strains in the gastric body leading to decreased acid production can also permit overgrowth of pH-sensitive bacteria, conversion of ingested *N*-nitrosamines to nitrites, and an increased risk for gastric cancer.

7. CONCLUSIONS

Gastric cancer is a highly lethal disease when diagnosed in the United States and establishment of *H. pylori* as a risk factor for this malignancy permits an approach to identify persons at increased risk; however, infection with this organism is extremely common and most colonized persons never develop cancer. Thus, techniques to identify high-risk subpopulations must use other biological markers. It is apparent from recent studies that cancer risk is the summation of the polymorphic nature of the bacterial population in the host, the host genotype, and environmental exposures, each affecting the level of long-term interactions between *H. pylori* and humans. Analytical tools now exist, however, including genome sequences (*H. pylori* and human), measurable phenotypes (CagA phosphorylation), and practical animal models, to discern the fundamental biological basis of *H. pylori*-associated neoplasia, which should have direct clinical applications. For example, identification of persons with polymorphisms associated with high levels of IL-1β expression, and who are colonized by *cag⁺ vacA* s1-type strains may be most likely to derive benefit from *H. pylori* eradication as such treatment could result in a substantially reduced cancer risk. It is important to gain more insight into the pathogenesis of *H. pylori*-induced gastric adenocarcinoma, not only to develop more effective treatments for this common cancer, but also because this model might serve as a paradigm for the role of chronic inflammation in the genesis of other malignancies that arise within the gastrointestinal tract.

REFERENCES

1. Coussens LM, Werb Z. Inflammation and cancer. Nature 2002; 420:860–867.
2. Peek RM, Jr., Blaser MJ. *Helicobacter pylori* and gastrointestinal tract adenocarcinomas. Nature Rev Cancer 2002; 2:28–37.
3. Correa P. *Helicobacter pylori* and gastric cancer: state of the art. Cancer Epidemiol Biomarkers Prev 1996; 5:477–481.
4. Sipponen P, Marshall BJ. Gastritis and gastric cancer. Western countries. Gastroenterol Clin North Am 2000; 29:579–592.
5. Peterson WL. *Helicobacter pylori* and peptic ulcer disease. N Engl J Med 1991; 324:1043–1048.
6. Karnes WE, Jr., Samloff IM, Siurala M, et al. Positive serum antibody and negative tissue staining for *Helicobacter pylori* in subjects with atrophic body gastritis. Gastroenterology 1991; 101:167–174.
7. Forman D, Newell DG, Fullerton F, et al. Association between infection with *Helicobacter pylori* and risk of gastric cancer: evidence from a prospective investigation. BMJ 1991; 302:1302–1305.
8. Nomura A, Stemmermann GN, Chyou PH, Kato I, Perez-Perez GI, Blaser MJ. *Helicobacter pylori* infection and gastric carcinoma among Japanese Americans in Hawaii. N Engl J Med 1991; 325:1132–1136.
9. Parsonnet J, Friedman GD, Vandersteen DP, et al. *Helicobacter pylori* infection and the risk of gastric carcinoma. N Engl J Med 1991; 325:1127–1131.
10. Watanabe Y, Kurata JH, Mizuno S, et al. *Helicobacter pylori* infection and gastric cancer. A nested case-control study in a rural area of Japan. Dig Dis Sci 1997; 42:1383–1387.
11. Siman JH, Forsgren A, Berglund G, Floren CH. Association between *Helicobacter pylori* and gastric carcinoma in the city of Malmo, Sweden. A prospective study. Scand J Gastroenterol 1997; 32:1215–1221.
12. Sipponen P, Kosunen TU, Valle J, Riihela M, Seppala K. *Helicobacter pylori* infection and chronic gastritis in gastric cancer. J Clin Pathol 1992; 45:319–323.
13. Hansson LE, Engstrand L, Nyren O, et al. *Helicobacter pylori* infection: independent risk indicator of gastric adenocarcinoma. Gastroenterology 1993; 105:1098–1103.
14. Hu PJ, Mitchell HM, Li YY, Zhou MH, Hazell SL. Association of *Helicobacter pylori* with gastric cancer and observations on the detection of this bacterium in gastric cancer cases. Am J Gastroenterol 1994; 89:1806–1810.
15. Kikuchi S, Wada O, Nakajima T, et al. Serum anti-*Helicobacter pylori* antibody and gastric carcinoma among young adults. Research Group on Prevention of Gastric Carcinoma among Young Adults. Cancer 1995; 75:2789–2793.
16. Kokkola A, Valle J, Haapiainen R, Sipponen P, Kivilaakso E, Puolakkainen P. *Helicobacter pylori* infection in young patients with gastric carcinoma. Scand J Gastroenterol 1996; 31:643–647.
17. Barreto-Zuniga R, Maruyama M, Kato Y, et al. Significance of *Helicobacter pylori* infection as a risk factor in gastric cancer: serological and histological studies. J Gastroenterol 1997; 32:289–294.
18. Miehlke S, Hackelsberger A, Meining A, et al. Histological diagnosis of *Helicobacter pylori* gastritis is predictive of a high risk of gastric carcinoma. Int J Cancer 1997; 73:837–839.
19. Gastric cancer and *Helicobacter pylori*: a combined analysis of 12 case control studies nested within prospective cohorts. Gut 2001; 49:347–353.
20. Uemura N, Okamoto S, Yamamoto S, et al. *Helicobacter pylori* infection and the development of gastric cancer. N Engl J Med 2001; 345:784–789.
21. Gobert AP, McGee DJ, Akhtar M, et al. *Helicobacter pylori* arginase inhibits nitric oxide production by eukaryotic cells: a strategy for bacterial survival. Proc Natl Acad Sci U S A 2001; 98:13844–13849.
22. Gewirtz AT, Navas TA, Lyons S, Godowski PJ, Madara JL. Cutting edge: bacterial flagellin activates basolaterally expressed TLR5 to induce epithelial proinflammatory gene expression. J Immunol 2001; 167:1882–1885.
23. Donnelly MA, Steiner TS. Two nonadjacent regions in enteroaggregative *Escherichia coli* flagellin are required for activation of Toll-like receptor 5. J Biol Chem 2002; 277:40456–40461.
24. Takeda K, Kaisho T, Akira S. Toll-like receptors. Annu Rev Immunol 2003; 21:335–376.

25. Perez-Perez GI, Shepherd VL, Morrow JD, Blaser MJ. Activation of human THP-1 cells and rat bone marrow-derived macrophages by *Helicobacter pylori* lipopolysaccharide. Infect Immun 1995; 63: 1183–1187.
26. Backhed F, Rokbi B, Torstensson E, et al. Gastric mucosal recognition of *Helicobacter pylori* is independent of Toll-like receptor 4. J Infect Dis 2003; 187:829–836.
27. Blaser MJ, Atherton JC. *Helicobacter pylori* persistence: biology and disease. J Clin Invest 2004; 113:321-33.
28. Lee SK, Stack A, Katzowitsch E, Aizawa SI, Suerbaum S, Josenhans C. *Helicobacter pylori* flagellins have very low intrinsic activity to stimulate human gastric epithelial cells via TLR5. Microbes Infect 2003; 5:1345–1356.
29. Gewirtz AT, Yu Y, Krishna US, Israel DA, Lyons SL, Peek RM, Jr. *Helicobacter pylori* flagellin evades Toll-like receptor 5-mediated innate immunity. J Infect Dis 2004; 189:1914–1920.
30. Aras RA, Fischer W, Perez-Perez GI, et al. Plasticity of repetitive DNA sequences within a bacterial (Type IV) secretion system component. J Exp Med 2003; 198:1349–1360.
31. Gebert B, Fischer W, Weiss E, Hoffmann R, Haas R. *Helicobacter pylori* vacuolating cytotoxin inhibits T lymphocyte activation. Science 2003; 301:1099–1102.
32. Boncristiano M, Paccani SR, Barone S, et al. The *Helicobacter pylori* vacuolating toxin inhibits T cell activation by two independent mechanisms. J Exp Med 2003; 198:1887–1897.
33. Sundrud MS, Torres VJ, Unutmaz D, Cover TL. Inhibition of primary human T cell proliferation by *Helicobacter pylori* vacuolating toxin (VacA) is independent of VacA effects on IL-2 secretion. Proc Natl Acad Sci U S A 2004; 101:7727–7732.
34. Zabaleta J, McGee DJ, Zea AH, Hernandez CP, Rodriguez PC, Sierra RA, Correa P, Ochoa AC. *Helicobacter pylori* arginase inhibits T cell proliferation and reduces the expression of the TCR ζ-chain (CD3ζ). J Immunol 2004; 173:586–593.
35. Goodwin CS, Armstrong JA, Marshall BJ. *Campylobacter pyloridis*, gastritis, and peptic ulceration. J Clin Pathol 1986; 39:353–365.
36. Mai UE, Perez-Perez GI, Allen JB, Wahl SM, Blaser MJ, Smith PD. Surface proteins from *Helicobacter pylori* exhibit chemotactic activity for human leukocytes and are present in gastric mucosa. J Exp Med 1992; 175:517–525.
37. Tufano MA, Rossano F, Catalanotti P, et al. Immunobiological activities of *Helicobacter pylori* porins. Infect Immun 1994; 62:1392–1399.
38. Yoshida N, Granger DN, Evans DJ, Jr., et al. Mechanisms involved in *Helicobacter pylori*-induced inflammation. Gastroenterology 1993; 105:1431–1440.
39. Byrne MF, Corcoran PA, Atherton JC, et al. Stimulation of adhesion molecule expression by *Helicobacter pylori* and increased neutrophil adhesion to human umbilical vein endothelial cells. FEBS Lett 2002; 532:411–414.
40. Crabtree JE, Shallcross TM, Heatley RV, Wyatt JI. Mucosal tumour necrosis factor alpha and interleukin-6 in patients with *Helicobacter pylori*-associated gastritis. Gut 1991; 32:1473–1477.
41. Fan XJ, Chua A, O'Connell MA, Kelleher D, Keeling PW. Interferon-gamma and tumour necrosis factor production in patients with *Helicobacter pylori* infection. Ir J Med Sci 1993; 162:408–411.
42. Crabtree JE, Peichl P, Wyatt JI, Stachl U, Lindley IJ. Gastric interleukin-8 and IgA IL-8 autoantibodies in *Helicobacter pylori* infection. Scand J Immunol 1993; 37:65–70.
43. Peek RM, Jr., Miller GG, Tham KT, et al. Heightened inflammatory response and cytokine expression *in vivo* to cagA+ *Helicobacter pylori* strains. Lab Invest 1995; 73:760–770.
44. Yamaoka Y, Kita M, Kodama T, Sawai N, Imanishi J. *Helicobacter pylori* cagA gene and expression of cytokine messenger RNA in gastric mucosa. Gastroenterology 1996; 110:1744–1752.
45. Eckmann L, Kagnoff MF. Cytokines in host defense against *Salmonella*. Microbes Infect 2001; 3: 1191–1200.
46. McCormick BA, Parkos CA, Colgan SP, Carnes DK, Madara JL. Apical secretion of a pathogen-elicited epithelial chemoattractant activity in response to surface colonization of intestinal epithelia by *Salmonella typhimurium*. J Immunol 1998; 160:455–466.
47. McCormick BA, Colgan SP, Delp-Archer C, Miller SI, Madara JL. *Salmonella typhimurium* attachment to human intestinal epithelial monolayers: transcellular signalling to subepithelial neutrophils. J Cell Biol 1993; 123:895–907.
48. McCormick BA, Hofman PM, Kim J, Carnes DK, Miller SI, Madara JL. Surface attachment of *Salmonella typhimurium* to intestinal epithelia imprints the subepithelial matrix with gradients chemotactic for neutrophils. J Cell Biol 1995; 131:1599–1608.

49. Jung HC, Eckmann L, Yang SK, et al. A distinct array of proinflammatory cytokines is expressed in human colon epithelial cells in response to bacterial invasion. J Clin Invest 1995; 95:55–65.
50. Crabtree JE, Lindley IJ. Mucosal interleukin-8 and *Helicobacter pylori*-associated gastroduodenal disease. Eur J Gastroenterol Hepatol 1994; 6 Suppl 1:S33–38.
51. Crabtree JE, Farmery SM, Lindley IJ, Figura N, Peichl P, Tompkins DS. CagA/cytotoxic strains of *Helicobacter pylori* and interleukin-8 in gastric epithelial cell lines. J Clin Pathol 1994; 47:945–950.
52. Crowe SE, Alvarez L, Dytoc M, et al. Expression of interleukin 8 and CD54 by human gastric epithelium after *Helicobacter pylori* infection in vitro. Gastroenterology 1995; 108:65–74.
53. Sharma SA, Tummuru MK, Miller GG, Blaser MJ. Interleukin-8 response of gastric epithelial cell lines to *Helicobacter pylori* stimulation in vitro. Infect Immun 1995; 63:1681–1687.
54. Aihara M, Tsuchimoto D, Takizawa H, et al. Mechanisms involved in *Helicobacter pylori*-induced interleukin-8 production by a gastric cancer cell line, MKN45. Infect Immun 1997; 65:3218–3224.
55. Casola A, Garofalo RP, Jamaluddin M, Vlahopoulos S, Brasier AR. Requirement of a novel upstream response element in respiratory syncytial virus-induced IL-8 gene expression. J Immunol 2000; 164: 5944–59851.
56. Peek RM, Jr. IV. *Helicobacter pylori* strain-specific activation of signal transduction cascades related to gastric inflammation. Am J Physiol Gastrointest Liver Physiol 2001; 280:G525–530.
57. Yamaoka Y, Kudo T, Lu H, Casola A, Brasier AR, Graham DY. Role of interferon-stimulated responsive element-like element in interleukin-8 promoter in *Helicobacter pylori* infection. Gastroenterology 2004; 126:1030–1043.
58. Verma IM, Stevenson JK, Schwarz EM, Van Antwerp D, Miyamoto S. Rel/NF-kappa B/I kappa B family: intimate tales of association and dissociation. Genes Dev 1995; 9:2723–2735.
59. Mercurio F, Zhu H, Murray BW, et al. IKK-1 and IKK-2: cytokine-activated IkappaB kinases essential for NF-kappaB activation. Science 1997; 278:860–866.
60. Keates S, Hitti YS, Upton M, Kelly CP. *Helicobacter pylori* infection activates NF-kappa B in gastric epithelial cells. Gastroenterology 1997; 113:1099–1109.
61. Sharma SA, Tummuru MK, Blaser MJ, Kerr LD. Activation of IL-8 gene expression by *Helicobacter pylori* is regulated by transcription factor nuclear factor-kappa B in gastric epithelial cells. J Immunol 1998; 160:2401–2407.
62. Maeda S, Yoshida H, Ogura K, et al. *Helicobacter pylori* activates NF-kappaB through a signaling pathway involving IkappaB kinases, NF-kappaB-inducing kinase, TRAF2, and TRAF6 in gastric cancer cells. Gastroenterology 2000; 119:97–108.
63. Ip YT, Davis RJ. Signal transduction by the c-Jun N-terminal kinase (JNK)—from inflammation to development. Curr Opin Cell Biol 1998; 10:205–219.
64. Garrington TP, Johnson GL. Organization and regulation of mitogen-activated protein kinase signaling pathways. Curr Opin Cell Biol 1999; 11:211–218.
65. Schaeffer HJ, Weber MJ. Mitogen-activated protein kinases: specific messages from ubiquitous messengers. Mol Cell Biol 1999; 19:2435–2444.
66. Keates S, Keates AC, Warny M, Peek RM, Jr., Murray PG, Kelly CP. Differential activation of mitogen-activated protein kinases in AGS gastric epithelial cells by *cag*+ and *cag*- *Helicobacter pylori*. J Immunol 1999; 163:5552–5559.
67. Naumann M, Wessler S, Bartsch C, et al. Activation of activator protein 1 and stress response kinases in epithelial cells colonized by *Helicobacter pylori* encoding the *cag* pathogenicity island. J Biol Chem 1999; 274:31655–31662.
68. Meyer-Ter-Vehn T, Covacci A, Kist M, Pahl HL. *Helicobacter pylori* activates mitogen-activated protein kinase cascades and induces expression of the proto-oncogenes *c-fos* and *c-jun*. J Biol Chem 2000; 275:16064–16072.
69. Keates S, Sougioultzis S, Keates AC, et al. *cag*+ *Helicobacter pylori* induce transactivation of the epidermal growth factor receptor in AGS gastric epithelial cells. J Biol Chem 2001; 276: 48127–48134.
70. Malinin NL, Boldin MP, Kovalenko AV, Wallach D. MAP3K-related kinase involved in NF-kappaB induction by TNF, CD95 and IL-1. Nature 1997; 385:540–544.
71. Evans DG, Evans DJ, Jr., Moulds JJ, Graham DY. N-acetylneuraminyllactose-binding fibrillar hemagglutinin of *Campylobacter pylori*: a putative colonization factor antigen. Infect Immun 1988; 56:2896–2906.
72. Perez-Perez GI, Dworkin BM, Chodos JE, Blaser MJ. *Campylobacter pylori* antibodies in humans. Ann Intern Med 1988; 109:11–17.

73. Crabtree JE, Shallcross TM, Wyatt JI, et al. Mucosal humoral immune response to *Helicobacter pylori* in patients with duodenitis. Dig Dis Sci 1991; 36:1266–1273.

74. Cover TL, Dooley CP, Blaser MJ. Characterization of and human serologic response to proteins in *Helicobacter pylori* broth culture supernatants with vacuolizing cytotoxin activity. Infect Immun 1990; 58:603–610.

75. Crabtree JE, Taylor JD, Wyatt JI, et al. Mucosal IgA recognition of *Helicobacter pylori* 120 kDa protein, peptic ulceration, and gastric pathology. Lancet 1991; 338:332–335.

76. Evans DJ, Jr., Evans DG, Graham DY, Klein PD. A sensitive and specific serologic test for detection of *Campylobacter pylori* infection. Gastroenterology 1989; 96:1004–1008.

77. Tosi MF, Czinn SJ. Opsonic activity of specific human IgG against *Helicobacter pylori*. J Infect Dis 1990; 162:156–162.

78. Gonzalez-Valencia G, Perez-Perez GI, Washburn RG, Blaser MJ. Susceptibility of *Helicobacter pylori* to the bactericidal activity of human serum. Helicobacter 1996; 1:28–33.

79. Negrini R, Lisato L, Zanella I, et al. *Helicobacter pylori* infection induces antibodies cross-reacting with human gastric mucosa. Gastroenterology 1991; 101:437–445.

80. Faller G, Steininger H, Kranzlein J, et al. Antigastric autoantibodies in *Helicobacter pylori* infection: implications of histological and clinical parameters of gastritis. Gut 1997; 41:619–623.

81. Vollmers HP, Dammrich J, Ribbert H, et al. Human monoclonal antibodies from stomach carcinoma patients react with *Helicobacter pylori* and stimulate stomach cancer cells in vitro. Cancer 1994; 74:1525–1532.

82. Go MF, Crowe SE. Virulence and pathogenicity of *Helicobacter pylori*. Gastroenterol Clin North Am 2000; 29:649–670.

83. Eaton KA, Mefford M, Thevenot T. The role of T cell subsets and cytokines in the pathogenesis of *Helicobacter pylori* gastritis in mice. J Immunol 2001; 166:7456–7461.

84. Roth KA, Kapadia SB, Martin SM, Lorenz RG. Cellular immune responses are essential for the development of *Helicobacter felis*-associated gastric pathology. J Immunol 1999; 163:1490–1497.

85. Macarthur M, Hold GL, El-Omar EM. Inflammation and Cancer II. Role of chronic inflammation and cytokine gene polymorphisms in the pathogenesis of gastrointestinal malignancy. Am J Physiol Gastrointest Liver Physiol 2004; 286:G515–520.

86. Bamford KB, Fan X, Crowe SE, et al. Lymphocytes in the human gastric mucosa during *Helicobacter pylori* have a T helper cell 1 phenotype. Gastroenterology 1998; 114:482–492.

87. Haeberle HA, Kubin M, Bamford KB, et al. Differential stimulation of interleukin-12 (IL-12) and IL-10 by live and killed *Helicobacter pylori in vitro* and association of IL-12 production with gamma interferon-producing T cells in the human gastric mucosa. Infect Immun 1997; 65:4229–4235.

88. Sawai N, Kita M, Kodama T, et al. Role of gamma interferon in *Helicobacter pylori*-induced gastric inflammatory responses in a mouse model. Infect Immun 1999; 67:279–285.

89. Smythies LE, Waites KB, Lindsey JR, Harris PR, Ghiara P, Smith PD. *Helicobacter pylori*-induced mucosal inflammation is Th1 mediated and exacerbated in IL-4, but not IFN-gamma, gene-deficient mice. J Immunol 2000; 165:1022–1029.

90. Sutton P, Kolesnikow T, Danon S, Wilson J, Lee A. Dominant nonresponsiveness to *Helicobacter pylori* infection is associated with production of interleukin 10 but not gamma interferon. Infect Immun 2000; 68:4802–4804.

91. Mohammadi M, Czinn S, Redline R, Nedrud J. *Helicobacter*-specific cell-mediated immune responses display a predominant Th1 phenotype and promote a delayed-type hypersensitivity response in the stomachs of mice. J Immunol 1996; 156:4729–4738.

92. Cui G, Houghton J, Finkel N, Carlson J, Wang TC. IFN-gamma infusion induces gastric atrophy, metaplasia, and dysplasia in the absence of *Helicobacter* infection- a role for immune response in *Helicobacter* disease. Gastroenterology 2003; 124:A19.

93. Sakagami T, Dixon M, O'Rourke J, et al. Atrophic gastric changes in both *Helicobacter felis* and *Helicobacter pylori* infected mice are host dependent and separate from antral gastritis. Gut 1996; 39:639–648.

94. Mohammadi M, Nedrud J, Redline R, Lycke N, Czinn SJ. Murine CD4 T-cell response to *Helicobacter* infection: TH1 cells enhance gastritis and TH2 cells reduce bacterial load. Gastroenterology 1997; 113:1848–1857.

95. Fox JG, Beck P, Dangler CA, et al. Concurrent enteric helminth infection modulates inflammation and gastric immune responses and reduces *helicobacter*-induced gastric atrophy. Nat Med 2000; 6:536–542.

96. Gupta RA, Dubois RN. Colorectal cancer prevention and treatment by inhibition of cyclooxygenase-2. Nat Rev Cancer 2001; 1:11–21.

97. Miyamoto T, Ogino N, Yamamoto S, Hayaishi O. Purification of prostaglandin endoperoxide synthetase from bovine vesicular gland microsomes. J Biol Chem 1976; 251:2629–2636.

98. Williams CS, Smalley W, DuBois RN. Aspirin use and potential mechanisms for colorectal cancer prevention. J Clin Invest 1997; 100:1325–1329.

99. Simmons DL, Levy DB, Yannoni Y, Erikson RL. Identification of a phorbol ester-repressible v-src-inducible gene. Proc Natl Acad Sci U S A 1989; 86:1178–1182.

100. Kujubu DA, Fletcher BS, Varnum BC, Lim RW, Herschman HR. TIS10, a phorbol ester tumor promoter-inducible mRNA from Swiss 3T3 cells, encodes a novel prostaglandin synthase/cyclooxygenase homologue. J Biol Chem 1991; 266:12866–12872.

101. Xie WL, Chipman JG, Robertson DL, Erikson RL, Simmons DL. Expression of a mitogen-responsive gene encoding prostaglandin synthase is regulated by mRNA splicing. Proc Natl Acad Sci U S A 1991; 88:2692–2696.

102. Romano M, Ricci V, Memoli A, et al. *Helicobacter pylori* up-regulates cyclooxygenase-2 mRNA expression and prostaglandin E2 synthesis in MKN 28 gastric mucosal cells in vitro. J Biol Chem 1998; 273:28560–28563.

103. Juttner S, Cramer T, Wessler S, et al. *Helicobacter pylori* stimulates host cyclooxygenase-2 gene transcription: critical importance of MEK/ERK-dependent activation of USF1/-2 and CREB transcription factors. Cell Microbiol 2003; 5:821–834.

104. Sawaoka H, Kawano S, Tsuji S, et al. *Helicobacter pylori* infection induces cyclooxygenase-2 expression in human gastric mucosa. Prostaglandins Leukot Essent Fatty Acids 1998; 59:313–316.

105. Fu S, Ramanujam KS, Wong A, et al. Increased expression and cellular localization of inducible nitric oxide synthase and cyclooxygenase 2 in *Helicobacter pylori* gastritis. Gastroenterology 1999; 116: 1319–13129.

106. Sung JJ, Leung WK, Go MY, et al. Cyclooxygenase-2 expression in *Helicobacter pylori*-associated premalignant and malignant gastric lesions. Am J Pathol 2000; 157:729–735.

107. Ristimaki A, Honkanen N, Jankala H, Sipponen P, Harkonen M. Expression of cyclooxygenase-2 in human gastric carcinoma. Cancer Res 1997; 57:1276–12780.

108. Farrow DC, Vaughan TL, Hansten PD, et al. Use of aspirin and other nonsteroidal anti-inflammatory drugs and risk of esophageal and gastric cancer. Cancer Epidemiol Biomarkers Prev 1998; 7:97–102.

109. Akre K, Ekstrom AM, Signorello LB, Hansson LE, Nyren O. Aspirin and risk for gastric cancer: a population-based case-control study in Sweden. Br J Cancer 2001; 84:965–968.

110. Pomorski T, Meyer TF, Naumann M. *Helicobacter pylori*-induced prostaglandin E(2) synthesis involves activation of cytosolic phospholipase A(2) in epithelial cells. J Biol Chem 2001; 276: 804–810.

111. Nardone G, Holicky EL, Uhl JR, et al. In vivo and in vitro studies of cytosolic phospholipase A(2) expression in *Helicobacter pylori* infection. Infect Immun 2001; 69:5857–5863.

112. Mannick EE, Bravo LE, Zarama G, et al. Inducible nitric oxide synthase, nitrotyrosine, and apoptosis in *Helicobacter pylori* gastritis: effect of antibiotics and antioxidants. Cancer Res 1996; 56: 3238–3243.

113. Baik SC, Youn HS, Chung MH, et al. Increased oxidative DNA damage in *Helicobacter pylori*-infected human gastric mucosa. Cancer Res 1996; 56:1279–1282.

114. Correa P, Malcom G, Schmidt B, et al. Review article: Antioxidant micronutrients and gastric cancer. Aliment Pharmacol Ther 1998; 12 Suppl 1:73–82.

115. Sobala GM, Schorah CJ, Shires S, et al. Effect of eradication of *Helicobacter pylori* on gastric juice ascorbic acid concentrations. Gut 1993; 34:1038–1041.

116. Tomb JF, White O, Kerlavage AR, et al. The complete genome sequence of the gastric pathogen *Helicobacter pylori*. Nature 1997; 388:539–547.

117. Alm RA, Ling LS, Moir DT, et al. Genomic-sequence comparison of two unrelated isolates of the human gastric pathogen *Helicobacter pylori*. Nature 1999; 397:176–180.

118. Go MF, Kapur V, Graham DY, Musser JM. Population genetic analysis of *Helicobacter pylori* by multilocus enzyme electrophoresis: extensive allelic diversity and recombinational population structure. J Bacteriol 1996; 178:3934–3938.

119. Salama N, Guillemin K, McDaniel TK, Sherlock G, Tompkins L, Falkow S. A whole-genome microarray reveals genetic diversity among *Helicobacter pylori* strains. Proc Natl Acad Sci U S A 2000; 97:14668–14673.

120. Israel DA, Salama N, Krishna U, et al. *Helicobacter pylori* genetic diversity within the gastric niche of a single human host. Proc Natl Acad Sci U S A 2001; 98:14625–14630.

121. Censini S, Lange C, Xiang Z, et al. *cag*, a pathogenicity island of *Helicobacter pylori*, encodes type I- specific and disease-associated virulence factors. Proc Natl Acad Sci U S A 1996; 93:14648–14653.

122. Akopyants NS, Clifton SW, Kersulyte D, et al. Analyses of the *cag* pathogenicity island of *Helicobacter pylori*. Mol Microbiol 1998; 28:37–53.

123. Peek RM, Jr., Miller GG, Tham KT, et al. Detection of *Helicobacter pylori* gene expression in human gastric mucosa. J Clin Microbiol 1995; 33:28–32.

124. Kuipers EJ, Perez-Perez GI, Meuwissen SG, Blaser MJ. *Helicobacter pylori* and atrophic gastritis: importance of the *cagA* status. J Natl Cancer Inst 1995; 87:1777–1780.

125. Crabtree JE, Wyatt JI, Sobala GM, et al. Systemic and mucosal humoral responses to *Helicobacter pylori* in gastric cancer. Gut 1993; 34:1339–1343.

126. Blaser MJ, Perez-Perez GI, Kleanthous H, et al. Infection with *Helicobacter pylori* strains possessing *cagA* is associated with an increased risk of developing adenocarcinoma of the stomach. Cancer Res 1995; 55:2111–2115.

127. Parsonnet J, Friedman GD, Orentreich N, Vogelman H. Risk for gastric cancer in people with CagA positive or CagA negative *Helicobacter pylori* infection. Gut 1997; 40:297–301.

128. Rudi J, Kolb C, Maiwald M, et al. Serum antibodies against *Helicobacter pylori* proteins VacA and CagA are associated with increased risk for gastric adenocarcinoma. Dig Dis Sci 1997; 42:1652–1659.

129. Queiroz DM, Mendes EN, Rocha GA, et al. *cagA*-positive *Helicobacter pylori* and risk for developing gastric carcinoma in Brazil. Int J Cancer 1998; 78:135–139.

130. Torres J, Perez-Perez GI, Leal-Herrera Y, Munoz O. Infection with CagA+ *Helicobacter pylori* strains as a possible predictor of risk in the development of gastric adenocarcinoma in Mexico. Int J Cancer 1998; 78:298–300.

131. Vorobjova T, Nilsson I, Kull K, et al. CagA protein seropositivity in a random sample of adult population and gastric cancer patients in Estonia. Eur J Gastroenterol Hepatol 1998; 10:41–46.

132. Shimoyama T, Fukuda S, Tanaka M, Mikami T, Munakata A, Crabtree JE. CagA seropositivity associated with development of gastric cancer in a Japanese population. J Clin Pathol 1998; 51:225–228.

133. Segal ED, Cha J, Lo J, Falkow S, Tompkins LS. Altered states: involvement of phosphorylated CagA in the induction of host cellular growth changes by *Helicobacter pylori*. Proc Natl Acad Sci U S A 1999; 96:14559–14564.

134. Odenbreit S, Puls J, Sedlmaier B, Gerland E, Fischer W, Haas R. Translocation of *Helicobacter pylori* CagA into gastric epithelial cells by type IV secretion. Science 2000; 287:1497–1500.

135. Stein M, Rappuoli R, Covacci A. Tyrosine phosphorylation of the *Helicobacter pylori* CagA antigen after *cag*-driven host cell translocation. Proc Natl Acad Sci U S A 2000; 97:1263–1268.

136. Asahi M, Azuma T, Ito S, et al. *Helicobacter pylori* CagA protein can be tyrosine phosphorylated in gastric epithelial cells. J Exp Med 2000; 191:593–602.

137. Backert S, Ziska E, Brinkmann V, et al. Translocation of the *Helicobacter pylori* CagA protein in gastric epithelial cells by a type IV secretion apparatus. Cell Microbiol 2000; 2:155–164.

138. Selbach M, Moese S, Hauck CR, Meyer TF, Backert S. Src is the kinase of the *Helicobacter pylori* CagA protein in vitro and in vivo. J Biol Chem 2002; 277:6775–6778.

139. Stein M, Bagnoli F, Halenbeck R, Rappuoli R, Fantl WJ, Covacci A. c-Src/Lyn kinases activate *Helicobacter pylori* CagA through tyrosine phosphorylation of the EPIYA motifs. Mol Microbiol 2002; 43:971–980.

140. Higashi H, Tsutsumi R, Muto S, et al. SHP-2 tyrosine phosphatase as an intracellular target of *Helicobacter pylori* CagA protein. Science 2002; 295:683–686.

141. Higashi H, Tsutsumi R, Fujita A, et al. Biological activity of the *Helicobacter pylori* virulence factor CagA is determined by variation in the tyrosine phosphorylation sites. Proc Natl Acad Sci U S A 2002; 99:14428–14433.

142. Tsutsumi R, Higashi H, Higuchi M, Okada M, Hatakeyama M. Attenuation of *Helicobacter pylori* CagA-SHP-2 signaling by interaction between CagA and C-terminal Src kinase. J Biol Chem 2003; 278: 3664–3670.

143. Tebbutt NC, Giraud AS, Inglese M, et al. Reciprocal regulation of gastrointestinal homeostasis by SHP2 and STAT-mediated trefoil gene activation in gp130 mutant mice. Nat Med 2002; 8: 1089–1097.

144. Judd LM, Alderman BM, Howlett M, et al. Gastric cancer development in mice lacking the SHP2 binding site on the IL-6 family co-receptor gp130. Gastroenterology 2004; 126:196–207.

145. Selbach M, Moese S, Hurwitz R, Hauck CR, Meyer TF, Backert S. The *Helicobacter pylori* CagA protein induces cortactin dephosphorylation and actin rearrangement by c-Src inactivation. EMBO J 2003; 22:515–528.

146. Mimuro H, Suzuki T, Tanaka J, Asahi M, Haas R, Sasakawa C. Grb2 is a key mediator of *Helicobacter pylori* CagA protein activities. Mol Cell 2002; 10:745–755.

147. Amieva MR, Vogelmann R, Covacci A, Tompkins LS, Nelson WJ, Falkow S. Disruption of the epithelial apical-junctional complex by *Helicobacter pylori* CagA. Science 2003; 300:1430–1434.

148. Tummuru MK, Sharma SA, Blaser MJ. *Helicobacter pylori picB*, a homologue of the *Bordetella pertussis* toxin secretion protein, is required for induction of IL-8 in gastric epithelial cells. Mol Microbiol 1995; 18:867–876.

149. Glocker E, Lange C, Covacci A, Bereswill S, Kist M, Pahl HL. Proteins encoded by the *cag* pathogenicity island of *Helicobacter pylori* are required for NF-kappaB activation. Infect Immun 1998; 66:2346–2348.

150. Crabtree JE, Kersulyte D, Li SD, Lindley IJ, Berg DE. Modulation of *Helicobacter pylori* induced interleukin-8 synthesis in gastric epithelial cells mediated by *cag* PAI encoded VirD4 homologue. J Clin Pathol 1999; 52:653–657.

151. Fischer W, Puls J, Buhrdorf R, Gebert B, Odenbreit S, Haas R. Systematic mutagenesis of the *Helicobacter pylori cag* pathogenicity island: essential genes for CagA translocation in host cells and induction of interleukin-8. Mol Microbiol 2001; 42:1337–1348.

152. Ogura K, Maeda S, Nakao M, et al. Virulence factors of *Helicobacter pylori* responsible for gastric diseases in Mongolian gerbil. J Exp Med 2000; 192:1601–1610.

153. Israel DA, Salama N, Arnold CN, et al. *Helicobacter pylori* strain-specific differences in genetic content, identified by microarray, influence host inflammatory responses. J Clin Invest 2001; 107: 611–620.

154. Cover TL, Blaser MJ. Purification and characterization of the vacuolating toxin from *Helicobacter pylori*. J Biol Chem 1992; 267:10570–10575.

155. Cover TL, Tummuru MK, Cao P, Thompson SA, Blaser MJ. Divergence of genetic sequences for the vacuolating cytotoxin among *Helicobacter pylori* strains. J Biol Chem 1994; 269:10566–10573.

156. Telford JL, Ghiara P, Dell'Orco M, et al. Gene structure of the *Helicobacter pylori* cytotoxin and evidence of its key role in gastric disease. J Exp Med 1994; 179:1653–1658.

157. Schmitt W, Haas R. Genetic analysis of the *Helicobacter pylori* vacuolating cytotoxin: structural similarities with the IgA protease type of exported protein. Mol Microbiol 1994; 12:307–319.

158. Phadnis SH, Ilver D, Janzon L, Normark S, Westblom TU. Pathological significance and molecular characterization of the vacuolating toxin gene of *Helicobacter pylori*. Infect Immun 1994; 62: 1557–1565.

159. Schistosomes, liver flukes and *Helicobacter pylori*. IARC Working Group on the Evaluation of Carcinogenic Risks to Humans. Lyon, 7-14 June 1994. IARC Monogr Eval Carcinog Risks Hum 1994; 61:1–241.

160. Leunk RD, Johnson PT, David BC, Kraft WG, Morgan DR. Cytotoxic activity in broth-culture filtrates of *Campylobacter pylori*. J Med Microbiol 1988; 26:93–99.

161. Tummuru MK, Cover TL, Blaser MJ. Mutation of the cytotoxin-associated *cagA* gene does not affect the vacuolating cytotoxin activity of *Helicobacter pylori*. Infect Immun 1994; 62:2609–2613.

162. Atherton JC, Cao P, Peek RM, Jr., Tummuru MK, Blaser MJ, Cover TL. Mosaicism in vacuolating cytotoxin alleles of *Helicobacter pylori*; Association of specific *vacA* types with cytotoxin production and peptic ulceration. J Biol Chem 1995; 270:17771–17777.

163. van Doorn LJ, Figueiredo C, Sanna R, et al. Expanding allelic diversity of *Helicobacter pylori vacA*. J Clin Microbiol 1998; 36:2597–2603.

164. van Doorn LJ, Figueiredo C, Megraud F, et al. Geographic distribution of *vacA* allelic types of *Helicobacter pylori*. Gastroenterology 1999; 116:823–830.

165. Letley DP, Atherton JC. Natural diversity in the N terminus of the mature vacuolating cytotoxin of *Helicobacter pylori* determines cytotoxin activity. J Bacteriol 2000; 182:3278–3280.

166. McClain MS, Cao P, Iwamoto H, et al. A 12-amino-acid segment, present in type s2 but not type s1 *Helicobacter pylori* VacA proteins, abolishes cytotoxin activity and alters membrane channel formation. J Bacteriol 2001; 183:6499–6508.

167. Rudi J, Kuck D, Strand S, et al. Involvement of the CD95 (APO-1/Fas) receptor and ligand system in *Helicobacter pylori*-induced gastric epithelial apoptosis. J Clin Invest 1998; 102:1506–1514.

168. Peek RM, Jr., Blaser MJ, Mays DJ, et al. *Helicobacter pylori* strain-specific genotypes and modulation of the gastric epithelial cell cycle. Cancer Res 1999; 59:6124–6131.

169. Galmiche A, Rassow J, Doye A, et al. The N-terminal 34 kDa fragment of *Helicobacter pylori* vacuolating cytotoxin targets mitochondria and induces cytochrome c release. EMBO J 2000; 19:6361–6370.

170. Cover TL, Krishna US, Israel DA, Peek RM, Jr. Induction of gastric epithelial cell apoptosis by *Helicobacter pylori* vacuolating cytotoxin. Cancer Res 2003; 63:951–957.

171. Willhite DC, Cover TL, Blanke SR. Cellular vacuolation and mitochondrial cytochrome c release are independent outcomes of *Helicobacter pylori* vacuolating cytotoxin activity that are each dependent on membrane channel formation. J Biol Chem 2003; 278:48204–48209.

172. Gerhard M, Lehn N, Neumayer N, et al. Clinical relevance of the *Helicobacter pylori* gene for blood-group antigen-binding adhesin. Proc Natl Acad Sci U S A 1999; 96:12778–12783.

173. Miehlke S, Kirsch C, Agha-Amiri K, et al. The *Helicobacter pylori vacA* s1, m1 genotype and *cagA* is associated with gastric carcinoma in Germany. Int J Cancer 2000; 87:322–327.

174. Miehlke S, Yu J, Schuppler M, et al. Helicobacter pylori *vacA*, *iceA*, and *cagA* status and pattern of gastritis in patients with malignant and benign gastroduodenal disease. Am J Gastroenterol 2001; 96: 1008–1013.

175. Louw JA, Kidd MS, Kummer AF, Taylor K, Kotze U, Hanslo D. The relationship between *Helicobacter pylori* infection, the virulence genotypes of the infecting strain and gastric cancer in the African setting. Helicobacter 2001; 6:268–273.

176. Atherton JC, Peek RM, Jr., Tham KT, Cover TL, Blaser MJ. Clinical and pathological importance of heterogeneity in *vacA*, the vacuolating cytotoxin gene of *Helicobacter pylori*. Gastroenterology 1997; 112:92–99.

177. Ghiara P, Marchetti M, Blaser MJ, et al. Role of the *Helicobacter pylori* virulence factors vacuolating cytotoxin, CagA, and urease in a mouse model of disease. Infect Immun 1995; 63:4154–4160.

178. Doig P, de Jonge BL, Alm RA, et al. *Helicobacter pylori* physiology predicted from genomic comparison of two strains. Microbiol Mol Biol Rev 1999; 63:675–707.

179. Solnick JV, Hansen LM, Salama NR, Boonjakuakul JK, Syvanen M. Modification of *Helicobacter pylori* outer membrane protein expression during experimental infection of rhesus macaques. Proc Natl Acad Sci U S A 2004; 101:2106–2111.

180. Ilver D, Arnqvist A, Ogren J, et al. *Helicobacter pylori* adhesin binding fucosylated histo-blood group antigens revealed by retagging. Science 1998; 279:373–377.

181. Mahdavi J, Sonden B, Hurtig M, et al. *Helicobacter pylori* SabA adhesin in persistent infection and chronic inflammation. Science 2002; 297:573–578.

182. Yamaoka Y, Kwon DH, Graham DY. A M(r) 34,000 proinflammatory outer membrane protein (oipA) of *Helicobacter pylori*. Proc Natl Acad Sci U S A 2000; 97:7533–7538.

183. Yamaoka Y, Kikuchi S, el-Zimaity HM, Gutierrez O, Osato MS, Graham DY. Importance of *Helicobacter pylori oipA* in clinical presentation, gastric inflammation, and mucosal interleukin 8 production. Gastroenterology 2002; 123:414–424.

184. Yamaoka Y, Kita M, Kodama T, et al. *Helicobacter pylori* infection in mice: Role of outer membrane proteins in colonization and inflammation. Gastroenterology 2002; 123:1992–2004.

185. Peek RM, Jr., Thompson SA, Donahue JP, et al. Adherence to gastric epithelial cells induces expression of a *Helicobacter pylori* gene, *iceA*, that is associated with clinical outcome. Proc Assoc Am Physicians 1998; 110:531–544.

186. Morgan RD, Camp RR, Wilson GG, Xu SY. Molecular cloning and expression of NlaIII restriction-modification system in *E. coli*. Gene 1996; 183:215–218.

187. van Doorn LJ, Figueiredo C, Sanna R, et al. Clinical relevance of the *cagA*, *vacA*, and *iceA* status of *Helicobacter pylori*. Gastroenterology 1998; 115:58–66.

188. Kidd M, Peek RM, Lastovica AJ, Israel DA, Kummer AF, Louw JA. Analysis of *iceA* genotypes in South African *Helicobacter pylori* strains and relationship to clinically significant disease. Gut 2001; 49:629–635.

189. Peek RM, Jr., van Doorn LJ, Donahue JP, et al. Quantitative detection of *Helicobacter pylori* gene expression in vivo and relationship to gastric pathology. Infect Immun 2000; 68:5488–5495.

190. Hansson LE, Nyren O, Hsing AW, et al. The risk of stomach cancer in patients with gastric or duodenal ulcer disease. N Engl J Med 1996; 335:242–249.

191. El-Omar EM. The importance of interleukin 1beta in *Helicobacter pylori* associated disease. Gut 2001; 48:743–747.

192. Noach LA, Bosma NB, Jansen J, Hoek FJ, van Deventer SJ, Tytgat GN. Mucosal tumor necrosis factor-alpha, interleukin-1 beta, and interleukin-8 production in patients with *Helicobacter pylori* infection. Scand J Gastroenterol 1994; 29:425–429.

193. Beales IL, Calam J. Interleukin 1 beta and tumour necrosis factor alpha inhibit acid secretion in cultured rabbit parietal cells by multiple pathways. Gut 1998; 42:227–234.

194. El-Omar EM, Carrington M, Chow WH, et al. Interleukin-1 polymorphisms associated with increased risk of gastric cancer. Nature 2000; 404:398–402.

195. Machado JC, Pharoah P, Sousa S, et al. Interleukin 1B and interleukin 1RN polymorphisms are associated with increased risk of gastric carcinoma. Gastroenterology 2001; 121:823–829.

196. Furuta T, El-Omar EM, Xiao F, Shirai N, Takashima M, Sugimurra H. Interleukin 1beta polymorphisms increase risk of hypochlorhydria and atrophic gastritis and reduce risk of duodenal ulcer recurrence in Japan. Gastroenterology 2002; 123:92–105.

197. Hwang IR, Kodama T, Kikuchi S, et al. Effect of interleukin 1 polymorphisms on gastric mucosal interleukin 1beta production in *Helicobacter pylori* infection. Gastroenterology 2002; 123:1793–1803.

198. Takashima M, Furuta T, Hanai H, Sugimura H, Kaneko E. Effects of *Helicobacter pylori* infection on gastric acid secretion and serum gastrin levels in Mongolian gerbils. Gut 2001; 48:765–773.

199. Fox JG, Wang TC, Rogers AB, et al. Host and microbial constituents influence *Helicobacter pylori*-induced cancer in a murine model of hypergastrinemia. Gastroenterology 2003; 124:1879–1890.

200. El-Omar EM, Rabkin CS, Gammon MD, et al. Increased risk of noncardia gastric cancer associated with proinflammatory cytokine gene polymorphisms. Gastroenterology 2003; 124:1193–1201.

201. Smith MG, Hold GL, Rabkin CS, et al. The *IL-8-251* promoter polymorphism is associated with high IL-8 production, severe inflammation, and increased risk of pre-malignant changes in *H. pylori*-positive subjects. Gastroenterology 2004; 126:A23.

202. Figueiredo C, Machado JC, Pharoah P, et al. *Helicobacter pylori* and interleukin 1 genotyping: an opportunity to identify high-risk individuals for gastric carcinoma. J Natl Cancer Inst 2002; 94:1680–1687.

203. Kirschner DE, Blaser MJ. The dynamics of *Helicobacter pylori* infection of the human stomach. J Theor Biol 1995; 176:281–290.

204. Xia HHX, Lam SK, Huang XR, et al. *Helicobacter pylori* infection is associated with increased expression of macrophage migratory inhibitory factor-by epithelial cells, T cells, and macrophages-in gastric mucosa. J Infect Dis 2004; 190:293–302.

2 HTLV-1, Cytokines, and Cancer

Michael Lairmore and Lee Ratner

CONTENTS

1. INTRODUCTION

Human T-cell lymphotropic virus type 1 (HTLV-1), is the causative agent of adult T-cell leukemia/lymphoma (ATLL) and a variety of immune-mediated disorders (Table 1). Currently, HTLV-1 infection occurs worldwide with endemic regions of higher prevalence. Natural transmission of these viruses occurs through cell-associated routes that include: orally from breast feeding, sexual contact, and by exposure to infected blood or whole cell blood products. While the molecular events of virus replication are beginning to be unraveled and knowledge about HTLV-1-associated diseases has increased, there remain many questions regarding the pathogenesis of the diseases associated with this complex retrovirus. In this chapter, we will focus on the pathogenesis and clinical presentation of ATLL with emphasis on new information regarding the viral etiology, pathologic lesions, patient susceptibility factors, host immune responses, and, in particular, the role of cytokines in the development of ATLL. The epidemiology and diseases associated with HTLV-1 are well known; however, the molecular mechanisms used by the virus to establish persistent infection and subsequently facilitate lymphocyte proliferation while circumventing immune elimination, remain less well defined.

From: *Cancer Drug Discovery and Development,*
Cytokines in the Genesis and Treatment of Cancer
Edited by: M. A. Caligiuri and M. T. Lotze © Humana Press Inc., Totowa, NJ

Table 1
HTLV-1 Associated Diseases

Strongly associated diseases	
Adult T-cell leukemia/ lymphoma (ATLL)	Aggressive T-cell malignancy—monoclonal expansion of CD3+/CD4+/CD8–/CD25+/HLA-DR+ T-cells *(5)*. One to 5% of early HTLV-1 infected individuals, develop ATLL after a prolonged incubation period ~ 20–30 years *(30,32)*. Clinically, patients present with malaise, fever, lymphadenopathy, hepatosplenomegaly, jaundice, drowsiness, weight loss, and opportunistic infections. Cutaneous nodules, lytic bone lesions, and hypercalcemia common. Diagnosis of ATLL includes proviral DNA in ATLL cells, positive serologic status for HTLV-1, marked leukocytosis, "flower cell" morphology of neoplastic T-cells, hypercalcemia, increased circulating levels of the IL-2 receptor α-chain (IL-2Rα/CD25), and elevated serum lactate dehydrogenase (LDL) levels *(30,31,34)*. Classified as: asymptomatic, preleukemic, chronic or smoldering and acute *(34–36)*.
HTLV-1-associated myelopathy/ tropical spastic paraparesis (HAM/TSP)	Slowly progressive lymphocyte-mediated myelopathy of pyramidal tracts *(17)*. Extremity weakness, back pain, incontinence, associated spasticity. Develops in ~1–5 % of HTLV-1 infected persons after moderate to prolonged latency. Long-term survival (months to years).
Associated diseases	
Reported diseases primarily in HTLV-1 endemic regions in Japan and Caribbean basin; role of HTLV-1 infection unclear, may initiate lesions through lymphocyte-mediated disorder, cytokine dysregulation, or alteration of immune reactivity	Polymyositis, polyarthritis, alveolitis, uveitis, dermatitits *(51)*.

The genome of HTLV-1 encodes structural (e.g., group specific core antigens, Gag) and enzymatic proteins (e.g., reverse transcriptase, RT), characteristic of all retroviruses. Additionally, HTLV-1, a complex retrovirus, utilizes an alternative splicing mechanism and internal initiator codons, to make several regulatory and accessory proteins encoded by four open reading frames (ORFs) of the pX region (pX ORF I to IV) (Table 2). ORF IV of HTLV-1 encodes the well-characterized Tax transactivating protein, while the ORF III encodes Rex, a key regulator of viral RNA transport. Tax is a 40 kDa nuclear-localizing phosphoprotein, which interacts with cellular transcription factors to activate transcription from the viral promoter (Tax responsive element, TRE), as well as the enhancer elements of various cellular genes associated with host cell proliferation or transformation. Rex is a 27 kDa, nucleolar-localizing phosphoprotein that functions to enhance nuclear export of

Table 2
Summary of HTLV-1 Regulatory and Accessory Proteins:
Role in Pathogenesis and Alteration of Cytokines

Protein*	PX ORF	Subcellular distribution	Functional activity
Tax	IV	Nuclear and cytoplasm	Transcriptional activator of px region, 40 kDa nuclear protein produced from a doubly spliced mRNA, transactivator of HTLV-1 gene transcription from the viral LTR (75,76). Binds to GC-rich sequences flanking the Tax responsive element 1 (TRE-1) and enhances CREB/ATF proteins to the TRE-1. Alters the expression of cellular genes by induction of NF-κB and SRF. Enhances cytokines including IL-2 (80), IL-3 (81), IL-4 (82), IL-6 (83), IL-8 (84), IL-2Rα (80), IL-1 (85), GM-CSF (86), TNFα (87), and TNFβ (88), transcription factors such as c-myc (89), c-fos (90), c-sis (91), erg-1 (92), c-rel (93), lck, (94) apoptosis related genes Bcl-x$_L$ and Bax (95–97) and DNA repair genes, proliferating cell nuclear antigen (PCNA) and β-polymerase (98).
Rex	III	Nuclear and nucleolar with shuttling	Rex, a nucleolar localizing 27 kD protein, responsible for nuclear export of unspliced (gag/pol) and singly spliced (env) viral RNA to cytoplasm. Not required for in vitro immortalization, but critical for infection in vivo (99).
p12^I	I	Endoplasmic reticulum and cis-Golgi	Calcium-mediated NFAT activation and decreases IL-2 requirement for T-cell activation. Abolished infectivity in rabbit model, reduced infectivity in nondividing primary human T-cells (246).
p13^{II}	II	Mitochondria and nucleus	Mitochondrial swelling and disruption of ΔΨ, sensitizes cells to apoptosis (222,247).
p30^{II}	II	Nuclear	Reduced viral load in rabbit model, transcriptional regulator, binds p300/CBP, post-transcriptional regulation of tax/rex RNA (214,246,248,249).

Tax and Rex are considered regulatory, p12^I, p13^{II}, and p30^{II} are considered accessory proteins.

unspliced or singly spliced viral RNA thus contributing to virus propagation. HTLV-1 infected cells, ATLL cells, and Tax transgenic mouse tumor cells express a wide range of cytokines that have been implicated in the development of ATLL. Constitutive expression of interleukin-2 (IL-2) or IL-15, and their receptor contributes to lymphoid cell proliferation and resistance to apoptosis. Production of a variety of chemokines and their receptors are likely to be important for tumor cell infiltration into skin, lymph nodes, and other tissues. Transforming growth factor beta (TGF-β) is expressed in ATLL cells, and may promote tumor cell growth in addition to altering the tumor stroma to enhance outgrowth or tissue invasion by transformed lymphocytes. Detailed analysis of cytokine expression in this disease has led to immunotherapeutic approaches directed against the IL-2 receptor, and opportunities for development of other novel approaches to altering cytokines activity. In addition, newly discovered roles for accessory gene products of the virus suggest new ways the virus exploits T-cells through disruption of cytokine-mediated events.

2. GEOGRAPHIC DISTRIBUTION AND TRANSMISSION OF HTLV-1

HTLV-1 was the first human retrovirus identified and subsequently associated with disease (1–3). Interestingly, HTLV-1 associated lymphoma was reported in 1977, before the isolation of the virus, as a unique and aggressive CD4+ T-cell malignancy in Japan classified as ATLL (4,5). In 1980, Drs. Poisez, Gallo and their colleagues detected type C retrovirus particles, later named HTLV-1, in T-cell lymphoblastoid cell lines and fresh peripheral blood lymphocytes from a patient with cutaneous T-cell lymphoma (classified originally as mycosis fungoides) (6). Similar type C retroviral particles were demonstrated in cell lines derived from Japanese patients diagnosed with ATLL (7–9). Subsequently additional sero-epidemiologic, immunologic, genetic, and molecular studies established the association between ATLL and HTLV-1 infection (1–3).

HTLV-1 infects approximately 15 to 25 million people worldwide (10). The virus is endemic in southern Japan (1), the Caribbean basin (11), central Africa (12), Central and South America (13,14), and among some Melanesian Islands in the Pacific basin (15). The seroprevalence of HTLV-1 varies between 0.1 and 30% of the population within endemic regions (10). The serious risk of HTLV-1 infection among susceptible groups in the United States, Japan, and Europe has led to public health intervention policies such as blood donor screening to prevent HTLV-1 contaminated blood from entering the blood supply (16–22).

HTLV-1 is a highly cell-associated virus and cell–cell contact between virus infected cells and target T-cells is required for efficient transmission (23). The principal route of HTLV-1 transmission in endemic areas is from mother to child through breastfeeding by transfer of infected milk-borne lymphocytes (24,25). HTLV-1 transmission also occurs by exposure to infected blood or whole-cell blood products and through the sharing of needles among intravenous drug users (26–28). Sexual transmission although less efficient is an important mode of transmission, in particularly between infected men and their sexual partners where transmission of the virus is approx four times as frequent (29).

3. ADULT T-CELL LEUKEMIA/LYMPHOMA

ATLL is an aggressive T-cell malignancy characterized by monoclonal expansion of CD3+/CD4+/CD8–/CD25+/HLA–DR+ T-cells (5). HTLV-1 proviral DNA is consistently demonstrated in ATLL cells and virtually all ATLL patients have antibodies against HTLV-1 (30,31). In general, 1–5 % of the HTLV-1 infected individuals, who acquire the virus before the age of 20 develop ATLL after a prolonged incubation period of around 20–30 years (30,32).

The clinical picture of ATLL is similar to non-Hodgkin's lymphoma. Affected patients present with malaise, fever, lymphadenopathy, hepatosplenomegaly, jaundice, drowsiness, weight loss, and opportunistic infections. These patients also exhibit a wide spectrum of cutaneous lesions (from large nodules to plaques and ulcers on the limbs, trunk, or face) and lytic bone lesions. Opportunistic fungal infections such as *Pneumocystis carinii* have been reported in some patients *(33)*. ATLL patients are usually hypercalcemic, with high serum concentrations of lactate dehydrogenase and elevated serum levels of soluble IL-2 receptor α chain (IL-2R/CD25). Neoplastic T-lymphocytes in ATLL patients have a characteristic convoluted multi-lobulated nuclei, which gives the appearance of "flower cells" *(34)*. Diagnosis of ATLL includes specific parameters including positive serologic status for HTLV-1, marked leukocytosis, "flower cell" morphology of neoplastic T-cells, T-cell immunophenotyping, hypercalcemia, increased circulating levels of IL-2Rα/CD25, and elevated serum lactate dehydrogenase (LDL) levels *(34)*. ATLL is classified into four somewhat overlapping types based on the clinical course of the disease namely asymptomatic, preleukemic, chronic or smoldering, and acute *(34–36)*. The chronic stage ATLL is characterized by leukocytosis, whereas the acute stage is characterized by the presence of flower cells, skin lesions, lymphadenopathy, and hepatosplenomegaly *(30)*.

The molecular mechanisms leading to ATLL have not been completely elucidated; however recent studies provide evidence of viral and host interactions that predict events leading to transformation. Like other retroviruses, HTLV-1 infects target cells by interactions between the viral envelope and cell surface receptors. Subsequent to uncoating and reverse transcription, the HTLV-1 provirus integrates randomly into the host cell chromosome *(37)*. Viral genome "replication" can occur in vivo indirectly through division of infected cells *(37)*, although it is well established that HTLV-1 is capable of typical replication via reverse transcription and production of new infectious viral particles. In ATLL, there is an initial polyclonal expansion of infected cells, followed by a progression to oligoclonal and then to monoclonal proliferation in vivo, which is achieved while the cells become IL-2 independent *(3,38,39)*. The long clinical latency and the small proportion of infected individuals developing ATLL strongly suggests a series of cellular alterations or mutations must occur before T-cell transformation *(40)*. HTLV-1 proteins such as Tax are believed to play a critical role in transformation of infected lymphocytes by altering critical cellular activation and death pathways. However, the presence of latent or defective proviruses in transformed cells indicates the possibility that viral protein expression is no longer needed for the maintenance of the transformed cell *(41,42)*.

4. OTHER DISEASES ASSOCIATED WITH HTLV-1-INFECTION

Gessain and colleagues first reported the association of tropical spastic paraparesis (TSP) with HTLV-1 infection in 1985 *(43)*. Another neurologic condition observed among HTLV-1-infected individuals, termed HTLV-1 associated myelopathy (HAM), having similar clinical findings as TSP patients was reported by Osame et al *(44)*. Subsequently, in 1988, the World Health Organization (WHO) declared HAM and TSP as the same disease, now known collectively as HAM/TSP. HAM/TSP is a progressive chronic myelopathy, predominantly of the thoracic spinal cord *(17,45–48)*. The development and progression to HAM/TSP is influenced by multiple risk factors including host genetic factors *(49)*, host immune response, high HTLV-1 proviral load *(50–54)*, route of infection (exposure via blood transfusion) *(55)*, and perhaps, by specific viral characteristics such as variations in the *tax gene (51,56–60)*. Although the pathogenesis of HAM/TSP is not completely resolved, immune- and cytokine-mediated damage is a widely accepted hypothesis supported by increased cellular and humoral immune responses observed in HAM/TSP patients. In addition to ATLL and HAM/TSP, HTLV-1 infection has been associated with many other disorders believed to be caused by immune-system dysfunction. These include uveitis *(61)*, HTLV-1-associated arthropathy *(62)*, Sjögren syndrome *(63)*, infective dermatitis *(64)*, polymyositis *(65)*, lymphadenitis *(66)*, chronic respiratory disease *(67)*, acute myeloid leukemia *(68)*, and conditions such as systemic sarcoidosis as well as increased susceptibility to *Strongyloides stercoralis* infection *(69)*. However, the direct role of HTLV-1 in the development of these conditions remains controversial.

5. HTLV-1 REPLICATION AND MECHANISMS OF CARCINOGENESIS

HTLV-1 is a complex retrovirus with type C retroviral morphology. The virus belongs to the deltaretrovirus group along with bovine leukemia virus (BLV) and Simian T lymphotropic virus (STLV). The HTLV-1 replication cycle starts when viral particles attach to the cell surface through an interaction between envelope and HTLV-1 receptors. Manel et al *(70)* have identified GLUT-1, a ubiquitous glucose transport protein, as a potential receptor for HTLV-1. When the viral envelope fuses with the cell membrane, components of the virion such as nucleocapsid and capsid enters the cytoplasm. In the cytoplasm, the viral genomic RNA is reverse transcribed to generate double-stranded DNA (dsDNA) using the virally encoded reverse transcriptase (RNA-dependent/ DNA-dependent polymerase). Viral dsDNA molecules together with cellular and viral proteins form a pre-integration complex *(71)*, which traffics to the nucleus and randomly integrates into the host genome using the viral encoded integrase. These processes are accomplished by the structural and enzymatic proteins packaged in the virions without de novo viral gene expression *(72)*.

Unlike simple retroviruses, complex retroviruses like HTLV-1 carry additional genes to encode for several regulatory and accessory proteins. As a complex retrovirus, HTLV-1 encodes regulatory proteins from the pX region (between *env* and 3′ LTR), by alternative splicing from four ORFs. ORF IV and ORF III encode regulatory proteins Tax and Rex, respectively *(73,74)*. Tax, (transcriptional activator of px region), a 40-kDa nuclear protein produced from a doubly spliced mRNA, is transactivator of HTLV-1 gene transcription from the viral LTR *(75,76)*. Tax binds to GC-rich sequences flanking the Tax responsive element 1 (TRE-1) for the transactivation of the LTR *(77,78)*. Tax enhances the binding of cyclic AMP response/activator of transcription (CREB/ATF) proteins to the TRE-1 and several basic leucine zipper (bZIP) proteins to the TRE-2 *(79)*. In addition, Tax regulates the expression of numerous cellular genes, predominantly by induction of the transcription factors nuclear factor kappa of B-cells (NF-κB) and serum response factor (SRF), independent of CREB activation. These cellular genes include cytokines such as IL-2 *(80)*, IL-3 *(81)*, IL-4 *(82)*, IL-6 *(83)*, IL-8 *(84)*, IL-1 *(85)*, GM-CSF *(86)*, TNFα *(87)*, and TNFβ *(88)*, IL-2Rα *(80)*, and transcription factors such as c-myc *(89)*, c-fos *(90)*, c-sis *(91)*, erg-1 *(92)*, c-rel *(93)*, lck, *(94)* apoptosis related genes Bcl-x$_L$ and Bax *(95–97)* and DNA repair genes proliferating cell nuclear antigen (PCNA) and β-polymerase *(98)*. Rex, a nucleolar localizing 27 kDa protein, is responsible for nuclear export of unspliced (*gag/pol*) and singly spliced (*env*) viral RNA to cytoplasm. Even though Rex is not required for in vitro immortalization by HTLV-1, Ye et al *(99)* reported that Rex is critical for efficient infection of cells and persistence in vivo.

6. ANIMAL MODELS TO UNDERSTAND THE ROLE
OF CYTOKINES IN HTLV-1 PATHOGENESIS

Since the initial discovery of the virus, a variety of animal models of HTLV-1 infection have been reported. However, the virus consistently infects only rabbits *(100,101)*, some nonhuman primates *(102,103)*, and to a lesser extent rats *(104,105)*. Viral transmission in mice using typical methods of infection produces inconsistent infections and limited virus expression in tissues *(50,106,107)*. Nonhuman primates have been infected with HTLV-1 and certain species have a natural infection with STLV-1 *(108–111)*. The squirrel monkey has been successfully infected with HTLV-1 and offers an attraction nonhuman primate model of HTLV-1 for vaccine testing *(112–114)*. Rats have been infected with HTLV-1 producing cells and offer a model of the neurologic disease associated with the viral infection *(115–118)*. Rats have also been used to test the role of cell-mediated immunity to the infection *(116,119)*. However, controversy exists regarding the reproducibility of the viral infection in rats *(105)*. Among these in vivo models the rabbit has been used the most extensively because of the ease and consistency of transmission of the infection to this species. Pioneering studies utilizing the rabbit model of HTLV-1 infection have provided important clues about transmission of the virus infection, body fluids likely to contain infectious virus, and effective means to prevent the transmission of the virus *(100,120,121)*.

The *Hu-PBL-SCID* mouse, developed by injection of primary human lymphocytes into the peritoneal cavity of mice homozygous for the SCID genetic defect *(122)*, provides a successful model of ATLL *(123–126)*. SCID mice inoculated with ATLL cells succumbed to lymphomas that retained characteristics of the leukemic cells from patients. There are substantial differences in ability to form tumors between patient derived ATLL cells and cells immortalized by HTLV in vitro, when inoculated into SCID mouse *(124)*, which is due, in part, to host natural killer cell activity in tumor formation *(123,127)*.

Transgenic mouse models of HTLV-1 have provided new understanding of the role of Tax in the pathogenesis of HTLV-1-associated lesions. Nerenberg et al *(128)* described neurofibromas associated with peripheral nerves in LTR-tax transgenic mice. Kitajima and Nerenberg *(129)* used antisense inhibition of NF-κB to demonstrate the importance of this transcription factor in the development of the tumors. Subsequently, this same group using the mouse Thy 1.2 promoter developed Tax transgenic mice that developed fibrosarcomas *(130)*. Iwakura et al. *(131)* generated LTR-Tax transgenic mice that have inflammatory arthropathy resembling the lesion associated with HTLV-1-infected subjects. Increased levels of nerve growth factor, GM-CSF, and IL-2Rα expression occur in some Tax transgenic mice *(132)*. To improve Tax expression in lymphoid compartments alternative promoters have been employed. HTLV-LTR-c-myc and immunoglobulin enhancer/promoter (Ig-enh)-Tax transgenic mice lines have been crossed resulting in the development of a variety of tumors in 100% of the offspring *(133)*. Our research group developed transgenic mice that specifically target the mature T-cell compartment by using the human granzyme B (GzmB) promoter *(134)*. This promoter limits expression to activated CD4+ and CD8+ T-cells, natural killer cells (NK) and lymphokine-activated killer (LAK) cells. Tumors composed of large granular lymphocytes developed in these mice on the tail, legs, and ears. Tax expression was restricted to the thymus, bone marrow, stomach, spleen, and tumor tissue. LGL lines cultured from these mice displayed surface markers indicating a pre-NK cell lineage (positive for FcγRII/III, CD122, CD44, Thy 1.2, 5E6) *(135)*.

In contrast, use of the human granzyme B promoter to regulate Tax expression (GzmB-Tax mice) resulted in large granular lymphocytic lymphoma/leukemia (LGL), and the penetrance was 100% *(134)*. The tumor cells have the cell surface phenotype of natural killer/T (NK/T) cells. The animals developed LGL at a median age of 6 months, and manifested up to 70% LGL cells in the blood and 40% LGL cells in the bone marrow. LGL tumors are first evident at peripheral sites, such as the tail, ears, or extremities, sites of trauma from tail clipping, ear labeling, or fighting. However, LGL cells are also present in the spleen, liver, lung, and mesenteric nodes. The GzmB-Tax mice have been used for studies of cytokine activation in LGL pathogenesis *(135)*. In studies of primary tumor cells, IL-1, IL-6, IL-10, and IL-15, GM-CSF, and IFN-γ were expressed, but not IL-2, IL-4, or IL-9 *(135)*. In contrast to primary tumor cells, tumor cell lines did not exhibit IL-1 expression, suggesting that IL-1 was expressed from a nonmalignant cell population infiltrating the LGL tumors. IL-1 can promote malignant cell growth and invasiveness, and also induce antitumor immunity *(136)*. High levels of GM-CSF in these transgenic mice are believed to initiate neutrophilia, a characteristic finding for this animal model. The roles of other cytokines in this model remain to be determined. IL-6 is a pleiotropic cytokine, acting as an acute-phase reactant that regulates differentiation, proliferation, and survival of a wide variety of cell types *(137)*. IL-10 suppresses inflammatory responses, and regulates the growth of NK and T-cells, and other cell types *(138–141)*. Thus, IL-10 could play an immunoevasion role for HTLV-1 infection.

The finding of high levels of IFN-γ expression in Tax transgenic mice is consistent with findings with ATLL cell lines *(138,142–145)*. The role of IFN-γ expression was investigated using GzmB-Tax mice with homozygous deletion of the IFN-γ gene (IFN-γ –/–). These mice exhibited accelerated tumor development, morbidity, and mortality *(146)*. Compared to IFN-γ +/+ mice, IFN-γ –/– mice had no significant alteration in CD4 or CD8 lymphocyte infiltration into tumors, cytotoxic T-cell (CTL) activity directed against tumors, or expression of MHC I or II proteins. However, IFN-γ –/– tumors, compared to IFN-γ +/+ tumors, exhibited enhanced angiogenesis, and gene array studies showed increased vascular endothelial growth factor and tenascin C and depressed tissue inhibitor of metalloproteinase-1 and tumor necrosis factor-α expression (L. Ratner, manuscript in preparation). Collectively these studies indicate that IFN-γ appears to be an important regulatory response for Tax-induced LGL tumors, inhibiting tumor angiogenesis.

7. CYTOKINE EXPRESSION IN RESPONSE TO HTLV-1 INFECTION

During HTLV-1 infection, a number of cytokines have been reported to be produced, including IL-1-α, IL-1-β, IL-2, 3, 4, 5, 6, 9, and 15, TGF-β, TNF-α, TNF-β, IFN-γ, and GM-CSF, as well as chemokines, such as IL-8, RANTES, and MIP-1-α *(138,144, 147–155)*. The mechanism of cytokine and chemokine induction in HTLV-1 infected cells has been primarily investigated in relationship to Tax activation of cellular gene expression. Tax activates gene expression through several different pathways, but activation through NF-κB appears to be most important for cytokine gene expression *(153,156–160)*. Activation of NF-κB occurs through multiple distinct cellular events triggered by Tax. First, Tax activates inhibitor-κ kinase (IKK) by direct binding to the

IKK-γ subunit *(160–162)*. Moreover, Tax physically interacts with mitogen activated protein kinase (MAPK) kinase kinase 1 (MEKK1) to enhance phosphorylation of IKK-α and β subunits *(163,164)*. In addition, Tax binds to the NF-κB p50 precursor protein, p100, and accelerates its proteolytic processing *(165)*. Most of the cytokines enumerated above have NF-κB binding sites in their promoters.

In contrast, Tax activates nuclear factor of activated transcription (NFAT) by inducing constitutive dephosphorylation *(166,167)*. NFAT is critical for induction of IL-2 and Fas ligand. Thus, Tax may directly or indirectly enhance the phosphatase calcineurin, which is required for dephosphorylation and thus nuclear translocation of NFAT. Moreover, Tax also induces activated protein-1 (AP-1) and c-Jun kinase (JNK) activities, although the mechanism of action is incompletely understood. This pathway has been implicated in the activation of TGF-β expression. In addition, Tax activates the CREB or ATF pathway through direct interactions with CREB-binding protein (CBP) and its homologous co-activator, p300 *(168,169)*. This pathway is involved in activation of the viral promoter. However, competition for CBP/p300 binding has been suggested as a means to depress TGF-β action *(170,171)*.

8. IL-2 AND IL-15 IN ATLL

IL-2 and IL-15 are structurally similar cytokines that function through the same IL-2R β and γ chains (common γ chain), but use distinct IL-2R and IL-15R-α chains *(172)*. Despite these similarities, IL-2 and IL-15 have distinct effects on NK and T-cells. IL-2 has a pivotal role in activation-induced T-cell death, whereas IL-15 stimulates the expression of CD8+ memory T-cells, and is critical for NK cell development and maintenance. ATLL cells constitutively express high levels of the IL-2Rα and many ATLL cell lines remain IL-2-dependent, suggesting a key role for IL-2 in the development of disease *(173–176)*. IL-15 and IL-15-specific binding receptor mRNA and protein levels are also increased in HTLV-1 infected cells *(157,177)*. This results from Tax expression and activation of NF-κB. Moreover other interleukin receptors that share the common γ chain, including those for IL-4 and IL-7, but notIL-9, are also over-expressed in ATLL cells.

The dependence of many ATLL cell lines for the IL-2/IL-2R system has resulted in the development of specific immunotherapy utilizing humanized antibodies to the IL-2Rα *(178)*. The most successful use of this therapeutic approach has been with humanized IL-2R antibody (anti-Tac) conjugated to α- or β-particle-emitting radionuclides. This approach has also been used for therapy in malignancies not associated with HTLV-1, but also characterized by exploitation of the IL-2/IL-2R system for proliferation. These have included anaplastic large cell, peripheral T-cell, cutaneous T-cell, and NK-cell lymphomas. In the ATLL-bearing SCID mouse model, humanized anti-Tac has resulted in antitumor responses *(179)*. These responses may be enhanced by co-administration of an antibody directed against pan-T-cell marker, CD2, using humanized antibody MEDI-507.

Transformation of T-cells by HTLV-1 may also result in IL-2 and 15-independence. Although, activation of the janus kinase 3 (JAK3) and transcription factor STAT5 pathway are essential for IL-2 and IL-15 induced proliferation of T-cells, this pathway is not required in IL-2-independent, HTLV-1 transformed cells *(176,180)*. This may provide an explanation for the resistance of some patients to anti-IL-2R immunotherapy. Thus, early stages of HTLV-1 immortalization involve polyclonal and then oligoclonal expansion of

CD4+ T-cells, which may involve autocrine or paracrine expression of IL-2, IL-15, and their receptors. Subsequent stages, however, result in uncoupling of the IL-2 and 15 pathways, resulting in Jak-3/Stat5 independence.

Several other interleukins, in addition to IL-2 and 15, may contribute to various aspects of ATLL. IL-6 is expressed in ATLL cells, and may contribute to hypercalcemia and osteolytic bone lesions (181,182). Transcriptional activation of IL-13 in HTLV-1 infected cells lines has also been described (144). IL-13 expression was directly related to levels of Tax expression. Because IL-13 has a key role in tumor immunosurveillance and central nervous system inflammation, it may contribute to the pathophysiology of HTLV-1 associated diseases. The Tax oncoprotein can also directly bind to the precursor of IL-16 (pro-IL-16) (183). This occurs through one of its PDZ domains, and inhibits the ability of pro-IL-16 to cause G1 cell cycle arrest. This may contribute to the effects of Tax in deregulation of T-cell proliferation.

9. CHEMOKINES AND HTLV-1-INDUCED CELL PROLIFERATION AND LYMPHOCYTE TRANSFORMATION

Chemokines play a role as leukocyte attractants, and chemokine expression by ATLL cells may enhance infiltration of malignant cells into skin and lymph nodes. Leukocyte migration from the circulation into tissues depends on integrin-mediated adhesion to endothelium. HTLV-1 infected cells express CC-chemokine receptors, CCR4, CCR5, and CCR7, as well as CCR5-binding chemokines MIP-1α, MIP-1β, and RANTES (159;184–194). In each case, Tax alone could reproduce these effects. Moreover, chemokine activation of G-protein coupled receptors and activation of phosphoinositide 3-kinases was found to be critical for cytoskeletal rearrangements critical to endothelial association (195). Tax was also shown to activate gene expression of human macrophage inflammatory protein-3α, also known as CCL20, as well as monocyte chemoattract protein-1 through the NF-kB pathway (186). IL-8 is activated through the AP-1 pathway in HTLV-1 infected cells (84). In addition, anti-apoptotic chemokine I-309, was also found to be expressed in ATLL cell cultures, and biologically active through its receptor CCR8 (191). HTLV-1 infected cells were also found to express stem cell-derived factor-1 (SDF-1) and its receptor, CXCR4, and migrated towards SDF-1 in chemotaxis assay (196).

10. TGF-β, TNF-α, AND HTLV-1-MEDIATED TRANSFORMATION

TGF-β suppresses premalignant lesions, but it is pro-oncogene in later stages of disease, and appears to contribute to metastasis (197,198). TGF-β acts as a tumor suppressor in premalignant lesions causing growth inhibition, induction of apoptosis, and genomic stability. In contrast, TGF-β in malignant lesions, contributes to tumor cell autonomy by promoting epithelial–mesenchymal transition, invasion, motility, and survival. TGF-β also has effects on tumor stroma including immunosuppression and angiogenesis. Intracellular signaling mediating TGF-β activities involve Smad-dependent and MAPK-dependent pathways (199,200).

The role of TGF-β in the induction or maintenance of ATLL is not entirely clear. Tax appears to promote the expression of TGF-β in Tax-transgenic mice (201). Tax transgenic mice with tumors in the submaxillary glands and skeletal muscle display high levels of Tax in combination with TGF-β mRNA and protein. Moreover, these investigators also reported that TGF-β stimulated the proliferation of neurofibromas derived from such Tax transgenic mice. In contrast to normal T-cells, ATLL cells are resistant to growth inhibitory effects of TGF-β. This effect has been explained by Tax activation of JNK, resulting in c-Jun phosphorylation, and formation of a c-Jun complex with Smad3 *(202)*. This abrogates DNA binding activity of Smad3. Other studies have shown direct interactions of Tax with several Smads, directly inactivating their DNA binding activity *(171)*. A third mechanism that has been proposed that involves Tax binding to transcriptional coactivators CBP/p300, competing for binding to Smads *(170)*. Collectively, these findings suggest a possible role of TGF-β in mediating Tax-induced tumorigenesis in ATLL.

Tax has also been shown to induce expression of TNF-α and to activate its transcription through the NF-κB pathway *(87)*. Another mechanism for TNF-α activation is through physical interaction of Tax with tristetrapolin, an immediate–early protein that enhances expression of TNF-α at a post-transcriptional level *(203)*. It is also interesting that a study of polymorphic germ line DNA loci associated with development of ATLL, after HTLV-1 infection, demonstrated that individuals with polymorphisms associated with high TNF-α expression were 2.3-fold more likely to develop ATLL, whereas no association was found with polymorphisms in anti-apoptotic genes breakpoint cluster region 2 (Bcl2), glutathione S transferase, or cytochrome P450 A1 *(204,205)*.

11. HTLV-1 ACCESSORY GENES IN CYTOKINE EXPRESSION AND T-CELL ACTIVATION

In addition to the regulatory proteins Tax and Rex, the HTLV-1 pX genome region encodes four accessory proteins, p12^{I}, p27^{I}, p13^{II}, and p30^{II} from alternatively spliced forms of mRNA in ORF I and II (Fig. 1) *(206–209)*. HTLV-1 accessory proteins were considered dispensable for viral replication *(210)*, however, recent findings have demonstrated the role of the HTLV-1 accessory proteins in viral infectivity, maintenance of high viral loads, host cell activation, and regulation of gene transcription *(211–224)*. Data from various studies provide strong evidence for the expression of these viral proteins during the natural viral infection *(208;209;225–227)*. HTLV-1 p12^{I} localizes in cellular endomembranes *(207)*, predominantly in the ER and cis-Golgi apparatus where it directly binds calreticulin and calnexin, two proteins in the ER associated with calcium storage and calcium-mediated cell signaling *(228)*. The binding of exogenously expressed p12^{I} to IL-2Rα chain correlates with a reduced cell-surface expression of the receptor and a decreased requirement of IL-2 to induce proliferation during suboptimal stimulation with anti-CD3 and anti-CD28 antibodies *(229)*. However, lymphocyte cell lines immortalized by the HTLV-1 proviral clone ablated for pX ORF I expression, ACH.p12^{I}, have intact IL-2R signaling pathways *(176)*. Nevertheless, p12^{I} does not appear to significantly alter the activation of the IL-2R-associated JAK1 and JAK3, or their downstream effectors STAT3 and STAT5, after immortalization. Collectively, these studies indicate that p12^{I} interacts with key cellular proteins involved in immune recognition and cellular proliferation to confer a growth advantage to infected cells during the early stages of infection, before immortalization. Future studies are necessary to characterize the interaction between p12^{I} and MHC-I in vivo and to understand the JAK3-independent pathway inducing STAT5 activation by p12^{I}.

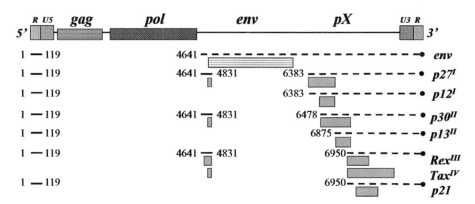

Fig. 1. Diagram of HTLV-1 genome and alternatively spliced mRNA and protein species from pX ORFs. Numbers correspond to nucleotide positions of exon splice acceptor and donor sites with respect to the full length HTLV-1 genome. Dotted lines indicate the mRNA while the boxes below the dotted lines indicate coding regions of each protein. Open reading frame from which each protein is produced is indicated as superscript, on the right of each protein.

11.1. Role of p12[I] in Calcium-Mediated T-cell Signaling

p12[I] specifically activates NFAT in synergy with Ras/MAP kinase activation stimulated by the phorbol ester, PMA. Reports from our laboratory demonstrated that p12[I] expression in Jurkat T-cells results in approx 20-fold activation of NFAT dependent gene expression, whereas AP-1 or NF-κB-mediated transcription remained unchanged *(212)*. Studies performed by inhibiting phospholipase C-γ (PLC-γ), LAT, calcineurin, and NFAT, narrowed the functional platform of p12[I] to be between PLC-γ and calcineurin *(212)*. Activation of NFAT by p12[I] was dependent on increase in cytosolic calcium and p12[I] functionally substituted for thapsigargin, a specific inhibitor of ER calcium ATPase, which specifically depletes the ER calcium store. In fact, p12[I] increases the base-line cytoplasmic calcium concentration, by release of calcium from ER stores and subsequent higher capacitative calcium entry *(213)*. Collectively, HTLV-1 p12[I] regulates the calcium homeostasis and activates NFAT-mediated transcription in lymphoid cells in a calcium-dependent manner.

Both the IP$_3$R, and calcium release activated calcium channels (CRAC), contribute to the NFAT activation by p12[I], strongly indicating the role of p12[I] on calcium homeostasis. Calcium release from the ER by p12[I] and subsequent activation of NFAT *(213)*, would be advantageous to the virus during the early stages of HTLV-1 infection. In addition, p12[I] mediated increase in NFAT activity could cause complete activation of cellular stimuli that would normally induce only partial activation of T-cells. These stimuli could be triggered by cytokines or chemokines released from infected neighboring cells or by direct contact between viral envelope proteins and certain cell surface receptors on newly targeted lymphocytes before viral entry *(230)*. Although localization of p12[I] to the ER appears to be essential for NFAT activation, *(231)*, direct binding between calreticulin and p12[I] does not correlate with the NFAT activation *(213)*. Interestingly, there is a functional similarity between p12[I] and a cellular protein CAML (Ca^{2+}-modulating cyclophilin ligand), which also contains two putative transmembrane domains and like p12[I] colocalizes with calreticulin in the ER, induces calcium release from the ER, and leads to NFAT activation *(232)*. Further studies are necessary to identify the significance of p12^I - calreticulin interaction in HTLV-1 infection and development of ATLL.

Expression of NFAT induces a highly permissive state to overcome the blockade at reverse transcription and permits HIV replication in primary CD4$^+$ T-cells. Therefore, it is possible that p12^I causes T-cells to be hypersensitive to T-cell receptor and CD28 stimulation and thus highly permissive for subsequent viral infection. Interestingly, susceptibility of these cells to HIV infection could be restored by mitogen treatment, likely owing to the phytohemagglutinin-induced upregulation of NFAT activity. This is similar to earlier reports from our laboratory that addition of mitogens can rescue the infectivity of a p12^I mutant viral clone in resting PBMC *(218)*, likely by overriding the requirement for p12^I-induced activation of NFAT.

p12^I competes with NFAT for calcineurin binding *(211)*. Interestingly, alanine substitution mutations in PxIxIT motif resulted in increased nuclear translocation and transcriptional activity (~2-fold) of NFAT *(211)*. Many calcineurin-binding proteins such as the anti-apoptotic protein Bcl-2, calcineurin B homologous protein, a kinase anchoring protein AKAP79, and myocyte-enriched calcineurin-interacting protein 1 inhibit either calcineurin phosphatase activity or its substrate NFAT transcriptional activity *(233–235)*. However, p12^I binding to calcineurin via a motif similar to PxIxIT did not inhibit calcineurin phosphatase activity, but instead influenced NFAT and calcineurin interaction by competing for binding with NFAT similar to artificial peptides representing this motif *(236)*.

The presence of calcineurin-binding motif in p12^I could regulate NFAT by either positive modulation via increasing cytosolic calcium concentration from ER stores or negative modulation by calcineurin binding. The significance of this mutually opposed regulatory functions of p12^I on NFAT transcriptional activity is unclear. Similar to another protein with similar binding properties such as Bcl-2, p12^I may act as an ion channel protein to increase ER calcium permeability and thereby affect apoptosis in HTLV-1-infected T-cells. Another ER membrane protein, CAML, activates NFAT by increasing calcium flux and binds with calcineurin indirectly, through its association with cyclophilin *(232)*. Overall, p12^I interacts with proteins involved in regulation of intracellular calcium levels such as calcineurin, mediated through a highly conserved PSLP(I/L)T motif, to further T-cell activation, and subsequently enhance viral infectivity.

In the case of HTLV-1, p12^I enhances the production of IL-2, a downstream gene of NFAT activation, in Jurkat T-cells and primary lymphocytes, in a calcium-dependent fashion *(231)*. This increase in IL-2 could account for the decrease in requirement for the cytokine in proliferation of human primary lymphocytes in the presence of p12^I *(229)*. Overall, p12^I expression hastens T-cell activation and likely facilitates viral replication and productive infection, which correlates with the indispensable nature of p12^I in viral infectivity in vivo *(219)*.

The mechanism by which calcium induces gene expression has been the focus of many investigations. Based on DNA microarray analysis, Feske et al *(237)* demonstrated that Ca^{2+} signals modulate the expression of various genes involved in transcription, including c-Myc, c-Jun, c-rel, STAT5B, STAT4, STAT-1, CREM, NFAT4, FosB, BRF2, E2F3, IRF-1, IRF-2, NF-IL3A, Fra-2, FLI1, MINOR, NOT, and SMBP2. Calcium-dependent activation of a wide variety of transcription factors, such as NFAT, NFκB, Elk-1, Nur77, AP-1, ATF-2, and CREB, is through calmodulin-dependent protein kinases and phosphatases *(238–240)*. Although a small transient spike of Ca^{2+} increase by store depletion activates signaling pathways and transcription factors such as NFκB and JNK (241), capacitative calcium entry and a sustained Ca^{2+} increase are necessary to activate other transcription factors, such as NFAT *(241–243)*.

Collectively, p12^{I} appears to be a key molecule required by HTLV-1 to replicate *(219)* and is a key molecule involved in modulation of cellular gene expression in a calcium-dependent manner. Future studies are needed to provide insight into how HTLV-1 uses accessory proteins to modulate their cellular environment for long-term cell survival setting the stage for lymphocyte transformation.

12. PERSPECTIVES OF HTLV-1 AND CYTOKINES

HTLV-1 infected cells, ATLL tumor cell lines, and Tax transgenic tumor cells are rich sources of cytokines, resulting from activated malignant T or NK cells. Technologies and model systems are now established to more fully define the role of cytokines in disease pathogenesis. Additional studies of antibodies, small molecules inhibitors, small interfering RNAs, dominant negative mutants, and genetic knockout strategies will be enlightening in defining the role of each cytokines in tumor initiation and progression. Exploitation of these findings for therapeutic development has already occurred with the use of antibodies to the IL-2R for ATLL *(178,244,245)*. Animal models and clinical studies will be critical to assess the efficacy and toxicity of these new approaches in order to improve the outcome of this aggressive malignancy. Lessons from HTLV-1 biology and ATLL pathogenesis will continue to be applicable to a much broader range of human malignancies.

ACKNOWLEDGMENTS

This work was supported by National Institute of Health (NIH) grants RR-14324 and CA-100730 awarded to M. Lairmore and subcontracted to Dr. Lee Ratner through CA100730, as well as NIH grants CA-70529 and CA-09338 awarded through The Ohio State University Comprehensive Cancer Center.

REFERENCES

1. Hinuma Y, Komoda H, Chosa T, et al. Antibodies to adult T-cell leukemia virus-associated antigen (ATLA) in sera from patients with ATL and controls in Japan: a nation-wide seroepidemiological study. Int J Cancer 1982; 29:631.
2. Yoshida M, Miyoshi I, Hinuma Y. Isolation and characterization of retrovirus from cell lines of human T-cell leukemia and its implication in the disease. Proc Natl Acad Sci USA 1982; 79:2031–2035.
3. Yoshida M, Seiki M, Yamaguchi K, Takatsuki K. Monoclonal integration of human T-cell leukemia provirus in all primary tumors of adult T-cell leukemia suggests causative role of human T-cell leukemia virus in the disease. Proc Natl Acad Sci U S A 1984; 81:2534–2537.
4. Takatsuki K, Uchiyama T, Sagawa K, Yodoi J. Adult T-cell leukemia in Japan. In: Seno S, Takaku F, Irino S, editors. Topics in Hematology. Amsterdam: Excerpta Medica, 1977: 73–77.
5. Uchiyama T, Yodoi J, Sagawa K, Takatsuki K, Uchino H. Adult T-cell leukemia: Clinical and hematologic features of 16 cases. Blood 1977; 50(3):481–492.
6. Poiesz BJ, Ruscetti FW, Gazdar AF, Bunn PA, Minna JD, Gallo RC. Detection and isolation of type C retrovirus particles from fresh and cultured lymphocytes of a patient with cutaneous T-cell lymphoma. Proc Natl Acad Sci USA 1980; 77(12):7415–7419.
7. Hinuma Y, Nagata K, Hanaoka M, et al. Adult T Cell Leukemia: Antigens in an ATL cell line and detection of antibodies to antigen in human sera. Proc Natl Acad Sci U S A 1981; 78:6476–6480.

8. Miyoshi I, Kubonishi I, Sumida M et al. A novel T-cell line derived from adult T-cell leukemia. Gann 1980; 71(1):155, 156.

9. Miyoshi I, Kubonishi I, Yoshimoto S, Shiraishi Y. A T-cell line derived from normal human cord leukocytes by co-culturing with human leukemic T-cells. Gann 1981; 72(6):978–981.

10. Gessain A, Mahieux R. A virus called HTLV-1. Epidemiological aspects. Presse Med 2000; 29(40): 2233–2239.

11. Blattner W, Kalyanaraman V, Robert-Guroff M et al. The human type-C retrovirus, HTLV, in blacks from the Caribbean region and relationchip to adult T-cell leukemia/lymphoma. Int J Cancer 1982; 30:257.

12. Saxinger WC, Blattner W, Levine P et al. Human T-cell leukemia virus (HTLV-I) antibodies in Africa. Science 1984; 225:1473.

13. Reeves W, Saxinger C, Brenes M, et al. Human T-cell lymphotropic virus type I (HTLV-I) and risk factors in metropolitan Panama. Am J Epidemiol 1988; 127:539.

14. Merino F, Robert-Guroff M, Clark J, Biondo-Bracho M, Blattner W, Gallo RC. Natural antibodies to human T-cell leukemia/lymphoma virus in healthy Venezuelan populations. Int J Cancer 1984; 34:501.

15. Asher DM, Goudsmit J, Pomeroy K, et al. Antibodies to HTLV-I in populations of the southwestern Pacific. J Med Virol 1988; 26:339.

16. Anderson DC, Epstein J, Pierik L, et al. Licensure of screening tests for antibody to human T-cell lymphotropic virus type I. Morb Mort Weekly Report 1988; 37:736.

17. Nagai M, Osame M. Human T-cell lymphotropic virus type I and neurological diseases. J Neurovirol 2003; 9(2):228–235.

18. Edlich RF, Arnette JA, Williams FM. Global epidemic of human T-cell lymphotropic virus type-I (HTLV-I). J Emerg Med 2000; 18(1):109–119.

19. Courouce AM, Pillonel J, Lemaire JM, Saura C. HTLV testing in blood transfusion. Vox Sang 1998; 74 Suppl 2:165–169.

20. Ferreira OC, Jr., Planelles V, Rosenblatt JD. Human T-cell leukemia viruses: Epidemiology, biology, and pathogenesis. Blood Rev 1997; 11(2):91–104.

21. Murphy EL, Glynn SA, Fridey J, et al. Increased incidence of infectious diseases during prospective follow-up of human T-lymphotropic virus type II- and I-infected blood donors. Arch Intern Med 1999; 159:1485–1491.

22. Schreiber GB, Murphy EL, Horton JA, et al. Risk factors for human T-cell lymphotropic virus types I and II (HTLV-I and -II) in blood donors: the Retrovirus Epidemiology Donor Study. NHLBI Retrovirus Epidemiology Donor Study. J Acquir Immune Defic Syndr Hum Retrovirol 1997; 14(3):263–271.

23. Yamamoto N, Okada M, Koyanagi Y, Kannagi M, Hinuma Y. Transformation of human Leukocytes by cocultivation with an adult T cell leukemia virus producer cell line. Science 1982; 217(20): 737–739.

24. Hino S, Yamaguchi K, Katamine S, et al. Mother-to-child transmission of human T-cell leukemia virus type-I. Jpn J Cancer Res 1985; 76(6):474–480.

25. Hino S. Milk-borne transmission of HTLV-I as a major route in the endemic cycle. Acta Paediatr Jpn 1989; 31(4):428–435.

26. Khabbaz RF, Douglas JM, Judson FN, et al. Seroprevalence of human T-lymphotropic virus type I or II in sexually transmitted disease clinic patients in the USA. J Infect Dis 1990; 162(1):241–244.

27. Khabbaz RF, Onorato IM, Cannon RO, et al. Seroprevalence of HTLV-1 and HTLV-2 among intravenous drug users and persons in clinics for sexually transmitted diseases. N Engl J Med 1992; 326(6):375–380.

28. Okochi K, Sato H, Hinuma Y. A retrospective study on transmission of adult T cell leukemia virus by blood transfusion: Seroconversion in recipients. Vox Sang 1984; 46(5):245–253.

29. Stuver SO, Tachibana N, Okayama A, et al. Heterosexual transmission of human T cell leukemia/lymphoma virus type I among married couples in southwestern Japan: an initial report from the Miyazaki Cohort Study. J Infect Dis 1993; 167:57–65.

30. Yamaguchi K, Takatsuki K. Adult T cell leukaemia-lymphoma. Clin Haematol 1993; 6(4):899–915.

31. Yamaguchi K. Human T-lymphotropic virus type I in Japan. Lancet 1994; 343(8891):213–216.

32. Cleghorn FR, Manns A, Falk R, et al. Effect of human T-lymphotropic virus type I infection on non-Hodgkin's lymphoma incidence. J Nat Cancer Inst 1995; 87:1009–1014.

33. White JD, Zaknoen SL, Kastensportes C, et al. Infectious complications and immunodeficiency in patients with human T-cell lymphotropic virus I-associated adult T- cell leukemia/lymphoma. Cancer 1995; 75:1598–1607.

34. Shimoyama M. Diagnostic criteria and classification of clinical subtypes of adult T-cell leukaemia-lymphoma. A report from the Lymphoma Study Group (1984–1987). Br J Haematol 1991; 79(3): 428–437.

35. Yamaguchi K, Nishimura H, Kohrogi H, Jono M, Miyamoto Y, Takatsuki K. A proposal for smoldering adult T-cell leukemia: a clinicopathologic study of five cases. Blood 1983; 62(4):758–766.

36. Kawano F, Yamaguchi K, Nishimura H, Tsuda H, Takatsuki K. Variation in the clinical courses of adult T-cell leukemia. Cancer 1985; 55(4):851–856.

37. Mortreux F, Gabet AS, Wattel E. Molecular and cellular aspects of HTLV-1 associated leukemogenesis in vivo. Leukemia 2003; 17(1):26–38.

38. Franchini G. Molecular mechanisms of human T-cell leukemia/lymphotropic virus type I infection. Blood 1995; 86(10):3619–3639.

39. Hollsberg P, Wucherpfennig KW, Ausubel LJ, Calvo V, Bierer BE, Hafler DA. Characterization of HTLV-1 In Vivo Infected T Cell Clones IL-2-independent Growth of Nontransformed T Cells. J Immunol 1992; 148:3256–3263.

40. Gatza ML, Watt JC, Marriott SJ. Cellular transformation by the HTLV-I Tax protein, a jack-of-all-trades. Oncogene 2003; 22(33):5141–5149.

41. Franchini G, Wong-Staal F, Gallo RC. Human T-cell leukemia virus (HTLV-I) transcripts in fresh and cultured cells of patients with adult T-cell leukemia. Proc Natl Acad Sci U S A 1984; 81(19):6207–6211.

42. Korber B, Okayama A, Donnelly R, Tachibana N, Essex M. Polymerase chain reaction analysis of defective human T-cell leukemia virus type 1 proviral genomes in leukemic cells of patients with adult T-cell leukemia. J Virol 1991; 65(10):5471–5476.

43. Gessain A, Barin F, Vernant J, et al. Antibodies to human T lymphotropic virus type 1 in patients with tropical spastic paresis. Lancet 1985; 2:407–410.

44. Osame M, Usuku K, Izumo S, et al. HTLV-I associated myelopathy, a new clinical entity. Lancet 1986; i:1031–1032.

45. Adedayo O, Grell G, Bellot P. Hospital admissions for human T-cell lymphotropic virus type-1 (HTLV-1) associated diseases in Dominica. Postgrad Med J 2003; 79(932):341–344.

46. Kasahata N, Shiota J, Miyazawa Y, Nakano I, Murayama S. Acute human T-lymphotropic virus type 1-associated myelopathy: A clinicopathologic study. Arch Neurol 2003; 60(6):873–876.

47. Furukawa Y, Kubota R, Eiraku N, et al. Human T-cell lymphotropic virus type I (HTLV-I)-related clinical and laboratory findings for HTLV-I-infected blood donors. J Acquir Immune Defic Syndr 2003; 32(3):328–334.

48. Kiwaki T, Umehara F, Arimura Y et al. The clinical and pathological features of peripheral neuropathy accompanied with HTLV-I associated myelopathy. J Neurol Sci 2003; 206(1):17–21.

49. Nagai M, Usuku K, Matsumoto W et al. Analysis of HTLV-I proviral load in 202 HAM/TSP patients and 243 asymptomatic HTLV-I carriers: High proviral load strongly predisposes to HAM/TSP. J Neurovirol 1998; 4(6):586–593.

50. Nitta T, Tanaka M, Sun B, Hanai S, Miwa M. The genetic background as a determinant of human T-cell leukemia virus type 1 proviral load. Biochem Biophys Res Commun 2003; 309(1):161–165.

51. Bangham CR. Human T-lymphotropic virus type 1 (HTLV-1): Persistence and immune control. Int J Hematol 2003; 78(4):297–303.

52. Bangham CR. The immune control and cell-to-cell spread of human T-lymphotropic virus type 1. J Gen Virol 2003; 84(Pt 12):3177–3189.

53. Yamano Y, Nagai M, Brennan M, et al. Correlation of human T-cell lymphotropic virus type 1 (HTLV-1) mRNA with proviral DNA load, virus-specific CD8(+) T cells, and disease severity in HTLV-1-associated myelopathy (HAM/TSP). Blood 2002; 99(1):88–94.

54. Kitze B, Usuku K. HTLV-1-mediated immunopathological CNS disease. Curr Top Microbiol Immunol 2002; 265:197–211.

55. Osame M, Janssen R, Kubota H et al. Nationwide survey of HTLV-I-associated Myelopathy in Japan: Association with blood transfusion. Ann Neurol 1990; 28:50–56.

56. Daenke S, Nightingale S, Cruickshank JK, Bangham CRM. Sequence variants of human T-cell lymphotropic virus type I from patients with tropical spastic paraparesis and adult T-cell leukemia do not distinguish neurological from leukemic isolates. J Virol 1990; 64(3):1278–1282.

57. Evangelista A, Maroushek S, Minnigan H, et al. Nucleotide sequence analysis of a provirus derived from an individual with tropical spastic paraparesis. Microb Pathog 1990; 8(4):259–278.

58. Gould KG, Bangham CR. Virus variation, escape from cytotoxic T lymphocytes and human retroviral persistence. Semin Cell Dev Biol 1998; 9:321–328.

59. Mahieux R, Ibrahim F, Mauclere P et al. Molecular epidemiology of 58 new African human T-cell leukemia virus type 1 (HTLV-1) strains: Identification of a new and distinct HTLV-1 molecular subtype in central Africa and in pygmies. J Virol 1997; 71(2):1317–1333.

60. Saito M, Furukawa Y, Kubota R, et al. Frequent mutation in pX region of HTLV-1 is observed in HAM/TSP patients, but is not specifically associated with the central nervous system lesions. J Neurovirol 1995; 1(3–4):286–294.

61. Mochizuki M, Watanabe T, Yamaguchi K, et al. HTLV-I Uveitis: A distinct clinical entity caused by HTLV-I. Jpn J Cancer Res 1992; 83:236–239.

62. Nishioka K, Maruyama I, Sato K, Kitajima I, Nakajima Y, Osame M. Chronic inflammatory arthropathy associated with HTLV-I [letter]. Lancet 1989; i(8635):441.

63. Terada K, Katamine S, Eguchi K, et al. Prevalence of serum and salivary antibodies to HTLV-1 in Sjogren's syndrome. Lancet 1994; 344:1116–1119.

64. Lagrenade L, Hanchard B, Fletcher V, Cranston B, Blattner W. Infective dermatitis of Jamaican children: a marker for HTLV-I infection. Lancet 1990; 336(8727):1345–1347.

65. Leonmonzon M, Illa I, Dalakas MC. Polymyositis in patients infected with human T-cell leukemia virus type I: The role of the virus in the cause of the disease. Ann Neurol 1994; 36:643-649.

66. Ohshima K, Kikuchi M, Masuda Y, et al. Human T-cell leukemia virus type I associated lymphadenitis. Cancer 1992; 69(1):239–248.

67. Kimura I, Tsubota T, Tada S, Sogawa J. Presence of antibodies against adult T cell leukemia antigen in the patients with chronic respiratory diseases. Acta Med Okayama 1986; 40(6):281–284.

68. Xu RZ, Gao QK, Wang SJ, et al. Human acute myeloid leukemias may be etiologically associated with new human retroviral infection. Leuk Res 1996; 20(6):449–455.

69. Yajima A, Kawada A, Aragane Y, Tezuka T. Detection of HTLV-I proviral DNA in sarcoidosis. Dermatology 2001; 203(1):53–56.

70. Manel N, Kim FJ, Kinet S, Taylor N, Sitbon M, Battini JL. The ubiquitous glucose transporter GLUT-1 is a receptor for HTLV. Cell 2003; 115(4):449–459.

71. Bukrinsky MI, Sharova N, Dempsey MP et al. Active nuclear import of human immunodeficiency virus type 1 preintegration complexes. Proc Natl Acad Sci U S A 1992; 89(14):6580-6584.

72. Green PL, Chen ISY. Regulation of human T cell leukemia virus expression. FASEB J 1990; 4:169–175.

73. Kiyokawa T, Seiki M, Iwashita S, Imagawa K, Shimizu F, Yoshida M. p27x-III and p21x-III, proteins encoded by the pX sequence of human T-cell leukemia virus type 1. Proc Natl Acad Sci USA 1985; 82:8359–8363.

74. Seiki M, Hikikoshi A, Taniguchi T, Yoshida M. Expression of the pX Gene of HTLV-1: General Splicing Mechanism in the HTLV Family. Science 1985; 228:1532–1534.

75. Felber BK, Paskalis H, Kleinmanewing C. The pX Protein of HTLV-1 is a Transcriptional Activator of its Long Terminal Repeats. Science 1985; 229:675–679.

76. Sodroski J, Rosen C, Goh WC, Haseltine W. A transcriptional activator protein encoded by the x-lor region of the human T-cell leukemia virus. Science 1985; 228(4706):1430–1434.

77. Kimzey AL, Dynan WS. Identification of a human T-cell leukemia virus type I tax peptide in contact with DNA. J Biol Chem 1999; 274:34226–34232.

78. Lenzmeier BA, Baird EE, Dervan PB, Nyborg JK. The tax protein-DNA interaction is essential for HTLV-I transactivation in vitro. J Mol Biol 1999; 291(4):731–744.

79. Perini G, Wagner S, Green MR. Recognition of bZIP proteins by the human T-cell leukaemia virus transactivator Tax. Nature 1995; 376:602–605.

80. Maruyama M, Shibuya H, Harada H et al. Evidence for aberrant activation of the interleukin-2 autocrine loop by HTLV-1-encoded p40x and T3/Ti complex triggering. Cell 1987; 48(2):343–350.

81. Wolin M, Kornuc M, Hong C, et al. Differential effect of HTLV infection and HTLV Tax on interleukin 3 expression. Oncogene 1993; 8(7):1905–1911.

82. Li-Weber M, Giaisi M, Chlichlia K, Khazaie K, Krammer PH. Human T cell leukemia virus type I Tax enhances IL-4 gene expression in T cells. Eur J Immunol 2001; 31(9):2623–2632.

83. Muraoka O, Kaisho T, Tanabe M, Hirano T. Transcriptional activation of the interleukin-6 gene by HTLV-1. Immunology Letters 1993; 37(2–3):159–165.

84. Mori N, Mukaida N, Ballard DW, Matsushima K, Yamamoto N. Human T-cell leukemia virus type I Tax transactivates human interleukin 8 gene through acting concurrently on AP-1 and nuclear factor-kappaB-like sites. Cancer Res 1998; 58(17):3993–4000.

85. Mori N, Prager D. Transactivation of the interleukin-1 alpha promoter by human T- cell leukemia virus type I and type II tax proteins. Blood 1996; 87(8):3410–3417.

86. Miyatake S, Seiki M, Malefijt RD et al. Activation of T cell-derived lymphokine genes in T cells and fibroblasts: effects of human T cell leukemia virus type I p40x protein and bovine papilloma virus encoded E2 protein. Nucleic Acids Res 1988; 16(14A):6547–6566.

87. Cowan EP, Alexander RK, Daniel S, Kashanchi F, Brady JN. Induction of tumor necrosis factor alpha in human neuronal cells by extracellular human T-cell lymphotropic virus type 1 Tax(1). J Virol 1997; 71(9):6982–6989.

88. Lindholm PF, Reid RL, Brady JN. Extracellular Tax Protein Stimulates Tumor Necrosis Factor-B and Immunoglobulin Kappa Light Chain Expression in Lymphoid Cells. J Virol 1992; 66:1294–1302.

89. Duyao MP, Kessler DJ, Spicer DB, et al. Transactivation of the c-myc Promoter by Human T Cell Leukemia virus Type 1 tax is Mediated by NFkB. J Biol Chem 1992; 267:16288–16291.

90. Fujii M, Sassone-Corsi P, Verma I. c-fos promotor trans-activation of cAMP on IL-2 stimulated gene expression. Proc Natl Acad Sci U S A 1988;8526–8530.

91. Ratner L. Regulation of expression of the c-sis proto-oncogene. Nucleic Acids Res 1989; 17(11): 4101–4115.

92. Fujii M, Tsuchiya H, Chuhjo T, Akizawa T, Seiki M. Interaction of HTLV-1 Tax1 with p67SRF causes the aberrant induction of cellular immediate early genes through CArG boxes. Genes Dev 1992; 6(11):2066–2076.

93. Li CC, Ruscetti FW, Rice NR et al. Differential expression of Rel family members in human T-cell leukemia virus type I-infected cells: Transcriptional activation of c-rel by Tax protein. J Virol 1993; 67:4205–4213.

94. Jeang KT, Widen SG, Semmes OJ, Wilson SH. HTLV-1 Trans-Activator Protein, Tax, Is a Trans-Repressor of the Human B-Ploymerase Gene. Science 1990; 247:1082, 1083.

95. Nicot C, Mahieux R, Takemoto S, Franchini G. Bcl-X(L) is up-regulated by HTLV-I and HTLV-II in vitro and in ex vivo ATLL samples. Blood 2000; 96(1):275–281.

96. Tsukahara T, Kannagi M, Ohashi T et al. Induction of Bcl-x(L) expression by human T-cell leukemia virus type 1 Tax through NF-kappaB in apoptosis-resistant T-cell transfectants with Tax. J Virol 1999; 73(10):7981–7987.

97. Lemasson I, Roberthebmann V, Hamaia S, Dodon MD, Gazzolo L, Devaux C. Transrepression of lck gene expression by human T-cell leukemia virus type 1-encoded p40(tax). J Virol 1997; 71(3):1975–1983.

98. Ressler S, Morris GF, Marriott SJ. Human T-cell leukemia virus type 1 Tax transactivates the human proliferating cell nuclear antigen promoter. J Virol 1997; 71(2):1181–1190.

99. Ye J, Silverman L, Lairmore MD, Green PL. HTLV-1 Rex is required for viral spread and persistence in vivo but is dispensable for cellular immortalization in vitro. Blood 2003; 102(12):3963–3969.

100. Akagi T, Takeda I, Oka T, Ohtsuki Y, Yano S, Miyoshi I. Experimental infection of rabbits with human T-cell leukemia virus type 1. Jpn J Cancer Res 1985; 76:86–94.

101. Lairmore MD, Roberts B, Frank D, Rovnak J, Weiser MG, Cockerell GL. Comparative biological responses of rabbits infected with human T-lymphotropic virus Type I isolates from patients with lymphoproliferative and neurodegenerative disease. Int J Cancer 1992; 50:124–130.

102. Murata N, Hakoda E, Machida H, et al. Prevention of human T cell lymphotropic virus type 1 infection in Japanese macaques by passive immunization. Leukemia 1996; 10(12):1971–1974.

103. Nakamura H, Hayami M, Ohta Y, et al. Protection of Cynomolgus Monkeys Against Infection by Human T-Cell leukemia Virus Type-1 by Immunization with Viral env Gene Products Produced in Escerichia coli. Int J Cancer 1987; 40:403–407.

104. Suga T, Kameyama T, Shimotohno K, et al. Infectiion of Rats with HTLV-1: A Small-Animal Model for HTLV-1 Carriers. Int J Cancer 1991; 49:764–769.

105. Ibrahim F, Fiette L, Gessain A, Buisson N, Dethe G, Bomford R. Infection of rats with human T-cell leukemia virus type-1: Susceptibility of inbred strains, antibody response and provirus location. Int J Cancer 1994; 58:446–451.

106. Furuta RA, Sugiura K, Kawakita S, et al. Mouse Model for the Equilibration Interaction between the Host Immune System and Human T-Cell Leukemia Virus Type 1 Gene Expression. J Virol 2002; 76(6):2703–2713.

107. Feng R, Kabayama A, Uchida K, Hoshino H, Miwa M. Cell-free entry of human t-cell leukemia virus type 1 to mouse cells. Jpn J Cancer Res 2001; 92(4):410–416.

108. Leendertz FH, Boesch C, Junglen S, Pauli G, Ellerbrook H. Characterization of a new simian T-lymphocyte virus type 1 (STLV-1) in a wild living chimpanzee (Pan troglodytes verus) from Ivory Coast: evidence of a new STLV-1 group? AIDS Res Hum Retroviruses 2003; 19(3):255–258.

109. Niphuis H, Verschoor EJ, Bontjer I, Peeters M, Heeney JL. Reduced transmission and prevalence of simian T-cell lymphotropic virus in a closed breeding colony of chimpanzees (Pan troglodytes verus). J Gen Virol 2003; 84(Pt 3):615–620.

110. Gabet AS, Gessain A, Wattel E. High simian T-cell leukemia virus type 1 proviral loads combined with genetic stability as a result of cell-associated provirus replication in naturally infected, asymptomatic monkeys. Int J Cancer 2003; 107(1):74–83.

111. Mahieux R, Chappey C, Georges-Courbot MC, et al. Simian T-cell lymphotropic virus type 1 from Mandrillus sphinx as a simian counterpart of human T-cell lymphotropic virus type 1 subtype D. J Virol 1998; 72(12):10316–10322.

112. Mortreux F, Kazanji M, Gabet AS, de Thoisy B, Wattel E. Two-step nature of human T-cell leukemia virus type 1 replication in experimentally infected squirrel monkeys (Saimiri sciureus). J Virol 2001; 75(2):1083–1089.

113. Kazanji M, Tartaglia J, Franchini G et al. Immunogenicity and protective efficacy of recombinant human T-cell leukemia/lymphoma virus type 1 NYVAC and naked DNA vaccine candidates in squirrel monkeys (Saimiri sciureus). J Virol 2001; 75(13):5939–5948.

114. Kazanji M. HTLV type 1 infection in squirrel monkeys (Saimiri sciureus): A promising animal model for HTLV type 1 human infection. AIDS Res Hum Retroviruses 2000; 16(16):1741–1746.

115. Hakata Y, Yamada M, Shida H. Rat CRM1 Is Responsible for the Poor Activity of Human T-Cell Leukemia Virus Type 1 Rex Protein in Rat Cells. J Virol 2001; 75(23):11515–11525.

116. Hanabuchi S, Ohashi T, Koya Y, et al. Development of human T-cell leukemia virus type 1-transformed tumors in rats following suppression of T-cell immunity by CD80 and CD86 blockade. J Virol 2000; 74(1):428–435.

117. Kasai T, Ikeda H, Tomaru U, et al. A rat model of human T lymphocyte virus type I (HTLV-I) infection: In situ detection of HTLV-I provirus DNA in microglia/macrophages in affected spinal cords of rats with HTLV-1-induced chronic progressive myeloneuropathy. Acta Neuropathol 1999; 97:107–112.

118. Sun B, Fang J, Yagami K, et al. Age-dependent paraparesis in WKA rats: evaluation of MHC k-haplotype and HTLV-1 infection. J Neurol Sci 1999; 167(1):16–21.

119. Hasegawa A, Ohashi T, Hanabuchi S, et al. Expansion of human T-cell leukemia virus type 1 (HTLV-1) reservoir in orally infected rats: inverse correlation with HTLV-1-specific cellular immune response. J Virol 2003; 77(5):2956–2963.

120. Kotani S, Yoshimoto S, Yamato K, et al. Serial transmission of human T-cell leukemia virus type 1 by blood transfusion in rabbits and its prevention by use of x-irradiated stored blood. Int J Cancer 1986; 37:843–847.

121. Uemura Y, Kotani S, Yoshimoto S, et al. Oral transmission of human T-cell leukemia Virus type-1 in the rabbit. Jpn J Cancer Res 1986; 77:970–973.

122. Mosier DE. Adoptive transfer of human lymphoid cells to severely immunodeficient mice: models for normal human immune function, autoimmunity, lymphomagenesis, and AIDS. Adv Immunol 1991; 50:303–325.

123. Feuer G, Stewart SA, Baird SM, Lee F, Feuer R, Chen IS. Potential role of natural killer cells in controlling tumorigenesis by human T-cell leukemia viruses. J Virol 1995; 69(2):1328–1333.

124. Liu Y, Dole K, Stanley JR, et al. Engraftment and tumorigenesis of HTLV-1 transformed T cell lines in SCID/bg and NOD/SCID mice. Leuk Res 2002; 26(6):561–567.

125. Takaorikondo A, Imada K, Yamamoto I, et al. Parathyroid hormone-related protein-induced hypercalcemia in SCID mice engrafted with adult T-cell leukemia cells. Blood 1998; 91:4747–4751.

126. Furlan R, Salazargrueso EF, Martino G, et al. Human T-cell lymphotropic virus type-I infection in the severe combined immunodeficiency mouse. J Med Virol 1996; 49(2):77–82.

127. Feuer G, Fraser JK, Zack JA, Lee F, Feuer R, Chen ISY. Human T-cell leukemia virus infection of human hematopoietic progenitor cells: Maintenance of virus infection during differentiation in vitro and in vivo. J Virol 1996; 70(6):4038–4044.

128. Nerenberg MI. An HTLV-I transgenic mouse model: role of the tax gene in pathogenesis in multiple organ systems. Curr Top Microbiol Immunol 1990; 160:121–128.

129. Kitajima I, Hanyu N, Kawahara K, et al. Ribozyme-based gene cleavage approach to chronic arthritis associated with human T cell leukemia virus type I - Induction of apoptosis in synoviocytes by ablation of HTLV- I tax protein. Arthritis Rheum 1997; 40:2118–2127.

130. Nerenberg MI, Minor T, Price J, Ernst DN, Shinohara T, Schwarz H. Transgenic thymocytes are refractory to transformation by the human T-cell leukemia virus type I tax gene. J Virol 1991; 65(6):3349–3353.

131. Iwakura Y, Saijo S, Kioka Y, et al. Autoimmunity induction by human T cell leukemia virus type 1 in transgenic mice that develop chronic inflammatory arthropathy resembling rheumatoid arthritis in humans. J Immunol 1995; 155(3):1588–1598.

132. Green JE. trans activation of nerve growth factor in transgenic mice containing the human T-cell lymphotropic virus type I tax gene. Mol Cellular Biol 1997; 11(9):4635–4641.

133. Benvenisty N, Ornitz DM, Bennett GL, et al. Brain tumours and lymphomas in transgenic mice that carry HTLV-I LTR/c- myc and Ig/tax genes. Oncogene 1992; 7(12):2399–2405.

134. Grossman WJ, Kimata JT, Wong FH, Zutter M, Ley TJ, Ratner L. Development of leukemia in mice transgenic for the tax gene of human T-cell leukemia virus type I. Proc Natl Acad Sci U S A 1995; 92(4):1057–1061.

135. Grossman WJ, Ratner L. Cytokine expression and tumorigenicity of large granular lymphocytic leukemia cells from mice transgenic for the tax gene of human T-cell leukemia virus type I. Blood 1997; 90(2):783–794.

136. Apte RN, Voronov E. Interleukin-1—a major pleiotropic cytokine in tumor-host interactions. Semin Cancer Biol 2002; 12(4):277–290.

137. Horn F, Henze C, Heidrich K. Interleukin-6 signal transduction and lymphocyte function. Immunobiology 2000; 202(2):151–167.

138. Carvalho EM, Bacellar O, Porto AF, Braga S, Galvao-Castro B, Neva F. Cytokine profile and immunomodulation in asymptomatic human T- lymphotropic virus type 1-infected blood donors. J Acquir Immune Defic Syndr 2001; 27(1):1–6.

139. Furuya T, Nakamura T, Fujimoto T, et al. Elevated levels of interleukin-12 and interferon-gamma in patients with human T lymphotropic virus type I associated myelopathy. J Neuroimmunol 1999; 95:185–189.

140. Scholz C, Hafler DA, Hollsberg P. Downregulation of IL-10 secretion and enhanced antigen-presenting abilities following HTLV-I infection of T cells. J Neuroscience Res 1996; 45:786–794.

141. Tsuruma T, Yagihashi A, Torigoe T, et al. Interleukin-10 inhibited the expression of tumor antigens and major histocompatibility complex antigen on EJ-ras oncogene transformants. Artificial Organs 1996; 20(8):895–897.

142. Hanon E, Goon P, Taylor GP, et al. High production of interferon gamma but not interleukin-2 by human T-lymphotropic virus type I-infected peripheral blood mononuclear cells. Blood 2001; 98(3):721–726.

143. Mitre E, Thompson RW, Carvalho EM, Nutman TB, Neva FA. Majority of interferon-gamma-producing CD4+ cells in patients infected with human T cell lymphotrophic virus do not express tax protein. J Infect Dis 2003; 188(3):428–432.

144. Chung HK, Young HA, Goon PK, et al. Activation of interleukin-13 expression in T cells from HTLV-1-infected individuals and in chronically infected cell lines. Blood 2003; 102(12): 4130–4136.

145. Pawelec G. Tumour escape: Antitumour effectors too much of a good thing? Cancer Immunol Immunother 2004; 53(3):262–274.

146. Mitra-Kaushik S, Harding JC, Hess J, Ratner L. Effects of the proteasome inhibitor PS-341 on tumor growth in HTLV-1 tax transgenic mice and tax tumor transplants. Blood 2004; 104(3): 802–809.

147. Persaud D, Munoz JL, Tarsis SL, Parks ES, Parks WP. Time course and cytokine dependence of human T-cell lymphotropic virus type 1 T-lymphocyte transformation as revealed by a microtiter infectivity assay. J Virol 1995; 69:6297–6303.

148. Tatewaki M, Yamaguchi K, Matsuoka M, et al. Constitutive overexpression of the L-selectin gene in fresh leukemic cells of adult T-cell leukemia that can be transactivated by human T-cell lymphotropic virus type 1 Tax. Blood 1995; 86:3109–3117.

149. Copeland KFT, Heeney JL. T helper cell activation and human retroviral pathogenesis. Microbiol Rev 1996; 60(4):722.

150. Biddison WE, Kubota R, Kawanishi T et al. Human T cell leukemia virus type I (HTLV-1)-specific CD8(+) CTL clones from patients with HTLV-I-associated neurologic disease secrete proinflammatory cytokines, chemokines, and matrix metalloproteinase. J Immunol 1997; 159(4):2018–2025.

151. Giraudon P, Buart S, Bernard A, Belin MF. Cytokines secreted by glial cells infected with HTLV-I modulate the expression of matrix metalloproteinases (MMPs) and their natural inhibitor (TIMPs): Possible involvement in neurodegenerative processes. [Review] [23 refs]. Molecular Psychiatry 1997; 2(2):107–10, 84.

152. Miyazato A, Kawakami K, Iwakura Y, Saito A. Chemokine synthesis and cellular inflammatory changes in lungs of mice bearing p40tax of human T-lymphotropic virus type 1. Clin Exp Immunol 2000; 120(1):113–124.

153. Li XH, Gaynor RB. Mechanisms of NF-kappaB activation by the HTLV type 1 tax protein. AIDS Res Hum Retroviruses 2000; 16(16):1583–1590.
154. Ng PW, Iha H, Iwanaga Y, et al. Genome-wide expression changes induced by HTLV-1 Tax: Evidence for MLK- 3 mixed lineage kinase involvement in Tax-mediated NF-kappaB activation. Oncogene 2001; 20(33):4484–4496.
155. Dodon MD, Li Z, Hamaia S, Gazzolo L. Tax protein of human T-cell leukaemia virus type 1 induces interleukin 17 gene expression in T cells. J Gen Virol 2004; 85(Pt 7):1921–1932.
156. Kuo YL, Tang Y, Harrod R, Cai P, Giam CZ. Kinase-inducible domain-like region of HTLV type 1 tax is important for NF-kappaB activation. AIDS Res Hum Retroviruses 2000; 16(16):1607–1612.
157. Mariner JM, Lantz V, Waldmann TA, Azimi N. Human T cell lymphotropic virus type I Tax activates IL-15R alpha gene expression through an NF-kappaB site. J Immunol 2001; 166(4):2602–2609.
158. Rivera-Walsh I, Waterfield M, Xiao G, Fong A, Sun SC. NF-kappaB signaling pathway governs TRAIL gene expression and human T- cell leukemia virus-I Tax-induced T-cell death. J Biol Chem 2001; 276(44):40385–40388.
159. Shimizu T, Kawakita S, Li QH, Fukuhara S, Fujisawa J. Human T-cell leukemia virus type 1 Tax protein stimulates the interferon-responsive enhancer element via NF-kappaB activity. FEBS Lett 2003; 539(1–3):73–77.
160. O'Mahony AM, Montano M, Van Beneden K, Chen LF, Greene WC. Human T-cell lymphotropic virus type 1 tax induction of biologically Active NF-kappaB requires IkappaB kinase-1-mediated phosphorylation of RelA/p65. J Biol Chem 2004; 279(18):18137–18145.
161. Sun SC, Harhaj EW, Xiao G, Good L. Activation of I-kappaB kinase by the HTLV type 1 tax protein: mechanistic insights into the adaptor function of IKKgamma. AIDS Res Hum Retroviruses 2000; 16(16):1591–1596.
162. Jeang KT. Functional activities of the human T-cell leukemia virus type I Tax oncoprotein: cellular signaling through NF-kappa B. Cytokine Growth Factor Rev 2001; 12(2-3):207–217.
163. Yin MJ, Christerson LB, Yamamoto Y, et al. HTLV-I tax protein binds to MEKK1 to stimulate I kappa B kinase activity and NF-kappa B activation. Cell 1998; 93:875–884.
164. Li XH, Murphy KM, Palka KT, Surabhi RM, Gaynor RB. The human T-cell leukemia virus type-1 Tax protein regulates the activity of the I kappa B kinase complex. J Biol Chem 1999; 274:34417–34424.
165. Suzuki T, Hirai H, Fujisawa J, Fujita T, Yoshida M. A trans-activator Tax of human T-cell leukemia virus type 1 binds to NF- kappa B p50 and serum response factor (SRF) and associates with enhancer DNAs of the NF-kappa B site and CArG box 5014. Oncogene 1993; 8(9):2391–2397.
166. Good L, Maggirwar SB, Harhaj EW, Sun SC. Constitutive dephosphorylation and activation of a member of the nuclear factor of activated T cells, NF-AT1, in Tax-expressing and type I human T-cell leukemia virus-infected human T cells 5284. J Biol Chem 1997; 272(3):1425–1428.
167. Rivera I, Harhaj EW, Sun SC. Involvement of NF-AT in type I human T-cell leukemia virus Tax-mediated Fas ligand promoter transactivation. J Biol Chem 1998; 273(35):22382–22388.
168. Georges SA, Giebler HA, Cole PA, Luger K, Laybourn PJ, Nyborg JK. Tax recruitment of CBP/p300, via the KIX domain, reveals a potent requirement for acetyltransferase activity that is chromatin dependent and histone tail independent. Mol Cell Biol 2003; 23(10):3392–3404.
169. Lemasson I, Polakowski NJ, Laybourn PJ, Nyborg JK. Transcription regulatory complexes bind the human T-cell leukemia virus 5' and 3' long terminal repeats to control gene expression. Mol Cell Biol 2004; 24(14):6117–6126.
170. Mori N, Morishita M, Tsukazaki T, et al. Human T-cell leukemia virus type I oncoprotein Tax represses Smad- dependent transforming growth factor beta signaling through interaction with CREB-binding protein/p300. Blood 2001; 97(7):2137–2144.
171. Lee DK, Kim BC, Brady JN, Jeang KT, Kim SJ. Human T-cell lymphotropic virus type 1 tax inhibits transforming growth factor-beta signaling by blocking the association of smad proteins with smad-binding element. J Biol Chem 2002; 277(37):33766–33775.
172. Yamada Y, Sugawara K, Hata T, et al. Interleukin-15 (IL-15) can replace the IL-2 signal in IL-2-dependent adult T-cell leukemia (ATL) cell lines: Expression of IL-15 receptor alpha on ATL cells. Blood 1998; 91:4265–4272.
173. Teshigawara K, Maeda M, Nishino K, et al. Adult T leukemia cells produce a lymphokine that augments interleukin 2 receptor expression. J Mol Cell Immunol 1985; 2(1):17–26.
174. Yodoi J, Tagaya Y, Masutani H, Maeda Y, Kawabe T. IL-2 receptor and Fc epsilon R2 gene activation in lymphocyte transformation: possible roles of ATL-derived factor. Int Symp Princess Takamatsu Cancer Res Fund 1988; 19:73–86.

175. Leung K, Nabel GJ. HTLV-1 transactivator induces interleukin-2 receptor expression through an NF-kappa B-like factor. Nature 1988; 333(6175):776–778.

176. Collins ND, D'Souza C, Albrecht B, et al. Proliferation response to interleukin-2 and Jak/Stat activation of T cells immortalized by human T-cell lymphotropic virus type 1 is independent of open reading frame I expression. J Virol 1999; 73(11):9642–9649.

177. Azimi N, Jacobson S, Leist T, Waldmann TA. Involvement of IL-15 in the pathogenesis of human T lymphotropic virus type I-associated myelopathy/tropical spastic paraparesis: Implications for therapy with a monoclonal antibody directed to the IL-2/15R beta receptor. J Immunol 1999; 163:4064–4072.

178. Waldmann TA. T-cell receptors for cytokines: targets for immunotherapy of leukemia/lymphoma. Ann Oncol 2000; 11 Suppl 1:101–106.

179. Zhang Z, Zhang M, Ravetch JV, Goldman C, Waldmann TA. Effective therapy for a murine model of adult T-cell leukemia with the humanized anti-CD2 monoclonal antibody, MEDI-507. Blood 2003; 102(1):284–288.

180. Kirken RA, Erwin RA, Wang L, Wang Y, Rui H, Farrar WL. Functional uncoupling of the janus kinase 3-stat5 pathway in malignant growth of human T cell leukemia virus type 1-transformed human T cells. J Immunol 2000; 165(9):5097–5104.

181. Roodman GD. Biology of osteoclast activation in cancer. J Clin Oncol 2001; 19(15):3562–3571.

182. Roodman GD, Choi SJ. MIP-1 alpha and myeloma bone disease. Cancer Treat Res 2004; 118:83–100.

183. Wilson KC, Center DM, Cruikshank WW, Zhang Y. Binding of HTLV-1 tax oncoprotein to the precursor of interleukin-16, a T cell PDZ domain-containing protein. Virology 2003; 306(1):60–67.

184. Moriuchi H, Moriuchi M, Fauci AS. Factors secreted by human T lymphotropic virus type I (HTLV-I)-infected cells can enhance or inhibit replication of HIV-1 in HTLV-I-uninfected cells: Implications for in vivo coinfection with HTLV-I and HIV-1. J Exp Med 1998; 187:1689–1697.

185. Calabresi PA, Martin R, Jacobson S. Chemokines in chronic progressive neurological diseases: HTLV-1 associated myelopathy and multiple sclerosis. J Neurovirology 1999; 5:102–108.

186. Mori N, Ueda A, Ikeda S, et al. Human T-cell leukemia virus type I tax activates transcription of the human monocyte chemoattractant protein-1 gene through two nuclear factor-kappaB sites. Cancer Res 2000; 60(17):4939–4945.

187. Hasegawa H, Nomura T, Kohno M et al. Increased chemokine receptor CCR7/EBI1 expression enhances the infiltration of lymphoid organs by adult T-cell leukemia cells. Blood 2000; 95(1):30–38.

188. Seki M, Higashiyama Y, Kadota J, et al. Elevated levels of soluble adhesion molecules in sera and BAL fluid of individuals infected with human T-cell lymphotropic virus type 1. Chest 2000; 118(6):1754–1761.

189. Lewis MJ, Gautier VW, Wang XP, Kaplan MH, Hall WW. Spontaneous production of C-C chemokines by individuals infected with human T lymphotropic virus type II (HTLV-II) alone and HTLV-II/HIV-1 coinfected individuals. J Immunol 2000; 165(7):4127–4132.

190. Sharma V, Lorey SL. Autocrine role of macrophage inflammatory protein-1 beta in human T- cell lymphotropic virus type-I tax-transfected Jurkat T-cells. Biochem Biophys Res Commun 2001; 287(4):910–913.

191. Ruckes T, Saul D, Van Snick J, Hermine O, Grassmann R. Autocrine antiapoptotic stimulation of cultured adult T-cell leukemia cells by overexpression of the chemokine I-309. Blood 2001; 98(4):1150–1159.

192. Yoshie O, Fujisawa R, Nakayama T, et al. Frequent expression of CCR4 in adult T-cell leukemia and human T-cell leukemia virus type 1-transformed T cells. Blood 2002; 99(5):1505–1511.

193. Imaizumi Y, Sugita S, Yamamoto K et al. Human T cell leukemia virus type-I Tax activates human macrophage inflammatory protein-3 alpha/CCL20 gene transcription via the NF-kappa B pathway. Int Immunol 2002; 14(2):147–155.

194. Mori N, Krensky AM, Ohshima K, et al. Elevated expression of CCL5/RANTES in adult T-cell leukemia cells: possible transactivation of the CCL5 gene by human T-cell leukemia virus type I tax. Int J Cancer 2004; 111(4):548-557.

195. Tanaka Y, Mine S, Figdor CG, et al. Constitutive chemokine production results in activation of leukocyte function-associated antigen-1 on adult T-cell leukemia cells. Blood 1998; 91(10):3909–3919.

196. Arai M, Ohashi T, Tsukahara T, et al. Human T-cell leukemia virus type 1 Tax protein induces the expression of lymphocyte chemoattractant SDF-1/PBSF. Virology 1998; 241:298–303.

197. Johnson AN, Newfeld SJ. The TGF-beta family: signaling pathways, developmental roles, and tumor suppressor activities. Scientific World Journal 2002; 2:892–925.

198. Wakefield LM, Roberts AB. TGF-beta signaling: positive and negative effects on tumorigenesis. Curr Opin Genet Dev 2002; 12(1):22–29.

199. Ellenrieder V, Buck A, Gress TM. TGFbeta-regulated transcriptional mechanisms in cancer. Int J Gastrointest Cancer 2002; 31(1–3):61–69.

200. Attisano L, Wrana JL. Signal transduction by the TGF-beta superfamily. Science 2002; 296(5573): 1646–1647.

201. Kim SJ, Winokur TS, Lee HD, et al. Overexpression of transforming growth factor-beta in transgenic mice carrying the human T-cell lymphotropic virus type I tax gene. Mol Cell Biol 1991; 11(10): 5222–5228.

202. Arnulf B, Villemain A, Nicot C, et al. Human T-cell lymphotropic virus oncoprotein Tax represses TGF-beta 1 signaling in human T cells via c-Jun activation: a potential mechanism of HTLV-I leukemogenesis. Blood 2002; 100(12):4129–4138.

203. Twizere JC, Kruys V, Lefebvre L, et al. Interaction of retroviral Tax oncoproteins with tristetraprolin and regulation of tumor necrosis factor-alpha expression. J Natl Cancer Inst 2003; 95(24):1846–1859.

204. Seki N, Yamaguchi K, Yamada A, et al. Polymorphism of the 5 '-flanking region of the tumor necrosis factor (TNF)-alpha gene and susceptibility to human T-cell lymphotropic virus type I (HTLV-I) uveitis. J INFEC DIS 1999; 180:880–883.

205. Tsukasaki K, Miller CW, Kubota T, et al. Tumor necrosis factor alpha polymorphism associated with increased susceptibility to development of adult T-cell leukemia/lymphoma in human T-lymphotropic virus type 1 carriers. Cancer Res 2001; 61(9):3770–3774.

206. Ciminale V, D'Agostino D, Zotti L, Franchini G, Felber BK, Chieco-Bianchi L. Expression and characterization of proteins produced by mRNAs spliced into the X region of the human T-cell leukemia/lymphotropic virus type II. Virology 1995; 209:445–456.

207. Koralnik IJ, Fullen J, Franchini G. The p12I, p13II, and p30II proteins encoded by human T-cell leukemia/lymphotropic virus type I open reading frames I and II are localized in three different cellular compartments. J Virol 1993; 67(4):2360–2366.

208. Koralnik IJ, Gessain A, Klotman ME, Lo MA, Berneman ZN, Franchini G. Protein isoforms encoded by the pX region of human T-cell leukemia/lymphotropic virus type I. Proc Natl Acad Sci U S A 1992; 89(18):8813–8817.

209. Berneman ZN, Gartenhaus RB, Reitz MS, et al. Expression of alternatively spliced human T-lymphotropic virus type 1 pX mRNA in infected cell lines and in primary uncultured cells from patients with adult T-cell leukemia/lymphoma and healthy carriers. Proc Natl Acad Sci USA 1992; 89:3005–3009.

210. Derse D, Mikovits J, Ruscetti F. X-I and X-II open reading frames of HTLV-I are not required for virus replication or for immortalization of primary T-cells in vitro. Virology 1997; 237:123–128.

211. Kim SJ, Ding W, Albrecht B, Green PL, Lairmore MD. A conserved calcineurin-binding motif in human T lymphotropic virus type 1 p12I functions to modulate nuclear factor of activated T cell activation. J Biol Chem 2003; 278(18):15550–15557.

212. Albrecht B, D'Souza CD, Ding W, Tridandapani S, Coggeshall KM, Lairmore MD. Activation of nuclear factor of activated T cells by human T- lymphotropic virus type 1 accessory protein p12(I). J Virol 2002; 76(7):3493–3501.

213. Ding W, Albrecht B, Kelley RE et al. Human T-cell lymphotropic virus type 1 p12(I) expression increases cytoplasmic calcium to enhance the activation of nuclear factor of activated T cells. J Virol 2002; 76(20):10374–10382.

214. Zhang W, Nisbet JW, Albrecht B et al. Human T-lymphotropic virus type 1 p30(II) regulates gene transcription by binding CREB binding protein/p300. J Virol 2001; 75(20):9885–9895.

215. Bartoe JT, Albrecht B, Collins ND et al. Functional role of pX open reading frame II of human T-lymphotropic virus type 1 in maintenance of viral loads in vivo. J Virol 2000; 74:1094–1100.

216. Lairmore MD, Albrecht B, D'Souza C, et al. In vitro and in vivo functional analysis of human T cell lymphotropic virus type 1 pX open reading frames I and II. AIDS Res Hum Retroviruses 2000; 16(16):1757–1764.

217. Zhang W, Nisbet JW, Bartoe JT, Ding W, Lairmore MD. Human T-lymphotropic virus type 1 p30(II) functions as a transcription factor and differentially modulates CREB-responsive promoters. J Virol 2000; 74(23):11270–11277.

218. Albrecht B, Collins ND, Burniston MT. et al. Human T-lymphotropic virus type 1 open reading frame I p12(I) is required for efficient viral infectivity in primary lymphocytes. J Virol 2000; 74(21): 9828–9835.

219. Collins ND, Newbound GC, Albrecht B, Beard JL, Ratner L, Lairmore MD. Selective ablation of human T-cell lymphotropic virus type 1 p12I reduces viral infectivity in vivo. Blood 1998; 91(12): 4701–4707.
220. Johnson JM, Franchini G. Retroviral proteins that target the major histocompatibility complex class I. Virus Res 2002; 88(1-2):119–127.
221. Dekaban GA, Peters AA, Mulloy JC, et al. The HTLV-I orfI protein is recognized by serum antibodies from naturally infected humans and experimentally infected rabbits. Virology 2000; 274(1): 86–93.
222. D'Agostino DM, Zotti L, Ferro T, Franchini G, Chieco-Bianchi L, Ciminale V. The p13II protein of HTLV type 1: comparison with mitochondrial proteins coded by other human viruses. AIDS Res Hum Retroviruses 2000; 16(16):1765–1770.
223. Ciminale V, Zotti L, Dagostino DM, et al. Mitochondrial targeting of the p13(II) protein coded by the x-II ORF of human T-cell leukemia/lymphotropic virus type I (HTLV-I). Oncogene 1999; 18:4505–4514.
224. Trovato R, Mulloy JC, Johnson JM, Takemoto S, de Oliveira MP, Franchini G. A lysine-to-arginine change found in natural alleles of the human T-cell lymphotropic/leukemia virus type 1 p12(I) protein greatly influences its stability. J Virol 1999; 73(8):6460–6467.
225. Ciminale V, Pavlakis GN, Derse D, Cunningham CP, Felber BK. Complex splicing in the human T-cell leukemia virus (HTLV) family of retroviruses: Novel mRNAs and proteins produced by HTLV type I. J Virol 1992; 66:1737–1745.
226. Furukawa K, Furukawa K, Shiku H. Alternatively spliced mRNA of the pX region of human T lymphotropic virus type I proviral genome. FEBS Lett 1991; 295(1-3):141–145.
227. Cereseto A, Berneman Z, Koralnik I, Vaughn J, Franchini G, Klotman ME. Differential expression of alternatively spliced pX mRNAs in HTLV-I-infected cell lines. Leukemia 1997; 11(6):866–870.
228. Ding W, Albrecht B, Luo R et al. Endoplasmic Reticulum and cis-Golgi Localization of Human T-Lymphotropic Virus Type 1 p12(I): Association with Calreticulin and Calnexin. J Virol 2001; 75(16): 7672–7682.
229. Nicot C, Mulloy JC, Ferrari MG et al. HTLV-1 p12(I) protein enhances STAT5 activation and decreases the interleukin-2 requirement for proliferation of primary human peripheral blood mononuclear cells. Blood 2001; 98(3):823–829.
230. Ballard DW. Molecular mechanisms in lymphocyte activation and growth. Immunol Res 2001; 23(2-3):157–166.
231. Ding W, Kim SJ, Nair AM et al. Human T-Cell Lymphotropic Virus Type 1 p12(I) Enhances Interleukin-2 Production during T-Cell Activation. J Virol 2003; 77(20):11027–11039.
232. von Bulow GU, Bram RJ. NF-AT activation induced by a CAML-interacting member of the tumor necrosis factor receptor superfamily. Science 1997; 278(5335):138–141.
233. Vogel KW, Briesewitz R, Wandless TJ, Crabtree GR. Calcineurin inhibitors and the generalization of the presenting protein strategy. Adv Protein Chem 2001; 56:253–291.
234. Crabtree GR. Calcium, calcineurin, and the control of transcription. J Biol Chem 2001; 276(4): 2313–2316.
235. Lewis RS. Calcium signaling mechanisms in T lymphocytes. Annu Rev Immunol 2001; 19:497–521.
236. Aramburu J, Yaffe MB, Lopez-Rodriguez C, Cantley LC, Hogan PG, Rao A. Affinity-driven peptide selection of an NFAT inhibitor more selective than cyclosporin A. Science 1999; 285(5436): 2129–2133.
237. Feske S, Giltnane J, Dolmetsch R, Staudt LM, Rao A. Gene regulation mediated by calcium signals in T lymphocytes. Nat Immunol 2001; 2(4):316–324.
238. Aramburu J, Rao A, Klee CB. Calcineurin: from structure to function. Curr Top Cell Regul 2000; 36:237–295.
239. Rao A, Luo C, Hogan PG. Transcription factors of the NFAT family: Regulation and function. Annu Rev Immunol 1997; 15:707–747.
240. Tokumitsu H, Enslen H, Soderling TR. Characterization of a Ca2+/calmodulin-dependent protein kinase cascade. Molecular cloning and expression of calcium/calmodulin-dependent protein kinase kinase. J Biol Chem 1995; 270(33):19320–19324.
241. Dolmetsch RE, Lewis RS, Goodnow CC, Healy JI. Differential activation of transcription factors induced by Ca2+ response amplitude and duration. Nature 1997; 386(6627):855–858.
242. Dolmetsch RE, Xu K, Lewis RS. Calcium oscillations increase the efficiency and specificity of gene expression. Nature 1998; 392(6679):933–936.

243. Li W, Llopis J, Whitney M, Zlokarnik G, Tsien RY. Cell-permeant caged InsP3 ester shows that Ca2+ spike frequency can optimize gene expression. Nature 1998; 392(6679):936–941.
244. Nyland SB, Cao C, Bai Y, Loughran TP, Ugen KE. Modulation of infection and type 1 cytokine expression parameters by morphine during in vitro coinfection with human T-cell leukemia virus type I and HIV-1. J Acquir Immune Defic Syndr 2003; 32(4):406–416.
245. Koga H, Imada K, Ueda M, Hishizawa M, Uchiyama T. Identification of differentially expressed molecules in adult T-cell leukemia cells proliferating in vivo. Cancer Sci 2004; 95(5):411–417.
246. Albrecht B, Lairmore MD. Critical role of human T-lymphotropic virus type 1 accessory proteins in viral replication and pathogenesis. Microbiol Mol Biol Rev 2002; 66(3):396–406.
247. Silic-Benussi M, Cavallari I, Zorzan T, et al. Suppression of tumor growth and cell proliferation by p13II, a mitochondrial protein of human T cell leukemia virus type 1. Proc Natl Acad Sci U S A 2004; 101(17):6629–6634.
248. Nicot C, Dundr M, Johnson JM, et al. HTLV-1-encoded p30II is a post-transcriptional negative regulator of viral replication. Nat Med 2004; 10(2):197–201.
249. Silverman LR, Phipps AJ, Montgomery A, Ratner L, Lairmore MD. Human T-cell lymphotropic virus type 1 open reading frame II-encoded p30II is required for in vivo replication: evidence of in vivo reversion. J Virol 2004; 78(8):3837–3845.

3 Herpesviruses, Cytokines, and Cancer

Frank J. Jenkins and Heather R. Hensler

CONTENTS

1. INTRODUCTION

Herpesviruses are large, enveloped, double-stranded DNA viruses, which are characterized by their ability to cause mild acute infections followed by lifelong latency in the host and periodic episodes of reactivation. The herpesviridae family is subdivided, based on their biologic properties, into the α-, β-, and γ-herpesvirinae and can be found in a wide variety of species (1). Of the eight human herpesviruses (HHV) identified to date, only two have been clearly shown to be oncogenic: Epstein-Barr virus (EBV, or HHV-4) and human herpesvirus 8 (HHV-8; also termed Kaposi's sarcoma-associated herpesvirus, KSHV). Both viruses belong to the γ-herpesvirus subfamily, but are further subdivided as a lymphocryptovirus (EBV) or a rhadinovirus (HHV-8). They can infect cells of lymphoid origin, particularly B-cells, but also have a tropism for other cell types, such as epithelial cells for EBV and endothelial cells for HHV-8. Infection of susceptible cells with either of these herpesviruses results in the triggering of both a humoral and cellular immune response, which includes the expression of numerous cellular cytokines. Interestingly, in addition to inducing host cytokines, both EBV and HHV-8 encode homologues to cellular cytokines and their expression is important in both modulation of the host's immune response to infection as well as viral-induced pathogenesis. In this chapter we will review cytokine responses, both virally encoded and cellular, that are produced as a result of EBV or HHV-8 infection focusing on those identified as having a potential role in carcinogenesis.

2. EBV

EBV is ubiquitous in the world's human population with a prevalence rate over 90% (2). Although the majority of primary EBV infections are believed to be asymptomatic,

From: *Cancer Drug Discovery and Development,*
Cytokines in the Genesis and Treatment of Cancer
Edited by: M. A. Caligiuri and M. T. Lotze © Humana Press Inc., Totowa, NJ

Table 1
EBV Gene Expression During Different Latency Programs

EBV latency program	Latent genes expressed	Associated cancers
Latency I	EBNA–1, EBERs	Burkitt's lymphoma
Latency II	EBNA–1, EBERs, LMP–1, –2A, –2B	Hodgkin's disease, nasopharyngeal carcinoma
Latency III	EBNA–1, –2, –3A, –3B, –3C, EBNA-LP, EBERs, LMP–1, –2A, –2B	Posttransplant lymphoproliferative disease

EBV infection in adolescents and young teens can result in infectious mononucleosis *(3)*. A primary EBV infection begins with the virus infecting the epithelial layer of the nasal and pharyngeal passages and spreading to nearby B-cells. As a result of viral replication, fever, pharyngitis, lymphadenopathy, splenomegaly, hepatocellular dysfunction, and oftentimes, skin rashes develop *(4)*. Normally, the immune response to EBV is aggressive, resulting in a rapid elimination of virus-infected cells. This aggressive immune response includes the activation of natural killer cells (NK), antibody-dependent cellular cytotoxicity (ADCC), and EBV-specific cytotoxic T-cells (CTL) *(5)*. The host's immune response controls viral replication, marking the end of the primary infection and forcing the virus into establishing a latent infection in B-cells *(5)*. The ability of EBV to establish latent infections in B-cells is believed to be directly responsible for the development of several different neoplasms including endemic Burkitt's lymphoma (BL), Hodgkin's disease (HD), post-transplant lymphoproliferative disease (PTLD), and undifferentiated nasopharyngeal carcinoma (NPC) *(6)*.

2.1. EBV-Induced Cancers

2.1.1. BURKITT'S LYMPHOMA

Burkitt's lymphoma (BL) presents in two forms: endemic, in which cases are >90% EBV positives, and nonendemic, which are only 15–30% EBV positive. The hallmark of this cancer is a translocation that displaces the *c-myc* gene on chromosome 8 with either the immunoglobulin heavy (chromosome 2) or light chains (chromosomes 14 or 22). The translocation is similar in both the endemic and nonendemic forms, but is thought to occur by different mechanisms. EBV infected BL have been shown to express the Latency I gene pattern (Table 1), which is described as expression of EBNA-1 (Epstein-Barr nuclear antigen 1) and the EBERs (Epstein-Barr virus-encoded small RNAs) *(6,7)*. The expression of these latent viral genes may contribute to the growth of BL cells, as EBER transcripts have been shown to induce human IL-10 (hIL-10) production *(8)*, which has been shown to induce the proliferation of activated B-cells (reviewed in Ref. *9*). The EBER transcripts may also have another role in tumorigenesis as they have been shown to block the IFN-α-activated apoptosis pathway by binding double-stranded RNA-activated protein kinase (PKR) *(10)*. Several studies have also looked at cytokine expression in AIDS-associated BL cells and found upregulation of IL-7, hIL-10, IL-12, IL-16, MIP-1α, and MIP-1β, suggesting a possible synergistic effect between HIV and EBV in tumor induction *(11)*.

2.1.2. HODGKIN'S DISEASE

Hodgkin's disease (HD) is a lymphoma characterized by the presence of Hodgkin/Reed-Sternberg (HRS) cells in a mass of nonmalignant immune cell infiltrate. The HRS cells, while rare, are present in the tumor and presumed to be the malignant cell and of B-cell lineage. Approximately 35% of all HD cases are EBV positive and of these cases, EBV is found in the HRS cells. EBV-related HD follows the Latency II pattern of EBV gene expression (Table 1) which is characterized by expression of EBNA-1 and the latent membrane proteins (LMP) LMP-1, LMP-2A, and LMP-2B (7).

Expression of the cytokines IL-5, IL-6, hIL-10, and IL-13 have been associated with the EBV-related HD. HD biopsies have been shown to express IL-6, but not IL-8, and have mixed expression of hIL-10 (12). Although one study has reported the downregulation of hIL-10 transcription in HRS cells (13), others have found IL-10 expression to be linked to LMP-1 expression. In these studies, patients with LMP-1 expressing HRS cells had higher serum hIL-10 levels and cellular IL-10 transcripts (14,15).

The levels of IL-5 and IL-13 transcripts have also been found to be up-regulated in EBV-related HD cells (13,16). The upregulation of IL-13 may act as growth factor for HRS cells. In a more recent report, Kapp and coworkers reported that neutralizing antibodies against IL-13, but not IL-5, suppressed the growth of HD-derived cell lines (16). Furthermore, IL-13 production seems confined to HRS cells in the tumor, while IL-13R expression was found on HRS cells, lymphocytes, histiocytes, fibroblasts, and endothelial cells (16,17). Therefore, it appears that IL-13 can act in a positive, autocrine manner on HRS cells, in addition to having a paracrine effect on other cells in the area of the tumor.

2.1.3. POST-TRANSPLANT LYMPHOPROLIFERATIVE DISEASE (PTLD)

Post-transplant lymphoproliferative disease (PTLD) is a category of EBV-related cancers that arise as a result of the immunosuppressive regimen used after organ transplant and usually show the latency III pattern of gene expression (Table 1), which is characterized by expression of all the EBNAs and EBERs along with expression of LMP-1 and LMP-2 (7). The immunosuppression associated with organ transplant can result in EBV reactivation from either the donor or organ recipient and subsequent expansion of EBV-infected lymphocytes. The risk for development of PTLD is greater in young patients and those with a seronegative status at the time of transplant who receive an organ from a seropositive donor. The level of EBV DNA in circulating lymphocytes has a predictive value in PTLD development and progression such that increasing levels predict the onset of PTLD (18). Treatment of PTLD primarily involves reduction in immunosuppression, but also includes antiviral therapy, interferon administration, and traditional cancer treatments.

As a large percentage of PTLDs regress upon reduction in immunosuppression (19), it appears the establishment, maintenance, and regression of this cancer is because of, to a significant degree, the host immune response. For example, studies have suggested that the cytokines IL-4 and hIL-10 are involved in PTLD initiation and progression whereas the cytokines IL-2, GM-CSF, IL-18 and IFN-gamma are involved in tumor regression.

PTLD tumors have been shown to express the Th2 type cytokines IL-4 and hIL-10, and are negative for production of IFN-γ and IL-2. Regression of these tumors was associated with a concomitant loss or reduction of IL-4 expression (20). Studies have also shown that neutralization of hIL-10 in cultures of spontaneous lymphoblastoid cell lines from PTLD patients by antibody or soluble IL-10R, results in decreased growth of these cells *(21)*. Thus both IL-4 and hIL-10 are implicated in tumor survival.

The cytokines IL-2, IL-18, GM-CSF, and IFN-γ have been implicated in the prevention or regression of PTLD tumors. In an animal model using SCID mice, PTLD development was prevented by administration of IL-2 and GM-CSF, which resulted in the recruitment of NK cells, CD8+ cells, and monocytes *(22)*. Recent studies have also focused on IL-18 as a factor in the resolution of PTLD as it appears that expression of this cytokine is higher in the serum of patients with regressing PTLD and its upregulation is owing to LMP-1 expression *(23,24)*. Expression of IL-18 results in the induction of IFN-γ and its related chemokines, IP-10 and Mig, which also have a role in tumor reduction *(25,26)*. As a result, therapeutic induction of IL-18 may have promise in the treatment and prevention of PTLD. The importance of IFN-γ induction in PTLD tumor regression is further corroborated by a preliminary study showing an association of PTLD development with an IFN-γ genetic polymorphism that results in lower IFN-γ production *(27)*.

2.1.4. Nasopharyngeal Carcinoma

Undifferentiated nasopharyngeal carcinoma (NPC), which occurs largely in middle-aged males, is a tumor of the epithelial cells lining the posterior nasopharynx. NPC is rare, but has a very high prevalence among Taiwanese and Inuit populations. Almost all undifferentiated NPC is EBV positive, whereas only a small proportion of other subtypes are positive. NPC is associated with EBV in the latency II pattern (EBNA-1, EBERs, LMP-1, LMP-2; Table 1) and a nonrandom deletion in chromosome 3 at 3p25 and 3p14 *(6,7)*. Several studies have shown the presence of both host and viral cytokines linked with NPC. It has been reported that serum hIL-10 is higher in NPC patients vs controls *(28)*. Also one study has demonstrated that whereas NPC biopsies are positive for IL-1α, IL-1β, and the viral IL-10 homologue (vIL-10; discussed below), control NP cells were negative or rarely positive by both in situ hybridization and RT-PCR. The IL-1 detected in these biopsies may be because of expression from both infiltrating CD4+ cells and infected epithelial tumor cells *(29)*. Infiltrating T-cells have also been shown to produce IFN-γ whereas infiltrating macrophages produce the chemokines MIP-1α and MCP-1, all of which attract additional lymphocytes into the tumor *(30)*. IL-8, which is known to increase angiogenesis, has also been demonstrated in NPC sections by immunohistochemistry and its presence is correlated both with microvessel count and LMP-1, VEGF, and bFGF expression. Furthermore, transfection of LMP-1 alone was enough to induce IL-8 production through an NFκB-dependent pathway *(31)*. However, contrasting results have also been reported, showing that EBV positive tumors are negative for IL-10 with IL-6 and IL-8 expression present in rare cases *(12)*. It is possible though, that because there appear to be multiple categories of NPC, which may or may not all be associated with EBV, and because there are many different types of cells in the tumor, these studies may actually be looking at different phenomena.

2.2. Viral IL-10 (vIL-10)

As discussed above, IL-10 is implicated as an important cytokine in the initiation and maintenance of EBV-related cancers. Human IL-10 is a type II cytokine produced by activated T-cells, B-cells, monocytes, and keratinocytes and has suppressive effects on macrophages, dendritic cells, NK cells, and T-cell functions such as antigen presentation, proliferation, and cytotoxicity. The expression of hIL-10 inhibits expression of Th1 cytokines such as IL-2, and IFN-γ, in addition to IL-3, GM-CSF, and TNF-α. A major function of hIL-10 is to inhibit Th1 functions and to limit and terminate inflammatory responses (reviewed in Ref. *32*). As a robust Th1 response is a critical component of the immune system's ability to fight tumorigenesis, the induction of hIL-10 by EBV-related cancers represents at least one method that the virus may use to circumvent the immune system leading to increased carcinogenesis.

Interestingly, in addition to using hIL-10 in the development of tumors, EBV also encodes an IL-10 homologue. The EBV open reading frame BCRF1 encodes a protein that is commonly referred to as vIL-10, as it shares 85% amino acid homology with hIL-10 and 70% nucleotide and amino acid sequence homology with murine IL-10 (mIL-10) *(33)*.

Recent crystallography experiments have shown the vIL-10 protein to be similar to hIL-10 with only slight conformational changes, which may be responsible for the differences in binding affinities of the IL-10 proteins to the IL-10 receptor (IL-10R) *(34)*. The vIL-10 protein binds hIL-10R with 1000-fold less affinity than the hIL-10 protein, but induces the proliferation of some IL-10R expressing cells to a greater degree than hIL-10 *(35)*. However, on some cell types, such as mast cells and thymocytes, vIL-10 lacks the immunostimulatory capacity of hIL-10 and this difference has been attributed to the lack of an isoleucine residue at 87aa *(36)*.

During an EBV infection, both IL-10 proteins are expressed. The vIL-10 protein was originally thought to be expressed late in the viral replication cycle, but has been demonstrated as early as 6 hours postinfection in B-lymphocytes, with expression of hIL-10 following 1 day later *(37)*.

The vIL-10 protein is thought to assist in transformation of B-cells by either increasing cell viability or by downregulation of the antiproliferative effects of IFN-γ *(38)*. Thus it is required for the transformation of B-cells with EBV *(37)* and suppresses the rejection of both allogeneic and syngeneic tumors in mice presumably through a localized immunosuppression function. This effect can be neutralized with anti-hIL-10 or administration of either IL-2 or IL-12. The immunosuppressive effect of vIL-10 is in contrast to mIL-10, which stimulates an immune response resulting in suppression of tumor growth *(39)*. In addition, Rapamycin, which inhibits hIL-10 secretion and signaling, also inhibits growth of B-cell lines from post-transplant lymoproliferative disorder (PTLD) patients and experimental PTLD in mice *(40)*. This effect appears to be complex, however, as others have determined that neutralization of hIL-10 in the huPBL-SCID model of EBV-PTLD did not reduce the occurrence of the disease *(41)*. Additionally, it has also been reported that both VIL-10 and hIL-10 reduced the growth of Burkitt's lymphoma cells in SCID mice via the blocking of VEGF and FGF production *(42)*. This suggests that EBV-related cancers may have different requirements for VIL-10 and hIL-10.

3. HUMAN HERPESVIRUS 8

Chang and colleagues in 1994, using representational difference analysis, described the detection of two DNA fragments associated uniquely with a KS lesion from a patient with AIDS *(43)*. The predicted amino acids encoded by these DNA sequences were found to share 39 and 51% identity to the capsid and tegument proteins of two transforming primate γherpesviruses, Epstein-Barr virus (EBV), and herpesvirus saimiri (HVS) respectively. The descriptive name of Kaposi's sarcoma-associated herpesvirus (KSHV) or the more formal name of human herpesvirus 8 (HHV-8) emerged. HHV-8 is a γherpesvirinae and member of the rhadinovirus subfamily *(44)*.

A primary HHV-8 infection among healthy adults has not been associated with a disease, syndrome, or significant clinical symptoms *(45)* although primary infections among immunocompetent children have been reported to manifest with a febrile maculopapular rash *(46)*.

Seroepidemiologic studies have suggested that HHV-8 can be transmitted by both sexual and nonsexual routes. HHV-8 DNA has been detected in PBMCs, semen, and saliva of infected patients, with detection in the saliva the most common site where virus is found *(47–52)*. The seroprevalence of HHV-8 varies among different populations and regions of the world. In the United States, seroprevalence ranges from 3–5.1% among blood donors (53) whereas in areas of Africa seroprevalence surpasses 50% *(54–56)*. Among homosexual men in the United States the seroprevalence rate ranges from 42% among HIV seronegative men to 63% among HIV-infected men (L.P. Jacobson and F.J. Jenkins, unpublished results) whereas among college students, the seroprevalence is approximately 10% *(57)*.

In the United States, among the general population, the seroprevalence of HHV-8 increases with age and sexual promiscuity. Thus HHV-8 infection among children under the age of 15 is rare but among individuals above the age of 15, ranges from 0 to 20% have been observed *(53,58–62)*. This is in contrast to other parts of the world where HHV-8 infection occurs at much earlier ages. In French Guiana, a strong familial aggregation in HHV-8 seroprevalence was found with high mother-child (odd ratio 2.8 [95% CI 1.6–5.0]) and sibling–sibling (3.8 [1.6–9.5]) correlations, supporting the spread of HHV-8 through casual intimate contact *(63)*.

3.1. HHV-8-Related Cancers

3.1.1. KAPOSI SARCOMA (KS)

Kaposi's sarcoma (KS) is neoplasm arising from vascular origins and is characterized by spindle-shaped cells with angiogenic properties surrounded by an inflammatory infiltrate. KS occurs frequently in HHV-8 and HIV co-infected persons (it is the most common AIDS-associated cancer and is an AIDS-defining illness), but also occurs in an endemic form in Africa, a classical form in older Mediterranean men and a post-solid organ transplant related form (termed iatrogenic KS). The AIDS-related KS often regresses with anti-HIV treatment while iatrogenic KS recedes with reduction in immunosuppression. This suggests a role for the host immune response in development and maintenance of KS and it follows that cytokine production may be involved in regulating this response. A role for cytokines in KS development is supported by early studies, which showed that treatment of KS with TNF-α *(64)* or IFN-γ *(65)* actually exacerbated KS disease. Isolated PBMC from KS patients have been reported to produce predominately Th1-type cytokines (IFN-γ, TNF-α, IL-1 and IL-6) with little or no Th2 cytokine production. *(66,67,68)*. In particular, IL-4 is rarely secreted by PBMCs from KS patients, while IFN-γ secretion is high and can be found in both PBMC and KS cell cultures *(69)*. Since a KS lesion is not a homogenous population, but rather a mixed population of spindle cells and immune infiltrate, it has been further shown that

IFN-γ production in a KS lesion is produced primarily by the infiltrating lymphocytes, particularly CD8+ T-cells, and monocytes/macrophages. It has been suggested that this IFN-γ production leads to angiogenesis in the KS lesion as IFN-γ activated endothelial cells have been shown to produce tumors in nude mice similar in morphologic appearance to early KS *(70)*. Additionally, IFN-γ has been implicated in the maintenance of HHV-8 infection of B-cells and monocytes in KS *(71)*.

Alternatively, it appears that IFN-α has the converse effect on growth of KS, as it has been shown to reduce HHV-8 viral load in cultured PBMC from KS patients *(72)*. Specifically, it has been proposed that the antiproliferative effects of IFN-α are owing to downregulation of *c-myc* expression. Furthermore, while PDGF-β has been shown to upregulate expression of *c-myc* and induces growth of KS cells, IFN-α inhibits these activities *(73)*. Because of this, IFN-α is frequently used with success in the treatment of classical and AIDS-KS *(74,75)*.

3.1.2. PLEURAL EFFUSION LYMPHOMAS (PEL)

Primary effusion lymphoma (PEL) is a rare type of non-Hodgkin's B-cell lymphoma characterized by the absence of a solid tumor mass, indeterminate immunophenotype, and frequent co-infection with EBV *(76)*. The largest proportion of PELs occur in AIDS patients, but in rare cases, arise in individuals who are only infected with HHV-8. Given its similarity to EBV-B-cell lymphomas, several studies have investigated the expression of IL-6 and IL-10 in PEL cell lines. Not surprisingly, all the PEL-derived cell lines studied (BC-1, -2, -3, BCBL-1, KS-1, BCP-1, etc.) have been shown to express both IL-6 and IL-10 by ELISA, RT-PCR and Western blot *(77–80)*. Additionally, one study has also demonstrated secretion of IL-6 (100%) and IL-10 (87.5%) in AIDS-PEL patient samples *(78)*. Similarly, these studies have also been able to show expression of the HHV-8 viral IL-6 homolog (vIL-6; discussed below) in these cells. Moreover, a role for these cytokines in PEL growth has also been shown. Soluble hIL-6R and IL-6 antisense oligonucleotides prevent the growth of PEL lines *(79,80)*, as does neutralization of IL-10, IL-6 and vIL-6 *(77)*. Along these lines, one study has shown both IFN-α and IFN-γ to be inhibitory with respect to clonal growth *(80)*. Interestingly, IFN-γ has been shown to reactivate latent HHV-8 as shown by viral gene expression *(81,82)*, while, on the other hand, IFN-α appears to have the opposite effect on HHV-8 gene induction and virus replication, and has further been shown to reduce viral load in infected PBMC *(72,83)*. It is unclear how the modes of action of these interferons differ in PEL cells, although more recent work suggests that IFN-α may induce apoptosis in these cells *(84)*.

3.1.3. MULTICENTRIC CASTLEMAN DISEASE

Multicentric Castleman Disease (MCD) is a lymphoproliferative disease characterized by the expansion of lymph node germinal centers, hypergammaglobulinemia, and B-cell expansion. The disorder exists in two forms, a vascular-hyaline variant and a plasma cell variant, but HHV-8 is only strongly associated with the plasma cell form. Several reports have confirmed the importance of IL-6 in the pathogenesis of MCD. It has been demonstrated that higher levels of human IL-6 can be found in the blood of patients with AIDS-related MCD and can be correlated with symptoms of exacerbated disease and HHV-8 viral load *(85)*. The viral IL-6 homologue is also found at high levels in MCD lesions as shown by immunohistochemistry and RT-PCR *(86)*. Furthermore, like the cellular IL-6, vIL-6 has also been found in the serum of an AIDS-MCD patient, could be correlated with HHV-8 viral load, and decreased with the implementation of Foscarnet treatment (87). It follows that anti-IL-6 therapy should be of use in the treatment of MCD, but so far reports are conflicting and it appears that treatment may work in some but not all cases (88–90). Alternatively, treatment involving IFN-α appears to have a strong effect on alleviation of MCD, likely through its antiviral activity, and it currently a mainstay of treatment for the disease (91–93).

3.2. Virally Encoded Genes

3.2.1. VIRAL IL-6 (vIL-6)

Human IL-6 is a key inflammatory, acute phase response cytokine. It binds to the hIL-6 binding receptor (IL-6Rα/gp80), producing a low affinity complex which then associates with the IL-6 signaling receptor, gp130. The binding of gp130 (by the IL-6/gp-80 complex) results in the triggering of an intracellular signaling cascade that includes activation of the JAK/STAT3 pathway as well as activation of the MAPK pathway (for review see ref. 94). Binding of hIL-6 to the gp80 receptor alone does not result in further signaling and the hIL-6 protein does not bind directly to the gp130 receptor. Thus, both the gp80 and gp130 receptors are necessary and important in hIL-6 signaling.

HHV-8 encodes a homologue for IL-6, vIL-6, which is encoded by open reading frame (ORF) K2. The protein has 204 amino acids with a predicted size of 23.4 kDa and shares 24.7% identity with the hIL-6 and 24.9% identity with mIL-6 (95). Comparison of the predicted amino acid sequences of vIL-6 and hIL-6 and mIL-6 shows strong homology to the region of the IL-6 protein involved in receptor binding (95). The vIL-6 protein has been shown to be capable of supporting the growth of an IL-6 dependent hybridoma cell line, B9 (96) and capable of binding to the gp80 receptor, activating the IL-6 signaling cascade. It has been reported that vIL-6 can stimulate all of the known hIL-6-induced signaling pathways (97). Interestingly, the vIL-6 protein can also bind to the gp130 homodimer, in the absence of gp80, resulting in downstream signaling (98). The affinity of vIL-6 to the IL-6 receptors appears to be lower than hIL-6. Nonetheless, the ability of the vIL-6 protein to bind directly to gp130 indicates that the viral protein can initiate IL-6 signaling without binding to the gp80 receptor. This would permit the vIL-6 protein to trigger signaling in a larger variety of cell types (including those that do not express the gp80 receptor, but do express gp130). In addition, the ability of vIL-6 to bind directly to gp130 would also result in continued signaling of the IL-6 pathways even if the cell attempts to shut down these pathways by down-regulation of gp80 expression (99).

Constitutive expression of the vIL-6 protein in a mouse model has been shown to result in hematopoiesis, plasmacytosis and angiogenesis (100). This study suggests that expression of vIL-6 is important for any tumorigenic effects. However, analysis of PEL and MCD cells as well as KS sections has indicated that vIL-6 can be detected in PEL and MCD cells but rarely in KS sections (86,101). Thus a role for vIL-6 in B-cell lymphomas such as PEL and MCD is apparent, while a role in KS is less clear.

3.2.2. VIRAL G-PROTEIN-COUPLED RECEPTOR (vGPCR)

ORF 74 of HHV-8 encodes a protein which homology to the cellular chemokine, IL-8 receptor (IL-8R), a member of a family of G-protein coupled receptors. As a result, ORF74 is often termed the viral G-protein coupled receptor (vGPCR). The vGPCR protein expresses constitutive signaling in the absence of ligand binding and this signaling has been shown to induce the production of several cytokines and chemokines. For example, expression of vGPCR has been shown to induce VEGF and an angioproliferative disease similar to KS in transgenic mice or nude mice injected with vGPCR-expressing NIH3T3 cells *(102,103)*. In addition, it's expression induces the production of several pro-inflammatory cytokines and chemokines such IL-6, Groα, MIP-1α and MIP-1β *(104)*. Furthermore, depending on the cell type, transfection of a vGPCR expressing plasmid has resulted in the production of IL-2, IL-4, IL-8, IL-1β, TNF-α, bFGF and MCP-1 *(105–107)*. This constitutive downstream signaling is mediated by the last five amino acids in the protein's cytoplasmic tail and activates the inositol phosphate phospholipase C pathways and the mitogen-activated protein (MAP) kinases/p38 and JNK/SAP *(105,108)*. The constitutive signaling by vGPCR, its ability to increase angiogenesis in vivo, and knowledge that it is expressed in KS lesions at very low levels, has lead the suggestion that it acts through a paracrine model for HHV-8-induced pathogenesis and carcinogenesis *(109)*.

3.2.3. Viral Interferon Regulatory Factors (vIRF)

HHV-8 encodes three proteins with homology to cellular interferon regulatory factors (IRF). vIRF-1 (ORF K9), -2 (ORF K11.1), and -3 (ORF 10.5/6, also called LANA-2), each functioning at different stages of interferon regulation. vIRF-1 inhibits transcription of genes regulated by both type I and type II interferons *(110); (111)*, particularly, those regulated by hIRF-1 *(112,113)*, and contributes to the transformation of cells. These studies have also shown that vIRF-1 does not bind DNA or IRF-1 directly, nor does it compete with hIRF-1 for binding of interferon consensus sequences. Furthermore, vIRF-1 is expressed primarily in B-cells as opposed to KS cells, and represses the antiviral activity of interferons in these cells. It has recently been shown that vIRF-1 interacts with retinoid-IFN-induced mortality 19 (GRIM19), both in vivo and in vitro, via its N-terminal region and downregulates GRIM19-induced cell death in the presence of IFN *(114)*. vIRF-1 also inhibits CD95L mediated activation induced cell death via hIRF-1, and to a lesser extent, that of TCR/CD3 activation *(115)*.

vIRF-2 is constitutively expressed at low levels in the nuclei of PEL-derived cell lines and recombinant protein has been shown to bind to NFκB binding sites. The protein interacts with hIRF-1 and hIRF-2, and the transcriptional proteins RelA and p300, but not hIRF-3, and as a result, can inhibit the transcriptional activation of the IFN-α promoter and RelA stimulated activity of the HIV LTR *(116)*. vIRF-2 also interacts with double-stranded RNA-activated protein kinase (PKR) to prevent autophosphoylation, and as a result downmodulates interferon-mediated antiviral effects *(117)*.

vIRF-3 (also termed LANA-2) is the most recently identified IRF in the HHV-8 genome, is latently expressed in the nucleus, and can be upregulated with TPA treatment. The protein shares homology to hIRF-4 and vIRF-2, and appears to inhibit the activities of hIRF-3 and -7 through direct interaction and the transcriptional activity of the IFN-α promoter, which prevents the production of interferons *(118,119)*.

4. SUMMARY

In summary, it appears that cytokines can contribute to the oncogenic nature of herpesviruses by influencing the proliferation of infected cells, suppressing cellular antiviral tactics and inhibiting apoptosis. In support of this, the human gamma-herpesviruses EBV and HHV-8, have evolutionarily captured cellular genes that add to their ability to subvert the immune response and use it for its own survival. Recent work in these fields also suggest that targeting of some of the viral or cellular cytokines may be advantageous in the treatment of herpesvirus-related cancers.

REFERENCES

1. McGeoch DJ. Molecular evolution of the gamma-Herpesvirinae. Philos Trans R Soc Lond B Biol Sci 2001; 356(1408):421–435.
2. Henle W, Henle G. Epidemiologic aspects of Epstein-Barr virus (EBV)-associated diseases. Ann N Y Acad Sci 1980; 354:326–331.
3. Straus SE, Cohen JI, Tosato G, Meier J. NIH conference. Epstein-Barr virus infections: biology, pathogenesis, and management. Ann Intern Med 1993; 118(1):45–58.
4. Straus SE, Cohen JI, Tosato G, Meier J. NIH conference. Epstein-Barr virus infections: biology, pathogenesis, and management. Ann Intern Med 1993; 118(1):45–58.
5. Ohga S, Nomura A, Takada H, Hara T. Immunological aspects of Epstein-Barr virus infection. Crit Rev Oncol Hematol 2002; 44(3):203–215.
6. Thompson MP, Kurzrock R. Epstein-Barr virus and cancer. Clin Cancer Res 2004; 10(3):803–821.
7. Young LS, Dawson CW, Eliopoulos AG. The expression and function of Epstein-Barr virus encoded latent genes. Mol Pathol 2000; 53(5):238–247.
8. Kitagawa N, Goto M, Kurozumi K, et al. Epstein-Barr virus-encoded poly(A)(-) RNA supports Burkitt's lymphoma growth through interleukin-10 induction. EMBO J 2000; 19(24):6742–6750.
9. Itoh K, Hirohata S. The role of IL-10 in human B cell activation, proliferation, and differentiation. J Immunol 1995; 154(9):4341–4350.
10. Nanbo A, Inoue K, Adachi-Takasawa K, Takada K. Epstein-Barr virus RNA confers resistance to interferon-alpha-induced apoptosis in Burkitt's lymphoma. EMBO J 2002; 21(5):954–965.
11. Sharma V. Current perspectives on cytokines for anti-retroviral therapy in AIDS related B-cell lymphomas. Curr Drug Targets Infect Disord 2003; 3(2):137–149.
12. Beck A, Pazolt D, Grabenbauer GG, et al. Expression of cytokine and chemokine genes in Epstein-Barr virus-associated nasopharyngeal carcinoma: comparison with Hodgkin's disease. J Pathol 2001; 194(2):145–151.
13. Ohshima K, Karube K, Hamasaki M, et al. Differential chemokine, chemokine receptor and cytokine expression in Epstein-Barr virus-associated lymphoproliferative diseases. Leuk Lymphoma 2003; 44(8):1367–1378.
14. Herling M, Rassidakis GZ, Medeiros LJ, et al. Expression of Epstein-Barr virus latent membrane protein-1 in Hodgkin and Reed-Sternberg cells of classical Hodgkin's lymphoma: associations with presenting features, serum interleukin 10 levels, and clinical outcome. Clin Cancer Res 2003; 9(6): 2114–2120.
15. Herbst H, Foss HD, Samol J, et al. Frequent expression of interleukin-10 by Epstein-Barr virus-harboring tumor cells of Hodgkin's disease. Blood 1996; 87(7):2918–2929.
16. Kapp U, Yeh WC, Patterson B, et al. Interleukin 13 is secreted by and stimulates the growth of Hodgkin and Reed-Sternberg cells. J Exp Med 1999; 189(12):1939–1946.
17. Ohshima K, Akaiwa M, Umeshita R, Suzumiya J, Izuhara K, Kikuchi M. Interleukin-13 and interleukin-13 receptor in Hodgkin's disease: possible autocrine mechanism and involvement in fibrosis. Histopathology 2001; 38(4):368–375.
18. Rowe DT, Webber S, Schauer EM, Reyes J, Green M. Epstein-Barr virus load monitoring: its role in the prevention and management of post-transplant lymphoproliferative disease. Transplant Infectious Disease 2001; 3(2):79–87.
19. Tsai DE, Hardy CL, Tomaszewski JE, et al. Reduction in immunosuppression as initial therapy for posttransplant lymphoproliferative disorder: analysis of prognostic variables and long-term follow-up of 42 adult patients. Transplantation 2001; 71(8):1076–1088.
20. Nalesnik MA, Zeevi A, Randhawa PS, et al. Cytokine mRNA profiles in Epstein-Barr virus-associated post-transplant lymphoproliferative disorders. Clin Transplant 1999; 13(1 Pt 1):39–44.
21. Beatty PR, Krams SM, Martinez OM. Involvement of IL-10 in the autonomous growth of EBV-transformed B cell lines. J Immunol 1997; 158(9):4045–4051.

22. Baiocchi RA, Ward JS, Carrodeguas L, et al. GM-CSF and IL-2 induce specific cellular immunity and provide protection against Epstein-Barr virus lymphoproliferative disorder. J Clin Invest 2001; 108(6):887–894.

23. Birkeland SA, Hamilton-Dutoit S, Bendtzen K. Long-term follow-up of kidney transplant patients with posttransplant lymphoproliferative disorder: duration of posttransplant lymphoproliferative disorder-induced operational graft tolerance, interleukin-18 course, and results of retransplantation. Transplantation 2003; 76(1):153–158.

24. Yao L, Setsuda J, Sgadari C, Cherney B, Tosato G. Interleukin-18 expression induced by Epstein-Barr virus-infected cells. J Leukoc Biol 2001; 69(5):779–784.

25. Sgadari C, Angiolillo AL, Cherney BW, et al. Interferon-inducible protein-10 identified as a mediator of tumor necrosis in vivo. Proc Natl Acad Sci U S A 1996; 93(24):13791–13796.

26. Sgadari C, Farber JM, Angiolillo AL, et al. Mig, the monokine induced by interferon-gamma, promotes tumor necrosis in vivo. Blood 1997; 89(8):2635–2643.

27. Vanbuskirk AM, Malik V, Xia D, Pelletier RP. A gene polymorphism associated with posttransplant lymphoproliferative disorder. Transplant Proc 2001; 33(1-2):1834.

28. Budiani DR, Hutahaean S, Haryana SM, Soesatyo MH, Sosroseno W. Interleukin-10 levels in Epstein-Barr virus-associated nasopharyngeal carcinoma. J Microbiol Immunol Infect 2002; 35(4): 265–268.

29. Huang YT, Sheen TS, Chen CL, et al. Profile of cytokine expression in nasopharyngeal carcinomas: a distinct expression of interleukin 1 in tumor and CD4+ T cells. Cancer Res 1999; 59(7):1599–1605.

30. Tang KF, Tan SY, Chan SH, et al. A distinct expression of CC chemokines by macrophages in nasopharyngeal carcinoma: implication for the intense tumor infiltration by T lymphocytes and macrophages. Hum Pathol 2001; 32(1):42–49.

31. Yoshizaki T, Horikawa T, Qing-Chun R, et al. Induction of interleukin-8 by Epstein-Barr virus latent membrane protein-1 and its correlation to angiogenesis in nasopharyngeal carcinoma. Clin Cancer Res 2001; 7(7):1946–1951.

32. Moore KW, de Waal MR, Coffman RL, O'Garra A. Interleukin-10 and the interleukin-10 receptor. Annu Rev Immunol 2001; 19:683–765.

33. Moore KW, Vieira P, Fiorentino DF, Trounstine ML, Khan TA, Mosmann TR. Homology of cytokine synthesis inhibitory factor (IL-10) to the Epstein-Barr virus gene BCRF1. Science 1990; 248:1230.

34. Zdanov A, Schalk-Hihi C, Menon S, Moore KW, Wlodawer A. Crystal structure of Epstein-Barr virus protein BCRF1, a homolog of cellular interleukin-10. J Mol Biol 1997; 268(2):460–467.

35. Liu Y, de Waal MR, Briere F, et al. The EBV IL-10 homologue is a selective agonist with impaired binding to the IL-10 receptor. J Immunol 1997; 158(2):604–613.

36. Ding Y, Qin L, Kotenko SV, Pestka S, Bromberg JS. A single amino acid determines the immunostimulatory activity of interleukin 10. J Exp Med 2000; 191(2):213–224.

37. Miyazaki I, Cheung RK, Dosch HM. Viral interleukin 10 is critical for the induction of B cell growth transformation by Epstein-Barr virus. J Exp Med 1993; 178(2):439–447.

38. Stuart AD, Stewart JP, Arrand JR, Mackett M. The Epstein-Barr virus encoded cytokine viral interleukin-10 enhances transformation of human B lymphocytes. Oncogene 1995; 11(9):1711–1719.

39. Suzuki T, Tahara H, Narula S, Moore KW, Robbins PD, Lotze MT. Viral interleukin 10 (IL-10), the human herpes virus 4 cellular IL-10 homologue, induces local anergy to allogeneic and syngeneic tumors. J Exp Med 1995; 182(2):477–486.

40. Nepomuceno RR, Balatoni CE, Natkunam Y, Snow AL, Krams SM, Martinez OM. Rapamycin inhibits the interleukin 10 signal transduction pathway and the growth of Epstein Barr virus B-cell lymphomas. Cancer Res 2003; 63(15):4472–4480.

41. Khatri VP, Caligiuri MA. A review of the association between interleukin-10 and human B-cell malignancies. Cancer Immunol Immunother 1998; 46(5):239–244.

42. Cervenak L, Morbidelli L, Donati D, et al. Abolished angiogenicity and tumorigenicity of Burkitt lymphoma by interleukin-10. Blood 2000; 96(7):2568–2573.

43. Chang Y, Cesarman E, Pessin MS, et al. Identification of herpesvirus-like DNA sequences in AIDS-associated Kaposi's sarcoma. Science 1994; 266:1865–1869.

44. Moore PS, Chang Y. Kaposi's sarcoma-associated herpesvirus. In: Knipe DM, Howley PM, editors. Fields Virology. Philadelphia: Lippincott Williams and Wilkins, 2001: 2803–2833.

45. Wang QJ, Jenkins FJ, Jacobson LP, et al. Primary human herpesvirus 8 infection generates a broadly specific CD8(+) T-cell response to viral lytic cycle proteins. Blood 2001; 97(8):2366–2373.

46. Andreoni M, Sarmati L, Nicastri E, et al. Primary human herpesvirus 8 infection in immunocompetent children. JAMA 2002; 287(10):1295–1300.

47. Blackbourn DJ, Lennette ET, Ambroziak J, Mourich DV, Levy JA. Human herpesvirus 8 detection in nasal secretions and saliva. J Infect Dis 1998; 177(1):213–216.

48. Martin JN. Diagnosis and epidemiology of human herpesvirus 8 infection. Semin Hematol 2003; 40(2):133–142.

49. Pauk J, Huang ML, Brodie SJ, et al. Mucosal shedding of human herpesvirus 8 in men. N Engl J Med 2000; 343(19):1369–1377.

50. Howard MR, Whitby D, Bahadur G, et al. Detection of human herpesvirus 8 DNA in semen from HIV-infected individuals but not healthy semen donors. AIDS 1997; 11(2):F15–F19.

51. Huang YQ, Li JJ, Poiesz BJ, Kaplan MH, Friedman-Kien AE. Detection of the herpesvirus-like DNA sequences in matched specimens of semen and blood from patients with AIDS-related Kaposi's sarcoma by polymerase chain reaction in situ hybridization. Am J Pathol 1997; 150(1):147–153.

52. Viviano E, Vitale F, Ajello F, et al. Human herpesvirus type 8 DNA sequences in biological samples of HIV- positive and negative individuals in Sicily. AIDS 1997; 11(5):607–612.

53. Pellett PE, Wright DJ, Engels EA, et al. Multicenter comparison of serologic assays and estimation of human herpesvirus 8 seroprevalence among US blood donors. Transfusion 2003; 43:1260–1268.

54. DeSantis SM, Pau CP, Archibald LK, et al. Demographic and immune correlates of human herpesvirus 8 seropositivity in Malawi, Africa. Int J Infect Dis 2002; 6(4):266–271.

55. Hladik W, Dollard SC, Downing RG, et al. Kaposi's sarcoma in Uganda: risk factors for human herpesvirus 8 infection among blood donors. J Acquir Immune Defic Syndr 2003; 33(2):206–210.

56. Olsen SJ, Chang Y, Moore PS, Biggar RJ, Melbye M. Increasing Kaposi's sarcoma-associated herpesvirus seroprevalence with age in a highly Kaposi's sarcoma endemic region, Zambia in 1985. AIDS 1998; 12(14):1921–1925.

57. Jenkins FJ, Hoffman LJ, Liegey-Dougall A. Reactivation of and primary infection with human herpesvirus 8 among solid-organ transplant recipients. J Infect Dis 2002; 185:1238–1243.

58. Hudnall SD, Chen T, Rady P, Tyring S, Allison P. Human herpesvirus 8 seroprevalence and viral load in healthy adult blood donors. Transfusion 2003; 43(1):85–90.

59. Ablashi D, Chatlynne L, Cooper H, et al. Seroprevalence of human herpesvirus-8 (HHV-8) in countries of Southeast Asia compared to the USA, the Caribbean and Africa. Br J Cancer 1999; 81(5):893–897.

60. Chatlynne LG, Ablashi DV. Seroepidemiology of Kaposi's sarcoma-associated herpesvirus (KSHV). Semin Cancer Biol 1999; 9(3):175–185.

61. Greenblatt RM, Jacobson LP, Levine AM, et al. Human herpesvirus 8 infection and Kaposi's sarcoma among human immunodeficiency virus-infected and -uninfected women. J Infect Dis 2001; 183(7): 1130–1134.

62. Hoffman LJ, Bunker CH, Pellett PE, et al. Elevated seroprevalence of human herpesvirus 8 among men with prostate cancer. J Infect Dis 2004; 189(1):15–20.

63. Bourboulia D, Whitby D, Boshoff C, et al. Serologic evidence for mother-to-child transmission of Kaposi sarcoma- associated herpesvirus infection. JAMA 1998; 280(1):31,32.

64. Aboulafia D, Miles SA, Saks SR, Mitsuyasu RT. Intravenous recombinant tumor necrosis factor in the treatment of AIDS-related Kaposi's sarcoma. J Acquir Immune Defic Syndr 1989; 2(1):54–58.

65. Krigel RL, Odajnyk CM, Laubenstein LJ, et al. Therapeutic trial of interferon-gamma in patients with epidemic Kaposi's sarcoma. J Biol Response Mod 1985; 4(4):358–364.

66. Oxholm A, Oxholm P, Permin H, Bendtzen K. Epidermal tumour necrosis factor alpha and interleukin 6-like activities in AIDS-related Kaposi's sarcoma. An immunohistological study. APMIS 1989; 97(6):533–538.

67. Miles SA, Rezai AR, Salazar-Gonzalez JF, et al. AIDS Kaposi sarcoma-derived cells produce and respond to interleukin 6. Proc Natl Acad Sci U S A 1990; 87(11):4068–4072.

68. Sturzl M, Brandstetter H, Zietz C, et al. Identification of interleukin-1 and platelet-derived growth factor-B as major mitogens for the spindle cells of Kaposi's sarcoma: a combined in vitro and in vivo analysis. Oncogene 1995; 10(10):2007–2016.

69. Sirianni MC, Vincenzi L, Fiorelli V, et al. gamma-Interferon production in peripheral blood mononuclear cells and tumor infiltrating lymphocytes from Kaposi's sarcoma patients: correlation with the presence of human herpesvirus-8 in peripheral blood mononuclear cells and lesional macrophages. Blood 1998; 91(3):968–976.

70. Fiorelli V, Gendelman R, Sirianni MC, et al. gamma-Interferon produced by CD8+ T cells infiltrating Kaposi's sarcoma induces spindle cells with angiogenic phenotype and synergy with human

immunodeficiency virus-1 Tat protein: an immune response to human herpesvirus-8 infection? Blood 1998; 91(3):956–967.

71. Monini P, Colombini S, Sturzl M, et al. Reactivation and persistence of human herpesvirus-8 infection in B cells and monocytes by Th-1 cytokines increased in Kaposi's sarcoma. Blood 1999; 93(12):4044–4058.

72. Monini P, Carlini F, Sturzl M, et al. Alpha interferon inhibits human herpesvirus 8 (HHV-8) reactivation in primary effusion lymphoma cells and reduces HHV-8 load in cultured peripheral blood mononuclear cells. J Virol 1999; 73(5):4029–4041.

73. Koster R, Blatt LM, Streubert M, et al. Consensus-interferon and platelet-derived growth factor adversely regulate proliferation and migration of Kaposi's sarcoma cells by control of c-myc expression. Am J Pathol 1996; 149(6):1871–1885.

74. Real FX, Oettgen HF, Krown SE. Kaposi's sarcoma and the acquired immunodeficiency syndrome: treatment with high and low doses of recombinant leukocyte A interferon. J Clin Oncol 1986; 4(4): 544–551.

75. Tur E, Brenner S, Michalevicz R. Low dose recombinant interferon alfa treatment for classic Kaposi's sarcoma. Arch Dermatol 1993; 129(10):1297–1300.

76. Ensoli B, Sturzl M, Monini P. Cytokine-mediated growth promotion of Kaposi's sarcoma and primary effusion lymphoma. Semin Cancer Biol 2000; 10(5):367–381.

77. Jones KD, Aoki Y, Chang Y, Moore PS, Yarchoan R, Tosato G. Involvement of interleukin-10 (IL-10) and viral IL-6 in the spontaneous growth of Kaposi's sarcoma herpesvirus-associated infected primary effusion lymphoma cells. Blood 1999; 94(8):2871–2879.

78. Aoki Y, Yarchoan R, Braun J, Iwamoto A, Tosato G. Viral and cellular cytokines in AIDS-related malignant lymphomatous effusions. Blood 2000; 96(4):1599–1601.

79. Drexler HG, Meyer C, Gaidano G, Carbone A. Constitutive cytokine production by primary effusion (body cavity- based) lymphoma-derived cell lines. Leukemia 1999; 13(4):634–640.

80. Asou H, Said JW, Yang R, et al. Mechanisms of growth control of Kaposi's sarcoma-associated herpes virus-associated primary effusion lymphoma cells. Blood 1998; 91(7):2475–2481.

81. Chang J, Renne R, Dittmer D, Ganem D. Inflammatory cytokines and the reactivation of Kaposi's sarcoma- associated herpesvirus lytic replication. Virology 2000; 266(1):17–25.

82. Blackbourn DJ, Fujimura S, Kutzkey T, Levy JA. Induction of human herpesvirus-8 gene expression by recombinant interferon gamma. AIDS 2000; 14(1):98, 99.

83. Chang J, Renne R, Dittmer D, Ganem D. Inflammatory cytokines and the reactivation of Kaposi's sarcoma-associated herpesvirus lytic replication. Virology 2000 Jan 5 266;17–25.

84. Toomey NL, Deyev VV, Wood C, et al. Induction of a TRAIL-mediated suicide program by interferon alpha in primary effusion lymphoma. Oncogene 2001; 20(48):7029–7040.

85. Oksenhendler E, Carcelain G, Aoki Y, et al. High levels of human herpesvirus 8 viral load, human interleukin-6, interleukin-10, and C reactive protein correlate with exacerbation of multicentric castleman disease in HIV-infected patients. Blood 2000; 96(6):2069–2073.

86. Staskus KA, Sun R, Miller G, et al. Cellular tropism and viral interleukin-6 expression distinguish human herpesvirus 8 involvement in Kaposi's sarcoma, primary effusion lymphoma, and multicentric Castleman's disease. J Virol 1999; 73(5):4181–4187.

87. Aoki Y, Tosato G, Fonville TW, Pittaluga S. Serum viral interleukin-6 in AIDS-related multicentric Castleman disease. Blood 2001; 97(8):2526, 2527.

88. Beck JT, Hsu SM, Wijdenes J, et al. Brief report: alleviation of systemic manifestations of Castleman's disease by monoclonal anti-interleukin-6 antibody. N Engl J Med 1994; 330(9):602–605.

89. Nishimoto N, Sasai M, Shima Y, et al. Improvement in Castleman's disease by humanized anti-interleukin-6 receptor antibody therapy. Blood 2000; 95(1):56–61.

90. Corbellino M, Bestetti G, Scalamogna C, et al. Long-term remission of Kaposi sarcoma-associated herpesvirus-related multicentric Castleman disease with anti-CD20 monoclonal antibody therapy. Blood 2001; 98(12):3473–3475.

91. Nord JA, Karter D. Low dose interferon-alpha therapy for HIV-associated multicentric Castleman's disease. Int J STD AIDS 2003; 14(1):61, 62.

92. Andres E, Maloisel F. Interferon-alpha as first-line therapy for treatment of multicentric Castleman's disease. Ann Oncol 2000; 11(12):1613, 1614.

93. Kumari P, Schechter GP, Saini N, Benator DA. Successful treatment of human immunodeficiency virus-related Castleman's disease with interferon-alpha. Clin Infect Dis 2000; 31(2):602–604.

94. Heinrich PC, Behrmann I, Haan S, Hermanns HM, Muller-Newen G, Schaper F. Principles of interleukin (IL)-6-type cytokine signalling and its regulation. Biochem J 2003; 374(Pt 1):1–20.

95. Neipel F, Albrecht JC, Ensser A, et al. Human herpesvirus 8 encodes a homolog of interleukin-6. J Virol 1997; 71(1):839–842.

96. Burger R, Neipel F, Fleckenstein B, et al. Human herpesvirus type 8 interleukin-6 homologue is functionally active on human myeloma cells. Blood 1998; 91(6):1858–1863.

97. Osborne J, Moore PS, Chang Y. KSHV-encoded viral IL-6 activates multiple human IL-6 signaling pathways. Hum Immunol 1999; 60(10):921–927.

98. Wan X, Wang H, Nicholas J. Human herpesvirus 8 interleukin-6 (vIL-6) signals through gp130 but has structural and receptor-binding properties distinct from those of human IL-6. J Virol 1999; 73(10):8268–8278.

99. Chatterjee M, Osborne J, Bestetti G, Chang Y, Moore PS. Viral IL-6-induced cell proliferation and immune evasion of interferon activity. Science 2002; 298(5597):1432–1435.

100. Aoki Y, Jaffe ES, Chang Y, et al. Angiogenesis and hematopoiesis induced by Kaposi's sarcoma-associated herpesvirus-encoded interleukin-6. Blood 1999; 93(12):4034–4043.

101. Cannon JS, Nicholas J, Orenstein JM, et al. Heterogeneity of viral IL-6 expression in HHV-8-associated diseases. J Infect Dis 1999; 180(3):824–828.

102. Yang TY, Chen SC, Leach MW, et al. Transgenic expression of the chemokine receptor encoded by human herpesvirus 8 induces an angioproliferative disease resembling Kaposi's sarcoma. J Exp Med 2000; 191(3):445–454.

103. Bais C, Santomasso B, Coso O, et al. G-protein-coupled receptor of Kaposi's sarcoma-associated herpesvirus is a viral oncogene and angiogenesis activator. Nature 1998; 391(6662):86–89.

104. Polson AG, Wang D, DeRisi J, Ganem D. Modulation of host gene expression by the constitutively active G protein-coupled receptor of Kaposi's sarcoma-associated herpesvirus. Cancer Res 2002; 62(15):4525–4530.

105. Sodhi A, Montaner S, Patel V, et al. The Kaposi's sarcoma-associated herpes virus G protein-coupled receptor up-regulates vascular endothelial growth factor expression and secretion through mitogen-activated protein kinase and p38 pathways acting on hypoxia-inducible factor 1alpha. Cancer Res 2000; 60(17):4873–4880.

106. Shepard LW, Yang M, Xie P, et al. Constitutive activation of NF-kappa B and secretion of interleukin-8 induced by the G protein-coupled receptor of Kaposi's sarcoma-associated herpesvirus involve G alpha(13) and RhoA. J Biol Chem 2001; 276(49):45979–45987.

107. Schwarz M, Murphy PM. Kaposi's sarcoma-associated herpesvirus G protein-coupled receptor constitutively activates NF-kappa B and induces proinflammatory cytokine and chemokine production via a C-terminal signaling determinant. J Immunol 2001; 167(1):505–513.

108. Arvanitakis L, Geras-Raaka E, Varma A, Gershengorn MC, Cesarman E. Human herpesvirus KSHV encodes a constitutively active G-protein- coupled receptor linked to cell proliferation. Nature 1997; 385(6614):347–350.

109. Pati S, Cavrois M, Guo HG, et al. Activation of NF-kappaB by the human herpesvirus 8 chemokine receptor ORF74: evidence for a paracrine model of Kaposi's sarcoma pathogenesis. J Virol 2001; 75(18):8660–8673.

110. Gao SJ, Boshoff C, Jayachandra S, Weiss RA, Chang Y, Moore PS. KSHV ORF K9 (vIRF) is an oncogene which inhibits the interferon signaling pathway. Oncogene 1997; 15(16):1979–1985.

111. Li M, Lee H, Guo J, et al. Kaposi's sarcoma-associated herpesvirus viral interferon regulatory factor. J Virol 1998; 72(7):5433–5440.

112. Zimring JC, Goodbourn S, Offermann MK. Human herpesvirus 8 encodes an interferon regulatory factor (IRF) homolog that represses IRF-1-mediated transcription. J Virol 1998; 72(1):701–707.

113. Flowers CC, Flowers SP, Nabel GJ. Kaposi's sarcoma-associated herpesvirus viral interferon regulatory factor confers resistance to the antiproliferative effect of interferon- alpha. Mol Med 1998; 4(6):402–412.

114. Seo T, Lee D, Shim YS, et al. Viral interferon regulatory factor 1 of Kaposi's sarcoma-associated herpesvirus interacts with a cell death regulator, GRIM19, and inhibits interferon/retinoic acid-induced cell death. J Virol 2002; 76(17):8797–8807.

115. Kirchhoff S, Sebens T, Baumann S, et al. Viral IFN-regulatory factors inhibit activation-induced cell death via two positive regulatory IFN-regulatory factor 1-dependent domains in the CD95 ligand promoter. J Immunol 2002; 168(3):1226–1234.

116. Burysek L, Yeow WS, Pitha PM. Unique properties of a second human herpesvirus 8-encoded interferon regulatory factor (vIRF-2). J Hum Virol 1999; 2(1):19–32.

117. Burysek L, Pitha PM. Latently expressed human herpesvirus 8-encoded interferon regulatory factor 2 inhibits double-stranded RNA-activated protein kinase. J Virol 2001; 75(5):2345–2352.

118. Lubyova B, Kellum MJ, Frisancho AJ, Pitha PM. Kaposi's sarcoma-associated herpesvirus-encoded vIRF-3 stimulates the transcriptional activity of cellular IRF-3 and IRF-7. J Biol Chem 2004; 279(9):7643–7654.

119. Lubyova B, Pitha PM. Characterization of a novel human herpesvirus 8-encoded protein, vIRF- 3, that shows homology to viral and cellular interferon regulatory factors. J Virol 2000; 74(17): 8194–8201.

II   CYTOKINES AND CARCINOGENESIS

4 Tumor Necrosis Factor and Cancer

Mark DeWitte, David J. Shealy,
Marian T. Nakada, and G. Mark Anderson

Contents

1. INTRODUCTION

Tumor necrosis factor α (TNF) is a potent, pleiotropic, proinflammatory cytokine that is produced by macrophages, neutrophils, fibroblasts, keratinocytes, NK, T- and B-cells and also by tumor cells. TNF binds to either of two receptors, TNF-R1 or TNF-R2, expressed on virtually all mammalian cell types. TNF was named because of its ability, when administered in pharmacologic doses, to cause necrosis of tumors in experimental models. Recombinant TNF is approved in Europe to be given locoregionally as a therapy for sarcoma. TNF produced by the body mediates host responses in acute and chronic inflammatory conditions and aids in host protection from infection and malignancy. The biology of the TNF/TNF-receptor system was reviewed by Palladino et al. 2003 *(1)*.

Emerging evidence suggests that the effects of endogenously produced TNF in cancer pathophysiology may be contrary to those observed with high-dose pharmacologic TNF therapy. The paradox that this cytokine can act as both a "tumor necrosis factor" and a "tumor promoting factor" is lucidly explored by Balkwill *(2)*. In contrast to causing tumor regression, TNF can also mediate tumor progression by causing the proliferation, invasion, and metastasis of tumor cells. Recent studies now support the notion that TNF secreted by tumors can actually promote tumor growth. This apparent conflict concerning

From: *Cancer Drug Discovery and Development,*
Cytokines in the Genesis and Treatment of Cancer
Edited by: M. A. Caligiuri and M. T. Lotze © Humana Press Inc., Totowa, NJ

the role of TNF in cancer perhaps can be explained by the differences in the levels of TNF in distinct settings. When TNF is administered therapeutically in extremely high, pharmacologic doses it can act as a vasculotoxic, tumor-regressing agent. In contrast, when TNF is produced by tumors and tumor-associated macrophages, the resulting lower concentrations of TNF can promote tumor progression by a variety of mechanisms that are only now beginning to be elucidated. This chapter will explore these various aspects of TNF biology as they relate to both the pathogenesis and therapy of cancer.

2. THE BIOLOGY OF TNF

The original endotoxin-induced serum factor described by Old and colleagues demonstrated a remarkable ability to lyse specific murine tumor cells and this biologic activity provided the name for this protein—tumor necrosis factor, or TNF *(3)*. Only in 1984, when the gene for TNF was cloned and recombinant protein was obtained, did numerous additional biologic functions become apparent *(4)*. In addition to triggering apoptosis of certain tumor cells, TNF was shown to mediate the inflammatory response and modulate immune function. Eventually, TNF and its two receptors, TNF-R1 (also known as p55 or CD120a) and TNF-R2 (p75 or CD120b), were recognized as the prototypes for the TNF superfamily of cytokines and their receptors *(5)*, which were capable of controlling cell differentiation, proliferation, and apoptosis necessary to control mammalian development, in particular immune function and hematopoeisis. In contrast to the normal functions of TNF, uncontrolled excessive production of TNF can lead to chronic disease *(6)*.

TNF is produced predominantly by macrophages upon lipopolysaccharide interaction with CD14 and the toll-like receptor 4 as part of the adaptive immune response *(7)*, as well as by T-cells, B-cells, NK cells, and granulocytes. Expressed on the cell surface as a 26-kDa type II membrane protein, three subunits self-associate to form a homotrimer that is eventually released as a soluble TNF homotrimer following proteolytic cleavage by TNF converting enzyme (TACE; also known as ADAM-17) *(8,9)*. The homotrimer is the bioactive form of both soluble and transmembrane TNF *(10,11)*. Figure 1 shows schematically the synthesis of TNF and the signals generated when the TNF-R1 and TNF-R2 receptors are engaged.

The extracellular domains of the TNF receptors show significant homology that allows both receptors to bind in the groove at the interface between TNF subunits. Hence when two or three receptors engage the three available binding sites on the TNF trimer, clustering of the receptor cytoplasmic domains initiates signaling. The existence of two receptors contributes significantly to the diversity of activities shown by TNF owing to their different tissue distribution and to their distinctly different modes of signaling following activation. Although TNF-R1 is constitutively expressed on virtually all enucleated cells, expression of TNF-R2 is limited to immune cells and endothelial cells *(5)*.

Early studies suggested that most of the activities attributed to TNF were mediated by TNF-R1, as it was shown to have a significantly higher affinity for soluble TNF than TNF-R2 *(12)*. The on/off kinetics of TNF binding to TNF-R2 even suggested that on cells expressing both receptors, TNF-R2 transiently bound TNF and then passed the ligand to the TNF-R1 receptor for signaling *(13)*. TNF-R2 does appear to have specific signaling functions in T-cells that lack the TNF-R1 receptor *(14)*. Another difference between the two receptors is the presence of a death domain on the cytoplasmic portion

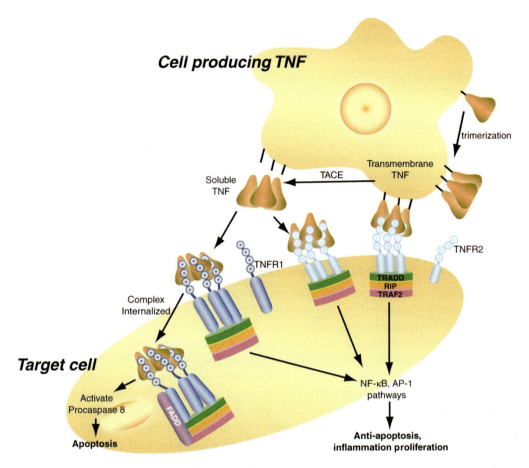

Fig. 1. Model demonstrating the multiple ways in which TNF can activate potential target cells. TNF can be presented as transmembrane TNF, which favors binding to TNF-R2, or it can be released as soluble TNF by TACE, which favors engagement of TNF-R1. TNF-R2 lacks a death domain and thus signaling is limited to activation of transcription factors in the NF-kB and AP-1 pathways that activate genes favoring inflammation, cell survival and proliferation. NF-κB also induces genes known to block apoptosis. Activation of TNF-R1 can lead to either apoptosis or NF-κB/AP-1 activation depending upon the presence of appropriate accessory proteins. It has been reported that the TNF/TNF-R1 complex must be internalized to signal apoptosis, a mechanism that might preclude signaling of apoptosis by transmembrane TNF.

of TNF-R1 that is not found on TNF-R2. After TNF binding, signaling through TNF-R1 proceeds by recruitment of the TNF-receptor associated death domain (TRADD), the receptor-interacting protein (RIP) and TNF-R-associated factor 2 (TRAF2) to the cyto-plasmic portion of TNF-R1. At this point, the presence in the cell of various accessory proteins determines whether signaling will lead to apoptosis or inhibition of apoptosis. Further recruitment of the Fas-associated death domain (FADD) leads to the binding and activation of procaspase 8, which in turn activates caspase 3 to induce apoptosis *(15)*. Alternatively, TRAF2 can recruit cellular inhibitors of apoptosis (cIAP-1 and cIAP-2) and activate signaling pathways leading to nuclear translocation of the anti-apoptotic NF-κB and activating protein-1 (AP-1) transcription factors, which upregulate genes necessary to increase inflammation and cell proliferation as well as block apoptosis *(16)*. Although TNF-R2 lacks the death domain and therefore cannot trigger apoptosis, it can still recruit TRAF2 and activate the NF-κB and AP-1 pathways. The path that a given cell takes is thus dependent on which receptor(s) is present and the constellation of other accessory proteins present owing to tissue specific gene expression patterns or the mutational status of the cell.

Several labs have reported that internalization of the TNF/TNF-R1 signaling complex is necessary for activation of apoptosis *(17,18)* whereas the clustering of the TNF/TNF-R1 signaling complex in lipid rafts results in the activation of the NF-κB and AP-1 pathways *(19)*. This means of regulating the decision between cell death or cell survival could in part be controlled by the form of TNF encountered by the cell. As noted above, the binding of soluble TNF is favored by TNF-R1 and therefore could signal either direction. However, the binding of transmembrane TNF to TNF-R2 would result in a complex that would not be able to internalize, and therefore would be unable to signal cell death.

2.1. TNF as a Therapy for Cancer

Systemically administered TNF was evaluated in the clinic in the 1980s as a therapy for solid tumors (reviewed in Lejeune 1998 *[20]*) and found to have severe toxicities, most notably hypotension and organ failure. These studies revealed that the maximally tolerated dose of TNF was significantly lower than that required to see antitumor effects in rodents. The delivery of locally high levels of TNF, without systemic exposure, is now accomplished by the technique of isolated limb perfusion where the circulation of the limb is surgically connected to a bypass circuit into which drugs are administered. Leakage into the systemic circulation is carefully monitored. After rinsing, the vessels are reattached. Isolated limb perfusion with TNF in combination with chemotherapy is currently approved in Europe for the treatment of locally advanced, unresectable, soft-tissue sarcomas and the clinical studies of isolated limb perfusion with TNF are summarized in Eggermont et al. 2003 *(21)*. Positive clinical data have been reported with this technique for TNF delivery for in-transit melanoma and drug-resistant bony sarcomas *(21)*. Although effective, this procedure is highly specialized and not widely used. The mechanism of action of TNF in this setting is believed to involve direct toxic effects on newly formed blood vessels supplying the tumor without affecting the normal vasculature. TNF causes vessel regression as well as hemorrhagic necrosis, as the apoptotic cells comprising the endothelium become procoagulant. The specific effect of TNF on angiogenic and not normal vasculature has been suggested from in vitro and in vivo studies to be caused by the deactivation of the angiogenesis-associated integrin αvβ3 by TNF in combination with interferon (IFN)γ leading to endothelial apoptosis *(22)*. TNF also causes enhanced vascular permeability, facilitating the uptake and accumulation of chemotherapeutic drugs such as melphalan and doxorubicin (21) as well as antibodies *(23)*. TNF alone is not effective when administered via isolated limb perfusion, suggesting that enhancement of drug exposure is the primary mechanism of action. An et al. *(24)* reported potent synergistic anticancer effects in vitro using the proteasome inhibitor bortezomib in combination with apoptotic stimuli such as TNF and tumor necrosis factor-related ligand (TRAIL). Bortezomib synergized with TNF and TRAIL to inhibit growth of prostate cancer cells but did not synergize with any of three selected cytotoxic chemotherapy agents. Noting the systemic toxicity of TNF compared to safe delivery of TRAIL to animals, it is warranted to test bortezomib plus TRAIL in vivo.

2.2. *Targeted Delivery of TNF*

A range of additional approaches are being undertaken to deliver therapeutic TNF specifically to tumors to avoid systemic toxicities. TNFerade is a gene therapy agent in clinical trials that is administered intratumorally. The TNF gene is controlled by a radiation-inducible promoter and is delivered via an adenoviral vector. TNFerade has been administered safely in a phase I trial *(25)*. Very low amounts of systemically administered TNF conjugated to peptides that bind angiogenic vessel targets aminopeptidase N (CD13) *(26)* or αv integrins *(27)* increase the penetration of doxorubicin and melphalan in tumor. This effect is observed in the absence of toxicity. TNF has also been fused with single-chain antibody fragments that bind angiogenic targets *(28)*.

3. ROLE OF TNF IN TUMOR METASTASIS AND ANGIOGENESIS

TNF may promote cancer progression by a variety of mechanisms, including mediation of tumor metastasis and angiogenesis. Several studies have demonstrated that TNF can promote metastatic behavior in cancer cells via diverse mechanisms. In in vitro assays TNF promotes melanoma cell migration and invasion, apparently due to the induction of cellular protease activity *(29)*. Breast cancer cells that are cultured in the presence of macrophages exhibit increased invasiveness owing to the presence of macrophage produced TNF *(30)*. Inhibitors of matrix metalloproteases or inhibition of TNF activity with neutralizing antibodies prevented the increased invasiveness, suggesting a model in which macrophage-produced TNF induces the production of proteases by tumor or stromal cells to promote metastasis. Interestingly, primary nontransformed breast epithelial cells did not respond to the same stimuli with an increase in invasive behavior. TNF has also been shown to promote metastasis of xenografted human gastric cancer cells in a mouse model through an unusual mechanism. The mesothelial cells lining the abdominal wall are relatively resistant to the adhesion and invasion of cancer cells. In this animal model TNF affects the mesothelial cells and triggers cytoskeletal changes that result in a loss of intercellular contact in the monolayer lining, exposing the underlying extracellular matrix. These exposed areas then allow the adherence of sloughed tumor cells and serve as foci for new metastatic growth on the abdominal wall *(31)*.

The effects of TNF on tumor angiogenesis appear to be complex and at times contradictory. TNF inhibits endothelial cell growth in vitro, yet it stimulates angiogenesis in a rabbit cornea model *(32)*. Fajardo et al. *(33)* demonstrated in mice that low doses of TNF induced angiogenesis in subcutaneously implanted pellets but that higher dose levels inhibited angiogenesis in the same assay. As with direct effects on tumor cells, it may be that the lower physiologic, and even patho-physiologic, concentrations of TNF produced locally in tumors support angiogenesis and tumor growth rather than suppress it. Additional experimentation is necessary to resolve this issue.

4. CLINICAL OBSERVATIONS AND ASSOCIATIONS IMPLICATING TNF IN CANCER PROGRESSION

As reviewed by Szlosarek and Balkwill *(34)*, much evidence from animal and in vitro experimentation supports the mechanistic connections between chronic inflammatory stimulation involving TNF and subsequent initiation or eventual promotion of malignancy. Chronic, dysregulated (nonself-limited) inflammation seems to provoke compensatory cellular over-replication, with increased chances for replication errors. Mutagenesis, neo-plastic growth, invasion, and metastasis involve TNF mediated production of nitric oxide, induction of angiogenic factors and matrix metalloproteinases (MMPs), modulation of chemokines and chemokine receptors controlling leukocyte infiltration of tumors, loss of hormonal responsiveness, and acquired resistance to cytotoxic chemotherapy. Similarly, in his review of cytokines in the pathogenesis and treatment of cancer, Dranoff *(35)* describes evidence that chemical carcinogens, immunodeficiency, chronic infection, and chronic inflammation all have been causally associated with tumorigenesis mediated by overpro-duction of cytokine growth factors. These imbalances and disease effects arise when cytokine function that is normally adaptive for response to mild injury induced by carcino-gens, pathogens, or environmental antigens is insufficient to limit cellular stress and the resultant cellular damage. The chronic inflammatory stimulation does not lead to repair, but instead leads to persistent and eventually dysregulated cellular function.

Several reports in the older literature have associated detection of abnormally high levels of circulating TNF in cancer patients with a wide range of tumor types *(36)* including pancreatic *(37)*, kidney *(38)*, breast *(39)*, lung (asbestosis-induced) *(40)*, and prostate cancers *(41,42)*. Within groups of patients with the same tumor type, higher levels of TNF have been correlated with tumor stage, extent of paraneoplastic compli-cations (such as the anorexia-cachexia syndrome), and shorter survival time. However, circulating TNF is not always detectable in cancer patients and may vary within indi-vidual patients over time and course of disease *(43)*. Indeed, tumor tissue levels may be more relevant than blood levels of TNF and its receptors in explaining protumorigenic associations such as those reported in head/neck squamous cell carcinoma *(44)*. Notably, significantly elevated preoperative TNF mRNA transcripts in pancreatic can-cer patients were reduced after tumor resection to levels similar to controls *(45)*.

Upregulated expression of TNF mRNA was not found in fresh pleural effusion sam-ples or tumor samples from patients with nonsmall cell lung cancer (NSCLC), but expression of interleukin (IL)-4, IL-10, transforming growth factor (TGF)α and TGF-β1 were upregulated, suggesting an immunosuppressive state of the cancer microenvi-ronment that facilitated escape from immunologic surveillance *(46)*. This supports an earlier study by Boldrini et al. *(47)* that reported expression of TNF and TGF-β mRNA in approximately half of 61 NSCLC tumor samples; TNF-R1 and TNF-R2 were PCR positive in a higher percentage. TNF levels correlated with lower microvessel count, high bcl-2 protein expression, and a better prognosis. The investigators suggest that the favorable association of positive TNF with clinical outcome could be related to inhibi-tion of neovascular development, mediated by bcl-2.

That result contrasts with the results reported by Wang et al. *(48)*. Elevated TNF was associated with disease severity and poor nutritional status; serum TNF correlated neg-atively with body fat mass and serum albumin. In 31 patients with hepatocellular carci-noma and 26 patients with cirrhosis, TNF levels in serum were significantly higher than in controls. However, elevated serum TNF in cirrhosis limits the use of this cytokine as an early marker of liver cancer.

In a prospective study of 80 patients with prostate cancer (localized or metastatic), but no evidence of active infection or inflammatory disease, serum levels of both IL-6 and TNF correlated directly with the extent of malignant disease. Both cytokines became elevated at the point of prostate-specific-antigen progression. IL-6 and TNF may prove valuable as prognostic markers for prostate cancer. There was a significantly greater elevation of TNF in patients with metastatic cancer compared to the level in patients with localized disease and in controls. The authors caution that association does not prove causality; studies that target these specific cytokines should determine if they contribute to malignant progression *(49)* and are reviewed in Chapter 23.

TNF has also been investigated extensively for genetic variation. Associations have been reported between malignancy and TNF polymorphisms in non-Hodgkin's lymphoma, myeloma, and prostate carcinoma. Similar associations were found between TNF microsatellites and colorectal carcinoma and also laryngeal carcinoma. Chronic inflammation of the bladder is a well-recognized risk factor for bladder cancer and inflammation associated with superficial bladder cancer is common; the importance of TNF in the pathogenesis of bladder cancer suggested that variation in the gene for TNF might affect its course. Marsh et al. *(50)* reported a significant association of TNF polymorphisms TNF+488A and TNF-859T and increased risk of bladder cancer, phenotype of the cancer, and subsequent tumor behavior. The investigators also found strong linkage disequilibrium between these two sites in bladder cancer patients, normal controls and melanoma patients. This study reported a significant association of these polymorphisms with grade of tumor at presentation; when TNF+488A or TNF-859T was present, generally, the tumors were less well differentiated. Notably, there was no association of the TNF+488A or TNF-859T polymorphisms with recurrence or progression, suggesting that other factors, such as oncogene upregulation, may be needed for progression. The polymorphism at position TNF+488 has also been associated with prostate cancer.

5. CLINICAL CANCER MODELS IMPLICATING TNF IN CANCER PROGRESSION

Do the pathophysiologic mechanisms of endometriosis and ovarian cancer characterize the same pathways along a continuum of malignant transformation and tumor promotion? Serum TNF has been reported, in a study of 77 women, to be associated significantly with endometriomas and ovarian cancer, but not with benign tumors *(51)*. Ness reviewed several inflammatory conditions associated with endometriosis and ovarian cancer including exposure to various exogenous irritants and also ovulation itself *(52)*. All were accompanied by cell proliferation, oxidative stress, vascular permeability, elevated prostaglandins, leukotrienes, and cytokines including TNF, IL-6 and IL-1. mRNA for these cytokines was found in epithelial ovarian tumors and its related ascites. TNF was also found consistently in the peritoneal fluid around endometrial foci. These cytokines attract platelets and macrophages that then secrete vascular endothelial growth factor (VEGF), MMP-9, and TGF-β, all of which promote infiltration of ectopic endometrium and/or invasion and metastasis of ovarian tumors. The invasive tissue of endometriosis is surrounded by an immune response ineffective in clearing it, just as ovarian tumors are surrounded by inflammatory cells that seem impotent against the neoplasia *(52)*. The host immune environment linked to mutagenesis involves a predominance of T-helper cell type 2 (TH2) cytokines over TH1 cytokines; although endometriosis and ovarian cancer generate TH1 predominance, chronic inflammation may invoke a switch from TH1-dominant to an eventual TH2-dominant microenvironment. In both disease states, progression may be modified by immune suppression suggesting a role for anti-inflammatory agents to treat endometriosis and potentially prevent ovarian cancer.

Esophageal metaplasia (Barrett esophagus; BM) is found in the setting of chronic inflammation and is a lesion often noted in progression through dysplasia to adenocarcinoma (Barrett adenocarcinoma; BA). Does its pathophysiology also involve TNF? This was thoroughly and elegantly studied in an in vitro model by Tselepis et al. *(53)*. The investigators showed in BA and BM that there is reduced expression of the cell adhesion molecule and tumor suppressor E-cadherin, resulting in decreased degradation of cytoplasmic/nuclear β-catenin. The latter protein activates transcription of oncogenes (e.g., *c-myc* and cyclin D1) by complexing with T-cell factors. Thus aberrant degradation of β-catenin can increase oncogene activation. Knowing that TNF can downregulate expression of E-cadherin, the investigators found that TNF induces *c-myc* via β-catenin mediated transcription in a mitogen activated protein kinase- (MAPK) dependent manner and independent of NF-κB activation. Epithelial TNF expression was absent in normal gastric and esophageal squamous mucosa, but increased stepwise from metaplasia through dysplasia to carcinoma. The chronic inflammation in nondysplastic BM had elevated TNF immunoreactivity, with the increase localized to mucosal regions of prominent lymphoid infiltrate, notably where metaplastic stem cells are located. Within individual glands, the most dysplastic cells expressed TNF, and TNF-R1 levels increased in abundance during disease progression, potentially amplifying the TNF signal. This study demonstrated a novel signaling pathway for oncogene activation by an inflammatory cytokine.

Japanese researchers reported evidence suggesting that TNF may be a tumor promoter in three premalignant, clinical disease settings *(54)*. Noting that lung cancer occurs in populations with a history of pulmonary tuberculosis at rates 5–10 times higher than in a normal population, the researchers found that mycoloyl glycolipids (a cord factor) from *Mycobacterium tuberculosis* injected into mice activated protein kinase C and increased TNF in serum and especially in lung tissue. Similarly, a cord factor from *Microsporum canis* increased TNF in the murine model, suggesting a mechanistic link between this prevalent fungus, endemic chronic bronchitis, and an unusually high incidence of lung cancer in Northern Thai women. In the third setting, gene products from *Helicobacter pylori* transfected into clonal cell lines induced TNF expression, and the cells rapidly produced tumors when transplanted subcutaneously in nude mice in the presence of v-H-*ras* gene initiation. Given that overexpression of H-K and N-*ras* gene mutations are found often in human gastric cancer, the association with *H. pylori*-induced TNF implies tumor promotion, or at least argues against antitumor effects of this cytokine in this context.

6. ANTI-TNF THERAPY IN CANCER

Supporting an approach that contrasts with the use of pharmacologic doses of TNF as antitumor therapy in combination with cytotoxic chemotherapeutic agents, evidence from animal models and the clinic increasingly point toward the use of anti-TNF therapies to treat cancer or its symptoms. Some of the most detailed work regarding the role of TNF as a tumor promoter was published in a series of papers from the laboratory of Fran Balkwill *(55–57)*. The authors used the induction of skin tumors in mice as a model system to dissect the contribution of TNF and its signaling pathways to skin tumor initiation. In this system 9, 10-dimethyl-1,2-benzanthracene (DMBA) is used as a topical DNA-damaging tumor inducer followed by the application of 12-*O*-tetradecanoylphorbol-13-acetate (TPA) as a tumor promoter. TNF was first implicated in tumor growth in this model by the observation that TNF knockout mice are highly resistant to the generation of skin tumors by this method. The presence of functional TNF has no effect on DNA mutation rates and therefore tumor initiation, but rather profoundly influences tumor promotion. TPA was shown to induce TNF in skin keratinocytes from wild-type mice. Activation of the AP-1 transcription factor pathway (due primarily to effects on the c-jun component) and the subsequent expression of AP-1 induced genes such as granulocyte-macrophage colony-stimulating factor (GM-CSF), MMP-3, and MMP-9 is important for the tumor promoting effect. Both TNF-R1 and TNF-R2 were shown to be critical for optimal skin tumor formation, with TNF-R1 contributing most to the effect. Similar TNF antitumor effects were observed following pharmacological intervention with a neutralizing anti-mouse TNF antibody. The potential role of TNF in the growth of human skin cancers, initiated largely by UV radiation, will be an important area for future investigation.

Increasing clinical evidence also suggests that TNF is an important anticancer target. Tsimberidou et al reviewed potential clinical indications for agents that block or inactivate TNF, specifically the soluble TNF receptor fusion protein, etanercept, and the anti-TNF monoclonal antibody (mAb) infliximab, with focus on the functions of TNF in multiple myeloma (MM), myelodysplastic syndrome (MDS), acute myelogenous leukemia (AML), and myelofibrosis *(58)*. The authors report evidence of limited therapeutic activity of monotherapy with anti-TNF molecules but advise on the need to optimize dose and schedule, to combine the anticytokine agent with other active biologic or cytotoxic agents and to better understand individual cancer patient proteomic patterns of disease and gene polymorphisms (profiling) that could predict response to blockade or neutralization of TNF *(59)*.

It is known that in addition to monocytes and macrophages, TNF is produced by stimulated T-, B-, and large granular lymphocytes. In chronic lymphocytic leukemia (CLL), neoplastic lymphocytes release TNF spontaneously in vitro, and leukemic lymphocytes are more proliferative and more viable when exposed in vitro to TNF. Is TNF a pro-leukemic cytokine? The prognostic and clinical significance of TNF was evaluated in 150 consecutive patients with CLL *(60)*. The mean plasma concentration of TNF (16.4 pg/mL) was significantly higher than the mean in 20 hematologically normal subjects (8.7 pg/mL; $P < 0.0001$). The results showed correlation of TNF with extent of disease, with serum β_2 microglobulin (β_2-M), and with low hemoglobin and low platelets. There was significantly higher TNF in patients with chromosomal abnormalities. Moreover, the TNF level was predictive of survival in a Cox multivariate analysis, independent of staging, β_2-M, hemoglobin (Hgb), white blood cell (WBC), and platelet count. Such association is provocative of the idea that inhibition of TNF could be of therapeutic value in CLL, potentially by blocking both a growth signal to the leukemic clone and a suppressive effect on other hematopoietic lineages.

Similar rationale underlies the evaluation of anti-TNF agents to inhibit the excessive apoptosis in hematopoietic cells suspected as the cause of cytopenias in MDS. The pathognomonic, hyperproliferative marrow of MDS, with excessive apoptosis and overexpression of TNF, compels intervention to modulate the dysregulated cytokine milieu in the hematopoietic tissues. In a short report *(61)*, Italian investigators described two cases of low/intermediate-risk MDS treated with infliximab. Both patients achieved sustained peripheral erythroid responses along with marrow response of increased erythroid progenitor cell by BFU-E assay and a clear decrease in the percentage of CD34+ cells expressing the apoptosis marker annexin V.

In a separate study, infliximab was given to 37 low-risk (international prognostic symptom score [IPSS] ≤1.0) MDS patients, 17 with normal karyotypes. Therapy was well tolerated and the side effects included slight myelosuppression, and moderate infusion reactions. Of 28 evaluable patients, 8 (29%) patients showed a partial response, including one patient with a trilineage response, one with a bilineage response, two with >100% increase in absolute neutrophil count (ANC), one with >1 Gm/dL increase in hemoglobin, one with decrease in bone marrow blasts from 7 to 1% changing the MDS classification (FAB) from refractory anemia with excess blasts (RAEB) to refractory anemia with ringed sideroblasts (RARS). Two patients had minor cytogenetic responses (one had >50% reduction in trisomy 8 cells and the other in 20q- cells) *(62)*. The pluripotent activity of TNF is implicated again by the variety of modulatory effects achieved by blocking TNF with the mAb, and suggests that the microenvironment of the marrow is more directly affected than are the dysplastic hematopoietic cells. A logical next evaluation could be use of a specific anti-TNF agent to modulate cell–cell signaling and stromal interactions in the marrow, combined with a cytotoxic agent known to be active against the clonal myelodysplastic cells.

Evidence supporting the use of anti-TNF regimens for the treatment of solid tumors is mounting as well. For example, immunotherapy using agents such as interferon α and IL-2 are the standard treatment options for patients with advanced renal cell carcinoma (RCC). However, these regimens have low response rates and cause considerable toxicity, related in large part to the high levels TNF and IL-6 that are induced. Phase II trials have achieved promising results in patients with advanced RCC using thalidomide *(63)*, which has demonstrated apoptotic, immunomodulatory, and anti-angiogenic effects. Thalidomide inhibits TNF gene activation by decreasing NF-κB binding *(64)*. On this basis, a single-arm, phase II study evaluated monotherapy with the anti-TNF mAb infliximab for advanced RCC in 19 patients who were refractory to prior treatments with IL-2, interferon and/or chemotherapy *(65)*. The antibody treatments were well tolerated. Three confirmed responses on study were reported, including a patient with reduction in the size of metastatic hepatic lesions, and one additional late responder. Further investigations in RCC should determine if a dose–response relationship exists, if baseline characteristics (cytokine profiles or gene polymorphisms) can predict response to an anti-TNF antibody, and if responses correlate with prolonged survival time. Combination therapy with IL-2 and an anti-TNF agent might allow a patient to receive more IL-2 if the TNF-mediated toxicity is abrogated. Anti-TNF therapy is also reviewed in Chapter 23.

7. POTENTIAL RISKS OF ANTI-TNF THERAPY

Because of the adaptive, protective purpose of inflammation, pharmacologic inhibition of this pro-inflammatory cytokine could have adverse effects in the host, unrelated to the target disease of the anti-TNF therapy. The risk of reactivation of latent tuberculosis is addressed in the prescribing information for infliximab (REMICADE® [infliximab] package insert. Centocor, Inc, Malvern, PA: 2006.) Pre-emptive systemic antifungal therapy is recommended for patients receiving infliximab for treatment of graft-vs-host disease (GVHD) *(66)*. Smith and Skelton reported cases of squamous cell carcinoma (SCC) that became evident and grew rapidly during an initial period of etanercept therapy for rheumatoid arthritis (RA) *(67)*. The tumors may have been present but occult and controlled before disruption of immunologic control. Etanercept could disable innate antitumor surveillance by blockade of both lymphotoxin α (TNF-β), and cytotoxic effects of TNF and/or by inhibition of the Th1 cytokine pattern and impairment of cytotoxic T-cells. All cases were in chronically UV-damaged, actinic skin predisposed to tumorigenesis by long-term, low level production of TNF. No new SCCs developed in patients who continued treatment for more than one year, suggesting prolonged anti-TNF therapy could be preventive of cutaneous malignancies.

Pharmacovigilance data on etanercept, infliximab, and adalimumab were reviewed by the FDA in 2003, with a focus on lymphoproliferative disease in patients treated with these anti-TNF agents, relative to the rate expected in populations with immune-mediated diseases *(68)*. The potential role of TNF-blocking therapy in the development of malignancies is not known. A prospective study of 18,572 RA patients treated with anti-TNF therapy plus methotrexate reported an increased standard incidence ratio (SIR) compared to patients not receiving methotrexate or biologicals, but confidence intervals overlapped for all treatments *(69)*. Patients with highly active disease and/or chronic exposure to immunosuppressant therapies may have several-fold higher risk for development of lymphoma, thus caution should be exercised when considering anti-TNF agents in patients with a history of malignancy or who develop malignancy during treatment.

The FDA reported on the risks of histoplasmosis *(70)*, lymphoma *(71)*, and/or listeriosis *(72)*. The Mayo clinic reviewed the safety of infliximab in 500 Crohn disease patients treated with infliximab *(73)*. The biologic basis of concern warrants heightened vigilance and consideration of the benefit to risk ratio when prescribing anti-TNF therapies.

8. SUPPORTIVE CARE

In addition to approaches aimed at the tumor, anti-TNF therapies are increasingly being tested for supportive care indications. The range of potential indications in this area is extremely broad and diverse owing to the pleiotropism of TNF action and includes cancer associated depression, fatigue, cachexia, treatment of toxicities caused by chemotherapy and radiotherapy, treatment of metastatic bone pain, and GVHD *(74,75)*.

A wealth of evidence implicates TNF as a mediator of cachexia. In fact, before its purification and cloning TNF was termed "cachectin" when it was identified as the soluble factor responsible for severe wasting in rodent models of disease. TNF has also been shown to be important in these processes at the cellular and molecular levels both by increasing destructive proteolysis in mature skeletal muscle and by inhibiting the differentiation of myoblasts necessary for the repair of damaged or stressed muscle tissue *(76)*. Clinical trials are now testing the ability of anti-TNF agents such as infliximab to inhibit wasting in cancer patients *(77,78)* and are reviewed in Chapter 23.

Cancer related pain remains a significant unmet medical need for too many patients. TNF appears to be important both for the pain signal itself in some situations and for the metastatic bone erosion that often underlies severe cancer pain. Past research has established that TNF stimulates osteoclastogenesis and osteoclast activation in a variety of immune mediated diseases and that TNF plays a role in tumor-induced osteolysis concomitant with metastatic invasion of bone. This presents an obvious opportunity for clinical application of anti-TNF agents to attenuate tumor-induced destruction of bone and associated neuropathic pain. Tobinick reported two cases of intractable pain from spinal lesions, uncontrolled by narcotics, which were treated with etanercept. One case was

Table 1
Drugs That Modulate TNF Function[a]

Class	Compound (Company)	Status/Indications
Biologic agonist		
Recombinant protein	Human TNF (Boehringer-Ingelheim)	Approved in Europe for isolated limb perfusion for soft tissue sarcomas.
Gene delivery	TNFerade (GenVec)	Under evaluation in cancer patients for nonresectable solid tumors undergoing radiation therapy (Phase II)
Biologic antagonist		
Monoclonal anti-TNF antibody	Infliximab (Centocor)	Approved in Europe and US for rheumatoid arthritis, Crohn's disease, ankylosing spondylitis; under evaluation in cancer patients for supportive care (Phase II; cachexia and GVHD) and for therapy of multiple myeloma (Phase I), renal cell carcinoma (Phase II), and MDS (Phase II).
	Adalimumab (Abbott)	Approved in Europe and US for rheumatoid arthritis.
TNF receptor-Ig fusion protein	Etanercept (Amgen)	Approved in Europe and US for rheumatoid arthritis, juvenile arthritis, ankylosing spondylitis, psoriatic arthritis, psoriasis; under evaluation in cancer patients for ovarian cancer and refractory multiple myeloma.
Pegylated anti-TNF antibody fragment	CDP-870 (Celltech)	Under evaluation for Crohn's disease (Phase III) and rheumatoid arthritis (Phase III).
DN-TNF inactive variant protein	(Xencor)	Preclinical

Small Molecule Antagonists

Inhibitors of TNF synthesis and signaling	Thalidomide (Celgene)	Approved in Europe and US for erythema nodosum leprosum; under evaluation in cancer patients for multiple myeloma (Phase III) and renal cell carcinoma (Phase II)
	Pentoxifylline (Aventis)	Approved in Europe and US for peripheral vascular disease; under evaluation in cancer patients for radiation-induced fibrosis (Phase II)
p38 MAP kinase inhibitor	SCIO-469 (Johnson & Johnson)	Under evaluation for rheumatoid arthritis (Phase IIa)
	BIRB796 (Boehringer Ingelheim)	Under evaluation for psoriasis (Phase IIb/III), rheumatoid arthritis (Phase IIa) and Crohn's disease (Phase IIa).
	SB-681323 (GlaxoSmithkline)	Under evaluation for rheumatoid arthritis (Phase I), COPD (Phase I) and artherosclerosis (Phase I)
	VX-702 (Vertex)	Under evaluation for acute coronary syndrome (Phase IIa).
TACE inhibitors	TMI-005 (Wyeth Research)	Under evaluation for rheumatoid arthritis (Phase I).
	IM491 (Bristol-Myers Squibb)	Preclinical
NF-kB inhibitors	IDDB30934 (GlaxoSmithkline)	Preclinical
	BMS-345541 (Bristol-Myers Squibb)	Preclinical

[a]Numerous biologic and small molecule compounds capable of modulating TNF function are either available commercially, or are under clinical evaluation. Only human TNF is currently approved for a cancer indication, but several of the TNF antagonists are approved for other indications and under investigation for supportive care or treatment of various malignancies.

of metastatic lung cancer and the other was the result of metastatic mammary ductal carcinoma. Relief of pain was reported to have occurred rapidly (5 minutes–1 hour), was complete within 24 hours, and had not recurred after 5 months (till death), and 11 months follow-up, respectively. PET scan evidence in the second patient showed diminution of neoplastic activity and restricted invasion *(79)*. Preliminary evidence such as this warrants the conduct of phase II studies followed by randomized, controlled, and blinded clinical trials to confirm the benefits of anti-TNF therapy for the relief of pain caused by skeletal metastases. Additional preclinical studies will also be necessary to understand the detailed mechanisms by which TNF promotes neuropathic pain and bone destruction.

Investigative and clinical uses of etanercept or infliximab in GVHD are based on the firmly established role of upregulated TNF as a critical effector cytokine in the multi-organ immunoreactivity to pretransplant conditioning regimens and/or allogeneic antigens *(80)*. Infliximab has been reported by transplant clinicians/researchers to be effective in some cases when added to ongoing treatment of refractory acute and chronic GVHD in both adult and pediatric hematopoietic stem cell transplant patients *(81)*. Added immunosuppression and risk of serious infections in these patients warrant vigilance when using anti-TNF agents in GVHD patients. Notably, no studies yet have elucidated an optimal dose and schedule of the anti-TNF mAb and its kinetics in GVHD patients, primarily because of especially high levels of TNF and often severe protein-losing enteropathy *(82,83)*.

TNF also appears to mediate many of the unwanted side effects of radiation therapy. Radiation induced production of TNF by tumor cells enhances the intended local pro-inflammatory effects of ionizing radiation, but also damages normal tissue. Cell lines derived from Ewing sarcoma were investigated in vitro as well as in vivo using established xenografts in mice, for production of TNF mRNA and protein in response to increasing doses of radiation. The induction of TNF was time and dose dependent; the expression of TNF from irradiated tumor cells was up to 2000 times higher than the maximal radiation induced release of TNF from normal lung tissue in pneumonic phase *(84)*. The cytotoxicity of the released cytokine was confirmed by a bioactivity assay in which all the activity could be blocked by anti-TNF mAb. The clinical implication is that extremely high levels of TNF produced by irradiated tumor cells can damage neighboring healthy tissue, negating some of the value of the precision with which the radiation is delivered.

The potential preventive and therapeutic effects of anti-TNF treatment have been evaluated in animal models of radiation toxicity and in the clinic. Pneumonitis limits radiation treatment of lung cancer; enteritis limits radiation treatment of rectal cancer; TNF is a key mediator of these iatrogenic inflammatory conditions. Pentoxifylline down-regulates TNF in response to noxious stimuli, inhibits granulocyte-mediated cytotoxicity after exposure to TNF, and inhibits TNF production from alveolar macrophages. Rube et al. *(85)* showed a pronounced reduction in release of TNF mRNA and TNF protein in animals given pentoxifylline plus radiation compared to animals given radiation alone.

Delanian et al. demonstrated in a randomized, double blind, placebo controlled clinical study that pentoxifylline plus vitamin E significantly reduced chronic and gradually worsening superficial dermal fibrosis caused by excessive external beam radiation or by interstitial brachytherapy boost in the area of mammary tumor excision *(86)*. In a separate study of the effects of pentoxifylline on late, radiation-induced fibrosis (1–29 years post-treatment) patients receiving pentoxifylline demonstrated improved active and passive range of motion (of limbs and spine), improved muscle strength and decreased limb edema and pain *(87)*. These provocative studies strongly suggest that TNF plays a role in mediating radiation-induced fibrosis and that anti-TNF therapies may be effective treatments for the prevention as well as reversal of fibrosis in this setting.

9. CURRENT AND FUTURE TNF-RELATED THERAPIES

The biologic anti-TNF therapies currently approved include etanercept, infliximab, and adalimumab (summarized in Table 1). While approvals are in chronic inflammatory diseases such as RA, Crohn's disease, and psoriasis, these agents are being extensively tested in several areas of cancer therapy and supportive care. Etanercept is a fusion protein consisting of the extracellular domain of TNF-R2 fused to immunoglobulin CH2 and CH3 constant domains, and hence it is capable of neutralizing both TNF and lymphotoxin. Both infliximab and the recently-approved adalimumab are monoclonal antibodies that neutralize only TNF and have no effect on lymphotoxin. In addition, several small molecule, oral TNF therapies are under development (reviewed in Palladino et al. 2003 *[1]*, Table 1) that act to inhibit TNF signaling and synthesis, including inhibitors of TACE (the protease that releases soluble TNF), p38 MAP kinase (known to be involved in signaling both TNF synthesis and activity), NF-κB (a major signaling pathway for TNF activity), and thalidomide (a TNF synthesis inhibitor).

10. CONCLUSION

The extraordinary success of anti-TNF therapies in treating debilitating inflammatory disorders such as RA and Crohn's disease has exceeded the hopes of even some of their most optimistic supporters. Understanding of the complex role that TNF plays in cancer and its associated conditions is in its infancy, but excitement surrounding TNF as a pharmacologic target for oncology is building. Already TNF therapy has proven its usefulness in specific settings and continued advances promise to widen its use. Early results suggest that anti-TNF therapies will find an important place in cancer treatment, both as antitumor agents and perhaps much more broadly for supportive care.

REFERENCES

1. Palladino MA, Bahjat FR, Theodorakis EA, Moldawer LL. Anti-TNF-alpha therapies: The next generation. Nat Rev Drug Discov 2003;2(9):736–746.
2. Balkwill F. Tumor necrosis factor or tumor promoting factor? Cytokine Growth Factor Rev 2002; 13(2):135–141.
3. Carswell EA, Old LJ, Kassel RL, Green S, Fiore N, Williamson B. An endotoxin-induced serum factor that causes necrosis of tumors. Proc Natl Acad Sci U S A 1975;72(9):3666–3670.
4. Pennica D, Nedwin GE, Hayflick JS, et al. Human tumour necrosis factor: Precursor structure, expression and homology to lymphotoxin. Nature 1984;312(5996):724–729.
5. Aggarwal BB. Signalling pathways of the TNF superfamily: A double-edged sword. Nat Rev Immunol 2003;3(9):745–756.
6. Feldmann M, Brennan FM, Paleolog E, et al. Anti-TNFalpha therapy of rheumatoid arthritis: What can we learn about chronic disease? Novartis Found Symp 2004;256:53–69; discussion -73, 106–111, 266–269.
7. Tapping RI, Akashi S, Miyake K, Godowski PJ, Tobias PS. Toll-like receptor 4, but not toll-like receptor 2, is a signaling receptor for Escherichia and Salmonella lipopolysaccharides. J Immunol 2000; 165(10):5780–5787.

8. Black RA, Rauch CT, Kozlosky CJ, et al. A metalloproteinase disintegrin that releases tumour-necrosis factor-alpha from cells. Nature 1997;385(6618):729–733.

9. Moss ML, Jin SL, Milla ME, et al. Cloning of a disintegrin metalloproteinase that processes precursor tumour-necrosis factor-alpha. Nature 1997;385(6618):733–736.

10. Smith RA, Baglioni C. The active form of tumor necrosis factor is a trimer. J Biol Chem 1987;262 (15):6951–6954.

11. Perez C, Albert I, DeFay K, Zachariades N, Gooding L, Kriegler M. A nonsecretable cell surface mutant of tumor necrosis factor (TNF) kills by cell-to-cell contact. Cell 1990;63(2):251–258.

12. Grell M, Wajant H, Zimmermann G, Scheurich P. The type 1 receptor (CD120a) is the high-affinity receptor for soluble tumor necrosis factor. Proc Natl Acad Sci U S A 1998;95(2):570–575.

13. Tartaglia LA, Pennica D, Goeddel DV. Ligand passing: The 75-kDa tumor necrosis factor (TNF) receptor recruits TNF for signaling by the 55-kDa TNF receptor. J Biol Chem 1993;268(25): 18542–18548.

14. Grell M, Becke FM, Wajant H, Mannel DN, Scheurich P. TNF receptor type 2 mediates thymocyte proliferation independently of TNF receptor type 1. Eur J Immunol 1998;28(1):257–263.

15. Ashkenazi A, Dixit VM. Death receptors: Signaling and modulation. Science 1998;281(5381): 1305–1308.

16. Baud V, Karin M. Signal transduction by tumor necrosis factor and its relatives. Trends Cell Biol 2001;11(9):372–377.

17. Schutze S, Machleidt T, Adam D, et al. Inhibition of receptor internalization by monodansylcadaverine selectively blocks p55 tumor necrosis factor receptor death domain signaling. J Biol Chem 1999;274(15):10203–10212.

18. Micheau O, Tschopp J. Induction of TNF receptor I-mediated apoptosis via two sequential signaling complexes. Cell 2003;114(2):181–190.

19. Legler DF, Micheau O, Doucey MA, Tschopp J, Bron C. Recruitment of TNF receptor 1 to lipid rafts is essential for TNFalpha-mediated NF-kappaB activation. Immunity 2003;18(5):655–664.

20. Lejeune FJ. Clinical use of TNF revisited: Improving penetration of anti-cancer agents by increasing vascular permeability. J Clin Invest 2002;110(4):433–435.

21. Eggermont AM, de Wilt JH, ten Hagen TL. Current uses of isolated limb perfusion in the clinic and a model system for new strategies. Lancet Oncol 2003;4(7):429–437.

22. Ruegg C, Yilmaz A, Bieler G, Bamat J, Chaubert P, Lejeune FJ. Evidence for the involvement of endothelial cell integrin alphaVbeta3 in the disruption of the tumor vasculature induced by TNF and IFN-gamma. Nat Med 1998;4(4):408–414.

23. Folli S, Pelegrin A, Chalandon Y, et al. Tumor-necrosis factor can enhance radio-antibody uptake in human colon carcinoma xenografts by increasing vascular permeability. Int J Cancer 1993;53(5): 829–836.

24. An J, Sun YP, Adams J, Fisher M, Belldegrun A, Rettig MB. Drug interactions between the proteasome inhibitor bortezomib and cytotoxic chemotherapy, tumor necrosis factor (TNF) alpha, and TNF-related apoptosis-inducing ligand in prostate cancer. Clin Cancer Res 2003;9(12):4537–4545.

25. Senzer N, Mani S, Rosemurgy A, et al. TNFerade biologic, an adenovector with a radiation-inducible promoter, carrying the human tumor necrosis factor alpha gene: A phase I study in patients with solid tumors. J Clin Oncol 2004;22(4):592–601.

26. Curnis F, Sacchi A, Corti A. Improving chemotherapeutic drug penetration in tumors by vascular targeting and barrier alteration. J Clin Invest 2002;110(4):475–482.

27. Curnis F, Gasparri A, Sacchi A, Longhi R, Corti A. Coupling tumor necrosis factor-alpha with alphaV integrin ligands improves its antineoplastic activity. Cancer Res 2004;64(2):565–571.

28. Borsi L, Balza E, Carnemolla B, et al. Selective targeted delivery of TNFalpha to tumor blood vessels. Blood 2003;102(13):4384–4392.

29. Katerinaki E, Evans GS, Lorigan PC, MacNeil S. TNF-alpha increases human melanoma cell invasion and migration in vitro: The role of proteolytic enzymes. Br J Cancer 2003;89(6):1123–1129.

30. Hagemann T, Robinson SC, Schulz M, Trumper L, Balkwill FR, Binder C. Enhanced invasiveness of breast cancer cell lines upon co-cultivation with macrophages is due to TNF-(R) dependent upregulation of matrix metalloproteases. Carcinogenesis 2004:bgh146.

31. Mochizuki Y, Nakanishi H, Kodera Y, et al. TNF-alpha promotes progression of peritoneal metastasis as demonstrated using a green fluorescence protein (GFP)-tagged human gastric cancer cell line. Clin Exp Metastasis 2004;21(1):39–47.

32. Frater-Schroder M, Risau W, Hallmann R, Gautschi P, Bohlen P. Tumor necrosis factor type alpha, a potent inhibitor of endothelial cell growth in vitro, is angiogenic in vivo. Proc Natl Acad Sci U S A 1987;84(15):5277–5281.

33. Fajardo LF, Kwan HH, Kowalski J, Prionas SD, Allison AC. Dual role of tumor necrosis factor-alpha in angiogenesis. Am J Pathol 1992;140(3):539–544.

34. Szlosarek PW, Balkwill FR. Tumour necrosis factor alpha: A potential target for the therapy of solid tumours. Lancet Oncol 2003;4(9):565–573.

35. Dranoff G. Cytokines in cancer pathogenesis and cancer therapy. Nat Rev Cancer 2004;4(1):11–22.

36. Mantovani G, Maccio A, Mura L, et al. Serum levels of leptin and proinflammatory cytokines in patients with advanced-stage cancer at different sites. J Mol Med 2000;78(10):554–561.

37. Karayiannakis AJ, Syrigos KN, Polychronidis A, Pitiakoudis M, Bounovas A, Simopoulos K. Serum levels of tumor necrosis factor-alpha and nutritional status in pancreatic cancer patients. Anticancer Res 2001;21(2B):1355–1358.

38. Yoshida N, Ikemoto S, Narita K, et al. Interleukin-6, tumour necrosis factor alpha and interleukin-1beta in patients with renal cell carcinoma. Br J Cancer 2002;86(9):1396–1400.

39. Leek RD, Landers R, Fox SB, Ng F, Harris AL, Lewis CE. Association of tumour necrosis factor alpha and its receptors with thymidine phosphorylase expression in invasive breast carcinoma. Br J Cancer 1998;77(12):2246–2251.

40. Partanen R, Koskinen H, Hemminki K. Tumour necrosis factor-alpha (TNF-alpha) in patients who have asbestosis and develop cancer. Occup Environ Med 1995;52(5):316–319.

41. Pfitzenmaier J, Vessella R, Higano CS, Noteboom JL, Wallace D, Jr., Corey E. Elevation of cytokine levels in cachectic patients with prostate carcinoma. Cancer 2003;97(5):1211–1216.

42. Nakashima J, Tachibana M, Ueno M, Miyajima A, Baba S, Murai M. Association between tumor necrosis factor in serum and cachexia in patients with prostate cancer. Clin Cancer Res 1998;4(7):1743–1748.

43. Bossola M, Muscaritoli M, Bellantone R, et al. Serum tumour necrosis factor-alpha levels in cancer patients are discontinuous and correlate with weight loss. Eur J Clin Invest 2000;30(12):1107–1112.

44. von Biberstein SE, Spiro JD, Lindquist R, Kreutzer DL. Enhanced tumor cell expression of tumor necrosis factor receptors in head and neck squamous cell carcinoma. Am J Surg 1995;170(5):416–422.

45. Ariapart P, Bergstedt-Lindqvist S, van Harmelen V, Permert J, Wang F, Lundkvist I. Resection of pancreatic cancer normalizes the preoperative increase of tumor necrosis factor alpha gene expression. Pancreatology 2002;2(5):491–494.

46. Li R, Ruttinger D, Si LS, Wang YL. Analysis of the immunological microenvironment at the tumor site in patients with non-small cell lung cancer. Langenbecks Arch Surg 2003;388(6):406–412.

47. Boldrini L, Calcinai A, Samaritani E, et al. Tumour necrosis factor-alpha and transforming growth factor-beta are significantly associated with better prognosis in non-small cell lung carcinoma: Putative relation with BCL-2-mediated neovascularization. Br J Cancer 2000;83(4):480–486.

48. Wang YY, Lo GH, Lai KH, Cheng JS, Lin CK, Hsu PI. Increased serum concentrations of tumor necrosis factor-alpha are associated with disease progression and malnutrition in hepatocellular carcinoma. J Chin Med Assoc 2003;66(10):593–598.

49. Michalaki V, Syrigos K, Charles P, Waxman J. Serum levels of IL-6 and TNF-alpha correlate with clinicopathological features and patient survival in patients with prostate cancer. Br J Cancer 2004;90(12):2312–2316.

50. Marsh HP, Haldar NA, Bunce M, et al. Polymorphisms in tumour necrosis factor (TNF) are associated with risk of bladder cancer and grade of tumour at presentation. Br J Cancer 2003;89(6):1096–1101.

51. Darai E, Detchev R, Hugol D, Quang NT. Serum and cyst fluid levels of interleukin (IL) -6, IL-8 and tumour necrosis factor-alpha in women with endometriomas and benign and malignant cystic ovarian tumours. Hum Reprod 2003;18(8):1681–1685.

52. Ness RB. Endometriosis and ovarian cancer: Thoughts on shared pathophysiology. Am J Obstet Gynecol 2003;189(1):280–294.

53. Tselepis C, Perry I, Dawson C, et al. Tumour necrosis factor-alpha in Barrett's oesophagus: A potential novel mechanism of action. Oncogene 2002;21(39):6071–6081.

54. Fujiki H, Suganuma M, Okabe S, Kurusu M, Imai K, Nakachi K. Involvement of TNF-alpha changes in human cancer development, prevention and palliative care. Mech Ageing Dev 2002;123(12):1655–1663.

55. Arnott CH, Scott KA, Moore RJ, et al. Tumour necrosis factor-alpha mediates tumour promotion via a PKC alpha- and AP-1-dependent pathway. Oncogene 2002;21(31):4728–4738.

56. Scott KA, Moore RJ, Arnott CH, et al. An anti-tumor necrosis factor-alpha antibody inhibits the development of experimental skin tumors. Mol Cancer Ther 2003;2(5):445–451.
57. Arnott CH, Scott KA, Moore RJ, Robinson SC, Thompson RG, Balkwill FR. Expression of both TNF-alpha receptor subtypes is essential for optimal skin tumour development. Oncogene 2004;23 (10):1902–1910.
58. Tsimberidou AM, Giles FJ. TNF-alpha targeted therapeutic approaches in patients with hematologic malignancies. Expert Rev Anticancer Ther 2002;2(3):277–286.
59. Liotta LA, Kohn EC, Petricoin EF. Clinical proteomics: Personalized molecular medicine. Jama 2001;286(18):2211–2214.
60. Ferrajoli A, Keating MJ, Manshouri T, et al. The clinical significance of tumor necrosis factor-alpha plasma level in patients having chronic lymphocytic leukemia. Blood 2002;100(4):1215–1219.
61. Stasi R, Amadori S. Infliximab chimaeric anti-tumour necrosis factor alpha monoclonal antibody treatment for patients with myelodysplastic syndromes. Br J Haematol 2002;116(2):334–337.
62. Raza A, Lisak LA, Tahir S, et al. Hematologic improvement in response to anti-tumor necrosis factor (TNF) therapy with Remicade® in patients with myelodysplastic syndromes (MDS). ASH 44th Annual Meeting; 6-10 December 2002; Philadelphia, PA.
63. Eisen T, Boshoff C, Mak I, et al. Continuous low dose Thalidomide: A phase II study in advanced melanoma, renal cell, ovarian and breast cancer. Br J Cancer 2000;82(4):812–817.
64. Turk BE, Jiang H, Liu JO. Binding of thalidomide to alpha1-acid glycoprotein may be involved in its inhibition of tumor necrosis factor alpha production. Proc Natl Acad Sci U S A 1996;93(15):7552–7556.
65. Maisey NR, Hall K, Lee C, et al. Infliximab: A phase II trial of the tumour necrosis factor (TNFα) monoclonal antibody in patients with advanced renal cell cancer (RCC). 40th ASCO Annual Meeting; June 5-8, 2004; New Orleans, LA.
66. Marty FM, Lee SJ, Fahey MM, et al. Infliximab use in patients with severe graft-versus-host disease and other emerging risk factors of non-Candida invasive fungal infections in allogeneic hematopoietic stem cell transplant recipients: A cohort study. Blood 2003;102(8):2768–2776.
67. Smith KJ, Skelton HG. Rapid onset of cutaneous squamous cell carcinoma in patients with rheumatoid arthritis after starting tumor necrosis factor alpha receptor IgG1-Fc fusion complex therapy. J Am Acad Dermatol 2001;45(6):953–956.
68. Kavanaugh A, Keystone EC. The safety of biologic agents in early rheumatoid arthritis. Clin Exp Rheumatol 2003;21(5 Suppl 31):S203–208.
69. Wolfe F, Michaud K. Lymphoma in rheumatoid arthritis: The effect of methotrexate and anti-TNF therapy in 18,572 patients. Arthritis Rheum. p. suppl. S242.
70. Lee JH, Slifman NR, Gershon SK, et al. Life-threatening histoplasmosis complicating immunotherapy with tumor necrosis factor alpha antagonists infliximab and etanercept. Arthritis Rheum 2002; 46(10):2565–2570.
71. Brown SL, Greene MH, Gershon SK, Edwards ET, Braun MM. Tumor necrosis factor antagonist therapy and lymphoma development: Twenty-six cases reported to the Food and Drug Administration. Arthritis Rheum 2002;46(12):3151–3158.
72. Slifman NR, Gershon SK, Lee JH, Edwards ET, Braun MM. Listeria monocytogenes infection as a complication of treatment with tumor necrosis factor alpha-neutralizing agents. Arthritis Rheum 2003;48(2):319–324.
73. Colombel JF, Loftus EV, Jr., Tremaine WJ, et al. The safety profile of infliximab in patients with Crohn's disease: The Mayo clinic experience in 500 patients. Gastroenterology 2004;126(1):19–31.
74. Kurzrock R. The role of cytokines in cancer-related fatigue. Cancer 2001;92(6 Suppl):1684-8.
75. Wichers M, Maes M. The psychoneuroimmuno-pathophysiology of cytokine-induced depression in humans. Int J Neuropsychopharmacol 2002;5(4):375–388.
76. Guttridge DC, Mayo MW, Madrid LV, Wang CY, Baldwin AS, Jr. NF-kappaB-induced loss of MyoD messenger RNA: Possible role in muscle decay and cachexia. Science 2000;289(5488): 2363–2366.
77. Tisdale MJ. Cachexia in cancer patients. Nat Rev Cancer 2002;2(11):862–871.
78. Argiles JM, Busquets S, Lopez-Soriano FJ. Cytokines in the pathogenesis of cancer cachexia. Curr Opin Clin Nutr Metab Care 2003;6(4):401–406.
79. Tobinick EL. Targeted etanercept for treatment-refractory pain due to bone metastasis: Two case reports. Clin Ther 2003;25(8):2279–2288.

80. Korngold R, Marini JC, de Baca ME, Murphy GF, Giles-Komar J. Role of tumor necrosis factor-alpha in graft-versus-host disease and graft-versus-leukemia responses. Biol Blood Marrow Transplant 2003;9(5):292–303.
81. Couriel DR, Saliba R, Hicks K, et al. TNF-Alpha Inhibition for the Treatment of Chronic GVHD. ASH 44th annual meeting; 6-10 December 2002; Philadelphia, PA.
82. Campos A, Vaz CP, Costa N, et al. Infliximab as Salvage Therapy for Patients with Acute Graft Versus Host Disease Refractory to Steroids. ASH 45th Annual Meeting; 6-9 December 2003; San Diego, CA.
83. Jacobsohn DA, Hallick J, Anders V, McMillan S, Morris L, Vogelsang GB. Infliximab for steroid-refractory acute GVHD: A case series. Am J Hematol 2003;74(2):119–124.
84. Rube CE, van Valen F, Wilfert F, et al. Ewing's sarcoma and peripheral primitive neuroectodermal tumor cells produce large quantities of bioactive tumor necrosis factor-alpha (TNF-alpha) after radiation exposure. Int J Radiat Oncol Biol Phys 2003;56(5):1414–1425.
85. Rube CE, Wilfert F, Uthe D, et al. Modulation of radiation-induced tumour necrosis factor alpha (TNF-alpha) expression in the lung tissue by pentoxifylline. Radiother Oncol 2002;64(2):177–187.
86. Delanian S, Porcher R, Balla-Mekias S, Lefaix JL. Randomized, placebo-controlled trial of combined pentoxifylline and tocopherol for regression of superficial radiation-induced fibrosis. J Clin Oncol 2003;21(13):2545–2550.
87. Okunieff P, Augustine E, Hicks JE, et al. Pentoxifylline in the treatment of radiation-induced fibrosis. J Clin Oncol 2004;22(11):2207–2213.

5

Transforming Growth Factor-β and Cancer

Alyssa R. Bonine-Summers, Brian K. Law, and Harold L. Moses

CONTENTS

1. TGF-β SIGNALING AND TUMORIGENESIS

Normal tissue homeostasis is maintained by strict regulation of interactions between cells and their microenvironment. How a cell responds to stimulatory and inhibitory signals it receives from the microenvironment will directly impact whether or not that particular cell will proceed through the cell cycle and proliferate or stop cell cycle progression and undergo assessment. When cells no longer respond to their microenvironmental cues and proliferate autonomously, tumors arise. The major known negative regulators of cell proliferation are the transforming growth factor βs (TGF-βs). The TGF-β signaling pathways are tumor suppressive, yet once tumors have developed, TGF-β signaling can enhance tumor progression.

The TGF-β signaling pathways regulate an important network of signals that control cellular growth, differentiation and migration *(1)*. TGF-β activates key signaling events that are either blocked in tumor cells to allow cellular proliferation or are used by tumor cells to promote metastasis *(2)*. TGF-β exists as three isoforms, TGF-β1, β2, and β3, that signal through cell surface serine/threonine kinase receptors designated TGF-β type I (TβRI) and TGF-β type II (TβRII). TβRII is a constitutively active protein kinase that is autophosphorylated upon TGF-β ligand binding. The TGF-β/TβRII phospho-complex

From: *Cancer Drug Discovery and Development,*
Cytokines in the Genesis and Treatment of Cancer
Edited by: M. A. Caligiuri and M. T. Lotze © Humana Press Inc., Totowa, NJ

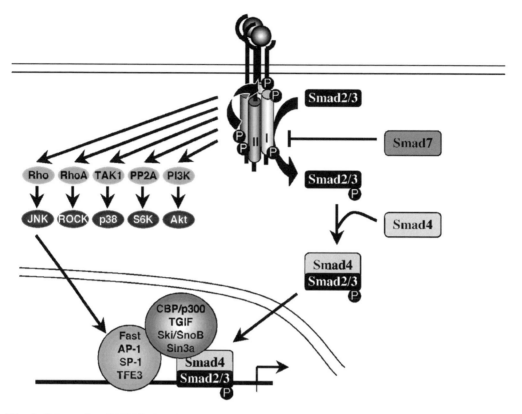

Fig. 1. Schematic of TGF-β signal transduction. A simplified schematic showing Smad signaling on the right, known to be necessary for growth inhibition and non-Smad signaling on the left, known to be involved in epithelial to mesenchymal transition (EMT) and motility. JNK, c-Jun amino-terminal kinase; ROCK, Rho-associated kinase.

recruits TβRI that when bound is phosphorylated by TβRII. Phosphorylated TβRI then propagates the signal by phosphorylating receptor-regulated Smad proteins (R-Smads) that consist of Smad2 and Smad3 proteins. Upon activation of the R-Smad proteins a common-mediator Smad (Co-Smad), designated Smad4, binds the R-Smad complex. The R-Smad/Co-Smad heteromeric complex then accumulates in the nucleus where it participates in transcriptional regulation of target genes *(3)* (Fig. 1).

The TGF-β receptor complex can also signal independently of Smad proteins. Secondary pathways include activation of the mitogen-activated protein kinase (MAPK) pathways. Activation of the RhoA pathway as well as the phosphatidylinositol 3 kinase (PI-3K) and Akt pathways have been shown to increase stress fiber formation and delocalization of cell adhesion molecules *(4,5)*. Moreover, the integrin1 and p38/MAPK pathway has been shown to be involved in epithelial motility *(6,7)*. In addition to cell motility, TGF-β receptors activate apoptosis related pathways through the mitochondrial pathway. Activation of the apoptosis related protein in TGF-β signaling (ARTS) blocks an inhibitor of a caspase degradation protein called XIAP *(8,9)*. These and other related pathways show the diversity of TGF-β signaling through activation of a plethora of effector proteins.

The diversity of the TGF-β network allows for complex signaling during tumor progression. Tumors have been shown to escape the effects of TGF-β through mutations of

TβRI, TβRII and/or Smad proteins, thereby ablating their tumor suppressive properties *(10,11)*. However, many cancers also use the TGF-β pathway to their benefit. Once established, as the tumor progresses, mutations accumulate that disrupt the suppressive effects of TGF-β. Tumors have then been found to elevate levels of the TGF-β ligand to promote an increased metastatic state *(12)*. Thus, TGF-β can act as a tumor suppressor or tumor promoter depending on the context of the tumor microenvironment.

2. TGF-β ACTIVATES A TUMOR SUPPRESSIVE PATHWAY

The protective effects of TGF-β against malignant transformation have been analyzed through the use of several transgenic mouse model systems. Initial studies using in vitro assays documented that the growth suppressive abilities of TGF-β are dominant over the tumor promoting effects of the mitogen TGF-α *(13)*. The protective effects of TGF-β were further verified by Pierce et al. *(14)* in vivo through the generation of transgenic mice constitutively expressing the TGF-β1 ligand using the promoter/enhancer MMTV to target mammary tissue. The MMTV/TGF-β1 mice were then crossed with transgenic mice over-expressing the mitogen TGF-α. Offspring from the MMTV/TGF-β1/TGF-α mice developed a significantly lower number of tumors compared to TGF-α mice alone. Furthermore, MMTV/TGF-β1 mice treated with the carcinogen DMBA (7,12-dimethylbenz[a]anthracene) showed marked resistance to the drug relative to their wild type counterparts. These data demonstrate the protective role that TGF-β1 plays during mammary carcinogenesis.

Further evidence for the tumor protective effects of TGF-β have been documented through epidemiologic studies looking at polymorphisms that increase serum levels of TGF-β. A polymorphism was detected that altered the common allele thymine (T) to a variant containing cytosine (C) thus substituting the amino acid leucine for a proline. Individuals that are homozygous for T/T alleles or heterozygous T/C alleles are more likely to develop breast cancer than homozygous C/C individuals. Further experiments determined that those patients with homozygous C/C genotypes had a higher circulating amount of TGF-β than individuals with the common T/T genotype *(15)*, thereby suggesting that an increase in circulating TGF-β is protective against human tumor formation.

Owing to the protective role played by TGF-β many tumors attempt to evade the TGF-β signaling pathway through perturbation of TGF-β receptor signaling through several mechanisms. One mechanism is loss of TGF-β ligand expression that has been suggested to be an early step in tumor progression. Studies using antisense TGF-β1 to reduce TGF-β autocrine function in a human colon carcinoma cell line demonstrated that loss of TGF-β1 expression drastically increased the ability of the colon cancer cells to form tumors in mice compared to wild type controls *(16,17)*. Another mechanism to evade TGF-β signaling is inactivating mutations of TGF-β receptors. Studies have shown that mice expressing dominant negative TβRII (dnTβRII) have enhanced tumorigenesis in lung, mammary tissue, and skin upon carcinogen treatment *(18,19)*. Furthermore, it was shown by Tu et al. *(20)* that mice expressing both the SV40 large T antigen and the dnTβRII transgene are more prone toward metastasis from primary prostate tumors than mice expressing the SV40 large T antigen alone. Recently, evidence has demonstrated that mice expressing dnTβRII in the mammary gland have an increased propensity for mammary carcinogenesis without a carcinogen inducing agent, though with a longer latency *(21)*.

Disruption of the downstream Smad proteins also dramatically increases the susceptibility to tumor formation in mouse models. Mice lacking functional Smad2, Smad3, or

Smad4 have been generated to examine any redundancy these proteins have in development and tumorigenesis. Mice with homozygous inactivating mutations of the *Smad2* or
Smad4 genes die in embryogenesis whereas Smad3 null mice are viable *(22)*. Data indicate that Smad3 is a tumor suppressor protein, because Smad3 null mice develop colon
cancer with a 100% incidence by 4–6 mo of age in the 129/Sv genetic background *(23)*.
Yet, other studies of Smad3 null mice did not show this dramatic phenotype perhaps due
to different targeting strategies used to knock out the *Smad3* gene *(24,25)*. In humans,
however, it was observed recently that 37.5% of human gastric cancers ablate Smad3
expression *(26)*. This suggests that *Smad3* is indeed a tumor suppressor gene.

Although homozygous Smad2 and Smad4 mouse mutants die as embryos *Smad2* and
Smad4 genes can be studied in heterozygous null mouse models. These studies have
identified both *Smad2* and *Smad4* genes as potent tumor suppressors. After a 1-yr
latency, heterozygous *Smad4* mutant mice develop malignant intestinal tumors that are
attributed to loss of heterozygosity and duplication of the mutant *Smad4* allele *(27,28)*.
In addition, mice carrying inactivation mutations of both *Smad4* and *APC* genes in a
heterozygous fashion develop highly metastatic intestinal tumors compared to mice carrying mutated *APC* alone *(29)*. *APC* mutations alone induce a high incidence of intestinal tumors but with a low incidence of malignancy *(30)*. The *APC* gene is frequently
inactivated in colon cancers and like the Smad4 protein the APC protein inhibits cellular proliferation through transcriptional regulation of target genes. Similar results have
been observed in *Smad2/APC* heterozygous mutant mice. Loss of Smad2, as with the
loss of Smad4, increases the invasiveness of existing APC induced tumors causing
accelerated tumor growth *(31)*. Clearly mutations in the *Smad2* or *Smad4* tumor suppressor genes enhance the effect of *APC* mutations to form a more aggressive tumor
phenotype. Overall these data provide substantial evidence for the physiologic importance of TGF-β signaling in tumor suppression.

3. GENETIC ALTERATIONS IN THE TGF-β
PATHWAY IN HUMAN CANCER

Although mouse models allow for detailed manipulation of tumor signaling pathways the final question is how relevant are these results to human cancer? As stated earlier, TGF-β plays a central role in the control of cellular growth and many tumors escape
the inhibitory function of TGF-β through mutational inactivation of genes within the
TGF-β signaling network. Striking evidence for the importance of TGF-β signaling in
human cancers comes from recent estimates that most pancreatic and colon cancers
have mutations that block the function of one or more components of the TGF-β signaling pathway *(32,33)*. It was first shown by Markowitz et al. *(34)* that the *Tgfbr2* gene is
frequently inactivated in mismatch repair (MMR) deficient sporadic colon cancers.
Cancers that are MMR deficient have an increased mutational rate through the addition
or deletion of nucleotides in regions of genes that contain long repeated sequences. The
Tgfbr2 gene contains a microsatellite region consisting of a 10-base-pair polyadenine
repeat (BAT-RII tract) encoding part of the extracellular domain of the TβRII receptor.
Mutations in the BAT-RII tract, caused by MMR deficiency, cause the introduction of
early stop codons that result in a truncated nonfunctional TβRII receptor. Subsequent
analyses also identified BAT-RII mutations in hereditary nonpolyposis colon cancer
(HNPCC), 68–91% of gastric cancers, 71% of gliomas and 50% of pancreatic-biliary

maljunction-associated biliary tract tumors *(35–40)*. The *Tgfbr2* gene is also inactivated by point mutations in head and neck carcinomas, gastric lymphoma, T-cell lymphoma, and ovarian carcinomas *(10,41–44)*.

Certain cancers have also been shown to have inactivation of the *TβRI* gene. The first evidence for TβRI mutations in human cancer was documented by Chen et al. *(45)*. A point mutation that results in a serine to tyrosine substitution (S387Y) in the *TβRI* gene was identified in secondary lymph metastases in breast carcinoma patients. These results suggest that *TβRI* mutations are more commonly associated with metastatic disease than primary tumor lesions. However, it has been proposed that the S387Y mutation in *TβRI* is perhaps not as likely a promoter of metastasis as initially thought because *TβRI* is not found to be commonly mutated in breast, lung, and colon metastases *(46)*. Nonetheless, *TβRI* mutations are clearly associated with many cancers. In nonsmall-cell lung cancers (NSCLC), a polymorphism located within intron 7 of the *TβRI* gene changes a guanine (G) nucleotide to adenine (A). Individuals homozygous for the A/A polymorphism had threefold higher incidence of NSCLC development than individuals with the more common G/G genotype *(47)*. In addition, Pasche et al. *(48)* identified a common polymorphism designated TβRI(6A) that contains a deletion of three alanine residues in the extracellular domain of the receptor and an uncommon polymorphism designated TβRI(10A) that contains an insertion of an alanine residue in the same domain. The TβRI(6A) mutation favors cell proliferation by disabling TGF-β growth suppressive effects. Furthermore an analysis of TβRI(6A) frequency in 12 case-control studies found a 70% increased colon cancer risk in individuals that were homozygous for the TβRI(6A) allele and a 19% increase in heterozygous individuals *(49)*. These data support the idea that TβRI plays a significant role in tumorigenesis and that TGF-β related epidemiologic predispositions are a critical evaluator in cancer progression.

As observed in mouse models, Smads play an important role in TGF-β signaling and are key suppressors of cancer progression. In human cancers the *Smad4* gene is mutated more commonly than *Smad2* or *Smad3*. The *Smad4* gene is a target for mutation in 50% of pancreatic cancers and 33% of metastatic colon cancers *(50,51)*. In addition to somatic mutations, *Smad4* germ-line mutations were also identified in patients with juvenile polyposis syndromes (JPS). These patients exhibit hamartomatous intestinal polyps with an increased risk of developing gastrointestinal cancer *(52)*. Interestingly, *Smad4* is frequently mutated in conjunction with other TGF-β signaling components. In biliary cancer both *Smad4* and *TβRI* genes are mutated, whereas certain colon cancers carry *Smad4/TβRII* double mutations *(32,33)*. *Smad4* mutations have also been found in conjunction with *Smad2* mutations in colon, lung, and pancreatic cancer *(53)*. Finally, *Smad2* mutations alone have been observed in colon and lung cancer, whereas *Smad3* mutations have been found associated with breast cancer, gastric cancer, and occur infrequently in colon cancer *(54–56)*. Together these data show that the Smad proteins are potent tumor suppressor proteins that are critical to the growth suppressive effects of TGF-β in human carcinogenesis.

4. MECHANISMS OF TGF-β MEDIATED CELL CYCLE ARREST

The ability of TGF-β to act as a tumor suppressor is, in part, owing to its capability to induce cell cycle arrest in most epithelial cells. The cell cycle is governed by a group of proteins called cyclins that are regulated at the transcriptional level by E2F-dependent

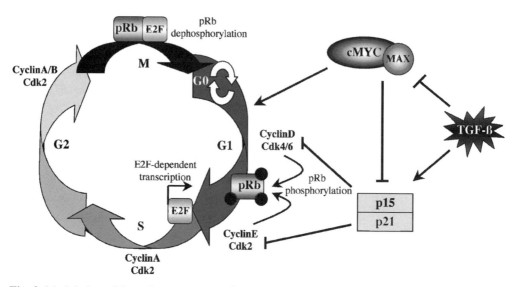

Fig. 2. Modulation of the cell cycle by TGF-β-G1 arrest: A basic diagram depicting the involvement of TGF-β in G1 cell cycle arrest. TGF-β through Smad transcriptional events induces p15 and p21, cdk inhibitors that block activation of the cyclin/cdk complexes. The retinoblastoma protein, pRb, then becomes dephosphorylated blocking E2F transcription factors. TGF-β also down-regulates c-Myc expression thus relieving p15 and p21 repression.

transcription and growth factors and at the protein level via phosphorylation by cyclin-dependent kinases (cdks) *(57)*. Cyclins and cdks are negatively regulated by cdk inhibitors (cdki). Cdki proteins block cell cycle progression by blocking the kinase activity of cyclin/cdk complexes *(58)*. There are two groups of cyclin proteins, those that govern the G_1–S phase of the cell cycle (cyclin D, E, and A) and those that govern the G_2–M transition (cyclin B). Each cyclin also has a corresponding cdk component. Both cyclin D/cdk4/6 and cyclin E/cdk2 complexes phosphorylate the retinoblastoma tumor suppressor protein (pRb). When pRb is hypophosphorylated it associates with E2F transcription factors and sequesters them from activating target genes required for cell cycle progression. However, upon hyperphosphorylation pRb disassociates from E2F, liberating E2F to activate genes required for cell cycle progression *(59,60)* (Fig. 2).

TGF-β primarily acts through proteins that regulate the G_1–S transition of the cell cycle. TGF-β affects cell cycle progression through a narrow window occurring 6–10 h after G_0 release, this is known as the restriction point. If TGF-β is added after the restriction point the cell will cycle through until the G1/S transition of the next cell cycle is reached and then undergo arrest *(60)*. TGF-β induces cytostasis by up-regulating the cdki proteins, p15 and p21. The p15 protein blocks cyclin D/cdk4/6 function whereas p21 blocks both cyclin D/cdk4/6 and cyclin E/cdk2 during G_1–S transition. Smads 2/3/4 are directly involved in transcriptional regulation of both p15 and p21 *(61,62)*. Evidence for the involvement of cdk inhibitors in the TGF-β cytostatic program has been demonstrated in cancers with mutated p15 because these cancers have been shown to be TGF-β insensitive and refractory toward TGF-β induced growth arrest *(63)*.

In addition to activating cell cycle inhibitors, TGF-β also down-regulates mitogenic proteins that stimulate cell growth. TGF-β down-regulates the potent mitogenic factor c-Myc. The c-Myc protein is involved in transcriptional regulation of many genes

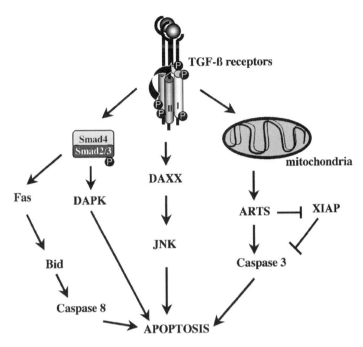

Fig. 3. TGF-β induced apoptotic pathways. There are two main apoptotic pathways in mammalian cells, the death receptor pathway and the mitochondrial pathway. In the death receptor pathway TGF-β induces apoptosis via Fas, DAXX, and DAPK. In the mitochondrial pathway TGF-β is known to affect the protein ARTS that signals through caspase-3. DAPK, death-associated protein kinase; ARTS, apoptosis-related protein in TGF-β signaling.

necessary for cell cycle progression as well as transcriptional repression of cdk inhibitors p15 and p21 *(64–66)*. Studies have shown that overexpression of c-Myc diminishes TGF-β growth-arrest capability *(67)*. Moreover, studies in breast cancer cell lines MCF-10A and MDA-MB-231 suggest that loss of TGF-β tumor-suppressive properties stem from the loss of TGF-β repression of c-*myc*. The Smad proteins that repress c-*myc* transcription are direct targets for mutational inactivation in breast cancer progression *(68)*. In addition, loss of c-*myc* repression is also correlated with ovarian cancer resistance to TGF-βs antiproliferative effects *(69)*.

5. MECHANISMS OF TGF-β MEDIATED APOPTOSIS

Besides the cytostatic properties of TGF-β mediated through cell-cycle arrest, TGF-β also has a pro-apoptotic effect. However, activation of apoptosis by TGF-β is variable depending on the cell and tissue type. Therefore a single pathway will not suffice to explain TGF-β's role in programmed cell death *(70)*. The microenvironment greatly influences how cells respond to apoptotic signals either from other cells or exogenous environmental signals. Deregulated apoptosis, like deregulated proliferation, is a key factor during carcinogenesis. When cells no longer undergo apoptosis appropriately upon DNA damage, tissues are more likely to become tumorigenic because of the accumulation of cell number as well as genetic mutations that may allow them to then proliferate autonomously. There are two major apoptosis pathways in mammalian cells, the death receptor pathway and the mitochondrial pathway *(71)* (Fig. 3).

TGF-β affects a multitude of apoptotic effector molecules within both the death receptor and the mitochondrial pathways. In the human gastric SNU-620 cell line it was recently shown that TGF-β induces apoptosis from the Fas death receptor pathway. Kim et al. *(72)* identified TGF-β as a Fas ligand-independent activator of Fas and subsequent activator of caspase-8 via Bid cleavage. Furthermore it is known that Smad transcriptional targets are important modulators of TGF-β mediated apoptosis as Smad3 knockdown in these cells abrogated the apoptotic phenotype. Other studies also demonstrate the requirement for Smad3 mediated transcription in the apoptotic pathway. Conery et al. *(73)* uncovered a novel function for Akt in apoptosis through its ability to cross-talk with Smad3. Independent of its kinase activity Akt binds and sequesters Smad3 to the cytoplasm thereby blocking Smad3-mediated transcription and apoptosis. This may be one mechanism that Akt uses to promote cellular survival. Other Smad induced factors related to TGF-β mediated apoptosis are the TGF-β early-response gene (TIEG1) and the death-associated protein kinase (DAPK) *(74,75)*. Both proteins are up-regulated upon TGF-β treatment and are some of the first TGF-β responsive genes to be identified as important mediators of TGF-β induced apoptosis *(1)*. TIEG1 mimics TGF-β by inducing cell-cycle arrest and has recently been shown to enhance TGF-β mediated apoptosis in OLI-neu cells *(76)*. TGF-β directly activates the *DAPK* gene via the Smad2/3/4 transcription factors and in turn DAPK sensitizes cells to TGF-β dependent apoptosis *(75)*. DAPK has been shown to be a critical evaluator of apoptosis as it is a target for alteration in lung cancer. Decreased DAPK expression has been correlated with epigenetic alteration in the promoter region of the gene in 44% of lung carcinoma cell lines and 37% of primary lung cancers *(77)*. Taken together these data strongly support the role of Smad proteins and their genetic targets as key players in the death receptor branch of apoptosis.

TGF-β receptors have also been shown to activate the death-receptor apoptotic pathway via the interaction between DAXX and TβRII. DAXX is a Fas-receptor associated protein that activates apoptosis via the JNK pathway and is a requirement for some cells to undergo apoptosis *(78)*. Consistent with the TβRII/DAXX interaction it was recently demonstrated that decreased TβRII expression correlates with prostate carcinogenesis and a decreased apoptotic index *(79)*. Together these data suggest that one mechanism for tumor survival is to evade TGF-β mediated apoptosis through the inactivation of TβRII and possible blockade of the DAXX signaling pathway.

In the mitochondrial pathway TGF-β receptors activate apoptosis via a newly discovered protein called ARTS (apoptosis-related protein in the TGF-β pathway). The ARTS protein was recently described as a mitochondrial related protein that down-regulates inhibitors of apoptosis proteins (IAPs) that negatively regulate the caspase cascade leading to apoptosis. Upon TGF-β treatment, ARTS induces caspase-3 by down regulation of an IAP called XIAP *(8,9)*. In summary, these data indicate that TGF-β is involved in mediating apoptosis through several mechanisms via both the death receptor and mitochondrial pathways.

6. TUMOR PROMOTING EFFECTS OF TGF-β

Evasion of TGF-β induced growth arrest and apoptosis is an early event during tumorigenesis. However, later, these same tumors often use the TGF-β pathway to their advantage during tumor progression. An example of this type of dichotomy is seen in human breast carcinoma. Frequently, cells derived from breast carcinomas express the TGF-β ligand, yet are refractory to TGF-β mediated growth inhibition *(80–82)*. This suggests that these cells have abrogated the growth inhibitory function of TGF-β, but retain the signaling pathways that lead to increased tumor invasiveness. Many studies have shown that increased levels of TGF-β expression during later stages of breast tumorigenesis correlates with poor prognosis *(83)*. Furthermore, it was observed that mice injected with MDA-MB-231 breast cancer cells expressing a dominant negative TβRII receptor formed less bone metastases and showed prolonged survival *(84)*. These studies suggest that tumors use TGF-β signaling during the later stages of carcinogenesis as a selection advantage leading to metastasis.

Mechanistically it has been proposed that TGF-β induces metastasis through increasing motility in epithelial cells. This phenomenon involves an epithelial to mesenchymal transition (EMT) and is thought to be a mechanism by which TGF-β increases cellular plasticity. Tumor cells may use this pathway to move away from the primary tumor site into the circulation, allowing tumors cells to metastasize and become established at a secondary site *(85)*. Studies have shown that TGF-β can induce morphological changes in nontransformed and transformed mammary epithelial cells through an EMT pathway. Cellular morphology changes from epithelial to mesenchymal in phenotype and key cell adhesion and cytoskeletal proteins are activated or repressed. TGF-β induced EMT is accompanied by actin cytoskeletal reorganization as well as up-regulation of the cytoskeletal marker vimentin. Furthermore, TGF-β down-regulates the expression of the cell adhesion molecules E-cadherin and ZO-1 *(86)* (Fig. 4).

Recently, the p38 mitogen-activated protein kinase (MAPK) pathway has been suggested to be critical for TGF-β mediated EMT. Bhowmick et al. *(6)* identified integrin-β1 as required for TGF-β to activate the p38MAPK pathway and induce EMT in mammary epithelial cells. These data were further verified by Bakin et al. *(7)* by demonstrating impaired TGF-β mediated morphologic cellular changes and decreased cytoskeletal reorganization in NmuMG cells upon treatment with a p38MAPK inhibitor, SB202190. These data support the model that TGF-β has the ability to induce cell motility through promoting EMT.

7. TUMOR PROGRESSION THROUGH ACTIVATION OF ANGIOGENESIS

In addition to tumor induced cell motility, tumors acquire new blood vessels that allow tumor cells to receive nutrients and oxygen for growth. Moreover, vascularized tumors are more likely to extravasate into the blood stream resulting in tumor progression leading to metastasis. Without tumor vascularization the growing tumor undergoes necrosis and has a more benign phenotype *(87,88)*. The formation and maintenance of blood vessels is critical in tumor progression and an important step to target in anticancer therapies.

There are two main cell types that are required for vessel formation, endothelial cells (ECs) and perimural cells. There are several distinct steps during angiogenesis *(89,90)*. First, angiogenic factors such as vascular endothelial growth factor (VEGF) are induced and activate a signaling cascade triggering angiogenesis. Matrix metalloproteinases (MMPs) are then activated and facilitate breakdown of the extracellular matrix (ECM). Endothelial cells then escape the capillary wall and migrate to the site of angiogenesis.

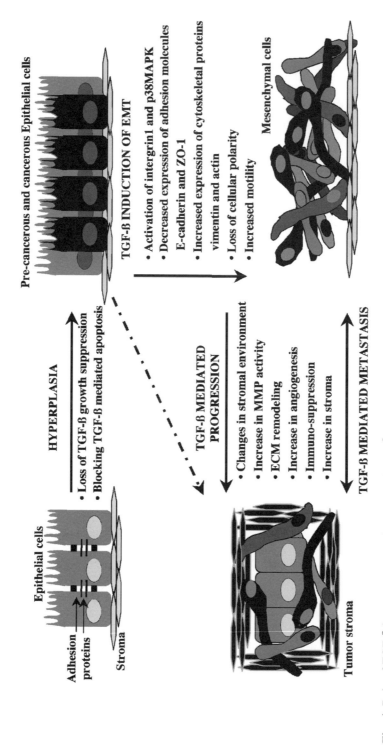

Fig. 4. Role of TGF-β in tumor progression. Loss of TGF-β signaling has been shown to promote increased cellular growth as well as deregulated apoptosis. As cells proliferate and acquire mutations they can either become transformed and begin to upregulate TGF-β and undergo morphologic changes. Through activation the p38/MAPK pathway and loss of adherens junctions epithelial cells undergo structural changes to a mesenchymal phenotype. Mesenchymal cells have increased motility and are more likely to metastasize. MMP, matrix metalloproteinase.

These ECs then release platelet derived growth factor β (PDGF-β) that in turn recruits pericytes and smooth muscle cells (SMCs). The SMCs then migrate to cover the vessel tube created by endothelial cells. In the resolution phase the SMCs cover the newly formed tube and stop proliferating upon differentiation, thus completing the newly formed blood vessel *(89,90)*. TGF-β primarily acts during the later stage of angiogenesis, in the resolution phase. TGF-β is thought to induce differentiation of the precursor perimural cells into pericytes and SMCs. The pericytes and SMCs have been suggested to act as stabilizers through the inhibition of proliferation and migration of the ECs forming the vessel tube *(89,91)*. Recently, interleukin-3 (IL-3) was shown to play a critical role in EC-mediated SMC recruitment through increasing the activity of TGF-β *(92)*. Together these data strongly support the role of TGF-β in blood vessel stabilization.

Several mouse studies have further demonstrated the importance of the TGF-β pathway in angiogenesis. Mutations in the *TGF-β1*, *TβRI*, and *TβRII* genes lead to death in midgestation of developing embryos owing to defects in vasculogenesis and blood vessel integrity *(93–95)*. These data support the role of TGF-β as a critical player during vascularization. Furthermore, TGF-β recruits the angiogenic factor VEGF that is involved in tumor vascularization *(96–98)*. TGF-β secondarily affects angiogenesis by acting as a chemoattractant for monocytes that release other angiogenic cytokines *(99)*. TGF-β induction of angiogenesis is correlated with cancer progression as seen in human cancers. In NSCLC increased TGF-β1 protein levels were strongly associated with microvessel density of the tumor and poor patient prognosis *(100)*. Together these data show that TGF-β can regulate angiogenesis at many levels during development and carcinogenesis.

8. TUMOR PROGRESSION VIA TGF-β IMMUNE SUPPRESSION

Another mechanism of TGF-β-induced tumor progression is immune suppression. The immune system is critical in fighting tumor development and tumor growth. However, tumors often have several mechanisms to avoid immune surveillance. One mechanism is to negatively regulate key players that would lead to an immune response.

TGF-β has been shown to negatively regulate the functions of both cytotoxic T-cells and natural killer (NK) cells allowing tumors to evade immunologic cell death *(101)*. These observations were demonstrated in experiments using TGF-β1 cDNA to overexpress TGF-β1 in a highly immunogenic tumor cell line. TGF-β expression resulted in abrogation of the host T-cell mediated cytotoxic response thus allowing tumor growth *(102)*. Other studies validate the importance of TGF-β in immune surveillance by blocking the TGF-β2 ligand from activating TβRI and TβRII. Using antisense TGF-β2 injected into rats with gliomas, researchers examined tumor regression. Results indicated a three- to fourfold higher incidence of cytotoxic T-cell response in rats injected with the antisense TGF-β2 than rats injected with a control vector. Furthermore, the tumors from the TGF-β2 injected rats were drastically reduced in size compared with the control rats *(103)*. These data suggest that loss of TGF-β mediated immunosuppression allows for increased tumor cell death by cytotoxic T-cells.

Additional studies have suggested that not only does TGF-β repress cytotoxic effector cells but that TGF-β may also activate a distinct type of T-cell that has immunosuppressive capabilities. Sakaguchi et al. *(104)* were first to identify CD4[+] T-lymphocytes that constitutively express the CD25 marker. These specialized T-lymphocytes are recognized as potent immunosuppressor cells. TGF-β has been suggested to positively regulate these CD4[+]/CD25[+] T-cells as demonstrated in experiments that have blocked TGF-β1 expression and reversed the repressive phenotype of these CD4[+]/CD25[+] T-cells in a dose-dependent manner. In addition, the CD4[+]/CD25[+] T-cells have been shown to produce increased levels of TβRII on the cell surface as well as the TGF-β ligand. CD4[+]/CD25[+] are thought to initiate cell contact with CD4[+] or CD8[+] cells via TβRII and inhibit the immune response of these T-lymphocytes *(105)*. Recent data have demonstrated that CD4[+]/CD25[+] T-cells also block the antigen-presenting dendritic cells *(106)*. These regulatory CD4[+]/CD25[+] T-cells are generally associated with suppression of self-reactive T-cells thus blocking autoimmune diseases. However, CD4[+]/CD25[+] T-cells are now being correlated with cancer progression via the blockade of the host-immune response to tumors. Increased CD4[+]/CD25[+] T-cell expression has been correlated with colon, breast, pancreas, and lung carcinomas *(107–109)*.

9. TGF-β AND THE STROMAL ENVIRONMENT

The TGF-β signaling pathway is a complex network of signals that produce different outcomes depending on the cell type. In epithelial cells, as we have discussed, TGF-β primarily acts as a growth suppressor. However, in many fibroblasts TGF-β acts as a mitogen and promotes cellular growth. During tumorigenesis epithelial and stromal fibroblasts are important partners in tumor progression. The majority of cancers arise from an epithelial origin; however, it is the stromal cells that are essential for epithelial maintenance. Upon induction of carcinogenesis, either by oncogenic mutations or loss of tumor suppressors, epithelial cells change. In addition, the stromal environment surrounding the newly formed epithelial cancer also changes to create a permissive and supportive environment *(110)*. One of the key cytokines involved in stromal remodeling is TGF-β (Fig. 5).

Tumor derived TGF-β1 has been implicated as an important molecule involved in directly differentiating stromal fibroblasts into myofibroblasts both in vitro and in vivo *(111)*. Myofibroblasts facilitate tumor progression through increased proliferation, increased extracellular matrix (ECM) remodeling, and acquisition of smooth muscle cell phenotype allowing greater motility *(112,113)*. Frequently, myofibroblasts are located at the invasion front of growing tumors as observed in colon, skin, breast, liver, lung, prostate, pancreas, and squamous carcinomas and contribute toward invasiveness *(114–121)*. Cross-talk between the tumor and stroma has been demonstrated through direct cell–cell contacts and through the release of cytokines and other important factors that constitute the tumor microenvironment. Tumor–stromal communication is critical to the survival of the tumor and its ability to metastasize *(110)*.

An example of tumor-stromal communication has recently been demonstrated in human melanomas that constitutively express TGF-β. Berking et al. *(115)* suggest that melanoma cells can directly modulate their microenvironment through the activation of the cytokine TGF-β to remodel the stromal compartment via changes in MMP and extracellular matrix proteins. Their data show that paracrine effects of TGF-β are associated with increased ECM deposition and decreased tumor necrosis and apoptosis. The TGF-β induced ECM-rich stromal cells are suggested to act as a scaffold for the tumor cells, resulting in increased migration and metastasis. In addition, studies of cervical cancer validate the assumption that tumors cells can modulate their stromal environment through the production of TGF-β. Hazelbag et al. *(122)* demonstrated that tumor-derived TGF-β

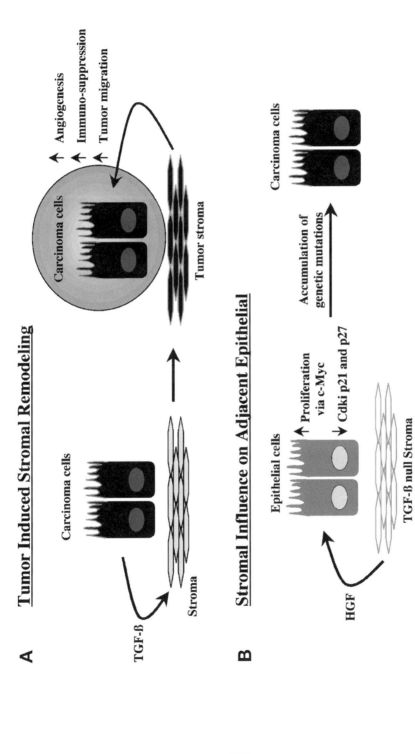

Fig. 5. TGF-β mediated epithelial and stromal interactions. (**A**) Tumor cells modulate their environment by altering the surrounding stromal cells. Altered stromal cells facilitate a more permissive tumor environment by promoting angiogenesis, immune-evasion and scaffolding for tumor invasion. (**B**) In addition, stromal cells lacking TGF-β signaling can influence the carcinogenic potential of adjacent epithelial cells via secretion of HGF, hepatocyte growth factor.

increases the deposition of the ECM proteins collagen IV, fibronectin, and laminin. The increase in ECM proteins was correlated with PAI-1 expression to verify TGF-β signaling and decreased staining for inflammatory cells. These data suggest that TGF-β can enhance immune evasion through increasing the amount of stroma surrounding the tumor.

Recent studies have further elaborated on the tumor–stroma cross-talk paradigm. Bhowmick et al. *(123)* has demonstrated that loss TGF-β signaling in fibroblasts can modulate epithelial cells by increasing their proliferation and carcinogenic potential. Mice were generated that conditionally knocked out the *Tgfbr2* gene in the fibroblasts. Homozygous TβRII null mice developed intraepithelial neoplasia in the prostate and invasive squamous cell carcinoma of the forestomach. Further experiments suggest that fibroblasts, through paracrine activation of the hepatocyte growth factor (HGF), contributed to cancer progression in these mice through an increase in proliferation of the adjacent epithelial cells. These data show that not only can epithelial tumor cells modulate their stromal environment but that the stroma has the potential to induce epithelial tumor potential.

10. THERAPEUTICS FOR TGF-β RESPONSIVE CARCINOMAS

A major goal in treating TGF-β-regulated tumors is to restore the suppressive properties of the TGF-β signaling pathway while blocking the multitude of tumor progressive effects. Given that tumors evade the tumor suppressive mechanisms of TGF-β differently it is essential that cancers be categorized into specific subgroups. For example, studies have shown that increased TGF-β1 in mouse models display varied results depending on the specific oncogene that is co-expressed. Data from MMTV-TGF-α × MMTV-TGF-β1 mice suggests that TGF-β1 is dominant over the oncogene TGF-α as demonstrated by lower tumor incidence than MMTV-TGF-α mice *(14)*. However, other TGF-β1 transgenic mice display different outcomes. MMTV-c-neu × MMTV-TGF-β1 and MMTV-PyVmt × MMTV-TGF-β1 mice develop the same number of tumors as mice expressing the oncogenes *neu* and *PyVmt* alone *(124,125)*. These data suggest that TGF-β1 associates with different factors during carcinogenesis depending of the context of the genetic mutations in the host. Thus, exogenous TGF-β1 as a therapeutic agent would be extremely context dependent. In addition to cooperation with certain oncogenes, TGF-β is tumor promoting during later stages of cancer progression. Therefore, analysis of tumor characteristics before administering exogenous TGF-β would be necessary. In sum, the use of exogenous TGF-β1 as a therapeutic agent for cancer treatment would be circumspect.

Other mechanisms of restoring TGF-β tumor suppression are through augmentation of the TGF-β signaling pathway by chemicals that mimic or cooperate with TGF-β signaling components. Several studies have used small molecule inhibitors that secondarily up-regulate TβRII expression. Given that many tumors decrease TβRII expression during tumor promotion these molecules have potentially interesting therapeutic properties. Some of the most promising molecules are histone deactylase inhibitors (HDACs) and farnesyl transferase inhibitors (FTIs) *(126,127)*. Another potential molecule is rapamycin and its derivatives RAD001 (Norvartis) and CCI-779 (Wyeth-Ayerst). These molecules are associated with restoring TGF-β growth suppression in cancer cell lines that were previously resistant to TGF-β growth arrest. Mechanistically, rapamycin cooperates with Smads and, in concert, inhibit cdk2 activity. Loss of cdk2 activity results in increased p21 and p27 cdk inhibitor proteins that block cell-cycle progression

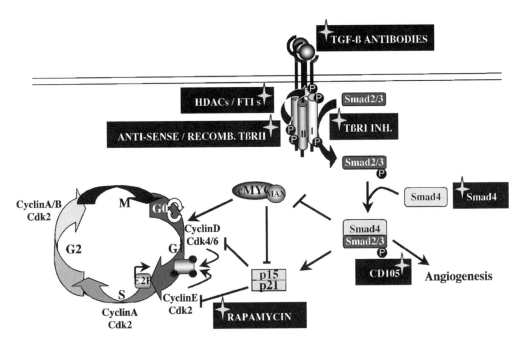

Fig. 6. TGF-β therapeutic targets. A simplified schematic showing where known therapeutics target the TGF-β signaling pathway. Therapeutics are shown in black boxes with a star.

(128). Thus, rapamycin has been shown to block autonomous tumor proliferation and restore TGF-β sensitivity (Fig. 6).

Another approach is to target the tumor promoting effects of TGF-β signaling. A number of antagonists have been identified and are in various stages of study. Several of the antagonists focus on depleting the amount of TGF-β ligand that is able to bind and activate the receptors. Antibodies that have been designed to block the TGF-β ligand include CAT-192 (Genzyme/CAT), CAT-152 (Genzyme/CAT), sTβRII/Fc (Biogen), 1D11(Genzyme/CAT), and 2G7(Genetech). In addition the TGF-β receptors have been targeted. The TβRI antagonists have been developed by various companies focusing on small molecule TβRI kinase inhibitors designated SB-431542 (GlaxoSmithKline), NPC 30345 (Scios, Inc.), and LY364947 (Lily Research). TβRII antagonists include antisense TβRII (Antisense Pharma) and a recombinant soluble TβRII (for review, *see* Reference *125*). Moreover, accessory proteins in the TGF-β receptor complex have become targets for blocking TGF-β induced tumor progression. One is the pleiotropic cytokine endoglin that is critically involved in angiogenesis. Recently it was shown that anti-CD105, an anti-endoglin monoclonal antibody, successfully blocks angiogenesis and tumor growth in vivo *(129)*. In contrast to blocking TGF-β signaling through antagonist, other studies have shown that restoration of TGF-β signaling is beneficial. Duda, et al. *(130)* show that restoration of the TGF-β pathway by restoration of Smad4 expression via gene therapy reverses the invasive phenotype in pancreatic adenocarcinoma cells.

The diversity of biologic responses of cancer cells to the TGF-β signaling pathway dictates that any therapeutic approach is context dependent. As stated earlier, it is extremely important to categorize tumors by their biologic response to TGF-β, as restoring signaling may promote carcinogenesis in some tumor types while inhibiting tumor progression in others. Moreover, the consideration of specificity of the therapeutic is an important issue given that TGF-β normally is required to maintain tissue homeostasis. Overall, the significance of TGF-β signaling in carcinogenesis is unquestionable, however; the best therapeutic approach still requires more study and a deeper understanding of the roles TGF-β plays in cancer progression.

REFERENCES

1. Siegel PM, Massague J. Cytostatic and apoptotic actions of TGF-beta in homeostasis and cancer. Nat Rev Cancer 2003;3(11):807–821.
2. Roberts AB, Wakefield LM. The two faces of transforming growth factor beta in carcinogenesis. Proc Natl Acad Sci U S A 2003;100(15):8621–8623.
3. Shi Y, Massague J. Mechanisms of TGF-beta signaling from cell membrane to the nucleus. Cell 2003;113(6):685–700.
4. Bakin AV, Tomlinson AK, Bhowmick NA, Moses HL, Arteaga CL. Phosphatidylinositol 3-kinase function is required for transforming growth factor beta-mediated epithelial to mesenchymal transition and cell migration. J Biol Chem 2000;275(47):36803–36810.
5. Bhowmick NA, Ghiassi M, Bakin A, et al. Transforming growth factor-beta1 mediates epithelial to mesenchymal transdifferentiation through a RhoA-dependent mechanism. Mol Biol Cell 2001; 12(1):27–36.
6. Bhowmick NA, Zent R, Ghiassi M, McDonnell M, Moses HL. Integrin beta 1 signaling is necessary for transforming growth factor-beta activation of p38MAPK and epithelial plasticity. J Biol Chem 2001;276(50):46707–46713.
7. Bakin AV, Rinehart C, Tomlinson AK, Arteaga CL. p38 mitogen-activated protein kinase is required for TGFbeta-mediated fibroblastic transdifferentiation and cell migration. J Cell Sci 2002;115 (Pt 15): 3193–3206.
8. Larisch-Bloch S, Danielpour D, Roche NS, et al. Selective loss of the transforming growth factor-beta apoptotic signaling pathway in mutant NRP-154 rat prostatic epithelial cells. Cell Growth Differ 2000;11(1):1–10.
9. Gottfried Y, Rotem A, Lotan R, Steller H, Larisch S. The mitochondrial ARTS protein promotes apoptosis through targeting XIAP. EMBO J 2004;23(7):1627–1635.
10. Kim SJ. [Molecular mechanism of inactivation of TGF-beta receptors during carcinogenesis]. Tanpakushitsu Kakusan Koso 2001;46(2):111–116.
11. Kretzschmar M. Transforming growth factor-beta and breast cancer: Transforming growth factor-beta/SMAD signaling defects and cancer. Breast Cancer Res 2000;2(2):107–115.
12. Miyazono K, Suzuki H, Imamura T. Regulation of TGF-beta signaling and its roles in progression of tumors. Cancer Sci 2003;94(3):230–234.
13. Coffey RJ, Jr., Sipes NJ, Bascom CC, et al. Growth modulation of mouse keratinocytes by transforming growth factors. Cancer Res 1988;48(6):1596–1602.
14. Pierce DF, Jr., Gorska AE, Chytil A, et al. Mammary tumor suppression by transforming growth factor beta 1 transgene expression. Proc Natl Acad Sci U S A 1995;92(10):4254–4258.
15. Ziv E, Cauley J, Morin PA, Saiz R, Browner WS. Association between the T29—>C polymorphism in the transforming growth factor beta1 gene and breast cancer among elderly white women: The Study of Osteoporotic Fractures. Jama 2001;285(22):2859–2863.
16. Wu SP, Theodorescu D, Kerbel RS, et al. TGF-beta 1 is an autocrine-negative growth regulator of human colon carcinoma FET cells in vivo as revealed by transfection of an antisense expression vector. J Cell Biol 1992;116(1):187–196.
17. Wu SP, Sun LZ, Willson JK, Humphrey L, Kerbel R, Brattain MG. Repression of autocrine transforming growth factor beta 1 and beta 2 in quiescent CBS colon carcinoma cells leads to progression of tumorigenic properties. Cell Growth Differ 1993;4(2):115–123.
18. Bottinger EP, Jakubczak JL, Haines DC, Bagnall K, Wakefield LM. Transgenic mice overexpressing a dominant-negative mutant type II transforming growth factor beta receptor show enhanced tumorigenesis in the mammary gland and lung in response to the carcinogen 7,12-dimethylbenz-[a]-anthracene. Cancer Res 1997;57(24):5564–5570.
19. Amendt C, Schirmacher P, Weber H, Blessing M. Expression of a dominant negative type II TGF-beta receptor in mouse skin results in an increase in carcinoma incidence and an acceleration of carcinoma development. Oncogene 1998;17(1):25–34.

20. Tu WH, Thomas TZ, Masumori N, et al. The loss of TGF-beta signaling promotes prostate cancer metastasis. Neoplasia 2003;5(3):267–277.
21. Gorska AE, Jensen RA, Shyr Y, Aakre ME, Bhowmick NA, Moses HL. Transgenic mice expressing a dominant-negative mutant type II transforming growth factor-beta receptor exhibit impaired mammary development and enhanced mammary tumor formation. Am J Pathol 2003;163(4):1539–1549.
22. Goumans MJ, Mummery C. Functional analysis of the TGFbeta receptor/Smad pathway through gene ablation in mice. Int J Dev Biol 2000;44(3):253–265.
23. Zhu Y, Richardson JA, Parada LF, Graff JM. Smad3 mutant mice develop metastatic colorectal cancer. Cell 1998;94(6):703–714.
24. Yang X, Letterio JJ, Lechleider RJ, et al. Targeted disruption of SMAD3 results in impaired mucosal immunity and diminished T cell responsiveness to TGF-beta. EMBO J 1999;18(5):1280–1291.
25. Datto MB, Frederick JP, Pan L, Borton AJ, Zhuang Y, Wang XF. Targeted disruption of Smad3 reveals an essential role in transforming growth factor beta-mediated signal transduction. Mol Cell Biol 1999;19(4):2495–2504.
26. Han SU, Kim HT, Seong do H, et al. Loss of the Smad3 expression increases susceptibility to tumorigenicity in human gastric cancer. Oncogene 2004;23(7):1333–1341.
27. Takaku K, Miyoshi H, Matsunaga A, Oshima M, Sasaki N, Taketo MM. Gastric and duodenal polyps in Smad4 (Dpc4) knockout mice. Cancer Res 1999;59(24):6113–6117.
28. Xu X, Brodie SG, Yang X, et al. Haploid loss of the tumor suppressor Smad4/Dpc4 initiates gastric polyposis and cancer in mice. Oncogene 2000;19(15):1868–1874.
29. Takaku K, Oshima M, Miyoshi H, Matsui M, Seldin MF, Taketo MM. Intestinal tumorigenesis in compound mutant mice of both Dpc4 (Smad4) and Apc genes. Cell 1998;92(5):645–656.
30. Oshima M, Oshima H, Kitagawa K, Kobayashi M, Itakura C, Taketo M. Loss of Apc heterozygosity and abnormal tissue building in nascent intestinal polyps in mice carrying a truncated Apc gene. Proc Natl Acad Sci U S A 1995;92(10):4482–4486.
31. Hamamoto T, Beppu H, Okada H, et al. Compound disruption of smad2 accelerates malignant progression of intestinal tumors in apc knockout mice. Cancer Res 2002;62(20):5955–5961.
32. Goggins M, Shekher M, Turnacioglu K, Yeo CJ, Hruban RH, Kern SE. Genetic alterations of the transforming growth factor beta receptor genes in pancreatic and biliary adenocarcinomas. Cancer Res 1998;58(23):5329–5332.
33. Grady WM, Myeroff LL, Swinler SE, et al. Mutational inactivation of transforming growth factor beta receptor type II in microsatellite stable colon cancers. Cancer Res 1999;59(2):320–324.
34. Markowitz S, Wang J, Myeroff L, et al. Inactivation of the type II TGF-beta receptor in colon cancer cells with microsatellite instability. Science 1995;268(5215):1336–1338.
35. Akiyama Y, Iwanaga R, Saitoh K, et al. Transforming growth factor beta type II receptor gene mutations in adenomas from hereditary nonpolyposis colorectal cancer. Gastroenterology 1997;112(1):33–39.
36. Myeroff LL, Parsons R, Kim SJ, et al. A transforming growth factor beta receptor type II gene mutation common in colon and gastric but rare in endometrial cancers with microsatellite instability. Cancer Res 1995;55(23):5545–5547.
37. Chung YJ, Song JM, Lee JY, et al. Microsatellite instability-associated mutations associate preferentially with the intestinal type of primary gastric carcinomas in a high-risk population. Cancer Res 1996;56(20):4662–4665.
38. Izumoto S, Arita N, Ohnishi T, et al. Microsatellite instability and mutated type II transforming growth factor-beta receptor gene in gliomas. Cancer Lett 1997;112(2):251–256.
39. Ohue M, Tomita N, Monden T, et al. Mutations of the transforming growth factor beta type II receptor gene and microsatellite instability in gastric cancer. Int J Cancer 1996;68(2):203–206.
40. Nagai M, Kawarada Y, Watanabe M, et al. Analysis of microsatellite instability, TGF-beta type II receptor gene mutations and hMSH2 and hMLH1 allele losses in pancreaticobiliary maljunction-associated biliary tract tumors. Anticancer Res 1999;19(3A):1765–1768.
41. Garrigue-Antar L, Munoz-Antonia T, Antonia SJ, Gesmonde J, Vellucci VF, Reiss M. Missense mutations of the transforming growth factor beta type II receptor in human head and neck squamous carcinoma cells. Cancer Res 1995;55(18):3982–3987.
42. Yasumi K, Guo RJ, Hanai H, et al. Transforming growth factor beta type II receptor (TGF beta RII) mutation in gastric lymphoma without mutator phenotype. Pathol Int 1998;48(2):134–137.
43. Knaus PI, Lindemann D, DeCoteau JF, et al. A dominant inhibitory mutant of the type II transforming growth factor beta receptor in the malignant progression of a cutaneous T-cell lymphoma. Mol Cell Biol 1996;16(7):3480–3489.

44. Lynch MA, Nakashima R, Song H, et al. Mutational analysis of the transforming growth factor beta receptor type II gene in human ovarian carcinoma. Cancer Res 1998;58(19):4227–4232.
45. Chen T, Carter D, Garrigue-Antar L, Reiss M. Transforming growth factor beta type I receptor kinase mutant associated with metastatic breast cancer. Cancer Res 1998;58(21):4805–4810.
46. Anbazhagan R, Bornman DM, Johnston JC, Westra WH, Gabrielson E. The S387Y mutations of the transforming growth factor-beta receptor type I gene is uncommon in metastases of breast cancer and other common types of adenocarcinoma. Cancer Res 1999;59(14):3363–3364.
47. Zhang HT, Fei QY, Chen F, et al. Mutational analysis of the transforming growth factor beta receptor type I gene in primary non-small cell lung cancer. Lung Cancer 2003;40(3):281–287.
48. Pasche B, Kolachana P, Nafa K, et al. TbetaR-I(6A) is a candidate tumor susceptibility allele. Cancer Res 1999;59(22):5678–5682.
49. Kaklamani VG, Hou N, Bian Y, et al. TGFBR1*6A and cancer risk: a meta-analysis of seven case-control studies. J Clin Oncol 2003;21(17):3236–3243.
50. Hahn SA, Schutte M, Hoque AT, et al. DPC4, a candidate tumor suppressor gene at human chromosome 18q21.1. Science 1996;271(5247):350–353.
51. Miyaki M, Iijima T, Konishi M, et al. Higher frequency of Smad4 gene mutation in human colorectal cancer with distant metastasis. Oncogene 1999;18(20):3098–3103.
52. Howe JR, Mitros FA, Summers RW. The risk of gastrointestinal carcinoma in familial juvenile polyposis. Ann Surg Oncol 1998;5(8):751–756.
53. Hata A, Shi Y, Massague J. TGF-beta signaling and cancer: structural and functional consequences of mutations in Smads. Mol Med Today 1998;4(6):257–262.
54. Eppert K, Scherer SW, Ozcelik H, et al. MADR2 maps to 18q21 and encodes a TGFbeta-regulated MAD-related protein that is functionally mutated in colorectal carcinoma. Cell 1996;86(4):543–552.
55. Riggins GJ, Thiagalingam S, Rozenblum E, et al. Mad-related genes in the human. Nat Genet 1996;13(3):347–349.
56. Arai T, Akiyama Y, Okabe S, Ando M, Endo M, Yuasa Y. Genomic structure of the human Smad3 gene and its infrequent alterations in colorectal cancers. Cancer Lett 1998;122(1-2):157–163.
57. Coqueret O. Linking cyclins to transcriptional control. Gene 2002;299(1-2):35–55.
58. Ortega S, Malumbres M, Barbacid M. Cyclin D-dependent kinases, INK4 inhibitors and cancer. Biochim Biophys Acta 2002;1602(1):73–87.
59. Gutierrez C, Ramirez-Parra E, Castellano MM, del Pozo JC. G(1) to S transition: more than a cell cycle engine switch. Curr Opin Plant Biol 2002;5(6):480–486.
60. Laiho M, DeCaprio JA, Ludlow JW, Livingston DM, Massague J. Growth inhibition by TGF-beta linked to suppression of retinoblastoma protein phosphorylation. Cell 1990;62(1):175–185.
61. Feng XH, Lin X, Derynck R. Smad2, smad3 and smad4 cooperate with Sp1 to induce p15(Ink4B) transcription in response to TGF-beta [In Process Citation]. EMBO J 2000;19(19):5178–5193.
62. Hu PP, Shen X, Huang D, Liu Y, Counter C, Wang XF. The MEK pathway is required for stimulation of p21(WAF1/CIP1) by transforming growth factor-beta. J Biol Chem 1999;274(50):35381–35387.
63. Batova A, Diccianni MB, Yu JC, et al. Frequent and selective methylation of p15 and deletion of both p15 and p16 in T-cell acute lymphoblastic leukemia. Cancer Res 1997;57(5):832–836.
64. Feng XH, Liang YY, Liang M, Zhai W, Lin X. Direct Interaction of c-Myc with Smad2 and Smad3 to Inhibit TGF-beta- Mediated Induction of the CDK Inhibitor p15(Ink4B). Mol Cell 2002;9(1):133–143.
65. Warner BJ, Blain SW, Seoane J, Massague J. Myc downregulation by transforming growth factor beta required for activation of the p15(Ink4b) G(1) arrest pathway. Mol Cell Biol 1999;19(9):5913–5922.
66. Wu S, Cetinkaya C, Munoz-Alonso MJ, et al. Myc represses differentiation-induced p21CIP1 expression via Miz-1-dependent interaction with the p21 core promoter. Oncogene 2003;22(3):351–360.
67. Alexandrow MG, Kawabata M, Aakre M, Moses HL. Overexpression of the c-Myc oncoprotein blocks the growth-inhibitory response but is required for the mitogenic effects of transforming growth factor beta 1. Proc Natl Acad Sci U S A 1995;92(8):3239–3243.
68. Chen CR, Kang Y, Massague J. Defective repression of c-myc in breast cancer cells: A loss at the core of the transforming growth factor beta growth arrest program. Proc Natl Acad Sci U S A 2001;98(3):992–999.
69. Baldwin RL, Tran H, Karlan BY. Loss of c-myc repression coincides with ovarian cancer resistance to transforming growth factor beta growth arrest independent of transforming growth factor beta/Smad signaling. Cancer Res 2003;63(6):1413–1419.

70. Schuster N, Krieglstein K. Mechanisms of TGF-beta-mediated apoptosis. Cell Tissue Res 2002; 307(1):1–14.

71. Joza N, Kroemer G, Penninger JM. Genetic analysis of the mammalian cell death machinery. Trends Genet 2002;18(3):142–149.

72. Kim SG, Jong HS, Kim TY, et al. Transforming growth factor-beta 1 induces apoptosis through Fas ligand-independent activation of the Fas death pathway in human gastric SNU-620 carcinoma cells. Mol Biol Cell 2004;15(2):420–434.

73. Conery AR, Cao Y, Thompson EA, Townsend CM, Jr., Ko TC, Luo K. Akt interacts directly with Smad3 to regulate the sensitivity to TGF-beta induced apoptosis. Nat Cell Biol 2004;6(4):366–372.

74. Tachibana I, Imoto M, Adjei PN, et al. Overexpression of the TGFbeta-regulated zinc finger encoding gene, TIEG, induces apoptosis in pancreatic epithelial cells. J Clin Invest 1997;99(10): 2365–2374.

75. Jang CW, Chen CH, Chen CC, Chen JY, Su YH, Chen RH. TGF-beta induces apoptosis through Smad-mediated expression of DAP-kinase. Nat Cell Biol 2002;4(1):51–58.

76. Bender H, Wang Z, Schuster N, Krieglstein K. TIEG1 facilitates transforming growth factor-beta-mediated apoptosis in the oligodendroglial cell line OLI-neu. J Neurosci Res 2004;75(3):344–352.

77. Toyooka S, Toyooka KO, Miyajima K, et al. Epigenetic down-regulation of death-associated protein kinase in lung cancers. Clin Cancer Res 2003;9(8):3034–3041.

78. Perlman R, Schiemann WP, Brooks MW, Lodish HF, Weinberg RA. TGF-beta-induced apoptosis is mediated by the adapter protein Daxx that facilitates JNK activation. Nat Cell Biol 2001;3(8): 708–714.

79. Zeng L, Rowland RG, Lele SM, Kyprianou N. Apoptosis incidence and protein expression of p53, TGF-beta receptor II, p27Kip1, and Smad4 in benign, premalignant, and malignant human prostate. Hum Pathol 2004;35(3):290–297.

80. Valverius EM, Bates SE, Stampfer MR, et al. Transforming growth factor alpha production and epidermal growth factor receptor expression in normal and oncogene transformed human mammary epithelial cells. Mol Endocrinol 1989;3(1):203–214.

81. Welch DR, Fabra A, Nakajima M. Transforming growth factor beta stimulates mammary adenocarcinoma cell invasion and metastatic potential. Proc Natl Acad Sci U S A 1990;87(19):7678–7682.

82. McCune BK, Mullin BR, Flanders KC, Jaffurs WJ, Mullen LT, Sporn MB. Localization of transforming growth factor-beta isotypes in lesions of the human breast. Hum Pathol 1992;23(1):13–20.

83. MacCallum J, Bartlett JM, Thompson AM, Keen JC, Dixon JM, Miller WR. Expression of transforming growth factor beta mRNA isoforms in human breast cancer. Br J Cancer 1994;69(6):1006–1009.

84. Yin JJ, Selander K, Chirgwin JM, et al. TGF-beta signaling blockade inhibits PTHrP secretion by breast cancer cells and bone metastases development. J Clin Invest 1999;103(2):197–206.

85. Thiery JP, Chopin D. Epithelial cell plasticity in development and tumor progression. Cancer Metastasis Rev 1999;18(1):31–42.

86. Miettinen PJ, Ebner R, Lopez AR, Derynck R. TGF-beta induced transdifferentiation of mammary epithelial cells to mesenchymal cells: involvement of type I receptors. J Cell Biol 1994;127(6 Pt 2): 2021–2036.

87. Folkman J. Angiogenesis in cancer, vascular, rheumatoid and other disease. Nat Med 1995;1(1):27–31.

88. O'Reilly MS, Holmgren L, Shing Y, et al. Angiostatin: a novel angiogenesis inhibitor that mediates the suppression of metastases by a Lewis lung carcinoma. Cell 1994;79(2):315–328.

89. Carmeliet P. Mechanisms of angiogenesis and arteriogenesis. Nat Med 2000;6(4):389–395.

90. Goumans MJ, Lebrin F, Valdimarsdottir G. Controlling the angiogenic switch: a balance between two distinct TGF-b receptor signaling pathways. Trends Cardiovasc Med 2003;13(7):301–307.

91. Pepper MS. Transforming growth factor-beta: vasculogenesis, angiogenesis, and vessel wall integrity. Cytokine Growth Factor Rev 1997;8(1):21–43.

92. Dentelli P, Rosso A, Calvi C, et al. IL-3 affects endothelial cell-mediated smooth muscle cell recruitment by increasing TGF beta activity: potential role in tumor vessel stabilization. Oncogene 2004;23(9):1681–1692.

93. Kulkarni AB, Huh CG, Becker D, et al. Transforming growth factor beta 1 null mutation in mice causes excessive inflammatory response and early death. Proc Natl Acad Sci U S A 1993;90(2): 770–774.

94. Larsson J, Goumans MJ, Sjostrand LJ, et al. Abnormal angiogenesis but intact hematopoietic potential in TGF-beta type I receptor-deficient mice. EMBO J 2001;20(7):1663–1673.

95. Oshima M, Oshima H, Taketo MM. TGF-beta receptor type II deficiency results in defects of yolk sac hematopoeisis and vasculogenesis. Dev Biol 1996;179(1):297–302.

96. Pertovaara L, Kaipainen A, Mustonen T, et al. Vascular endothelial growth factor is induced in response to transforming growth factor-beta in fibroblastic and epithelial cells. J Biol Chem 1994; 269(9):6271–6274.

97. Benjamin LE, Golijanin D, Itin A, Pode D, Keshet E. Selective ablation of immature blood vessels in established human tumors follows vascular endothelial growth factor withdrawal. J Clin Invest 1999; 103(2):159–165.

98. Damert A, Machein M, Breier G, et al. Up-regulation of vascular endothelial growth factor expression in a rat glioma is conferred by two distinct hypoxia-driven mechanisms. Cancer Res 1997; 57(17):3860–3864.

99. Sunderkotter C, Goebeler M, Schulze-Osthoff K, Bhardwaj R, Sorg C. Macrophage-derived angiogenesis factors. Pharmacol Ther 1991;51(2):195–216.

100. Hasegawa Y, Takanashi S, Kanehira Y, Tsushima T, Imai T, Okumura K. Transforming growth factor-beta1 level correlates with angiogenesis, tumor progression, and prognosis in patients with nonsmall cell lung carcinoma. Cancer 2001;91(5):964–971.

101. Tada T, Ohzeki S, Utsumi K, et al. Transforming growth factor-beta-induced inhibition of T cell function. Susceptibility difference in T cells of various phenotypes and functions and its relevance to immunosuppression in the tumor-bearing state. J Immunol 1991;146(3):1077–1082.

102. Torre-Amione G, Beauchamp RD, Koeppen H, et al. A highly immunogenic tumor transfected with a murine transforming growth factor type beta 1 cDNA escapes immune surveillance. Proc Natl Acad Sci U S A 1990;87(4):1486–1490.

103. Chen Y, Lebrun JJ, Vale W. Regulation of transforming growth factor beta- and activin-induced transcription by mammalian Mad proteins. Proc Natl Acad Sci U S A 1996;93(23):12992–12997.

104. Sakaguchi S, Sakaguchi N, Asano M, Itoh M, Toda M. Immunologic self-tolerance maintained by activated T cells expressing IL-2 receptor alpha-chains (CD25). Breakdown of a single mechanism of self-tolerance causes various autoimmune diseases. J Immunol 1995;155(3):1151–1164.

105. Chen W, Wahl SM. TGF-beta: the missing link in CD4+CD25+ regulatory T cell-mediated immunosuppression. Cytokine Growth Factor Rev 2003;14(2):85–89.

106. Misra N, Bayry J, Lacroix-Desmazes S, Kazatchkine MD, Kaveri SV. Cutting Edge: Human CD4+CD25+ T cells restrain the maturation and antigen-presenting function of dendritic cells. J Immunol 2004;172(8):4676–4680.

107. Somasundaram R, Jacob L, Swoboda R, et al. Inhibition of cytolytic T lymphocyte proliferation by autologous CD4+/CD25+ regulatory T cells in a colorectal carcinoma patient is mediated by transforming growth factor-beta. Cancer Res 2002;62(18):5267–5272.

108. Liyanage UK, Moore TT, Joo HG, et al. Prevalence of regulatory T cells is increased in peripheral blood and tumor microenvironment of patients with pancreas or breast adenocarcinoma. J Immunol 2002;169(5):2756–2761.

109. Woo EY, Yeh H, Chu CS, et al. Cutting edge: Regulatory T cells from lung cancer patients directly inhibit autologous T cell proliferation. J Immunol 2002;168(9):4272–4276.

110. De Wever O, Mareel M. Role of tissue stroma in cancer cell invasion. J Pathol 2003;200(4):429–447.

111. Tuxhorn JA, Ayala GE, Rowley DR. Reactive stroma in prostate cancer progression. J Urol 2001;166(6):2472–2483.

112. Sieuwerts AM, Klijn JG, Henzen-Logmand SC, et al. Urokinase-type-plasminogen-activator (uPA) production by human breast (myo) fibroblasts in vitro: influence of transforming growth factor-beta(1) (TGF beta(1)) compared with factor(s) released by human epithelial-carcinoma cells. Int J Cancer 1998;76(6):829–835.

113. Serini G, Gabbiani G. Mechanisms of myofibroblast activity and phenotypic modulation. Exp Cell Res 1999;250(2):273–283.

114. Dimanche-Boitrel MT, Vakaet L, Jr., Pujuguet P, et al. In vivo and in vitro invasiveness of a rat colon-cancer cell line maintaining E-cadherin expression: an enhancing role of tumor-associated myofibroblasts. Int J Cancer 1994;56(4):512–521.

115. Berking C, Takemoto R, Schaider H, et al. Transforming growth factor-beta1 increases survival of human melanoma through stroma remodeling. Cancer Res 2001;61(22):8306–8316.

116. Ronnov-Jessen L, Petersen OW, Koteliansky VE, Bissell MJ. The origin of the myofibroblasts in breast cancer. Recapitulation of tumor environment in culture unravels diversity and implicates converted fibroblasts and recruited smooth muscle cells. J Clin Invest 1995;95(2):859–873.

117. Neaud V, Faouzi S, Guirouilh J, et al. Human hepatic myofibroblasts increase invasiveness of hepa-tocellular carcinoma cells: evidence for a role of hepatocyte growth factor. Hepatology 1997;26(6): 1458–1466.
118. Doucet C, Jasmin C, Azzarone B. Unusual interleukin-4 and -13 signaling in human normal and tumor lung fibroblasts. Oncogene 2000;19(51):5898–5905.
119. Lewis MP, Lygoe KA, Nystrom ML, et al. Tumour-derived TGF-beta1 modulates myofibroblast dif-ferentiation and promotes HGF/SF-dependent invasion of squamous carcinoma cells. Br J Cancer 2004;90(4):822–832.
120. Gerdes MJ, Larsen M, Dang TD, Ressler SJ, Tuxhorn JA, Rowley DR. Regulation of rat prostate stro-mal cell myodifferentiation by androgen and TGF-beta1. Prostate 2004;58(3):299–307.
121. Lohr M, Schmidt C, Ringel J, et al. Transforming growth factor-beta1 induces desmoplasia in an experimental model of human pancreatic carcinoma. Cancer Res 2001;61(2):550–555.
122. Hazelbag S, Gorter A, Kenter GG, van den Broek L, Fleuren G. Transforming growth factor-beta1 induces tumor stroma and reduces tumor infiltrate in cervical cancer. Hum Pathol 2002;33(12): 1193–1199.
123. Bhowmick NA, Chytil A, Plieth D, et al. TGF-beta signaling in fibroblasts modulates the oncogenic potential of adjacent epithelia. Science 2004;303(5659):848–851.
124. Muraoka RS, Koh Y, Roebuck LR, et al. Increased malignancy of Neu-induced mammary tumors overexpressing active transforming growth factor beta1. Mol Cell Biol 2003;23(23):8691–8703.
125. Dumont N, Arteaga CL. Targeting the TGF beta signaling network in human neoplasia. Cancer Cell 2003;3(6):531–536.
126. Lee BI, Park SH, Kim JW, et al. MS-275, a histone deacetylase inhibitor, selectively induces trans-forming growth factor beta type II receptor expression in human breast cancer cells. Cancer Res 2001;61(3):931–934.
127. Adnane J, Bizouarn FA, Chen Z, et al. Inhibition of farnesyltransferase increases TGFbeta type II receptor expression and enhances the responsiveness of human cancer cells to TGFbeta. Oncogene 2000;19(48):5525–5533.
128. Law BK, Chytil A, Dumont N, et al. Rapamycin potentiates transforming growth factor beta-induced growth arrest in nontransformed, oncogene-transformed, and human cancer cells. Mol Cell Biol 2002;22(23):8184–8198.
129. Fonsatti E, Altomonte M, Arslan P, Maio M. Endoglin (CD105): a target for anti-angiogenetic cancer therapy. Curr Drug Targets 2003;4(4):291–296.
130. Duda DG, Sunamura M, Lefter LP, et al. Restoration of SMAD4 by gene therapy reverses the inva-sive phenotype in pancreatic adenocarcinoma cells. Oncogene 2003;22(44):6857–6864.

6 Interleukin-1 Family of Cytokines and Cancer

Michael T. Lotze

CONTENTS

1. INTRODUCTION

The interleukin (IL)-1 extended family (IL-1Fx) of beta trefoil cytokines now includes a total of 11 members, many of which have been identified as being produced by dendritic cells (DC)s and acting on natural killer (NK) and T-cells. Their major role in immunity remains not fully explored but based on expression data and studies done over the last two decades it is expected that they are important for the initial critical events in NK cell/DC and T-cell/DC interactions, serving as cytokine danger signals or Signal 0s alerting the host to damage or injury. They are likely important, following the delivery of antigen/MHC Signal 1 and B7/CD28 Signal 2s during polarization (Signal 3) of the immune response and during the effector phase, as potential Signal 4s associated with tissue specific signaling and homing, driving either inflammation or healing and

From: *Cancer Drug Discovery and Development,*
Cytokines in the Genesis and Treatment of Cancer
Edited by: M. A. Caligiuri and M. T. Lotze © Humana Press Inc., Totowa, NJ

the fibroblastic response, mediated by IL-1β during the effector phase of the immune response as Signal 5s *(1,2)*. Alternatively they deliver activation signals across the immunologic synapse to T-cells and NK cells *(3–9)*. A careful analysis of these factors and their role in NK cell/DC cross talk has not been performed, although analysis of these individual dendrikines in murine models and in vitro human studies suggest that at least IL-18 and a novel factor, IL-1F7b may play important antitumor roles. We will carefully extend observations with these IL-1s to other family members (IL-1Fx), determine how they and their inhibitors regulate NK/DC interactions, and promote the adaptive immune response to tumor.

2. IL-1 FAMILY MEMBERS

The role of the IL-1 family members in the initiation of immunity has been recognized for quite some time *(10–13)*. Recently, several new members have been added to the β trefoil IL-1 family, many of them identified as products of activated DCs. Four new IL-1 homologues termed IL-1H1(IL-1F9), IL-1H2 (IL-1F8), IL-1H3(IL-1F5), and IL-1H4 (IL-1F7) were identified at SmithKline Beecham *(14,15)* as well as at Immunex *(16)*. Three more recent additional factors *(17)*, brings the total number to eleven (with the addition of IL-33, *see* the following). The exon/intron structure and exon splicing of these novel members is shown in Fig. 1 as well as their accession numbers. The precise function of these and other new members and what their role might be in the initiation or maintenance of the immune response remains unclear. The IL-1 family members are proinflammatory cytokines that initiate the innate immune response by activating a set of transcription factors including NF-κB and AP-1 *(18)*. The better-studied members of the IL-1 family IL-1F1(IL-1α), IL-1F2 (IL-1β), IL-1F3 (IL-1RA), and IL-1F4 (IL-18), as well as the fibroblast growth factors are structurally related as β trefoil cytokines *(19–21)* that are secreted without signal peptides and do not follow the typical secretion pathways. It has been hypothesized that only apoptotic cells producing IL-1 and IL-18 can release these cytokines into the local milieu *(21)* but this appears only to be associated with caspase-1 activation. Recently, secretion of IL-1β, IL-18, and likely other family members in the form of rapidly shed microvesicles budding off of the plasma membrane has been identified as a method for secretion and this appears to be true for other members of the IL-1 family including IL-18, as well as the novel factor high mobility group 1 (HMGB1) released during necrotic cell death and secreted by activated monocytes *(3–6,9)*. Interestingly, IL-1β and IL-18 secretion by DCs occurs via exocytosis of pro-IL-1s containing secretory lysomes which are calcium dependent and induced by antigen specific interactions with T-cells. This group also demonstrated that CD40 ligation by CD4+ cells will induce secretion but not the reduction in intracellular IL-1/IL-18 which requires another, presumably antigen specific signal delivered by CD8+ cells. Release of IL-1 is mediated by signals other than activation of caspase 1 *(4)*. IL-18 is constitutively produced by DCs but its synthesis and secretion are not affected by stimuli inducing maturation *(8)*.

2.1. IL-1F1 and IL-1F2

IL-1α and IL-1β bind the type I IL-1 receptor (IL-1R) with subsequent recruitment of a signaling component, the IL-1R accessory protein (IL-1Racp *[22,23]*); both are potently secreted by DCs *(23)*. IL-1β can increase CD40L-induced cytokine secretion by monocyte-derived DC, CD34+-derived DC, and peripheral blood DC and secretion

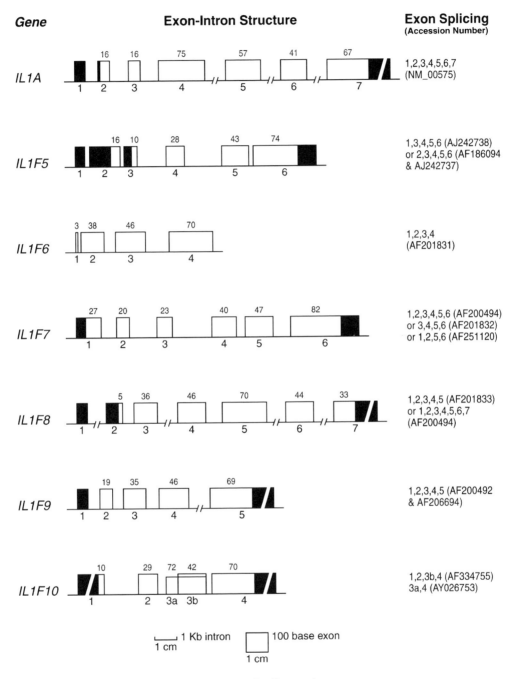

Fig. 1. IL-1 family members.

is increased in response to bacteria, CD40L, and IFN-γ *(24–26)*. Interestingly neither CD34+-derived DC nor peripheral blood DC produce IL-1β, distinguishing these DCs in an important way. Similar signaling through a unique pair of cellular receptors but apparently common intracellular events is found in IL-18 *(27)*. After the complex forms, a common adapter molecule My88 binds to the cytosolic portion of the IL-1R, which in turn activates IRAK to phosphorylate TRAF-6 and distally IκB kinase (IKK). IKK phosphorylation of IκB, results in release of NF-κB and transport to the nucleus. Downstream NF-κB then promotes cell survival and effector functions including secreting several other proinflammatory cytokines.

2.2. IL-1F3 and IL-1F4-F10

IL-1F3 (IL-1RA) also binds the type I receptor but does not recruit IL-1Racp, thereby preventing signaling by IL-1F1 (IL-1α) or IL-1F2 (IL-1β) (28,29). The type II IL-1R is a molecular decoy of IL-1 activity, binding IL-1 without signaling (30–32). IL-1F4 (IL-18) is a T helper type 1 (Th1) inducing dendrikine promoting IFN-γ production from T-cells, B-cells, and NK cells, especially in synergy with IL-12 (33–35). IL-1F4 (IL-18) has a similar signaling pathway to IL-1α and IL-1β but uses its own unique receptor, IL-1R related protein (IL-1Rrp) and a nonbinding chain, IL-1R accessory protein-like (IL-1RAcPL) cell surface molecule, both members of the IL-1R family (27,36). Anti-IL-1RAcPL mAb inhibited the IL-18-induced activation of NF-κB and the subsequent production of IFN-γ by Th1 cells (37). Quantitative PCR revealed that Th1 but not Th2 cells co-express IL-1Rrp1 and IL-1RAcPL. The six additional novel IL-1 family members identified expand the IL-1 family to 10 members (IL-1α, IL-1β, IL-1ra, IL-18, IL-1H1, IL-1H2, IL-1H3, IL-1H4, FIL1ε, and IL-1HY2) (15,38–43). Interestingly, the novel genes form a cluster with the other IL-1 family members on the long arm of human chromosome 2. The most distantly related members of the family, both IL-18 and its binding protein, are located on the long arm of human chromosome 11 (43). Very limited information exists about the other novel IL-1Fxs. IL-1F5 does not bind IL-1R but rather antagonizes the NF-κB inducing activity of IL-1F9 ligand signaling through the IL-1R6 (37,44). IL-1F9 is constitutively expressed in the placenta, skin and the squamous epithelium of esophagus. It is induced in vitro in keratinocytes following IFN-γ and TNF-α treatment. IL-1F8 has been detected in human bone marrow, tonsil, heart, placenta, lung, testis, and colon. As would be expected with a proinflammatory cytokine, IL-1F7 expression is upregulated by PMA treatment of PBMC. IL-1F7 specifically binds the IL-18 receptor with low affinity, but does not bind the putative IL-18 receptor accessory protein IL-1RacpL, suggesting the possibility of yet another co-receptor waiting to be identified. We have tested the IL-1F7 by creating adenoviral vectors expressing the mature cleaved form (45). The cytokine's activity is diminished only in IL-12 deficient mice but not in nude mice, SCID mice, NKT cell-deficient, IFN-γ, or Fas ligand deficient mice. Thus IL-1F7 mediates a mix of IL-12 and IL-18-like effects, placing it potentially more proximal in the inflammatory cascade. IL-1HY2 (IL-1F10) is expressed in skin and activated B-cells of human tonsil. IL-1HY2 binds to the sIL-1RI demonstrating the profound interaction of these closely related members of the IL-1 family.

2.3. IL-1F4 (IL-18)

IL-18 is a distantly related member of the IL-1 family, first identified as an IFN-γ inducing factor (46–50). It is upregulated in mature DCs (51) and present as proIL-18 in monocytes and immature DCs (iDCs). Mature DCs restimulated by soluble CD154 and IFN-γ, as would occur during interaction with T-cells, produce less IL-12 and more IL-18 than iDCs. Increased expression of IL-18 has been observed in several autoimmune diseases including rheumatoid arthritis (52) synovium (where it may induce fibroblast chemokine production), hemophagocytic lymphohistiocytosis (53), herpes hominis virus six (HHV6) infection *(54)*, sarcoidosis *(55)*, experimental myasthenia gravis *(56)*, tumors including squamous cell cancers and melanomas of the skin *(57)*, gastric cancers *(58)*, cutaneous T-cell lymphoma and NK cell lymphoma *(59)*, and in the unstable plaques of patients with atheromatous lesions *(60–62)*. In experimental models of atheroma, expression of the IL-18BP prevents plaque progression and rupture. IL-18 has modest effects by itself but in concert with individual cytokines present during an immune response modulates both Th1 and Th2 responses. IL-18 is elevated in the serum during bacterial infections, particularly those affecting the liver *(63)* and during acute graft-vs-host disease (GVHD) *(64)*. In the setting of a murine bone marrow transplantation model, blockade of IL-18 accelerates mortality whereas administration of IL-18 reduced serum TNF-α and LPS levels and resulted in improved survival only in animals with normal FasL suggesting that IL-18 modified the survival of self-reactive donor T-cells. Whether DCs use IL-18 to promote their own survival during the initiation of an immune response is conjectural. IL-18 appears to be even more potent than either IL-12 or IFN-γ for protection against *Listeria*, enhancing bacterial clearance in the complete absence of IFN-γ but in its presence promoting the optimal Th1 response *(65)*. An IL-18 binding protein located on the same chromosome and produced largely by the same cells with several pox virus homologues has also been identified *(66–69)*. Our studies suggested that the antitumor effects of IL-18 were mediated by critical interactions of T-cells, NK cells, and DCs *(70)*.

2.4. IL-1F5 (IL-1H3/FIL1δ/IL-1H3/IL-1RP3/IL-1L1/IL-1δ)

Concurrently identified by multiple groups *(16,38,39,44,71–76)*, it was suggested that IL-1F5 like IL-1Ra, is an antagonist but recent crystallization studies and evaluation of critical loop structures compared with IL-1β and IL-1Ra, suggest that it is an agonist *(77)*. IL-1F5 message is highly abundant in embryonic tissue and epithelial tissues (i.e., skin, lung, and stomach) as well as spleen, lymph node, tonsil, bone marrow, fetal brain, leukocytes, and various human cell lines *(77)*. RT-PCR from isolated skin cells revealed that only keratinocytes but not fibroblasts, endothelial cells, or melanocytes expressed IL-1F5 and IL-1F9, with IL-1F5 10 times greater than IL-1F9 *(44)*. Keratinocyte stimulation with IL-1β/TNF-α significantly up-regulated both IL-1F5 and IL-1F9 mRNA. Although NF-κB activation through IL-1Rrp2 was claimed for IL-F9, this was antagonized by IL-F5. In psoriatic skin increased mRNA expression of both IL-1F5 and IL-F9 as well as IL-1Rrp2 are increased when compared with healthy skin. Thus IL-1F5 and IL-1F9 may be important in the skin suggesting a potential unique role for the other IL-1 homologues within other epithelia.

3. DEMONSTRATION OF THE ROLE OF HMGB1/RAGE INTERACTIONS

HMGB1 protein is a critical nuclear protein, loosely associated with chromatin serving to cause DNA binding and bending, enhancing access to a variety of transcriptional factor complexes. Following acetylation on abundant lysine residues within the nuclear localization signals, HMGB1 can be translocated to the cytosol and be actively secreted by activated monocytes. Within the cell nucleus it promotes protein assembly, for example with the steroid/steroid receptor complex. Outside the cell, it binds with high affinity to RAGE (the receptor for advanced glycation end products), as well as TLR2 and

TLR4, potently enhancing inflammation *(78–81)*. HMGB1 is secreted by activated macrophages, and is released passively by necrotic cells. HMGB1$^{-/-}$ necrotic cells have a greatly reduced ability to promote inflammation *(9)*. Apoptotic cells do not release HMGB1 and bind it firmly to chromatin. Interestingly, cells undergoing apoptosis are limited in their ability to release this molecule. Activation of myeloid cells results in the redistribution of HMGB1 from the nucleus to the cytoplasm within organelles, presumably endolysosomes. Interestingly this is characteristic of both IL-1 and IL-18 as well although their secretion is induced earlier by ATP. Human DCs release IL-1β following specific interaction with alloreactive T-lymphocytes following induction of intracellular calcium increases *(3–9)*. Specific CD8$^+$ T-cells generate a Ca^{++} influx in DCs with enrichment in endolysosomes containing IL-1β and cathepsin D at the immunologic synapse with T-cells, allowing polarized delivery to the T-cell. Interestingly, HMGB1 secretion is generated later in the inflammatory setting *(9)*. Many studies have evaluated biochemical, immunologic, or other quantitative blood assays that might reflect the prognosis of patients with cancer *(82–100)*. We have recently demonstrated that HMGB1 can be detected in the serum of advanced cancer (melanoma, colorectal, and pancreatic cancer) patients to levels far exceeding that observed in normal patients with sepsis where such elevations have previously been identified. HMGB1 has recently been reported by Anna Rubartelli's group to be released into the immunologic synapse (personal communication, submitted) with DCs and our group and that of Bianchi and Tracey have reported that HMGB1 directly matures myeloid DCs *(101–102)*.

4. SIGNAL TRANSDUCTION IN DCs FOLLOWING INTERACTION WITH IL-1FX

DCs react to changes in their environment in various ways. Depending on the stimulus and developmental stage, DCs may proliferate, differentiate, mature, perform various effector functions including the release of dendrikines or mediate cytolytic activity, or ultimately, die an apoptotic death. The information from the environment is received via various receptors expressed on the cell surface. Binding of a ligand to its cell surface receptor creates a signal that is in turn transmitted to the cell nucleus by specific intracellular agents. The signal transduction pathways usually include various protein kinases and transcription factors, which regulate the gene expression in the cell. Signals can be mediated by soluble ligands or counter-receptors expressed on cells including NK cells, and many of these drive NFκB signaling pathways, promoting cell activation and survival.

NF-κB represents a group of five structurally related proteins (c-Rel, RelA, RelB, NF-κB 1, and NF-κB 2) which play a critical and evolutionary conserved role in the triggering of both innate and adaptive immune responses in a variety of different cells. The genes regulated by NFκB include cytokines (IL-1β, IL-2, IL-6, IL-12, TNF-α), molecules important for adaptive immune responses (MHC-antigens, T-cell costimulatory molecules), chemokines (IL-8, MIP-1α, RANTES), adhesion molecules (ICAM, VCAM and E-selectin), and several acute phase proteins *(103,104)*. Although recent evidence suggests that there is a continuous transit between cytoplasmic and nuclear NF-κB, a classic paradigm is that in resting cells NF-kB is bound to IκB and retained in the cytoplasm *(105)*. NF-κB activating signals result in activation of a specific IKK. Phosphorylated IκB is rapidly degraded by the proteasome, thereby freeing NF-κB, which in turn enters the nucleus, binds to DNA and activates transcription.

The NF-κB family of transcription factors has turned out to be very important, particularly for DC development and function. Of these RelB is crucial for the development of myeloid DCs. RelB-deficient mice lack thymic DCs, have greatly reduced number of myeloid splenic DCs and impaired antigen presenting function *(106,107)*. Increase in expression and nuclear translocation of RelB is correlated with DCs activation, maturation and function *(108–110)*. Activation of the NF-κB pathway in DC can be T-cell dependent (CD40-CD40L, RANK-RANKL) or independent, in which case signals are transmitted to DCs via "danger" mimics including LPS (binds toll-like receptors in DCs), proinflammatory cytokines (IL-1/TNF-α), and necrotic cells. Specific inhibition of NF-κB translocation to nucleus in GM-CSF/IL-4 cultured immature DCs significantly reduced the LPS or TNF-α induced upregulation of CD80, CD83, CD86 and DR, and production of IL-12p70, demonstrating the importance of NF-κB pathway also in DC-function and maturation *(109)*.

Mitogen activated protein kinases (MAPKs) play important roles in cellular responses including growth factor-induced cell proliferation, differentiation and survival. Three groups of MAPKs have been identified in mammals: the extracellular signal-regulated protein kinases (ERKs), the c-Jun terminal kinases, and the p38MAPKs. These kinases are activated by upstream MAPKs *(111)*. The ERK pathway appears mainly to respond to mitogens and growth factors that regulate cell proliferation and differentiation, including the IL-1 family members. Transient low-magnitude activation of ERK favors proliferation and sustained high magnitude stimulation inhibits growth, perhaps through RhoA *(112)*. Despite the presence of multiple mitogen-activated pathways, the temporally coordinated combination of just three is sufficient to drive cells through G1 and into S-phase *(113–115)*. ERKs (and c-Myc) are critically required near the onset of G1 but are dispensable later on during the G1 phase, when the PI3K (phosphoinositide-3 kinase) pathway is required. The other MAPKs are predominantly activated by stress, such as osmotic changes and heat shock, but also by proinflammatory cytokines such as IL-1β and TNF-α. The p38 MAPK pathway is involved in regulation of innate and adaptive immune responses, and promotes production of IL-12p70 in macrophages and DCs *(116)*. p38 MAPK phosphorylates several downstream targets, but it may also interfere with the NF-κB signaling pathway. A subset of cytokine and chemokine genes responding to NF-κB are dependent on p38MAPK-mediated histone-H3 phosphorylation, which enhanced the accessibility of NF-κB binding sites located within their promoter region *(117)*. Proinflammatory cytokines and agents (LPS, CpG-DNA) often activate p38MAPK in DCs and macrophages, to regulate IL-12 production and expression of several important T-cell costimulatory signals. Presence of p38MAPK inhibitors in DCs block the upregulation of CD80, CD83 and CD86 in response to LPS, but not that of CD40 and HLA-DR *(109)*.

PI3K is a key mediator of many cellular responses, including the movement of organelle membranes, alteration of cellular morphology through rearrangement of cytoskeletal structures, cell growth and proliferation, survival, and chemotaxis *(118)*. Similarly to NF-kB and p38MAPK, the PI3K-pathway is activated by IL-1Fx, mitogens, LPS and apoptotic cells *(119)*. PI3K phosphorylates Akt, which in turn promotes survival of DCs, but it also interferes with p38MAPK pathway in a negative fashion. In the presence of PI3K inhibitors or in PI3K knock-out mice, p38MAPK activity was upregulated and IL-12 production enhanced *(116)*. Together with p38MAPK, PI3K and NF-κB, ERK activity is usually upregulated in response to DC-activating/maturing factors. If DCs are activated either with TNF-α or LPS, ERK is upregulated, and cells undergo maturation.

However, if ERK specific inhibitors are present, DCs show increased expression of MHC-molecules, and costimulatory molecules, loss of mannose-receptor-mediated endocytic activity, NF-kB DNA binding activity, release of IL-12p40, and IL-12p70 *(120)*.

5. INTEGRATED BIOLOGY OF IL-1FX IN CANCER

We have been working quite diligently to study the immunobiology of cancer, DCs and NK cells as well as the critical role of IL-1 family members for more than 20 years. We have been defining the penultimate step *of the initiation of* adaptive immunity, the critical interactions between NK cells and DCs. This was in large part prompted by murine studies done here showing that IL-18 antitumor effects were NK cell dependent and, based on in vitro studies, dependent on DCs promoting a specific T-cell response *(70)*. Most recently we have studied the IL-1F7 homologue *(45)*, using what is for us conventional murine tumor models and demonstrated that it had, like IL-18, rather interesting antitumor activity when administered with an adenoviral vector, prompting us to consider a more detailed analysis of this cytokine in man. Delivery of IL-18 as a recombinant protein or with adenoviral vectors is associated with antitumor effects in several advanced tumor models including MOPC315 plasmacytoma, the MC38 colorectal adenocarcinoma and the methylcholanthrene induced sarcoma and can be abrogated by depleting NK cells with anti-asialoGM1 (Fig. 2). The immunity is long-lived and animals reject a subsequent challenge with tumor. Rejection of tumor is NK cell dependent but NKT cell independent; FasL dependent but perforin independent; and both IL-12 and IFN-γ only partially/minimally dependent. We have evaluated IL-18 initially at the University of Pittsburgh at comparable doses to what we had used with IL-12, i.e. up to 1μg/d for up to 7 d. Above, only when coupled with direct injection of DCs, was IL-18 as a gene therapy using adenovirus successful in eliminating the local and uninjected tumor. These too showed marginal efficacy and we then evaluated high dose IL-18 (Fig. 3) in a variety of tumor models including the MOPC-315 plasmacytoma *(121)*. This revealed profound antitumor effects at doses of 10 μg/d or greater and surprisingly, when treatment of this highly aggressive tumor was stopped, tumor recurrence and then spontaneous regression occurred without additional therapy. Based on these and other studies, dose escalating trials of rIL-18 to man have recently been completed and phase II studies begun. Interestingly Taqman analysis revealed a number of different cytokines induced in vitro that included not just IFN-γ but also a 20-fold increase in IL-1α, IL-1β, GM-CSF, IL-13, and IFN-γ after treatment of murine splenocytes or human PBMC for 24 h. Based on a series of knockout animals, we have established *(63,122,123)* that there is differential biology of IL-12 and IL-18 with IL-12 effects clearly more IFN-γ dependent than those of IL-18. It also suggests that DC provision of IL-12 and presumably, later IL-18, could mediate substantial synergy in enhancing a Th1 response with fundamentally different effector mechanisms. Surrogate markers of response were limited but included increased NK cell cytolytic activity from murine splenocytes and increased neopterin concentrations consistent with the evoked IFN-γ. When IL-18 is delivered by adenoviral vectors in conjunction with direct delivery of DCs into subcutaneous tumors of mice, both the injected and the uninjected lesions regress, suggesting that IL-18 and DCs, possibly through enhanced IL-12 production, synergize in mediating antitumor effects. This is one of now several demonstrations from our group and others showing that intratumoral injection of DCs *(124)*, when

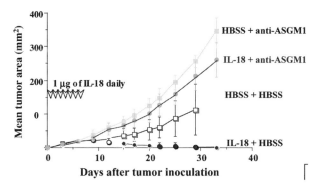

Fig. 2. Abrogation of antitumor effects of rIL-18 by anti-ASGM-1 administration, which eliminates NK cells.

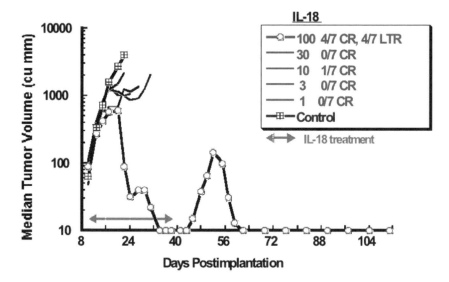

Fig. 3. High-dose IL-18 induces regression of advanced MOPC-315 plasmacytoma.

transfected with Th1 promoting cytokines such as IL-12, IL-18 or expression of chemokines such as CCL19 or CCL20 *(125)* provides profound antitumor immunity.

Delivery of the novel IL-1H4/IL-1F7b family member by multiple injections of adenoviral vectors encoding it is associated with tumor rejection. The biology of IL-1H4 was poorly defined although it had initially been thought to regulate the Th1/Th1 switch. Expression was limited to the spleen and tonsil and what appeared to be DC like cells at those sites. It is cleaved from a pro-peptide requiring cleavage by caspase 1 or 4 *(45)*. We created adenoviral vectors to express human IL-1H4/IL-1F7 and were able to demonstrate an appropriate broad band of the mature form by Western blotting (Fig. 4). In murine tumor models, we were able to demonstrate that a single injection of adenovirus expressing this cytokine was capable of mediating significant suppression when compared with the control Ad-Ψ5 vector. When multiple injections were carried out, complete suppression of tumor growth was noted in two of five animals with rejection in these animals of a subsequent challenge with tumor. Immunity is long-lived and animals reject a subsequent challenge with tumor. Rejection of the tumor is IL-12, FasL,

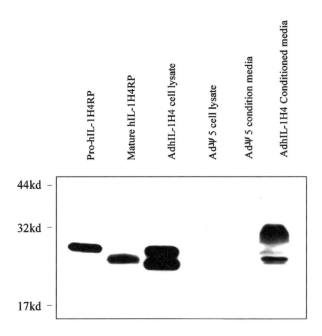

Fig. 4. Western blot for IL-1H4.

and IFN-γ dependent but NKT cell independent based on knockout experiments. This suggests that this cytokine has unusual biologic effects and warrants additional investigation. Like many of the other novel IL-1Fx members, this one has greatest homology with IL-1RA and preliminary data from another laboratory suggests that IL-1H4/IL-1F7 may pair with the IL-18BP and interact with the IL-18R to inhibit IL-18 binding (S. Kumar, personal communication). Its physiologic role will need to be clarified by understanding its potential in human in vitro studies.

6. IL-FX PROMOTED GENERATION OF SPECIFIC T-CELL RESPONSES

Murine coculture of T-cells, NK cells from nude mice spleen, tumor (MCA-205 or MC38), IL-18, and DCs cultured from CD4+, CD8+, B220 depleted bone marrow facilitate generation of exquisitely specific T-cells recognizing tumor (70). Recapitulation of the events believed to occur in vivo with therapy in vitro with the MC38 colorectal carcinoma or the MCA 205 sarcoma, the addition of IL-18, NK cells, DCs, tumor to naïve T-cells is associated with rapid generation of extraordinarily tumor-specific T-cells. This requires the presence of each element of culture noted (Fig. 5A); elimination of any of them is associated with marked diminution in the resultant T-cell response. Human studies have yet to be performed to replicate these findings and are planned in experiments with allogeneic and autologous human tumors. The cytotoxic activity of effector cells was examined from cocultures containing each of the various components, including live tumor cells, NK cells, DCs, T-cells, and IL-18. On day 4 of coculture, effector cells were collected and cytolytic activity was assessed against MCA205 cells at various E:T ratios. The data shown represent the mean ± SD of cytotoxicity. There is a statistically significant difference among the group that contained all components vs all others lacking an

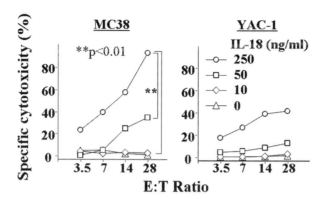

Fig. 5. Enhanced cytolytic activity generated against murine tumors in an IL-18 dose-dependent manner. When coculturing DCs autologous naive T-cells, tumor, low concentrations of IL-2 (100 U/mL) and IL-18 (shown in ng/mL), against the MC38 sarcoma **(left panel)** or the NK-sensitive YAC-1 lymphoma **(right panel)**, a dose-dependent enhancement of specific cytolytic activity was observed when culturing from 10–250 ng/mL. Some nonspecific lysis was observed at the higher concentrations.

individual element (**, $P < 0.01$ for all). In Fig. 5, panel B, effector cells were obtained from coculture separating either NK cells or DCs using a transwell system. On day 4 of coculture, effector cells were collected and cytolytic activity was assessed against MCA205 cells and the syngeneic NK cell sensitive target, YAC-1 cells at various E:T ratios. UC, upper chamber separated cells. Data represent the mean ± SD of cytotoxicity. There is a statistically significant difference between the group with no separation and a group with either NK cells or DCs separated (**, $P < 0.01$). Extraordinary specificity of these T-cells was noted with minimal or no cytotoxicity against a large panel of H2 targets tested in a ^{51}Cr release assay but with appropriate blocking of specific cytotoxicity when antibodies to H2K^b were used but not H2K^d. The development of this coculture system to initiate specific T-cells recognizing tumor targets has great potential utility with the ability to rapidly expand rare populations within naïve T-cells, enabling potential application in antigen discovery strategies. It is critical that it now be tested in human culture systems.

7. HUMAN IL-18 DRAMATICALLY SYNERGIZES WITH IL-2 TO ENHANCE CYTOLYTIC ACTIVITY, IFN-γ PRODUCTION, AND PROLIFERATION OF NEGATIVELY SORTED FRESH HUMAN NK CELLS *(126)*

This is associated with IL-18 induced upregulation of the IL-2Rα chain. Negatively separated human NK cells from normal healthy donors were cultured in the presence of IL-2 +/- IL-18 to evaluate ability to enhance NK cell cytolytic activity, NK cell production of IFN-γ, and proliferation. Substantial synergy in all assays was noted consistent with the ability of IL-18 to promote enhanced cytolytic activity with IL-2 and IL-12 as well (Fig. 6). Surprisingly little cytotoxicity is observed when one uses IL-18 alone.

In the right panel (Fig. 6), synergistic proliferation of PBMCs and NK cells is noted with IL-18 and IL-2. In the middle panel of Fig. 6 is shown the synergy in IFN-γ production.

Clearly enhanced NK cell function is noted with this combination. Exploration of the combination of IL-18 and the other IL-1 homologues with IL-2 to enhance NK for the purpose of interaction with iDC is based on the dramatic synergy observed with IL-2 and IL-18.

8. IL-18 CAN BE DETECTED AS WELL AS THE IL-18BP IN THE SERUM OF PATIENTS WITH MELANOMA, COLORECTAL CARCINOMA, AND SEVERAL OTHER TUMORS

Serum or plasma for IL-18 and IL-18BP were measured using Origen Technology and an Origen analyzer in Pittsburgh. Primary antibodies against each cytokine allows coupling to Oritag, a ruthenium tribipyridyl compound, which will emit chemolumines-cence after being excited at the surface of an electrode. The benefit of this technology is a very low background and wide dynamic range. Normal donors ($n = 19$) had a mean +/– SD of 0.46 +/–0.541 ng/mL of IL-18 and more than 50-fold greater IL-18BP with 26.3 +/– 27.8 ng/mL. This contrasted with serum levels which were somewhat depressed in melanoma patients ($n = 9$), with IL-18 0.197 ng/mL and comparable 19.7 +/– 22.4 ng/mL IL-18BP. When comparing serum IL-6, IFN-γ, and TNF-α in the serum of 57 patients and controls measured here, it was clear that there was a direct correla-tion of IL-18 at levels >1 ng/mL with heightened levels of each of these cytokines, con-sistent with a relationship to inflammation. Interestingly if one examines LPS stimulation of total PBMC in 19 normal controls, IL-12 was only 2.3 pg/mL, IL-18 30 pg/mL, IL-1β of 603.1 pg/mL, and TNF-α of 76.5 pg/mL. This suggests an exuberant response for some of the proinflammatory cytokines to bacterial stimuli. In melanoma patients (127) recently treated with IL-12, enhanced serum levels of IL-18BP were observed at presentation ranging from 6-28 ng/mL to a high of 95 ng/mL after treatment with IL-12. Baseline levels and induced levels following treatment tended to decrease with time, coincident with diminished response to IL-12 (tachyphylaxis) and less of an increase in serum IFN-γ levels. Thus, IL-18 and IL-18BP clearly circulate in normal individuals, in individuals with melanoma, and in stress.

9. IL-1F5 MEDIATES ENHANCED CYTOKINE PRODUCTION AND CYTOLYTIC ACTIVITY AGAINST MELANOMA CELL LINES

Interestingly, like our published studies with IL-1β and IL-18, IL-1F5 enhances pro-duction of IFN-γ with HMGB1 and IL-2, whereas this was not apparent on repeated study with the other novel homologues. This has, interestingly, a partial dependency on IL-2 and an absolute dependency on the presence of HMGB1 (this is endotoxin free by HPLC). As shown in Fig. 7, IL-1F5, like IL-1α and IL-1β, in the presence but not the absence (data not shown) of HMGB1 promote production of IL-6 peaking at 20–44 h. In the presence of IL-2, IFN-γ is also induced, suggesting a complex interaction of these cytokines, as we have shown requiring both a myeloid cell and NK cells (appendix; *see* ref. 128). We have recently received 10 carefully studied and prepared melanoma and melanoycte cell lines from the Wistar Institute. These are listed below: 451Lu (lung metastases; correlates with WM164), WM3211 (radial growth phase), WM1366 (vertical growth phase), WM1232 (metastatic melanoma; familial melanoma), WM793 (vertical growth phase melanoma), Sbcl2 (radial growth phase melanoma), WM35

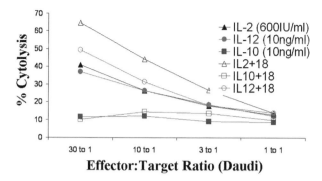

Fig. 6. Synergy of IL-2 and IL-18 on negatively separated NK cells (ENK, enriched NK) and PBMC in cytolytic activity. ENK were cultured with 50 ng/mL of IL-18 and IL-2 or IL-10 at the concentrations alone. Both IL-2 and IL-12 (at doses comparably increasing gamma interferon production) increased cytolytic activity against the Daudi NK-sensitive target in a four ^{51}Cr release assay.

(radial growth phase), WM9 (metastatic melanoma), WM115 (vertical growth phase), WM3248 (vertical growth phase), WM164 (also separate metastases) as well as two melanocyte lines. These have been expanded and are now characterized as to assessment of TRAIL receptors, BCL2, BCLxL, PUMA, NOXA, p53 by Western blot. Melanocytes are cultured in the presence of growth factors, bFGF, insulin (which substitutes for the more expensive IGF-1), SCF (c-kit ligand), endothelin-3, and FCS. The melanoma cells grow only with 2% FCS and insulin and basal medium. This should enable us to compare lysis of primary, presumably apoptotic sensitive nonimmortalized melanocyte lines, cultured primary melanoma cell lines, and melanoma lines obtained from metastatic lesions. These have been carefully defined as to their growth requirements, sensitivity to bFGF, and expression of ras/raf pathway mutations *(129–133)* by Meenhard Herlyn who kindly provided these well-characterized and studied lines. We have assessed release of HMGB1 into the media spontaneously by these various cell lines (*n* = 2 melanocyte cell lines, 2 early melanoma cell lines, 2 metastatic melanoma cell lines; total of 6 MM lines) and, are using Western blots to assess the relative abundance of HMGB1 within the nucleus (data not shown).

10. ABILITY OF ANK[IL-1FX] TO GENERATE DC1

We have prepared routine DCs with GM-CSF and IL-4 and demonstrated that they translocated NFκB by imaging cytometry in two different donors (nuclear to cytoplasmic translocation). The ability of IL-1 family members to modify the phenotype and function of DCs has now been tested in several experiments. IL-1β and TNF-α separately or together, markedly enhance the mature DC1 phenotype as defined by CD83, CD86, and class II expression.

11. HMGB1 PROMOTES MACROPHAGE DEPENDENT PRODUCTION OF IFN-γ BY HUMAN NK CELL

We have explored the application of the bioactive truncated B-box domain of HMGB1 (previously shown to contain the pro-inflammatory portion of the full-length molecule) for its capacity to modulate the inflammatory response in the context of in vitro cell

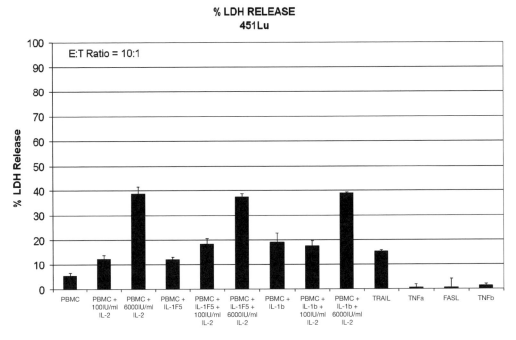

Fig. 7. Enhanced killing at low doses of IL-2 of melanoma cell line 451Lu by IL-1F5. Modest increases at 10:1 E:T ratio of cytolytic activity without IL-2 (red arrow) and at modest (100 U/mL IL-2) incubation. At higher doses of IL-2 (6000 U/mL), it is not possible to reveal greater cytolytic activity as measured in an LDH release assay. PBMC were incubated for 48 hrs before assay.

cultures. We have shown that in combination with IL-2, HMGB1 can synergize with known modulators of IFN-γ (IL-1α, IL-1β, IL-18) in Fig. 8. Shown are the day 1 and day 5 results from two separate donors, representative of over 8 separate experiments. IL-12 enhances the production of IFN-γ from PBMC cultures, with the most profound effect seen with the combination of IL-1 and IL-2 or IL-2 and IL-12. This effect is dependent on the presence of CD14+ cells and can be observed in cocultures of isolated CD14+ selected monocytes and negatively selected NK cells. In addition to enhancement of IFN-γ production, we found that HMGB1 induces TNF-α from PBMC and shows significant synergy in conditions that contained IL-1β (or IL-18) and IL-2. We speculate that in the presence of suitable pro-inflammatory mediators, HMGB1 may serve to amplify adaptive inflammatory responses mediated through monocytes/macrophages in vivo. We plan on examining the critical role of HMGB1 released from target cells and contrast the role of NK cell and monocyte/macrophage/DCs to respond in the presence of IL-1 family members. Furthermore IL-2 and IL-18 or IL-2 and IL-12 provided a similar synergy with HMGB1 stimulation consistent with this "danger" signal serving to enhance responsiveness to NK cell/macrophage autologous cocultures. Isolated, purified NK cells alone were not responsive to the addition of HMGB1.

12. SUMMARY

The understanding of the complexity of cytokines launched with the initial definition of the prototypic IL-1 and IL-2, could not have foretold the disclosure of literally

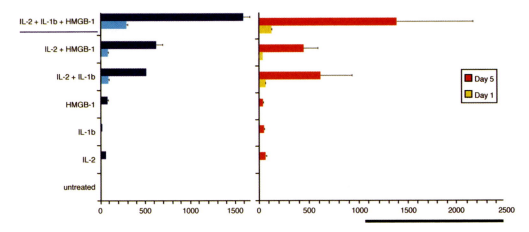

Fig. 8. HMGB1 enhances PBMC response with IFN-γ production in response to proinflammatory stimuli (IL-1+IL-2). Left donor1, Right donor 2.

hundreds of cytokines, now including 32 ILs, several TNF family members, chemokines, and defensins. The unusual aspects of the IL-1 family members detailed here include their ability to signal and initiate inflammation, promote the interface between the innate immune response and the adaptive immune response, and the specialized secretory lyso-some strategies employed to drive extracellular production of these cytokines. Emergent applications of these cytokines in cancer therapy include the apparent utility of IL-18 and possibly IL-1F7b. Limiting production of some of the cytokines including IL-1F1 and F2 may help prevent the initiation of chronic inflammation, reparative cell growth, and expansion of the neoplastic clones early in the process of cancer growth. Most recently, the novel IL-1 family member, IL-33, has been identified as the caspase 1-processed ligand for ST2, an orphan member of the IL-1R family, promoting Th2 responses *(134,135)*. Targeting caspase-1 itself may also have important pharmacologic roles.

REFERENCES

1. Kolb M, Margetts PJ, Anthony DC, Pitossi F, Gauldie J. Transient expression of IL-1beta induces lung injury and chronic repair leading to pulmonary fibrosis. J Clin Invest 2001;107:1529–1536.
2. Li M, Carpio DF, Zheng Y, et al. An essential role of the NF-kappa B/toll-like receptor pathway in induction of inflammatory and tissue-repair gene expression by necrotic cells. J Immunol 2001; 166:7128–7135.
3. Gardella S, Andrei C, Costigliolo S, Poggi A, Zocchi MR, Rubartelli A. Interleukin-18 synthesis and secretion by dendritic cells are modulated by interaction with antigen-specific T cells. J Leukocyte Biol 1999;66:237–241.
4. Gardella S, Andrei C, Costigliolo S, Olcese L, Zocchi MR, Rubartelli A. Secretion of bioactive inter-leukin-1beta by dendritic cells is modulated by interaction with antigen specific T cells. Blood 2000; 95:3809–3815.
5. Gardella S, Andrei C, Poggi A, Zocchi MR, Rubartelli A. Control of interleukin-18 secretion by den-dritic cells: Role of calcium influxes. FEBS Letter 2000;481:245–248.
6. Gardella S, Andrei C, Lotti LV, et al. CD8+ T lymphocytes induce polarized exocytosis of secretory lysosomes by dendritic cells with release of interleukin-1beta and cathepsin D. Blood 2001;98: 2152–2159.
7. Poggi A, Carosio R, Spaggiari GM, et al. NK cell activation by dendritic cells is dependent on LFA-1-mediated induction of calcium-calmodulin kinase II: Inhibition by HIV-1 Tat C-terminal domain. J Immunol 2002;168:95–101.

8. Angelini G, Gardella S, Ardy M, et al. Antigen-presenting dendritic cells provide the reducing extra-cellular microenvironment required for T lymphocyte activation. Proc Natl Acad Sci USA 2002; 2002:1491–1496.

9. Gardella S, Andrei C, Ferrera D, et al. The nuclear protein HMGB1 is secreted by monocytes via a non-classical, vesicle-mediated secretory pathway. EMBO Reports 2002;3(10):995–1001.

10. Dinarello CA. Interleukin-1. Cytokine Growth Factor Rev 1997;8:253–265.

11. Dinarello CA. Interleukin-1, interleukin-1 receptors and interleukin-1 receptor antagonist. Int Rev Immunol 1998;16:457–499.

12. Dinarello CA, Novick D, Puren AJ, et al. Overview of interleukin-18; more than an interferon-gamma inducing factor. J Leukocyte Biol 1998;63:658–664.

13. O'Neill LA, Greene C. Signal transduction pathways activated by the IL-1 receptor family: Ancient signaling machinery in mammals, insects, and plants. J Leukocyte Biol 1998;63:650–657.

14. Kumar S, McDonnell PC, Lehr R, et al. Identification and initial characterization of four novel members of the interleukin-1 family. J Biol Chem 2000;275:10,308–10,314.

15. Sims JE, Nicklin MJ, Bazan JF, et al. A new nomencalture for IL-1 family genes. Trends Immunol 2001;22:536–537.

16. Smith DE, Renshaw BR, Ketchem RR, Kubin M, Garka KE, Sims JE. Four new members expand the interleukin-1 superfamily. J Biol Chem 2000;275:1169–1175.

17. Dunn E, Sims JE, Nicklin MJ, O'Neill LA. Annotating genes with potential roles in the immune system: Six new members of the IL-1 family. Trends Immunol 2001;22:533–536.

18. Sims JE, March CJ, Cosman D, et al. cDNA expression cloning of the IL-1 receptor, a member of the immunoglobulin superfamily. Science 1988;241:585–589.

19. Schreuder H, Tardif C, Trump-Kallmeyer S, et al. A new cytokine-receptor binding mode revealed by the crystal structure of the IL-1 receptor with an antagonist. Nature 1997;386:194–200.

20. Xu X, Weinstein M, Li C, Deng C. Fibroblast growth factor receptors (FGFRs) and their roles in limb development. Cell Tissue Res 1999;296:33–43.

21. Le Feuvre RA, Brough D, Iwakura Y, Takeda K, Rothwell NJ. Printing of macrophages with lippolysaccharide potentiates P2X7-mediated cell death via a caspase-1-dependent mechanism, independently of cytokine production. J Biol Chem 2002;277:3210–3218.

22. Greenfeder SA, Nunes P, Kwee L, Labow M, Chizzonite RA, Ju G. Molecular cloning and characterization of a second subunit of the interleukin 1 receptor complex. J Biol Chem 1995;270:13, 757–13,765.

23. Cullinan EB, Kwee L, Nunes P, et al. IL-1 receptor accessory protein is an essential component of the IL-1 receptor. J Immunol 1998;161:5614–5620.

24. Wesa AK, Galy A. IL-1 beta induces dendritic cells to produce IL-12. Int Immunol 2001;13: 1053–1061.

25. Wesa AK, Galy A. Regulation of T cell cytokine production by dendritic cells generated in vitro from hematopoietic progenitor cells. Cell Immunol 2001;208:115–124.

26. Luft T, Luetjens P, Hochrein H, et al. IFN-alpha enhances CD40 ligand-mediated activation of immature monocyte-dervied dendritic cells. Int Immunol 2002;14:367–380.

27. Robinson D, Shibuya K, Mui A, et al. IGIG does not drive Th1 development but synergizes with IL-12 for interferon-gamma production and activates IRAK and NKkappaB. Immunity 1997;7:571–581.

28. Hannum CH, Wilcox CJ, Arend WP, et al. Interleukin-1 receptor antagonist activity of a human interleukin-1 inhibitor. Nature 1990;343:336–340.

29. Eisenberg SP, Evans RJ, Arend WP, et al. Primary structure and functional expression from complementary DNA of a human interleukin-1 receptor antagonist. Nature 1990;343:341–346.

30. Re F, Sironi M, Muzio M, et al. Inhibition of interleukin-1 responsiveness by type II receptor gene transfer: A surface "receptor" with anti-interleukin-1 function. J Exp Med 1996;183:1841–1850.

31. Colotta F, Saccani S, Giri JG, et al. Regulated expression and release of the IL-1 decoy receptor in human mononuclear phagocytes. J Immunol 1996;156:2534–2541.

32. Colotta F, Orlando S, Fadlon EJ, Sozzani S, Matteucci C, Mantovani A. Chemoattractants induce rapid release of the interleukin 1 type II decoy receptor in human polymorphonuclear cells. J Exp Med 1995;181:2181–2186.

33. Okamura H, Tsutsui H, Kashiwamura S, Yoshimoto T, Nakanishi K. Interleukin-18: A novel cytokine that augments both innate and acquired immunity. Adv Immunol 1998;70:281–312.

34. Ahn HJ, Mauro S, Tomura M, et al. A mechanism underlying synergy between IL-12 and IFN-γ-inducing factor in production of IFN-γ. J Immunol 1997;159:2125–2131.

35. Okamura H, Tsutsui H, Komatsu T, et al. Cloning of a new cytokine that induces IFN-gamma production by T cells. Nature 1995;378:88–91.
36. Thomassen E, Bird TA, Renshaw BR, Kennedy K, Sims JE. Binding of interleukin-18 to the interleukin-1 receptor homologous receptor IL-1Rrp1 leads to activation of signaling pathways similar to those used by interleukin-1. J Interferon Cytokine Res 1998;18:1077–1088.
37. Debets R, Timans JC, Churakowa T, et al. IL-18 receptors, their role in ligand binding and function: Anti-IL-1RAcPL antibody, a potent antagonist of IL-18. J Immunol 2000;165:4950–4956.
38. Mulero JJ, Nelken ST, Ford JE. Organization of the human interleukin-1 receptor antagonist gene IL1HY1. Immunogenetics 2000;51:425–428.
39. Mulero JJ, Pace AM, Nelken ST, et al. IL1HY1: A novel interleukin-1 receptor antagonist gene. Biochem Biophys Res Commun 1999;263:702–706.
40. Busfield SJ, Comrack CA, Yu G, et al. Identification and gene organization of three novel members of the IL-1 family on human chromosome 2. Genomics 2000;66:213–216.
41. Lin H, Ho AS, Haley-Vicente D, et al. Cloning and characterization of IL-1HY2, a novel interleukin-1 family member. J Biol Chem 2001;276:20,597–20,602.
42. Pan G, Risser P, Mao W, et al. IL-1H, an interleukin 1-related protein that binds IL-18 receptor/IL-1Rrp. Cytokine Growth Factor Rev 2001;13:1–7.
43. Nolan KF, Greaves DR, Waldmann H. The human interleukin gene IL-18 maps to 11q22.2-q22.3, closely linked to the DRD2 gene locus and distinct from mapped IDDM loci. Genomics 1998;51: 161–163.
44. Debets R, Timans JC, Homey B, et al. Two novel IL-1 family members, IL-1 delta and IL-1 epsilon, function as an antagonist and agonist of NF-kappaB activation through the orphan IL-1 receptor-related protein 2. J Immunol 2001;167:1440–1446.
45. Kumar S, Hanning CR, Brigham-Burke MR, et al. Interleukin-1F7B (IL-1H4/IL-1F7) is processed by caspase-1 and mature IL-1F7B binds to the IL-18 receptor but does not induce IFN-gamma production. Cytokine 2002;18:61–71.
46. Micallef MJ, Tanimoto T, Kohno K, Ikeda M, Kurimoto M. Interleukin 18 induces the sequential activation of natural killer cells and cytotoxic T lymphocytes to protect syngeneic mice from transplantation with Meth A sarcoma. Cancer Res 1997;57:4557–4563.
47. Micallef MJ, Yoshida K, Kawai S, et al. In vivo antitumor effects of murine interferon-gamma-inducing factor/interleukin-18 in mice bearing syngeneic Meth A sarcoma malignant ascites. Cancer Immunol Immunother 1997;43:361–367.
48. Micallef MJ, Ohtsuki T, Kohno K, et al. Interferon-gamma-inducing factor enhances T helper 1 cytokine production by stimulated human T cells: Synergism with interleukin -12 for interferon-gamma production. Eur J Immunol 1996;26:1647–1651.
49. Akiram S. The role of IL-18 in innate immunity. Curr Opin Immunol 2000;12:59–63.
50. Yoshimoto T, Takeda K, Tanaka T, et al. IL-12 up-regulates IL-18 receptor expression on T cells, Th1 cells, and B cells: Synergism with IL-18 for IFN-gamma production. J Immunol 1998;161:3400–3407.
51. Demeure CE, Tanaka H, Mateo V, Rubio M, Delespesse G, Sarfati M. CD47 engagement inhibits cytokine production and maturation of human dendritic cells. J Immunol 2000;164:2193–2199.
52. Morel JC, Park CC, Kumar P, Koch AE. Interleukin-18 induces rhematoid arthritis synovial fibroblast CXC chemokine production through NFkappaB activation. Lab Invest 2001;81:1371–1383.
53. Takada H, Nomura A, Ohga S, Hara T. Interleukin-18 in hempphagocytic lymphohistiocytosis. Leuk Lymphoma 2001;42:21–28.
54. Mayne M, Cheadle C, Soldan SS, et al. Gene expression profile of herpes virus-infected T cells obtained using immunomicroarrays: Induction of proinflammatory mechanisms. J Virol 2001;75: 11,641–11,650.
55. Fukami T, Miyazaki E, Matsumoto T, Kumamoto T, Tsuda T. Elevated expression of interleukin-18 in the granulomatous lesions of muscular sarcoidosis. Clin Immunol 2001;101:12–20.
56. Im SH, Barchan D, Maiti PK, Raveh L, Souroujon MC, Fuchs S. Suppression of experimental myasthenia gravis, a B cell-mediated autoimmune disease, by blockade of IL-18. FASEB J 2001;15: 2140–2148.
57. Park H, Byun D, Kim TS, et al. Enhanced IL-18 expression in common skin tumors. Immunol Lett 2001;79:215–219.
58. Kawabata T, Ichikura T, Majima T, et al. Preoperative serum interleukin-18 level as a postoperative prognostic marker in patients with gastric carcinoma. Cancer 2001;92:2050–2055.
59. Amo Y, Ohta Y, Hamada Y, Katsuoka K. Serum levels of interleukin-18 are increased in patients with cutaneous T-cell lymphoma and cutaneous natural killer cells lymphoma. Br J Dermatol 2001;145:674–676.

60. Mallat Z, Silvestre JS, Ricousse-Roussanne S, et al. Interleukin-18/interleukin-18 binding protein signaling modulates ischemia-induced neovascularization in mice hind limb. Circ Res 2002;91:441–448.
61. Mallat Z, Corbaz A, Scoazec A, et al. Expression of interleukin-18 in human atherosclerotic plaques and relation to plaque instability. Circulation 2001;104:1598–1603.
62. Mallat Z, Corbaz A, Scoazec A, et al. Interleukin-18/interleukin-18 binding protein signaling modulates atherosclerotic lesion development and stability. Circ Res 2001;89:E41–E5.
63. Hashimoto W, Osaki T, Okamura H, et al. Differential antitumor effects of administration of recombinant IL-18 or recombinant IL-12 are mediated primarily by Fas-Fas ligand- and perforin-induced tumor apoptosis, respectively. J Immunol 1999;163:583–589.
64. Reddy P, Teshima T, Kukuruga M, et al. Interleukin-18 regulates acute graft-versus-hot disease by enhancing Fas-mediated donor T cell apoptosis. J Exp Med 2001;194:1433–1440.
65. Nomura T, Kawamura I, Tsuchiya K, et al. Essential role of interleukin-12 (IL-12) and IL-18 for gamma interferon production induced by listeriolysin O in mouse spleen cells. Infect Immun 2002;70:1049–1055.
66. McCart JA, Ward JM, Lee J, et al. Systemic cancer therapy with a tumor-selective vaccinia virus mutant lacking thymidine kinase and vaccinia growth factor genes. Cancer Res 2001;61:8751–8757.
67. Xiang Y, Moss B. Correspondence of the functional epitopes of poxvirus and human interleukin-18-binding proteins. J Virol 2001;75:9947–9954.
68. Calderara S, Xiang Y, Moss B. Orthopoxvirus IL-18 binding proteins: Affinities and antagonist activities. Virology 2001;279:22–26.
69. Xiang Y, Moss B. IL-18 binding and inhibition of interferon gamma induction by human poxvirus-encoded proteins. Proc Natl Acad Sci 1999;96:11,537–11,542.
70. Tanaka F, Hashimoto W, Okamura H, Robbins PD, Lotze MT, Tahara H. Rapid generation of potent and tumor-specific cytotoxic T lymphocytes by interleukin 18 using dendritic cells and natural killer cells. Cancer Res 2000;60:4838–4844.
71. Barton JL, Herbst R, Bosisio D, Higgins L, Nicklin MJ. A tissue specific IL-1 receptor antagonist homolog from the IL-1 cluster lacks IL-1, IL-1ra, IL-18 and IL-18 antagonist activities. Eur J Immunol 2000;30:3299–3308.
72. Berglof E, Andre R, Renshaw BR, et al. IL-1Rrp2 expression and IL-1F9 (IL-1H1) actions in brain cells. J Neuroimmunol 2003;139:36–43.
73. Born TL, Smith DE, Garka KE, Renshaw BR, Bertles JS, Sims JE. Identification and characterization of two members of a novel class of the interleukin-1 receptor (IL-1R) family. Delineation of a new class of IL-1R-related proteins based on signaling. J Biol Chem 2000;275:29,946–29,954.
74. Busfield SJ, Comrack CA, Yu G, et al. Identification and gene organization of three novel members of the IL-1 family on human chromosome 2. Genomics 2000;66:213–216.
75. Radons J, Gabler S, Wesche H, Korherr C, Hofmeister R, Falk W. Identification of essential regions in the cytoplasmic tail of interleukin-1 receptor accessory protein critical for interleukin-1 signaling. J Biol Chem 2002;277:16,456–16,463.
76. Towne JE, Garka KE, Renshaw BR, Virca GD, Sims JE. Interleukin (IL)-1F6, IL-1F8, and IL-1F9 signal through IL-1Rrp2 and IL-1RAcP to activate the pathway leading to NF-kappaB and MAPKs. J Biol Chem 2004;279:13,677–13,688.
77. Kumar J. Interleukin 1 Family (F5-F10). In: Lotze MT, ed. The Cytokine Handbook, 4th ed. London: Academic Press; 2003:735–745.
78. Bucciarelli LG, Wendt T, Rong L, et al. RAGE is a multiligand receptor of the immunoglobulin superfamily: Implications for homeostasis and chronic disease. Cell MolLife Sci 2002;59:1117–1128.
79. Stern DM, Yan SD, Yan SF, Schmidt. AM. Receptor for advanced glycation endproducts (RAGE) and the complications of diabetes. Ageing Res Rev 2002;1:1–15.
80. Schmidt AM, Stern. DM. Receptor for age (RAGE) is a gene within the major histocompatibility class III region: Implications for host response mechanisms in homeostasis and chronic disease. Front Biosci 2001;6:D1151–D1160.
81. Schmidt AM, Yan SD, Yan SF, Stern. DM. The multiligand receptor RAGE as a progression factor amplifying immune and inflammatory responses. J Clin Invest 2001;108:949–955.
82. Dinarello CA. Induction of interleukin-1 and interleukin-1 receptor antagonist. Semin Oncol 1997;24:S9.
83. Acland K, Evans AV, Abraha H, et al. Serum S100 concentrations are not useful in predicting micrometastatic disease in cutaneous malignant melanoma. Br J Dermatol 2002;146:832–835.

84. Hunzelmann N, Kurschat P, Hani N, Jarisch A, Mauch. C. Applicability of reference values for the determination of serum S100 protein as a marker of malignant melanoma in children. Br J Dermatol 2002;146:536, 537.

85. Djukanovic D, Hofmann U, Sucker A, Schadendorf. D. Melanoma tumour markers S100B and MIA: Evaluation of stability in serum and blood upon storage and processing. Br J Dermatol 2001;145:1030, 1031.

86. Ghanem G, Loir B, Morandini R, et al. On the release and half-life of S100B protein in the peripheral blood of melanoma patients. Int J Cancer 2001;94:586–590.

87. Krahn G, Kaskel P, Sander S, et al. S100 beta is a more reliable tumor marker in peripheral blood for patients with newly occurred melanoma metastases compared with MIA, albumin and lactate-dehydrogenase. Anticancer Res 2001;21:1311–1316.

88. Mohammed MQ, Abraha HD, Sherwood RA, MacRae K, Retsas. S. Serum S100beta protein as a marker of disease activity in patients with malignant melanoma. Med Oncol 2001;18:109–120.

89. Huttunen HJ, Kuja-Panula J, Sorci G, Agneletti AL, Donato R, Rauvala. H. Coregulation of neurite outgrowth and cell survival by amphoterin and S100 proteins through receptor for advanced glycation end products (RAGE) activation. J Biol Chem 2000;275:40,096–40,105.

90. Schmidt S, Linington C, Zipp F, et al. Multiple sclerosis: Comparison of the human T-cell response to S100 beta and myelin basic protein reveal parallels to rat experimental autoimmune panencephalitis. Brain 1997;120:1437–1445.

91. Ilg EC, Sch%efer BW, Heizmann. CW. Expression pattern of S100 calcium-binding proteins in human tumors. Int J Cancer 1996;68:325–332.

92. Zeid NAaHKM. S100 positive dendritic cells in human lung tumors associated with cell differentiation and enhanced survival. Pathology 1993;25:338.

93. Balch CM, Soong SJ, Gershenwald JE, et al. Prognostic factors analysis of 17,600 melanoma patients: Validation of the American Joint Committee on Cancer melanoma staging system. J Clin Oncol 2001;19:3622–3634.

94. Balch CM, Buzaid AC, Soong SJ, et al. Final version of the American Joint Committee on Cancer staging system for cutaneous melanoma. J Clin Oncol 2001;19:3635–3648.

95. Plate KH, Isau. W. Angiogenesis in malignant gliomas. GLIA 1995;15:339–347.

96. Glumac N, Hocevar M, Snoj M, Novakovic. S. Detection of tyrosinase mRNA by an optimised nested RT-PCR in the peripheral blood of patients with advanced malignant melanoma. J Exp Clin Cancer Res 2001;20:529–536.

97. Tsao H, Nadiminti U, Sober AJ, Bigby. M. A meta-analysis of reverse transcriptase-polymerase chain reaction for tyrosinase mRNA as a marker for circulating tumor cells in cutaneous melanoma. Arch Dermatol 2001;137:325–330.

98. Brownbridge GG, Gold J, Edward M, MacKie. RM. Evaluation of the use of tyrosinase-specific and melanA/MART-1-specific reverse transcriptase-coupled—polymerase chain reaction to detect melanoma cells in peripheral blood samples from 299 patients with malignant melanoma. Br J Dermatol 2001;144.

99. Fernandez NC, Lozier A, Flament C, et al. Dendritic cells directly trigger NK cell functions: Cross-talk relevant in innate anti-tumor immune responses in vivo. Nature Med 1999;5:405–411.

100. Schmitz C, Brenner W, Henze E, Christophers E, Hauschild. A. Comparative study on the clinical use of protein S-100B and MIA (melanoma inhibitory activity) in melanoma patients. Anticancer Res 2000;20:5059–5063.

101. Messmer D, Yang H, Telusma G, et al. High mobility group box protein 1: An endogenous signal for dendritic cell maturation and Th1 polarization. J Immunol 2004;173:307–313.

102. Rovere-Querini P, Capobianco A, Scaffidi P, et al. HMGB1 is an endogenous immune adjuvant released by necrotic cells. EMBO Rep 2004;5:825–830.

103. Ghosh S, Karin M. Missing pieces in the NF-kappaB puzzle. Cell 2002;109:S81–96.

104. Ghosh S, May MJ.Kopp EB. NF-kappa B and Rel proteins: Evolutionarily conserved mediators of immune responses. Annu Rev Immunol 1998;16:225–260.

105. Baeuerle PA, Baltimore D. Activation of DNA-binding activity in an apparently cytoplasmic precursor of the NF-kappa B transcription factor. Cell 1988;53:211–217.

106. Burkly L, Hession C, Ogata L, et al. Expression of relB is required for the development of thymic medulla and dendritic cells. Nature 1995;373:531–56.

107. Weih F, Carrasco D, Durham SK, et al. Multiorgan inflammation and hematopoietic abnormalities in mice with a targeted disruption of RelB, a member of the NF-kappa B/Rel family. Cell 1995;80: 331–340.

108. Ammon C, Mondal K, Andreesen R, Krause SW. Differential expression of the transcription factor NF-kappaB during human mononuclear phagocyte differentiation to macrophages and dendritic cells. Biochem Biophys Res Commun 2000;268:99–105.

109. Ardeshna KM, Pizzey AR, Devereux S, Khwaja A. The PI3 kinase, p38 SAP kinase, and NF-kappaB signal transduction pathways are involved in the survival and maturation of lipopolysaccharide-stimulated human monocyte-derived dendritic cells. Blood 2000;96:1039–1046.

110. Pettit AR, Quinn C, MacDonald KP, et al. Nuclear localization of RelB is associated with effective antigen-presenting cell function. J Immunol 1997;159:3681–3691.

111. Boulton TG, Yancopoulos GD, Gregory JS, et al. An insulin-stimulated protein kinase similar to yeast kinases involved in cell cycle control. Science 1990;249:64–67.

112. Kaiser GC, Yan F, Polk DB. Conversion of TNF alpha from antiproliferative to proliferative ligand in mouse intestinal epithelial cells by regulating mitogen-activated protein kinase. Exp Cell Res 1999;249:349–358.

113. Jones SM, Kazlauskas A. Connecting signaling and cell cycle progression in growth factor-stimulated cells. Oncogene 2000;19:5558–5567.

114. Jones SM, Kazlauskas A. Growth-factor-dependent mitogenesis requires two distinct phases of signalling. Nat Cell Biol 2001;3:165–172.

115. Jones SM, Klinghoffer R, Prestwich GD, Toker A, Kazlauskas A. PDGF induces an early and a late wave of PI 3-kinase activity, and only the late wave is required for progression through G1. Curr Biol 1999;9:512–521.

116. Fukao T, Tanabe M, Terauchi Y, et al. PI3K-mediated negative feedback regulation of IL-12 production in DCs. Nat Immunol 2002;3:875–881.

117. Saccani S, Pantano S, Natoli G. p38-Dependent marking of inflammatory genes for increased NF-kappa B recruitment. Nat Immunol 2002;3:69–75.

118. Downward J. Mechanisms and consequences of activation of protein kinase B/Akt. Curr Opin Cell Biol 1998;10:262–267.

119. Reddy SM, Hsiao KH, Abernethy VE, et al. Phagocytosis of apoptotic cells by macrophages induces novel signaling events leading to cytokine-independent survival and inhibition of proliferation: Activation of Akt and inhibition of extracellular signal-regulated kinases 1 and 2. J Immunol 2002;169:702–713.

120. Puig-Kroger A, Relloso M, Fernandez-Capetillo O, et al. Extracellular signal-regulated protein kinase signaling pathway negatively regulates the phenotypic and functional maturation of monocyte-derived human dendritic cells. Blood 2001;98:2175–2182.

121. Jonak ZL, Trulli S, Maier C, et al. High-Dose Recombinant Interleukin-18 Induces an Effective Th1 Immune Response to Murine MOPC-315 Plasmacytoma. J Immunother 2002;25 Suppl 1:S20–S7.

122. Osaki T, Peron JM, Cai Q, et al. IFN-gamma-inducing factor/IL-18 administration mediates IFN-gamma- and IL-12-independent antitumor effects. J Immunol 1998;160:1742–1749.

123. Osaki T, Hashimoto W, Gambotto A, et al. Potent antitumor effects mediated by local expression of the mature form of the interferon-gamma inducing factor, interleukin-18 (IL-18). Gene Ther 1999;6: 808–815.

124. Nishioka Y, Hirao M, Robbins PD, Lotze MT, Tahara. H. Induction of systemic and therapeutic antitumor immunity using intratumoral injection of dendritic cells genetically modified to express interleukin 12. Cancer Res 1999;59:4035–4041.

125. Kirk CJ, Hartigan-O'Connor D, Nickoloff BJ, et al. T cell-dependent antitumor immunity mediated by secondary lymphoid tissue chemokine: Augmentation of dendritic cell-based immunotherapy. Cancer Res 2001;61:2062–2070.

126. Son YI, Dallal RM, Mailliard RB, Egawa S, Jonak ZL, Lotze. MT. Interleukin-18 (IL-18) synergizes with IL-2 to enhance cytotoxicity, interferon-γ production, and expansion of natural killer cells. Cancer Res 2001;61:884–888.

127. Veenstra KG, Jonak ZL, Trulli S, Gollob. JA. IL-12 induces monocyte IL-18 binding protein expression via IFN-gamma. J Immunol 2002;168:2282–2287.

128. DeMarco RA, Fink MP, Lotze MT. Monocytes promote natural killer cell interferon gamma production in response to the endogenous danger signal HMGB1. Molecular Immunology 2005;42: 433–444.

129. Berking C, Takemoto R, Satyamoorthy K, et al. Induction of melanoma phenotypes in human skin by growth factors and ultraviolet B. Cancer Res 2004;64:807–811.

130. Herlyn M, Shih IM. Interactions of melanocytes and melanoma cells with the microenvironment. Pigment Cell Res 1994;7:81–88.

131. Satyamoorthy K, Li G, Gerrero MR, et al. Constitutive mitogen-activated protein kinase activation in melanoma is mediated by both BRAF mutations and autocrine growth factor stimulation. Cancer Res 2003;63:756–759.

132. Schaider H, Oka M, Bogenrieder T, et al. Differential response of primary and metastatic melanomas to neutrophils attracted by IL-8. Int J Cancer 2003;103:335–343.

133. Wang E, Miller LD, Ohnmacht GA, et al. Prospective molecular profiling of melanoma metastases suggests classifiers of immune responsiveness. Cancer Res 2002;62:3581–3586.

134. Schmitz J, Owyang A, Oldham E, et al. IL-33, an interleukin-1-like cytokine that signals via the IL-1 receptor-related protein ST2 and induces T helper type 2-associated cytokines. Immunity. 2005 Nov;23(5):479–490.

135. Dinarello CA. An IL-1 family member requires caspase-1 processing and signals through the ST2 receptor. Immunity. 2005 Nov;23(5):461–462.

7 Interleukin-4/13 and Cancer

Koji Kawakami and Raj K. Puri

CONTENTS

INTRODUCTION
EFFECTS OF IL-4 AND IL-13 ON CANCER CELLS AND THEIR ROLE
   IN CANCER THERAPY
STRUCTURE AND FUNCTION OF IL-4/13 RECEPTORS ON CANCER CELLS
TARGETING OF IL-4/13 RECEPTORS FOR CANCER THERAPY
CONCLUSIONS
ACKNOWLEDGMENTS
REFERENCES

1. INTRODUCTION

Both interleukin-4 (IL-4) and interleukin-13 (IL-13) are predominantly T-helper-2 (Th2) derived cytokines and share many structural and functional characteristics with each other. Both cytokines are also shown to be produced by mast cells and basophils *(1–3)*. IL-4 was first identified in 1980s as a B-cell growth factor *(4)*, and shown to mediate many effects on numerous cell types including T-cells, B-cells, monocytes, mast cells, endothelial cells, fibroblasts, astrocytes, and osteoblasts *(5,6)*.

IL-13 was identified in 1990s and has also been shown to be produced by neutrophils, dendritic cells, natural killer (NK), renal cell carcinoma, and Hodgkin's Reed-Sternberg tumor cells *(7–16)*. Unlike IL-4, IL-13 has not been found to have any effect on the growth and differentiation of T-cells. Similar to IL-4, IL-13 inhibits the production of inflammatory cytokines (including IL-1, IL-6, IL-10, IL-12, TNF-α, and GM-CSF); chemokines (including IL-8, MCP-3, MIP-1, and RANTES); upregulates MHC class II and CD23 expression on monocytes; enhances proliferative responses to anti-IgM and anti-CD40 antibodies; induces anti-CD40-dependent IgE class switch; and induces IgG and IgM synthesis in B-cells *(1–3,7,8,17–21)*. These properties of IL-13 were further confirmed in IL-13 transgenic and knockout mouse models *(22–24)*. It has also been reported that IL-13 plays a role in various inflammatory diseases including bronchial asthma, allergic rhinitis, and atopic dermatitis *(3,25–30)*.

The biologic effects of IL-4/13 occur through specific plasma membrane receptors on target cells. IL-4/13 can mediate direct and indirect antitumor effects in vitro and in vivo. Recent studies have identified the role of IL-13 in tumor immune surveillance and

From: *Cancer Drug Discovery and Development,*
Cytokines in the Genesis and Treatment of Cancer
Edited by: M. A. Caligiuri and M. T. Lotze © Humana Press Inc., Totowa, NJ

immunity. In this chapter, the role of IL-4/13 and their receptors in cancer and targeting of these receptors by cytotoxins for cancer therapy is summarized.

2. EFFECTS OF IL-4 AND IL-13 ON CANCER CELLS AND THEIR ROLE IN CANCER THERAPY

2.1. Effects of IL-4 on Cancer Cells and its Role in Cancer Therapy

IL-4 has been shown to have significant antiproliferative activity against many human hematologic tumor cells including acute T-cell leukemia (31), acute lymphocytic leukemia (32), chronic myelomonocytic leukemia (33), B-type chronic lymphocytic leukemia (34,35), multiple myeloma (36), lymphoma (37), non-Hodgkin's lymphoma (38), acute myeloblastic leukemia (39), and histiocytic lymphoma (40). Interestingly, IL-4 was also found to have mitogenic activity towards human T-cell leukemia cells (41) and B-type chronic lymphocytic leukemia (B-CLL) cells (42,43). In B-CLL cells, IL-4 was found to be a survival factor and inhibited apoptosis of these cells (42,44).

IL-4 has direct antiproliferative activity against various solid tumor cancer cell lines including gastric cancer, renal cell carcinoma, lung cancer, malignant melanoma, and breast cancer (45–48). IL-4 was found to upregulate intracellular adhesion molecule-1 (ICAM-1) and potentiates the antitumor effects of TNF or IFN-γ on a variety of tumor cell lines (49–52). The antitumor effects of IL-4 and IFN-γ are mediated, in part, by nitric oxide production (53). IL-4 can also enhance androgen receptor-mediated prostate-specific antigen (PSA) expression through the Akt signaling pathway, thus sensitizing these cells to an immune response in the host (54). Similar to some effects on hematologic cancers, IL-4 can also stimulate growth of some head and neck cancer cell lines (55). Some cancer cell lines, such as thyroid cancer cell lines, can produce IL-4 and IL-10 and these autocrine cytokines can upregulate anti-apoptotic proteins resulting in resistance to chemotherapeutic drugs (56). A recent study has suggested that p73β-transfected tumor cells are sensitive to IL-4-mediated apoptosis (57). Taken together, in vitro studies suggest that IL-4 can mediate both antitumor and mitogenic activities on cancer cells. However, antitumor activities are predominant. Despite the realization of antitumor activities for the past 20 years, the detailed mechanism is still not completely known.

IL-4 has also been found to have significant antitumor activity in vivo (6,48,58,59). IL-4 was found to enhance cytotoxic activity of tumor infiltrating lymphocytes (TIL) and antitumor effects in vivo (60,61). IL-2 upregulated IL-4 receptors in TIL enhancing their activity (62). Later, Tepper et al. demonstrated that antitumor activity of IL-4 was predominantly mediated by eosinophils and macrophages as these cells were found to infiltrate into the tumor mass (58,59). Additional studies demonstrated that host CTL also played a major role in tumor response (63). It has also shown that antitumor effect of IL-4 on rat glioma (9L) model could be reversed by dexamethasone (64). Based on these results, IL-4 was tested in a number of clinical trials as a single agent (65–71) or combination with granulocyte macrophage-colony stimulating factor (72,73) (Table 1). However, clinical trials using systemic or local IL-4 administration in patients with primary and metastatic cancer did not exhibit promising results.

Recently, Okada et al. have investigated the use of autologous brain tumor vaccine transduced with IL-4 HSV-tk gene (74) or IL-4-transduced fibroblasts (75–77). Preclinical data and results from phase-I trials demonstrated that these transduced cells

Table 1
Clinical Trials With IL-4 in Cancer Patients[a]

Cancer type	Number of patients	Route	MTD	DLT	Biological effects	Reference
Refractory solid tumor	10	iv	10–15 µg/kg tid	Diarrhea, nausea, vomiting, fatigue, anorexia, headache, CLS	↓lymphocytes, CD16+and CD14+ cells ↑Hct, PT/PTT, sCD23	65
GI solid tumors and myeloma	9	sc	5 µg/kg/day	Flulike symptoms, ↑liver enzymes	↑neutrophils, platelets, PTT pain in lymph nodes	66
Advanced solid tumors	19	iv	400 µg/m²/day	Flulike symptoms, GI hemorrhage, CLS, ↑liver enzymes	Transient antitumor response in 2 patients	67
Advanced solid tumors	15	sc with IL-2	Not determined (tested up to 300 µg/m²/day)	Fatigue, fever, nausea/vomiting, anorexia, headache, nasal stuffiness	Eosinophilia, ↑T-cell subsets	68
Recurrent nonsmall cell lung cancer	63 (phase-II)	sc	Not determined (tested up to 1 µg/kg/day)	Not determined (Vomiting, dyspnea, fatigue, duodenal ulcer observed)	1/55 PR	69
NHL	39 (phase-II)	sc	3 µg/kg/day	Arhralgia/myalgia, fatigue, fever, headache, rigors/chills	1/39 PR	70
Advanced renal cell carcinoma	49 (phase-II)	sq	5 µg/kg/day	Nausea, vomiting, diarrhea, headache, malaise	No CR/PR	71
Advanced metastatic cancer	21	sc with GM-CSF	6 µg/kg/day (plus GM-CSF 2.5 µg/kg/day)	↑liver enzymes, dyspnea, headache, thrombocytopenia	↑number and function of APC	73

137

[a]GI, gastrointestinal; NHL, non-Hodgkin's lymphoma; Hct, hematocrit; CLS, capillary leak syndrome; GM-CSF, granulocyte-macrophage colony-stimulating factor; MTD, maximum tolerated dose; DLT, dose limiting toxicity; tid, three times a day; APC, antigen-presenting cells; CR, complete response; and PR, partial response.

successfully produced IL-4 in a local, sustained manner without autoimmune responses. Further investigation will reveal the efficacy of IL-4 transduced cells in cancer therapy.

2.2. Effects of IL-13 on Cancer Cells and Its Role in Cancer Therapy

The effects of IL-13 on solid cancer cells have been reported. IL-13 has a modest inhibitory effect on in vitro cell proliferation of low grade astrocytoma, renal cell carcinoma, breast cancer, pancreatic cancer, and ovarian cancer (16,78–82). Blais et al. reported that IL-13 can stimulate spermidine uptake by increasing total transport capacity and stimulate gross cystic disease fluid protein-15 (GCDFP-15) release, which may decrease estrogen-induced breast cancer cell proliferation (83,84). Lebel-Binay et al. demonstrated a gene therapy approach in which transplanted lung (3LL) and mastocytoma (P815) tumor cells engineered to produce IL-13 at the local site mediated in vivo antitumor activity (85). Our studies have demonstrated that IL-13 can mediate moderate antitumor activity in IL-13Rα2 chain-transfected breast (MDA-MB-231) tumors in xenograft nude mice model (9). In addition to direct growth modulatory activity in vitro and in vivo, IL-13 has also been found to exhibit an inhibitory effect on colon cancer cell–cell adhesion by down regulation of E-cadherin and carcinoembryonic antigen (CEA) (86). IL-13 can stimulate the enzyme activity of aminopeptidase N (APN) and dipeptidylpeptidase IV (DPIV) in renal cell carcinoma cells (87). The study of Huang et al. demonstrated that nonsmall cell lung cancer (NSCLC) derived cells express IL-13, however, its significance is unclear (88). We have found that IL-13 can augment expression of vascular cell adhesion molecule 1 (VCAM-1) on glioblastoma cells (A172) in vitro (89). Finally, Volpert et al. demonstrated that not only IL-4 but IL-13 can also inhibit tumor angiogenesis in vivo rat model, implicating that IL-13 may play a role in the inhibition of tumorigenicity as well as metastasis of the established cancer (90).

In hematologic malignancies, IL-13 has also been shown to mediate biologic activities. It can inhibit constitutive secretion of various cytokines by acute myelogenous leukemia (AML) blast cells although it does not have any effect on the proliferation of AML cells (91,92). Other reports have shown that IL-13 can mediate a differential effect on in vitro growth of B-lineage acute lymphoblastic leukemia cells (BCP-ALL) (93). Although IL-13 expression was found in B-cell lymphoid malignant tissues and in serum from AML, Hodgkin's lymphoma, non-Hodgkin's lymphoma, and chronic lymphocytic leukemia patients, its role in these malignancies is unclear (12–15,30,94,95). More recently, IL-13 was found to be autocrine growth factor in Hodgkin's lymphoma cells (12–15).

Using STAT6 knock out mice, Kacha et al. and Ostrand-Rosenberg et al. have demonstrated spontaneous rejection of tumors in these mice because of a shift from Th2 phenotype to a dominant Th1 phenotype (96,97). Later it was demonstrated that immunosurveillance in STAT6 knock out mice requires an IFN-γ dependent pathway to facilitate survival against metastatic cancer (98). Furthermore, Terabe et al. reported that treatment of tumor bearing mice with "IL-13 inhibitor" (sIL-13Rα2-Fc) resulted in resistance to the 15-12RM cell derived-tumor recurrence (99). It was hypothesized that IL-13 produced by natural killer T (NKT) cells uses STAT6 pathway which is necessary for down-regulation of tumor immunosurveillance. Later studies revealed that transforming growth factor-β (TGF-β) made by CD11b⁺Gr-1⁺ myeloid cells is necessary for down-regulation of tumor immunosurveillance in such system (100). Because Th1/Th2 balance is important in the tumor environment (80,101,102) and IL-13 can modulate

Th1/Th2 balance, it is hypothesized that IL-13 plays a critical role in host immune surveillance and tumor immunity.

Although limited direct antitumor activity of IL-13 has been reported in vitro and in vivo, no clinical trials using IL-13 as an antitumor agent have been conducted. Because IL-13 is possibly involved in tumor immunosurveillance and tumorigenicity (80,99), tumor immunotherapy approaches targeting IL-13 or IL-13R could be an effective modality for cancer therapy. Recently, Okano et al. identified CTL epitopes derived from human IL-13Rα2 chain (103). They have successfully shown that IL-13Rα2 peptide (WLPFGFILI) induced a CD8+ T-cell line, which specifically produced IFN-γ in response to HLA-A0201+ T2 cells pulsed with the relevant peptide and lysed target cells. These observations indicate that the IL-13Rα2 chain on cancer cells may be a target for the immune system.

3. STRUCTURE AND FUNCTION OF IL-4/13 RECEPTORS ON CANCER CELLS

Receptors for IL-4 (IL-4R) and IL-13 (IL-13R) share at least two subunits with each other. The two subunits are IL-4Rα and IL-13Rα1 chains. IL-4Rs are comprised of a 140 kDa protein termed IL-4Rα chain (also known as IL-4Rβ). It contains a WSXWS motif and four cysteine residues at the fixed location in the extracellular domain (104). The second subunit of IL-4R system was identified as a component of the IL-2 receptor system, the γ chain (105,106). Because IL-2Rγ chain was also shown to be a component of IL-7, IL-9, IL-15, and IL-21 receptor systems, it was named the common γ chain (γ_c) (107,108). In solid cancer cell lines, IL-13Rα1 chain (also known as IL-13Rα' chain) (109) forms a productive complex with the IL-4Rα chain instead of the γ_c chain (Fig. 1). This IL-4R subunit structure in cancer cells was confirmed by affinity cross-linking, Northern analysis, RT-PCR, and immunoprecipitation studies (110–114). When IL-4Rα forms a heterodimer with the γ_c chain or the IL-13Rα1 chain, IL-4 can mediate a biologic signal through these complexes. Both IL-4Rs and IL-13Rs use the JAK-STAT pathway to mediate biologic signaling (115–118).

Two predominant types of IL-13Rs have been identified in solid cancer cells. As shown in Fig. 1, the type I IL-13R complex is composed of the IL-13Rα1, IL-13Rα2, and IL-4Rα chains. The IL-13Rα1 chain (109,119,120) binds IL-13 with low affinity but when coupled with the IL-4Rα chain, the heterodimer binds IL-13 with high affinity and mediates IL-13 induced signaling (116–118). The IL-13Rα1 chain also interacts with the protein termed MIP-T3 (microtubule interacting protein that associates with tumor necrosis factor receptor associating factor-3 [TRAF-3]) (121). Another IL-13R chain, IL-13Rα2 (also known as IL-13Rα) has been cloned from human renal cell carcinoma (Caki-1) and malignant glioblastoma (U251) cell lines (89,122). This chain shares ~50% homology with the IL-5R at the DNA level, it contains a very short intracellular domain, and binds IL-13 with high affinity (122,123). Although IL-13Rα2 chain is expressed on solid tumor cell lines including renal cell carcinoma, malignant glioma, AIDS-associated Kaposi's sarcoma, some ovarian, and head and neck cancers (78,79,124–128), the significance of its expression is still unknown (9,128). The IL-13Rα2 chain not only can inhibit IL-13-mediated signaling but can also inhibit IL-4-mediated signaling in glioma cell lines (129,130). Although IL-13 binds to all three chains, only IL-13Rα1 and IL-4Rα chains form a productive complex. Because of the

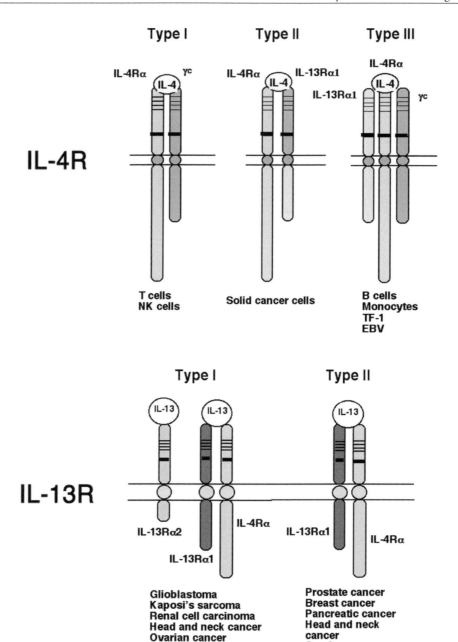

Fig. 1. Model of IL-4R and IL-13R. The significance of type III IL-4R is not confirmed, however, all three chains exist on cells.

presence of IL-13Rα2 chain, IL-13 binds to these cells more strongly. In the type II IL-13R system, IL-13Rα2 does not participate and the IL-13Rα1 chain forms a complex with IL-4Rα chain. This type of receptor is present in many tumor cell lines and normal immune cells. In contrast to the IL-4R system, γ_c chain does not bind IL-13 directly

Table 2
IL-4R Expression in Human Cancer Cell Lines

Cell type	IL-4 binding sites/cell	KDa (pM)	Reference
Renal cell carcinoma	1400–4000	100–300	45,110
Malignant melanoma	1200–1400	360–550	111
Ovarian carcinoma	300–1400	330	111
Kaposi's sarcoma	600–2200	19–160	142,143
Epidermoid carcinoma	1000	300	unpublished data
Breast cancer	700–4600	200–1000	111,144
Glioblastoma	1000–3000	100–700	135
Colon cancer	2000	77	48
Head and neck cancer	6100–13,000	–	167,184
Gastric cancer	–[a]	–	46
Lung cancer	10,600	2400	47,146
Prostate cancer	12,000	266	148

[a]Flow cytometric analysis

and is not involved in the IL-13R system. However, it affects IL-13 binding and function in some cell types (113,131,132).

4. TARGETING OF IL-4/13 RECEPTORS FOR CANCER THERAPY

4.1. IL-4 Cytotoxins

Because IL-4R and IL-13R are overexpressed on many solid cancer cell lines (Table 2), two receptor-directed therapeutic agents IL-4- and IL-13- cytotoxins have been developed. A cytotoxic chimeric protein composed of IL-4 and *Pseudomonas* exotoxin (PE) was first developed in 1991. PE is a 66 kDa protein produced by *Pseudomonas aeruginosa*. It has three domains; domain Ia binds to PE receptors, domain II catalyzes the translocation of the toxin into cytosol, and domain III inhibits protein synthesis and eventually kills the cells by ADP ribosylation of elongation factor-2 of the protein synthesis pathway (133). By replacing the binding domain of PE by IL-4, IL-4 cytotoxins were generated (134–137). Because IL-4 cytotoxin bound to IL-4 in glioma cells with 37-fold less affinity than native IL-4, a circularly permuted IL-4 cytotoxin, termed IL4 (38-37)-PE38KDAEL or cpIL4-PE was generated (138–141). This purified toxin was found to be highly cytotoxic to IL-4R positive cancer cells. cpIL4-PE was 3- to 30-fold more cytotoxic to cancer cell lines including glioblastoma cells compared to the first generation IL-4 cytotoxins (Table 3). The cytotoxicity of cpIL4-PE was also tested on normal human bone marrow-derived cells, EBV-transformed B-cells, promonocytic (U937) cells, H9 T-cells, and normal endothelial cells. Consistent with the expression of low numbers of IL-4R, cpIL4-PE was either not cytotoxic or only slightly cytotoxic to these resting human cells (141,142).

cpIL4-PE mediated profound antitumor activity in athymic nude mice with subcutaneously developed human tumors, e.g., glioblastoma, AIDS Kaposi's sarcoma, prostate, breast, lung, and head and neck cancer (143–149). cpIL4-PE also prolonged survival of mice orthotopically implanted with human pancreatic tumors (150).

Based on these preclinical results and its safety profile (136,140,143), a phase-I clinical trial to determine the safety and tolerability of cpIL4-PE was initiated in patients

Table 3
Cytotoxicity of IL4(38-37)-PE38KDAEL to Human Solid Cancer Cell Lines

Cells	$IC_{50}{}^a$	Cells	$IC_{50}{}^a$	Reference
Renal cell carcinoma				*141*
PM-RCC	0.30	MA-RCC	0.50	
WS-RCC	0.15	HL-RCC	0.12	
RC-2	3.0	Caki-1	40	
Kaposi's sarcoma				*142,143*
KSY-1	8.0	KS-imm	10	
KS248	1.7	NCB-59	6.2	
KS54A	41	KS220B	43	
Breast cancer				*144*
MCF-7	0.40	R-BT	0.20	
BT-20	75	ZR75-1	7.0	
MDA-MB-231	1.8			
Glioblastoma				*140*
T98G	1.0	A172	1.0	
SN19	9.0	U-373MG	2.0	
U251	6.5			
Colon cancer				*139*
HT-29	0.40	LS174T	9.0	
Colo-201	0.45	Colo-205	0.80	
SW1116	8.5	SW403	6.5	
Pancreatic cancer				*150*
PANC-1	0.35			
Head and neck cancer				*184*
KB	0.15	RPMI2650	92	
A253	<0.1	HN12	0.40	
YCUM862	0.75	KCCT873	0.70	
Prostate cancer				*148*
LNCaP	4.5	DU145	6.5	
Lung cancer				*146*
H226	<0.1	H322	2	
H358	<0.1	H460	>1000	
N417	35	H526	48	

$^a IC_{50}$, represents concentration of IL4(38-37)-PE38KDAEL at which 50% inhibition of protein synthesis is observed compared to untreated cells.

with recurrent human malignant glioblastoma *(151)*. In this trial, patients received intratumoral infusion of cpIL4-PE by convection-enhanced delivery (CED). CED is a local delivery method in which pressure gradient or bulk flow is used to control an infusate through the extracellular fluid compartment *(152,153)*. Six of nine patients receiving cpIL4-PE showed tumor necrosis. Of six patients, one patient remained disease free for >18 months after the procedure. Based on these initial clinical results, additional clinical trials were subsequently initiated at multiple centers in the United States and Germany to determine the maximum dose related to volume and safety of this agent when injected stereotactically *(154–156)*. cpIL4-PE is also being tested in systemic cancers when injected by intravenous routes for renal cell carcinoma *(157)*. Initial results

Table 4
IL-13R Expression in human cancer cell lines

Cell type	IL-13 binding (sites/cell)[a]	KDa (nM)[a]	Ref
Renal cell carcinoma			
MA-RCC	5000	0.1	*113*
PM-RCC	26,500	0.4	*113*
HL-RCC	150,000	3.1	*113*
WS-RCC	2100	0.2	*113*
Caki-1	140	–[b]	*178*
Ovarian carcinoma			
IGROV-1	1300	0.7	*79*
PA-1	70	–	*185*
Glioblastoma			
A172	23,000	1.6	*162*
U251MG	28,000	2.1	*162*
T98G	550	1.0	*162*
U373MG	16,000	1.8	*162*
U87MG	3000	–	*165*
Kaposi's sarcoma			
KS Y-1	4600	0.9	*164*
KS-imm	9500	3.7	*164*
KS-248	14,000	0.36	*127*
NCB-59	8000	0.53	*127*
Prostate cancer			
PC-3	UD[c]	0.16	*158*
DU145	30	–	*179*
Head and neck cancer			
HN12	5800	–	*126*
SCC-25	7800	–	*167*
KCCT873	7600	–	*167*
A253	190	–	*167*
YCUT891	20	–	*167*
Pancreatic cancer			
PANC-1	160	–	*179*
BxPC3	190		*182*

[a]Data are obtained from the results of binding studies using radiolabeled IL-13.

[b]Not done.

[c]UD, undetectable.

indicate that cpIL4-PE is well tolerated with MTD of 0.016 mg/m^2 in repeated cycles. Reversible transaminitis was observed at higher doses.

4.2. IL-13 Cytotoxins

To target IL-13R on cancer cells *(78,79,124–128,158)* (Table 4), a recombinant fusion IL-13 cytotoxin termed IL13-PE38QQR, IL13-PE38, or IL13-PE was developed *(126,159–161)*. This protein is composed of human IL-13 and a mutated form of

Table 5
Cytotoxicity of IL13-PE38QQR to Human Cancer Cell Lines

Cells (References)	$IC_{50}{}^a$	Cells	IC_{50}
Renal cell carcinoma (160)			
HL-RCC	0.03	MA-RCC	0.34
PM-RCC	0.09	WS-RCC	17.5
Caki–1	350		
Glioblastoma (162,165,179)			
A172	<1	U251MG	<1
T98G	>1000	U373MG	<1
U87MG	600		
Kaposi's sarcoma (127,164)			
KS Y–1	27	KS-imm	380
KS–248	3	NCB-59	8
ARL–13	270		
Prostate cancer (158,179)			
PC–3	50	DU145	750
LNCaP	200		
Head and neck cancer (163,167)			
SCC–25	2.4	KCCT873	4.0
A253	200	YCUT891	520
HN12	<10		
Pancreatic cancer (179,182)			
PANC–1	63	BxPC-3	>1000
CFPAC–1	>1000		

^{a}IC$_{50}$ represents a concentration of IL13-PE38QQR (ng/mL) at which 50% inhibition of protein synthesis is observed compared to untreated cells.

Pseudomonas exotoxin. IL-13 cytotoxins have a potent antitumor activity in IL-13R-expressing tumor cells in vitro *(126,127,158–163)* and in vivo *(164–168)*. In vitro cytotoxic activity of IL-13 cytotoxin is summarized in Table 5. It has been also shown that IL-13 cytotoxin induces apoptotic tumor cell death in immunodeficient mice xenografted with human head and neck tumors and gliomas *(169,170)*. In addition, Li et al. has developed IL-13-diphtheria fusion cytotoxin to target glioma cells *(171)*. Based on encouraging preclinical results, three phase-I/II clinical trials have been initiated to test the tolerability, safety, and effect of IL13-PE38QQR in adults with recurrent malignant glioma *(172–176)*. The first clinical trial involves convection-enhanced delivery (CED) of IL-13 cytotoxin into recurrent unresectable malignant glioma. So far, this route of IL-13 cytotoxin administration appears to be very well tolerated with no neurotoxicity *(172)*. The second clinical trial involves a preresection CED of IL-13 cytotoxin followed by postresection infusion into the brain adjacent to the resection cavity *(173–175)*. This novel route of IL-13 cytotoxin delivery in 27 patients is also well tolerated. In the third clinical trial, IL-13 cytotoxin is infused directly into tumors by CED followed by tumor resection *(176)*. This clinical trial has enrolled 19 patients and this route of IL-13 cytotoxin administration also appears to be safe. All three clinical trials are currently ongoing.

Because we later discovered that low-IL-13R expressing cancer cells lacked the expression of IL-13Rα2 chain, a critical IL-13 binding and internalization component

(129,177), we hypothesized that if cancer cells acquire IL-13Rα2 chain artificially, cytotoxicity of IL-13 cytotoxin to these cancer cells would be increased. To address this, we transiently or stably transfected various cancer cells with cDNA for IL-13Rα2 *(167,178,179)*. Cancer cells transfected with IL-13Rα2 cells acquired highly increased binding avidity to ligand (IL-13) compared with vector only transfected control cells. Consequently, antitumor activity of IL-13 cytotoxin to IL-13Rα2 chain-transfected cancer cells was enhanced in vitro and in vivo *(167,178,179)*. In addition, liposome-mediated direct gene transfer of IL-13Rα2 into prostate, pancreatic, breast, or head and neck tumors in vivo followed by systemic or intratumoral IL-13 cytotoxin therapy in immunodeficient mice demonstrated highly increased tumor killing *(180–183)*. Further studies will be performed to investigate various cancer therapy approaches in which the IL-13Rα2 chain is involved.

5. CONCLUSIONS

In this review article, we have summarized (1) the expression and characteristics of IL-4/13R on human cancer cell lines, (2) effect of IL-4 on cancer cells, (3) effect of IL-13 on cancer cells, and (4) the role of IL-13 in tumor immunity. In addition, cancer therapies utilizing IL-4 or IL-4R-targeted cytotoxin, and IL-13R-targeted cytotoxin are documented. IL-4 and IL-13 share two receptor chains to mediate biologic activities, and both cytokines have direct effects on cancer cells. However, it seems that only IL-13 has a possible role in tumorigenicity and tumor immunity. IL-4R- or IL-13R-directed therapeutic cytotoxins may have a significant role in the treatment of human cancer.

ACKNOWLEDGMENTS

We thank past and current members of the Laboratory of Molecular Tumor Biology, Division of Cellular and Gene Therapies, CBER/FDA for their contributions in various published studies. We are grateful to Drs. S. Rafat Husain and Keith Wonnacott for critical reading of this article.

REFERENCES

1. Minty A, Chalon P, Deroq JM, et al. Interleukin 13 is a new lymphokine regulating inflammatory and immune responses. Nature, 362: 248–250, 1993.
2. Zurawski G, de Vries J. Interleukin 13, an interleukin 4-like cytokine that acts on monocytes and B cells, but not on T cells. Immunol Today, 15: 19–26, 1994.
3. Brombacher F. The role of interleukin-13 in infectious diseases and allergy. BioEssays, 22: 646–656, 2000.
4. Howard M, Farrar J, Hilfiker M, et al. Identification of a T cell-derived B cell stimulatory factor distinct from IL-2. J Exp Med, 155: 914–923, 1982.
5. Paul WE. Interleukin-4: A prototypic immunoregulatory lymphokine. Blood, 77:1859–1870, 1990.
6. Puri RK. Structure and function of interleukin 4 and its receptors. *In:* Cytokines: Interleukins and their receptors. Kurzrock R, Talpaz M, eds., Kluwer Academic Publishers, Norwell, MA, 143–186, 1995.
7. McKenzie ANJ, Culpepper JA, de Waal Malefyt R, et al. Interleukin 13, a T cell-derived cytokine that regulates human monocytes and B-cell function. Proc Natl Acad Sci USA, 90: 3735–3739, 1993.
8. Boulay JJ, Paul WE. The interleukin-4-related lymphokines and their binding to hematopoietin receptors. J Biol Chem, 267: 20525–20528, 1992.
9. Kawakami K, Kawakami M, Snoy PJ, et al. In vivo over-expression of IL-13 receptor α2 chain inhibits tumorigenicity of human breast and pancreatic tumors in immunodeficient mice. J Exp Med, 194: 1743–1754, 2001.

10. de Saint Vis B, Fugier VI, Massacrier C, et al. The cytokine profile expressed by human dendritic cells is dependent on cell subtype and mode of activation. J Immunol, 160: 1666–1676, 1998.

11. Hoshino T, Winkler-Pickett RT, Mason AT, et al. IL-13 production by NK cells: IL-13 producing NK cells are present *in vivo* in the absence of IFN-γ. J Immunol, 162: 51–59, 1999.

12. Kaap U, Yeh W-C, Patterson B, et al. Interleukin 13 is secreted by and stimulates the growth of Hodgkin and Reed-Sternberg cells. J Exp Med, 189: 1939–1945, 1999.

13. Skinnider BF, Elia AJ, Gascoyne RD, et al. Interleukin 13 and interleukin 13 receptor are frequently expressed on Hodgkin and Reed-Sternberg cells of Hodgkin lymphoma. Blood, 97: 250–255, 2001.

14. Ohshima K, Akaiwa M, Umeshita R, et al. Interleukin-13 and interleukin-13 receptor in Hodgkin's disease: Possible autocrine mechanism and involvement in fibrosis. Histopathology, 38: 368–375, 2001.

15. Oshima Y, Puri RK. Suppression of an IL-13 autocrine growth loop in a human Hodgkin/Reed-Sternberg tumor cell line by a novel IL-13 antagonist. Cell Immunol, 211: 37–42, 2001.

16. Obiri NI, Husain SR, Debinski W, et al. Interleukin 13 inhibits growth of human renal cell carcinoma cells independently of the p140 interleukin 4 receptor chain. Clin Cancer Res, 2: 1743–1749, 1996.

17. Zurawski SM, Vega F, Huyghe B, et al. Receptors for interleukin-13 and interleukin-4 are complex and share a novel component that functions in signal transduction. EMBO J, 12: 2663–2670, 1993.

18. de Waal Malefyt R, Figdor CG, Huijbens R, et al. Effect on IL-13 on phenotype, cytokine production, and cytokine function of human monocytes: Comparison with IL-4 and modulation by IFN-γ or IL-10. J Immunol, 151: 6370–6381, 1993.

19. Defrance T, Carayon P, Billian G, et al. Interleukin 13 is a B cell stimulating factor. J Exp Med, 179: 135–143, 1994.

20. Cooks BG, de Waal Malefyt R, Galizzi JP, et al. IL-13 induces proliferation and differentiation of human B cells activated by the CD40 ligand. Int Immunol, 5: 657–663, 1993.

21. Punnonen J, Aversa G, Cooks BG, et al. Interleukin 13 induces interleukin 4-independent IgG_4 and IgE synthesis and CD23 expression by human B cells. Proc Natl Acad Sci USA, 90: 3730–3734, 1993.

22. McKenzie GJ, Emson CL, Bell SE, et al. Impaired development of Th2 cells in IL-13-deficient mice. Immunity, 9: 423–432, 1998.

23. McKenzie GJ, Fallon PG, Emson CL, et al. Simultaneous disruption of interleukin(IL)-4 and IL-13 defines individual roles in T helper cell type 2-mediated responses. J Exp Med, 189: 1565–1572, 1999.

24. McKenzie, A. N. J. Experimental models/tools for the analysis of IL-13 function. In: Brombacher F, ed. *Interleulin-13*. Landes Bioscience, Georgetown, TX. pp. 14–22, 2003.

25. Wills-Karp M, Luyimbazi J, Xu X, et al. Interleukin-13: central mediator of allergic asthma. Science, 282: 2258–2260, 1998.

26. Chiaramonte MG, Donaldson DD, Cheever AW, et al. An IL-13 inhibitor blocks the development of hepatic fibrosis during a T-helper type 2-dominated inflammatory response. J Clin Invest, 104: 777–785, 1999.

27. Li Y, Simons FER, HayGlass KT. Environmental antigen-induced IL-13 responses are elevated among subjects with allergic rhinitis, are independent of IL-4, and are inhibited by endogenous IFN-γ synthesis. J Immunol, 161: 7004–7014, 1998.

28. Pawankar R, Okuda M, Yssel H, et al. Nasal mast cells in perennial allergic rhinitics exhibit increased expression of the FcεRI, CD40L, IL-4, and IL-13, and can induce IgE synthesis in B cells. J Clin Invest, 99: 1492–1499, 1997.

29. AkDais CA, AkDais M, Trautmann A, et al. Immune response in atopic dermatitis. Curr Opin Immunol, 12: 641–646, 2000.

30. Wynn TA. IL-13 effector functions. Annu Rev Immunol, 21: 425–456, 2003.

31. Torigoe T, O'Connor R, Fagard R, et al. Interleukin-4 inhibits IL-2 induced proliferation of a human T-leukemia cell line without interfering with p56-lck kinase activation. Cytokine, 4: 369–376, 1992.

32. Manabe A, Coustan-Smith E, Kumagai M-A, et al. Interleukin-4 induces programmed cell death (apoptosis) in cases of high-risk acute lymphoblastic leukemia. Blood, 83: 1731–1737, 1994.

33. Akashi K, Shibuya T, Harada M, et al. Interleukin 4 suppresses the spontaneous growth of chronic myelomonocytic leukemia cells. J Clin Invest, 88: 223–230, 1991.

34. Luo H, Rubio M, Biron G, et al. Antiproliferative effect of interleukin-4 in B chronic lymphocytic leukemia. J Immunother, 10: 418–425, 1991.

35. Kooten CV, Rensink I, Aarden L, et al. Interleukin-4 inhibits both paracrine and autocrine tumor necrosis factor-α-induced proliferation of B chromic lymphocytic leukemia cells. Blood, 80: 1299–1306, 1992.

36. Andreeff FHM, Gruss H-J, Brach MA, et al. Interleukin-4 inhibits growth of multiple myelomas by suppressing IL-6 expression. Blood, 78: 2070–2074, 1991.
37. Taylor CW, Grogan TM, Salmon SE. Effects of interleukin-4 on the in vitro growth of human lymphoid and plasma cell neoplasms. Blood, 75: 1114–1118, 1990.
38. Defrance T, Fluckiger A-C, Rossi J-F, et al. Antiproliferative effects of IL-4 on freshly isolated non-Hodgkin malignant B-lymphoma cells. Blood, 79: 990–996, 1992.
39. Wagteveld AJ, Zanten AKV, Esselink MT, et al. Expression and regulation of IL-4 receptors on human monocytes and acute myeloblastic leukemia cells. Leukemia, 5: 782–788, 1991.
40. Totpal K, Aggarwal BB. Interleukin-4 potentiates the antiproliferative effects of tumor necrosis factor on various tumor cell lines. Cancer Res, 51: 4266–4270, 1991.
41. Mori N, Yamashita U, Tanaka Y, et al. Interleukin-4 induces proliferation of adult T-cell leukemia cells. Eur J Hematol, 50: 133–140, 1993.
42. Dancescu M, Rubio-Trujillo M, Biron G, et al. Interleukin-4 protects chronic lymphocytic leukemic B cells from death by apoptosis and upregulates Bcl-2 expression. J Exp Med, 176: 1319–1326, 1992.
43. Kay NE, Pittner BT. IL-4 biology: impact on normal and leukemic CLL B cells. Leuk Lymphoma, 44: 897–903, 2003.
44. Pu QQ, Bezwoda WR. Interleukin-4 prevents spontaneous in-vitro apoptosis in chronic lymphatic leukaemia but sensitizes B-CLL cells to melphalan cytotoxicity. Br J Haematol, 98: 413–417, 1997.
45. Obiri NI, Hillman G, Haas GP, et al. Expression of high affinity interleukin-4 receptors on human renal cell carcinoma cells and inhibition of tumor cell growth in vitro by interleukin-4. J Clin Invest, 91: 88–93, 1993.
46. Morisaki T, Yuzuki DH, Lin RT, et al. Interleukin-4 receptor expression and growth inhibition of gastric carcinoma by interleukin-4. Cancer Res, 52: 6059–6065, 1992.
47. Topp MS, Koenigsmann M, Mire-Sluis A, et al. Recombinant human interleukin-4 inhibits growth of some human lung tumor cell lines in vitro and in vivo. Blood, 82: 2837–2844, 1993.
48. Toi M, Bicknel R, Harris AL. Inhibition of colon and breast carcinoma cell growth by interleukin-4. Cancer Res, 52: 275–279, 1992.
49. Obiri NI, Tandon N, Puri RK. Upregulation of intracellular adhesion molecule-1 on human renal cell carcinoma cells by interleukin-4. Int J Cancer, 61: 635–642, 1995.
50. Hillman GG, Puri RK, Kukuruga MA, et al. Growth and major histocompatibility antigen expression regulation by interleukin 4, interferon γ, and tumor necrosis factor α on human renal cell carcinoma. Clin Exp Immunol, 96: 476–483, 1994.
51. Hoon DSB, Banez M, Okun E, et al. Modulation of human melanoma cells by interleukin-4 and in combination with γ-interferon or α-tumor necrosis factor. Cancer Res, 51: 2002–2008, 1991.
52. Hoon DSB, Okun E, Benez M, et al. Interleukin 4 alone with γ-interferon or tumor necrosis factor inhibits cell growth and modulates cell surface antigens on human renal cell carcinomas. Cancer Res, 51: 5687–5693, 1991.
53. Levesque MC, Misukonis MA, O'Loughlin CW, et al. IL-4 and interferon gamma regulate expression of inducible nitric oxide synthase in chronic lymphocytic leukemia cells. Leukemia, 17: 442–450, 2003.
54. Lee SO, Lou W, Hou M, et al. Interleukin-4 enhances prostate-specific antigen expression by activation of the androgen receptor and Akt pathway. Oncogene, 22: 7981–7988, 2003.
55. Myers JN, Yasumura S, Suminami Y, et al. Growth stimulation of human head and neck squamous cells carcinoma cell lines by interleukin 4. Clin Cancer Res, 2: 127–135, 1996.
56. Stassi G, Todaro M, Zerilli M, et al. Thyroid cancer resistance to chemotherapeutic drugs via autocrine production of interleukin-4 and interleukin-10. Cancer Res, 63: 6784–6790, 2003.
57. Sasaki Y, Mita H, Toyota M, et al. Identification of the interleukin 4 receptor α gene as a direct target for p73. Cancer Res, 63: 8145–8152, 2003.
58. Tepper RI, Pattengale PK, Leder P. Murine interleukin-4 displays potent anti-tumor activity in vivo. Cell, 57: 503–512, 1989.
59. Tepper RI, Coffman RL, Leder P. An eosinophil-dependent mechanism for the anti-tumor effect of interleukin-4. Science, 257: 548–551, 1992.
60. Kawakami Y, Rosenberg SA, Lotze MT. Interleukin 4 promotes the growth of tumor-infiltrating lymphocytes cytotoxic for human autologous melanoma. J Exp Med, 168: 2183–2191, 1988.
61. Mule JJ, Smith CA, Rosenberg SA. Interleukin 4 (B cell stimulatory factor 1) can mediate the induction of lymphokine-activated killer cell activity directed against fresh tumor cells. J Exp Med, 166: 792–797, 1987.

62. Puri RK, Finbloom DS, Leland P, et al. Expression of high-affinity IL-4 receptors on murine tumour infiltrating lymphocytes and their up-regulation by IL-2. Immunology, 70: 492–497, 1990.

63. McAdam AJ, Pulaski BA, Storozynsky E, et al. Analysis of the effect of cytokines (interleukins 2, 3, 4, and 6, granulocyte-monocyte colony-stimulating factor, and interferon-gamma) on generation of primary cytotoxic T lymphocytes against a weakly immunogenic tumor. Cell Immunol, 165: 183–192, 1995.

64. Benedetti S, Pirola B, Poliani PL, et al. Dexamethasone inhibits the anti-tumor effect of interleukin 4 on rat experimental gliomas. Gene Ther, 10: 188–192, 2003.

65. Atkins MB, Vachino G, Tilg H, et al. Phase I evaluation of the daily intravenous bolus interleukin-4 in patients with refractory malignancy. J Clin Oncol, 10: 1802–1809, 1992.

66. Gilleece MH, Scarffe JH, Ghosh A, et al. Recombinant human interleukin 4 (IL-4) given as daily subcutaneous injections-a phase I dose escalation toxicity trial. Br J Cancer, 66: 204–210, 1992.

67. Prendiville J, Thatcher N, Lind M, et al. Recombinant human interleukin 4 (IL-4) administered by the intravenous and subcutaneous injections-a phase I toxicity study and pharmacokinetics analysis. Eur J Cancer, 29: 1799–1807, 1993.

68. Whitehead RP, Friedman KDA, Clark DA, et al. Phase I trial of simultaneous administration of interleukin 2 and interleukin 4 subcutaneously. Clin Cancer Res, 1: 1145–1152, 1995.

69. Vokes EE, Figlin R, Hochster H, et al. A phase II study of recombinant human interleukin-4 for advanced or recurrent non-small cell lung cancer. Cancer J Sci Am, 4: 46–51, 1998.

70. Taylor CW, LeBlanc M, Fisher RI, et al. Phase II evaluation of interleukin-4 in patients with non-Hodgkin's lymphoma: A Southwest Oncology Group trial. Anti-Cancer Drugs, 11: 695–700, 2000.

71. Whitehead RP, Lew D, Flanigan RC, et al. Phase II trial of recombinant human interleukin-4 in patients with advanced renal cell carcinoma: A southwest oncology group study. J Immunother, 25: 352–358, 2002.

72. Kiertscher SM, Gitlitz BJ, Figlin RA, et al. Granulocyte/macrophage-colony stimulating factor and interleukin-4 expand and activate type-1 dendritic cells (DC1) when administered in vivo to cancer patients. Int J Cancer, 107: 256–261, 2003.

73. Gitlitz BJ, Figlin RA, Kiertscher SM, et al. Phase I trial of granulocyte macrophage-colony stimulating factor and interleukin-4 as a combined immunotherapy for patients with cancer. J Immunother, 26: 171–178, 2003.

74. Okada H, Pollack IF, Lotze MT, et al. Gene therapy of malignant gliomas: A phase I study of IL-4-HSV-TK gene-modified autologous tumor to elicit an immune response. Hum Gene Ther, 11: 637–653, 2000.

75. Okada H, Pollack IF, Lieberman F, et al. Gene therapy of malignant gliomas: A pilot study of vaccination with irradiated autologous glioma and dendritic cells mixed with IL-4 transduced fibroblasts to elicit an immune response. Hum Gene Ther, 12: 575–595, 2001.

76. Okada H, Lieberman FS, Edington HD, et al. Autologous glioma cell vaccine admixed with interleukin-4 gene transfected fibroblasts in the treatment of recurrent glioblastoma: Preliminary observations in a patient with a favorable response to therapy. J Neuro-Oncol, 64: 13–20, 2003.

77. Okada H, Kuwashima N. Gene therapy and biologic therapy with interleukin-4. Curr Gene Ther, 2: 437–450, 2002.

78. Liu H, Jacobs BS, Liu J, et al. Interleukin-13 sensitivity and receptor phenotypes of human glial cell lines: Non-neoplastic glia and low-grade astrocytoma differ from malignant glioma. Cancer Immunol Immunother, 49: 319–324, 2000.

79. Murata T, Obiri NI, Puri RK. Human ovarian-carcinoma cell lines express IL-4 and IL-13 receptors: Comparison between IL-4- and IL-13-induced signal transduction. Int J Cancer, 70: 230–240, 1997.

80. Hu HM, Urba WJ, Fox BA. Gene-modified tumor vaccine with therapeutic potential shifts tumor-specific T cell response from a type 2 to a type 1 cytokine profile. J Immunol, 161: 3033–3041, 1998.

81. Bernard J, Treton D, Vermot-Desroches C, et al. Expression of interleukin 13 receptor in glioma and renal cell carcinoma: IL13Rα2 as a decoy receptor for IL13. Lab Invest, 81: 1223–1231, 2001.

82. Serve H, Oelmann E, Herweg A, et al. Inhibition of proliferation and clonal growth of human breast cancer cells by interleukin 13. Cancer Res, 56: 3583–3588, 1996.

83. Blais Y, Zhao C, Huber M, et al. Growth-independent induction of spermidine transport by IL-4 and IL-13 in ZR-75-1 human breast cancer cells. Int J Cancer, 67: 532–538, 1996.

84. Blais Y, Gingras S, Haagensen DE, et al. Interleukin-4 and interleukin-13 inhibit estrogen-induced breast cancer cell proliferation and stimulate GCDFP-15 expression in human breast cancer cells. Mol Cell Endocrinol, 121: 11–18, 1996.

85. Lebel-Binay S, Laguerre B, Quintin-Colonna F, et al. Experimental gene therapy of cancer using tumor cells engineered to secrete interleukin-13. Eur J Immunol, 25: 2340–2348, 1995.

86. Kanai T, Watanabe M, Hayashi A, et al. Regulatory effect of interleukin-4 and interleukin-13 on colon cancer cell adhesion. Br J Cancer, 82: 1717–1723, 2000.

87. Riemann D, Kehlen A, Langner J. Stimulation of the expression and the enzyme activity of aminopeptidase N/CD13 and dipeptidylpeptidase IV/CD26 on human renal cell carcinoma cells and renal tubular epithelial cells by T cell-derived cytokines, such as IL-4 and IL-13. Clin Exp Immunol, 100: 277–283, 1995.

88. Huang M, Wang J, Lee P, et al. Human non-small cell lung cancer cells express a type 2 cytokine pattern. Cancer Res, 55: 3847–3853, 1995.

89. Kawakami M, Leland P, Kawakami K, et al. Mutation and functional analysis of IL-13 receptors in human malignant glioma cells. Oncol Res, 12: 459–467, 2001.

90. Volpert OV, Fong T, Koch AE, et al. Inhibition of angiogenesis by interleukin 4. J Exp Med, 188: 1039–1046, 1998.

91. Bruserud O. Effects of interleukin-13 on cytokine secretion by human acute myelogenous leukemia blasts. Leukemia, 10: 1497–1503, 1996.

92. Bruserud O, Pawelec G. Interleukin-13 secretion by normal and posttransplant T lymphocytes; in vitro studies of cellular immune responses in the presence of acute leukemia blast cells. Cancer Immunol Immunother, 45: 45–52, 1997.

93. Benard N, Duvert V, Banchereau J, et al. Interleukin-13 inhibits the proliferation of normal and leukemic human B-cell precursors. Blood, 84: 2253–2260, 1994.

94. Fior R, Vita N, Raphael M et al. Interleukin-13 gene expression by malignant and EBV-transformed human B lymphocytes. Eur Cytokine Netw, 5: 593–600, 1994.

95. Denizot Y, Turlure P, Bordessoule D, et al. Serum IL-10 and IL-13 concentrations in patients with haematological malignancies. Cytokine, 11: 634–635, 1999.

96. Kacha AK, Fallarino F, Markiewicz MA, et al. Spontaneous rejection of poorly immunogenic P1.HTR tumors by Stat-6 deficient mice. J Immunol, 165: 6024–6028, 2000.

97. Ostrand-Rosenberg S, Grusby MJ, Clements VK. STAT6-deficient mice have enhanced tumor immunity to primary and metastatic mammary carcinoma. J Immunol, 165: 6015–6019, 2000.

98. Ostrand-Rosenberg S, Clements VK, Terabe M, et al. Resistance to metastatic disease in STAT6-deficient mice requires hemopoietic and nonhemopoietic cells and is IFN-gamma dependent. J Immunol, 169: 5796–5804, 2002.

99. Terabe M, Matsui S, Noben-Trauth N, et al. NKT cell-mediated repression of tumor immunosurveillance by IL-13 and the IL-4R-STAT6 pathway. Nat Immunol, 1: 515–520, 2000.

100. Terabe M, Matsui S, Park JM, et al. Transforming growth factor-β production and myeloid cells are an effector mechanism through which CD1d-restricted T cells block cytotoxic T lymphocyte-mediated tumor immunosurveillance: Abrogation prevents tumor recurrence. J Exp Med, 198: 1741–1752, 2003.

101. van Sandick JW, Boermeester MA, Gisbertz SS, et al. Lymphocyte subsets and Th1/Th2 immune responses in patients with adenocarcinoma of the oesophagus or oesophagogastric junction: Relation to pTNM stage and clinical outcome. Cancer Immunol Immunother, 52: 617–624, 2003.

102. Ito N, Nakamura H, Tanaka Y, et al. Lung carcinoma: Analysis of T helper type 1 and 2 cells and T cytotoxic type 1 and 2 cells by intracellular cytokine detection with flow cytometry. Cancer, 85: 2359–2367, 1999.

103. Okano F, Storkus WJ, Chambers WH, et al. Identification of a novel HLA-A*0201-restricted, cytotoxic T lymphocyte epitope in a human glioma-associated antigen, interleukin 13 receptor α2 chain. Clin Cancer Res, 8: 2851–2855, 2002.

104. Idzerda RL, March CJ, Mosley B, et al. Human interleukin 4 receptor confers biological responsiveness and defines a novel receptor superfamily. J Exp Med, 171: 861–873, 1990.

105. Russell SM, Keegan AD, Harada N, et al. Interleukin-2 receptor gamma chain: A functional component of the interleukin-4 receptor. Science, 262: 1880–1883, 1993.

106. Kondo M, Takeshita T, Ishii N, et al. Sharing of interleukin-2 (IL-2) receptor gc chain between receptors for IL-2 and IL-4. Science, 262: 1874–1877, 1993.

107. Noguchi M, Nakamura Y, Russell SM, et al. Interleukin-2 receptor γ chain: A functional component of interleukin-7 receptor. Science, 262: 1877–1880, 1993.

108. Giri JG, Ahdieh M, Eisenman J, et al. Utilization of beta and gamma chains of the IL-2 receptor by novel cytokine IL-15. EMBO J, 13: 2822–2830, 1994.

109. Aman MJ, Tayebi N, Obiri NI, et al. cDNA cloning and characterization of the human interleukin-13 receptor α chain. J Biol Chem, 271: 29,265–29,270, 1996.

110. Obiri NI, Puri RK. Characterization of interleukin-4 receptors expressed on human renal cell carcinoma cells. Oncol Res, 6: 419–427, 1994

111. Obiri NI, Siegel JP, Varricchio F, et al. Expression and function of high affinity interleukin-4 receptors on human melanoma, ovarian and breast carcinoma cells. Clin Exp Immunol, 95: 148–155, 1994.

112. Murata T, Noguchi PD, Puri RK. Receptors for interleukin (IL) -4 do not associate with the common γ chain, and IL-4 induce the phosphorylation of JAK2 tyrosine kinase in human colon carcinoma cells. J Biol Chem, 270: 30,829–30,836, 1995.

113. Obiri NI, Debinski W, Leonard WJ, et al. Receptor for interleukin 13: Interaction with interleukin 4 by a mechanism that does not involve the common γ chain shared by receptors for interleukins 2, 4, 7, 9, and 15. J Biol Chem, 270: 8797–8804, 1995.

114. Murata T, Taguchi J, Puri RK. Interleukin-13 receptor α′ chain but not α chain: A functional component of interleukin-4 receptor. Blood, 91: 3884–3891, 1998.

115. Nelms K, Keegan AD, Zamorano J, et al. The IL-4 receptor: Signaling mechanisms and biologic functions. Annu Rev Immunol, 17: 701–738, 1999.

116. Murata T, Obiri NI, Puri RK. Structure of and signal transduction through interleukin 4 and interleukin 13 receptors. Int J Mol Med, 1: 551–557, 1998.

117. Kelly-Welch AE, Hanson EM, Boothby MR, et al. Interleukin-4 and interleukin-13 signaling connections maps. Science, 300: 1527, 1528, 2003.

118. Hölscher C. Interleukin-13: Genes, receptors and signal transduction. In: Interleukin-13, Ed. Brombacher F. Landes Bioscience, Georgetown, TX. pp. 1–8, 2003.

119. Hilton DJ, Zhang JG, Metcalf D, et al. Cloning and characterization of a binding subunit of the interleukin 13 receptor that is also a component of the interleukin 4 receptor. Proc Natl Acad Sci USA, 93: 497–501, 1996.

120. Miloux B, Laurent P, Bonnin O, et al. Cloning of the human IL-13Rα1 chain and reconstitution with the IL-4Rα of a functional IL-4/IL-13 receptor complex. FEBS Lett, 401: 163–166, 1997.

121. Niu Y, Murata T, Watanabe K, et al. MIP-T3 associates with IL-13Rα1 and suppress STAT6 activation in response to IL-13 stimulation. FEBS Lett, 550: 139–143, 2003.

122. Caput D, Laurent P, Kaghad M, et al. Cloning and characterization of a specific interleukin (IL)-13 binding protein structurally related to the IL-5 receptor α chain. J Biol Chem, 271: 16,921–16,926, 1996.

123. Donaldson DD, Whitters MJ, Fitz LJ, et al. The murine IL-13 receptor α2: Molecular cloning, characterization, and comparison with murine IL-13 receptor α1. J Immunol, 161: 2317–2324, 1998.

124. Kawakami K, Puri RK. Interleukin-13 and cancer. In: Interleukin-13, Ed. Brombacher F, Landes Bioscience, Georgetown, TX, pp. 65–78, 2003.

125. Joshi BH, Plautz GE, Puri RK. IL-13 receptor α chain: A novel tumor associated transmembrane protein in primary explants of human malignant gliomas. Cancer Res, 60: 1168–1172, 2000.

126. Joshi BH, Kawakami K, Leland P, et al. Heterogeneity in interleukin-13 receptor expression and subunit structure in squamous cell carcinoma of head and neck: Differential sensitivity to chimeric fusion proteins comprised of interleukin-13 and a mutated form of Pseudomonas exotoxin. Clin Cancer Res, 8: 1948–1956, 2002.

127. Husain SR, Obiri NI, Gill P, et al. Receptor for interleukin 13 on AIDS-associated Kaposi's sarcoma cells serves as a new target for a potent Pseudomonas exotoxin-based chimeric toxin protein. Clin Cancer Res, 3: 151–156, 1997.

128. Kawakami M, Kawakami K, Kasperbauer JL, et al. Interleukin-13 receptor α2 chain in human head and neck cancer serves as a unique diagnostic marker. Clin Cancer Res, 9: 6381–6388, 2003.

129. Kawakami K, Taguchi J, Murata T, et al. The interleukin-13 receptor α2 chain: An essential component for binding and internalization but not for interleukin-13-induced signal transduction through the STAT6 pathway. Blood, 97: 2673–2679, 2001.

130. Rahaman SO, Sharma P, Harbor PC, et al. IL-13Rα2, a decoy receptor for IL-13 acts as an inhibitor of IL-4-dependent signal transduction in glioblastoma cells. Cancer Res, 62: 1103–1109, 2002.

131. Obiri NI, Murata T, Debinski W, et al. Modulation of interleukin (IL)-13 binding and signaling by the γ_c chain of the IL-2 receptor. J Biol Chem, 272: 20,251–20,258, 1997.

132. Kuznetsov VA, Puri RK. Kinetic analysis of high affinity forms of interleukin (IL)-13 receptors: suppression of IL-13 binding by IL-2 receptor γ chain. Biophys J, 77: 154–172, 1999.

133. Pastan I, Chaudhary V, FitzGerald DJ. Recombinant toxins as novel therapeutic agents. Annu Rev Biochem, 61: 331–354, 1992.

134. Puri RK, Ogata M, Leland P, et al. Expression of high affinity IL4 receptors on murine sarcoma cells and receptor mediated cytotoxicity of tumor cells to chimeric protein between IL-4 and Pseudomonas extoxin. Cancer Res, 51: 3011–3017, 1991.

135. Puri RK, Leland P, Kreitman RJ, et al. Human neurological cancer cells express interleukin-4 (IL-4) receptors which are targets for the toxic effects of IL4-Pseudomonas exotoxin chimeric protein. Int J Cancer, 58: 574–581, 1994.

136. Kawakami K, Kawakami M, Puri RK. Overexpressed cell surface interleukin-4 receptor molecules can be successfully targeted for anti-tumor cytotoxin therapy. Crit Rev Immunol, 21: 299–310, 2001.

137. Kawakami M, Kawakami K, Puri RK. Interleukin-4-Pseudomonas exotoxin chimeric fusion protein for malignant glioma therapy. J Neuro-Oncol, 65: 15–25, 2003.

138. Kreitman RJ, Puri RK, Pastan I. A circularly permuted recombinant interleukin 4 toxin with increased activity. Proc Natl Acad Sci USA, 91: 6889–6893, 1994.

139. Kreitman RJ, Puri RK, Pastan I. Increased anti-tumor activity of a circularly permuted interleukin 4-toxin in mice with interleukin 4 receptor-bearing human carcinoma. Cancer Res, 55: 3357–3363, 1995.

140. Puri RK, Hoon DS, Leland P, et al. Preclinical development of a recombinant toxin containing circularly permuted interleukin-4 and truncated Pseudomonas exotoxin for therapy of malignant astrocytoma, Cancer Res, 56: 5631–5637, 1996.

141. Puri RK, Leland P, Obiri NI, et al. An improved circularly permuted interleukin 4-toxin is highly cytotoxic to human renal cell carcinoma cells. Cell Immunol, 171: 80–86, 1996.

142. Husain SR, Gill P, Kreitman RJ, et al. Interleukin-4 receptor expression on AIDS-associated Kaposi's sarcoma cells and their targeting by a chimeric protein comprised of circularly permuted interleukin-4 and Pseudomonas exotoxin. Mol Med, 3: 327–338, 1997.

143. Husain SR, Kreitman RJ, Pastan I, et al. Interleukin-4 receptor-directed cytotoxin therapy of AIDS-associated Kaposi's sarcoma tumors in xenografted model. Nat Med, 5: 817–822, 1999.

144. Leland P, Taguchi J, Husain SR, et al. Human breast carcinoma cells express type II IL-4 receptors and are sensitive to anti-tumor activity of a chimeric IL-4-Pseudomonas exptoxin fusion protein in vitro and in vivo. Mol Med, 6: 165–178, 2000.

145. Husain SR, Behari N, Kreitman RJ, et al. Complete regression of established human glioblastoma tumor xenograft by interleukin-4 toxin therapy. Cancer Res, 58: 3649–3653, 1998.

146. Kawakami M, Kawakami K, Stepensky VA, et al. Interleukin 4 receptor on human lung cancer: A molecular target for cytotoxin therapy. Clin Cancer Res, 8: 3503–3511, 2002.

147. Strome SE, Kawakami K, Alejandro D, et al. Interleukin 4 receptor-directed cytotoxin therapy for human head and neck squamous cell carcinoma in animal models. Clin Cancer Res, 8: 281–286, 2002.

148. Husain SR, Kawakami K, Kawakami M, et al. Interleukin-4 receptor-targeted cytotoxin therapy of androgen-dependent and -independent prostate carcinoma in xenograft models. Mol Cancer Ther, 2: 245–254, 2003.

149. Kawakami K, Kawakami M, Husain SR, et al. Effect of interleukin-4 cytotoxin on breast tumor growth after in vivo gene transfer of IL-4Rα chain. Clin Cancer Res, 9: 1826–1836, 2003.

150. Kawakami K, Kawakami M, Husain SR, et al. Targeting interleukin-4 receptors for effective pancreatic cancer therapy. Cancer Res, 62: 3575–3580, 2002.

151. Rand RW, Kreitman RJ, Patronas N, et al. Intratumoral administration of recombinant circularly permuted Interleukin-4-Pseudomonas exotoxin in patients with high-grade glioma. Clin Cancer Res, 6: 2157–2165, 2000.

152. Bobo RH, Laske DW, Akbasak A, et al. Convection-enhanced delivery to macromolecules in the brain. Proc Natl Acad Sci USA, 91: 2076–2080, 1994.

153. Laske DW, Youle RJ, Oldfield EH. Tumor regression with regional distribution of the targeted toxin TF-CRM107 in patients with malignant brain tumors. Nat Med, 3: 1362–1368, 1997.

154. Weber F, Asher A, Bucholz R, et al. Safety, tolerability, and tumor response of IL4-Pseudomonas exotoxin (NBI-3001) in patients with recurrent malignant glioma. J Neuro-Oncol, 64: 125–137, 2003.

155. Weber FW, Floeth F, Asher A, et al. Local convection enhanced delivery of IL4-Pseudomonas exotoxin (NBI-3001) for treatment of patients with recurrent malignant glioma. Acta Neurochir Suppl, 88: 93–103, 2003.

156. Rainov NG, Heidecke V. Long term survival in a patient with recurrent malignant glioma treated with intratumoral infusion of an IL4-targeted toxin (NBI-3001). J Neuro-Oncol, 66; 197–201, 2004.

157. Garland L, Gitlitz B, Ebbinghaus S, et al. Phase I trial of intravenous IL-4 Pseudomonas exotoxin protein (NBI-3001) in patients with advanced solid tumors that express the IL-4 receptor. J Immunother 28: 376–381, 2005.

158. Maini A, Hillman G, Haas GP, et al. Interleukin-13 receptors on human prostate carcinoma cell lines represent a novel target for a chimeric protein composed of IL-13 and a mutated form of Pseudomonas exotoxin. J Urol, 158: 948–953, 1997.

159. Debinski W, Obiri NI, Pastan I, et al. A novel chimeric protein composed of interleukin 13 and Pseudomonas exotoxin is highly cytotoxic to human carcinoma cells expressing receptors for interleukin 13 and interleukin 4. J Biol Chem, 270: 16,775–16,780, 1995.

160. Puri RK, Leland P, Obiri NI, et al. Targeting of interleukin-13 receptor on human renal cell carcinoma cells by a recombinant chimeric protein composed of interleukin-13 and a truncated form of Pseudomonas exotoxin A (PE38QQR). Blood, 87: 4333–4339, 1996.

161. Husain SR, Puri RK. Interleukin-13 receptor-directed cytotoxin for malignant glioma therapy: From bench to bedside. J Neuro-Oncol, 65: 37–48, 2003.

162. Debinski W, Obiri NI, Powers SK, et al. Human glioma cells overexpress receptors for interleukin 13 and are extremely sensitive to a novel chimeric protein composed of interleukin 13 and pseudomonas exotoxin. Clin Cancer Res, 1: 1253–1258, 1995.

163. Kawakami M, Kawakami K, Puri RK. Apoptotic pathways of cell death induced by an interleukin-13 receptor-targeted recombinant cytotoxin in head and neck cancer cells. Cancer Immunol Immunother, 50: 691–700, 2002.

164. Husain SR, Puri RK. Interleukin-13 fusion cytotoxin as a potent targeted agent for AIDS-Kaposi's sarcoma xenograft. Blood, 95: 3506–3513, 2000.

165. Husain SR, Joshi BH, Puri RK. Interleukin-13 receptor as a unique target for anti-glioblastoma therapy. Int J Cancer, 92: 168–175, 2001.

166. Ishii KJ, Kawakami K, Gursel I, et al. Anti-tumor therapy with bacterial DNA and toxin: Complete regression of established tumor by liposomal CpG ODN plus IL-13 cytotoxin. Clin Cancer Res, 9: 6516–6522, 2003.

167. Kawakami K, Kawakami M, Joshi BH, et al. Interleukin-13 receptor targeted cancer therapy in an immunodeficient animal model of human head and neck cancer. Cancer Res, 61: 6194–6200, 2001.

168. Kawakami K, Husain SR, Kawakami M, et al. Improved anti-tumor activity and safety of interleukin-13 receptor targeted cytotoxin by systemic continuous administration in head and neck cancer xenograft model. Mol Med, 8: 487–492, 2002.

169. Kawakami M, Kawakami K, Puri RK. Intratumoral administration of interleukin 13 receptor-targeted cytotoxin induces apoptotic cell death in human malignant glioma tumor xenografts. Mol Cancer Ther, 1: 999–1007, 2002.

170. Kawakami M, Kawakami K, Puri RK. Tumor regression mechanisms by interleukin-13 receptor-targeted cancer therapy involve apoptotic pathways. Int J Cancer, 103: 45–52, 2003.

171. Li C, Hall WA, Jin N, et al. Targeting glioblastoma multiforme with an IL-13/diphtheria toxin fusion protein in vitro and in vivo in nude mice. Protein Eng, 15: 419–427, 2002.

172. Weingart J, Strauss LC, Grossman SA, et al. Phase I/II study: intratumoral infusion of IL13-PE38QQR cytotoxin for recurrent supratentorial malignant glioma. Neuro-oncol, 4: 379, 2002.

173. Prados M, Lang F, Strauss L, et al. Pre and post-resection interstitial infusions of IL13-PE38QQR cytotoxin: Phase I study in recurrent respectable malignant glioma. First Qudrennial meeting- World Federation of Neuro-Oncology, Washington, DC, November 15–17, 2001.

174. Lang F, Kunwar S, Strauss L, et al. A clinical study of convection-enhanced delivery of IL13-PE38QQR cytotoxin pre- and post-resection of recurrent GBM. 70th annual meeting of the American Association of Neurological Surgeons (AANS), Chicago, IL, April 6–11, 2002.

175. Kunwar S, Prados M, Chang S, et al. Peritumoral convection-enhanced delivery of IL13-PE38QQR in patients with recurrent malignant glioma – Phase I interim results. Society of Neuro-oncology annual meeting, 2003.

176. Ram Z, Mehdorn M, Westphal M, et al. Phase I/II study of intratumoral convection-enhanced delivery of IL13-PE38QQR cytotoxin for recurrent malignant glioma followed by planned tumor resection. Society of Neuro-oncology annual meeting, Abstract. 403, 2003.

177. Kawakami K, Takeshita F, Puri RK. Identification of distinct roles for a dileucine and a tyrosine internalization motif in the interleukin (IL)-13 binding component IL-13 receptor α2 chain. J Biol Chem, 276: 25,114–25,120, 2001.

178. Kawakami K, Joshi BH, Puri RK. Sensitization of cancer cells to interleukin-13-Pseudomonas exotoxin induced cell death by gene transfer of IL-13 receptor α chain. Hum Gene Ther, 11: 1829–1835, 2000.

179. Kawakami K, Husain SR, Bright RK, et al. Gene transfer of interleukin 13 receptor α2 chain dramatically enhances the anti-tumor effect of IL-13 receptor-targeted cytotoxin in human prostate cancer xenografts. Cancer Gene Ther, 8: 861–868, 2001.

180. Kawakami K, Kawakami M, Puri RK. Cytokine receptor as a sensitizer for targeted cancer therapy. Anti-Cancer Drugs, 13: 693–699, 2002.

181. Kawakami K, Kawakami M, Puri RK. Interleukin-13 receptor-targeted cytotoxin cancer therapy leads to complete eradication of tumors with the aid of phagocytic cells in nude mice model of human cancer. J Immunol, 169: 7119–7126, 2002.

182. Kawakami K, Kawakami M, Husain SR, et al. Potent anti-tumor activity of IL-13 cytotoxin in human pancreatic tumors engineered to express IL-13 receptor α2 chain in vivo. Gene Ther, 10: 1116–1128, 2003.

183. Kawakami K, Kawakami M, Puri RK. Specifically targeted killing of interleukin-13 receptor-expressing breast cancer by IL-13 fusion cytotoxin in animal model of human disease. Mol Cancer Ther, 3: 137–147, 2003.

184. Kawakami K, Leland P, Puri RK. Structure, function, and targeting of interleukin 4 receptors on human head and neck carcinoma cells. Cancer Res, 60: 2981–2987, 2000.

185. Obiri N, Leland P, Murata T, et al. The IL-13 receptor structure differs on various cell types and may share more than one component with IL-4 receptor. J Immunol, 158: 756–764, 1997.

8   Interleukin-6 and Castleman's Disease

Norihiro Nishimoto

CONTENTS

1. INTRODUCTION

In 1956, Castleman et al. reported 13 patients who had localized mediastinal lymph node hyperplasia resembling thymoma *(1)*. The characteristic features of the hyperplastic lymph nodes were follicular hyperplasia with a large germinal center penetrated by branching hyaline blood vessels and proliferation of hyaline capillaries with endothelial hyperplasia in the interfollicular areas. Thereafter, Flendrig et al. and Keller et al. independently reported another morphologic type of the benign giant lymph node characterized by hyperplastic germinal centers and intervening sheets of plasma cells *(2,3)*. The former is referred to as the hyaline-vascular type (HV type) and the latter as the plasma cell type (PC type) of Castleman's disease.

"Multicentric" variant of Castleman's disease features the involvement of multiple lymphoid sites. The variant was reported as "multicentric" giant lymph node hyperplasia, "multicentric" angiofollicular lymph node hyperplasia, or angiofollicular and plasmacytic polyadenopathy *(4,5,6,7)*. Most of multicentric Castleman's disease (MCD) have been shown to be PC type and frequently associated with systemic manifestations.

Interleukin-6 (IL-6) is a pleiotropic cytokine with a wide range of biological activities in the immune regulation, hematopoiesis, inflammation, and oncogenesis *(8)*. PC type of Castleman's disease has been reported to be associated with deregulated overproduction of IL-6 *(9,10,11)* and the overproduction of IL-6 is responsible for the systemic manifestation of the disease.

From: *Cancer Drug Discovery and Development,*
Cytokines in the Genesis and Treatment of Cancer
Edited by: M. A. Caligiuri and M. T. Lotze © Humana Press Inc., Totowa, NJ

Table 1
Clinical Abnormalities in PC Type Castleman's Disease

Clinical signs
   Lymphadenopathy
   Fever
   General fatigue
   Body weight loss
   Anorexia
   Night sweats
   Splenomegaly
   Interstitial pneumonia
   Skin disorder
   AA amyloidosis
Laboratory findings
   Acceleration of ESR
   Elevation of acute phase proteins (CRP, fibrinogen, SAA, etc.)
   Hypoalbuminemia
   Anemia
   Low cholesterol levels
   Thrombocytosis
   Hyper γ-globulinemia
   Proteinuria
   Autoantibodies

1.1. Clinical Features of Castleman's disease

The relationship between HV type and PC type of Castleman's disease remains unclear. In addition to the morphological differences, HV type is characterized as an asymptomatic slowly growing mass, while PC type is associated with systemic inflammatory symptoms. Thus, some say the two types may be distinct. On the other hand, a mixed hyaline–vascular and plasma cell type or transitional form is also observed. Therefore, others say the PC type and HV type diseases may represent either two consecutive stages or two different expressions of the same inflammatory process *(2,3,12)*.

Although HV type of Castleman's disease is mostly asymptomatic, patients with PC type Castleman's disease, regardless of localized or multicentric form, are frequently associated with systemic manifestations such as slight fever, fatigue, appetite loss, body weight loss, peripheral neuropathy, skin rashes and abnormal laboratory findings such as hypochromic anemia, hypoalbuminemia, hypergammaglobulinemia, and an increase in acute phase proteins *(2,3,6,13,14)*. They are often complicated with nephritic syndrome, amyloidosis, Kaposi's sarcoma, and non-Hodgkin's lymphoma. Lymphocytic interstitial pneumonia was also frequently associated *(15; see* Table 1.)

Polyneuropathy organomegaly endocrinopathy M-protein skin change (POEMS) syndrome (also known as Takatsuki's disease or Crow-Fukase syndrome) intersects multicentric Castleman's disease according to both the pathological and clinical findings *(16)*, although PC type Castleman's disease usually presents polyclonal hypergammaglobulinemia while POEMS syndrome has a monoclonal gammopathy. In some reports, molecular genetic analysis has revealed rearrangement of immunoglobulin genes in lymph nodes of PC type Castleman's disease suggesting a transition from nonmalignant B-cell proliferation to malignant lymphoma *(6,17,18)*.

Localized Castleman's disease is more frequently reported in younger ages while multicentric Castleman's disease is more commonly seen in middle-age or older individuals *(3,19)*. In cases of localized Castleman's disease, various clinical abnormalities often resolve after excision of the affected lymph nodes *(9,11)*. On the other hand, the multicentric Castleman's disease requires systemic therapy such as corticosteroids, cytotoxic agents, or combination of them, although very limited information for the treatment is available *(6,13,14,20,21)*. Patients with multicentric Castleman's disease are often refractory to the treatment, and consequently the prognosis for such patients is poor.

2. IL-6 AND PC TYPE OF CASTLEMAN'S DISEASE

2.1. Pleiotropic Function of IL-6

IL-6 was originally identified as an antigen nonspecific B-cell differentiation factor in the culture supernatants of mitogen- or antigen-stimulated peripheral blood mononuclear cells which induced B-cells to produce immunoglobulins *(22,23)*, and then named B-cell stimulatory factor-2 (BSF-2). The cDNA encoding human BSF-2 was cloned in 1986 *(24)*. Simultaneously, interferon $\beta2$ *(25,26)* and a 26kDa protein *(27)* in fibroblasts were independently cloned by different groups and found to be identical to BSF-2. Later, a hybridoma/plasmacytoma growth factor *(28,29)* and a hepatocyte stimulating factor *(30,31,32)* were also proven to be the same molecule as BSF-2. Various names were initially used for this molecule because of its multiple biological activities, and thereafter, the common name of IL-6 was adopted.

IL-6 has been shown to be produced by T-cells, B-cells, monocytes, fibroblasts, endothelial cells, and several kinds of tumor cells, and also has a wide range of biological activities on various target cells *(8)*. IL-6 is a differentiation factor not only for B-cells but also for T-cells *(33)* and macrophages *(34)*. It differentiates megakaryocytes to produce platelets *(35)* and acts on hematopoietic stem cells synergistically with IL-3 to support the formation of multi-lineage blast cell colonies *(36,37)*. IL-6 stimulates hepatocytes to produce acute phase proteins such as C-reactive protein (CRP), fibrinogen, α1-antitrypsin, and serum amyloid A (SAA), while it simultaneously suppresses production of albumin *(30,31,32)*. It induces leukocytosis and fever when it is administered *in vivo (38)*. IL-6 also acts as a growth factor for mesangial cells *(39)*, and various tumor cells such as malignant lymphoma cells *(40)*, multiple myeloma cells *(41)*, and Kaposi's sarcoma cells *(42)*.

2.2. Mouse Models for Multicentric Castleman's Disease

IL-6 transgenic mice were produced by the introduction of the human IL-6 gene into C57BL/6 mice under the transcriptional control of the immunoglobulin μ heavy chain enhancer (Eμ) *(43)* or histocompatibility class I (H2-Ld) promoter *(44)*. The IL-6 transgenic mice showed hypergammaglobulinemia with massive plasmacytosis in the spleen and lymph nodes, increase in serum acute phase proteins such as fibrinogen, decrease in serum albumin, increase in the number of megakaryocytes in the bone marrow, mesangial proliferative glomerulonephritis *(43,44)*, and lymphocytic interstitial pneumonia *(45)*. These abnormalities are very consistent with those of multicentric Castleman's disease in humans. This evidence strongly suggested that IL-6 overproduction is responsible for the systemic manifestations of multicentric Castleman's disease.

In addition, mice lacking C/EBP beta (nuclear factor-IL6, NF-IL6), a key element of IL-6 signaling as well as an important transcriptional regulator of the IL-6 gene *(46)*,

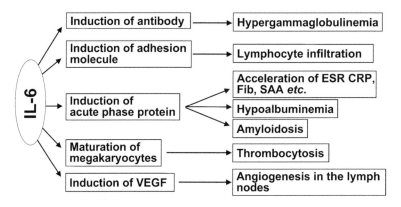

Fig. 1. Pathological roles of IL-6 in multicentric Castleman's disease.

showed increase in serum IL-6 and a nearly identical phenotype to that of multicentric Castleman's disease *(47)*. The finding also suggests the involvement of IL-6 overproduction in Castleman's disease although it is unknown whether or not the abnormality in the C/EBP beta exists in human disease.

2.3. Pathologic Significance of IL-6 in Castleman's Disease

The clinical and laboratory features of PC type Castleman's disease and the observation that clinical abnormalities disappear after the resection of the affected lymph nodes *(3,9,11,13)*, suggesting that a pro-inflammatory cytokine produced within the diseased nodes might be involved in this process. Yoshizaki et al. reported that large amounts of IL-6 were produced by the activated B-cells in the germinal centers of hyperplastic lymph nodes in patients with PC type of Castlemen's disease, without any significant production of other cytokines. Furthermore, in a patient with localized form of Castleman's disease, serum IL-6 level was immediately normalized after excision of the affected lymph node. There was correlation between serum IL-6 levels and lymphadenopathy, hypergammaglobulinemia, increase in acute phase proteins and clinical symptoms *(9)*. Thus, the constitutive production of IL-6 by B-cells in germinal centers of hyperplastic lymph nodes of Castleman's disease were thought to be responsible for the various clinical abnormalities (Fig. 1). Therapeutic strategies aimed at inhibiting IL-6 at the cellular level are described below and support this notion.

3. KAPOSI'S SARCOMA-ASSOCIATED HERPESVIRUS AND CASTLEMAN'S DISEASE

Kaposi's sarcoma-associated herpesvirus (also known as human herpesvirus type 8, KSHV/HHV-8) was identified from the skin lesion of the Kaposi's sarcoma patients *(48)*. The virus was etiologically associated not only with Kaposi's sarcoma but also with Castleman's disease *(49,50,51)*, predominantly in patients infected with human immunodeficiency virus (HIV). This KSHV/HHV-8 viral genome is a linear double-stranded DNA containing numerous open reading frames including genes homologous to cellular genes *(52)*. An interesting fact is that the K2 gene of KSHV/HHV-8 encodes a protein (viral IL-6, vIL-6), that has 24.8% homology with human IL-6 *(53,54,55)* and possesses biologic activities reminiscent of human IL-6. IL-6 is a growth factor for

Kaposi's sarcoma cells *(42)* and also a key factor for Castleman's disease. Together with the evidence that Kaposi's sarcoma is frequently associated with Castleman's disease *(6,13,14,56,57,58)*, KSHV/HHV-8 and its vIL-6 product have been thought to be an etiologic agent for Castleman's disease.

When vIL-6 is expressed in mice, it accelerates hematopoiesis and also induces vascular endothelial growth factor production resulting in the enhanced angiogenesis *(59,60)* that was implicated in the pathogenesis of Kaposi's sarcoma and Castleman's disease.

KSHV/HHV-8 positive cells are arrayed around the periphery of the germinal centers of the lymph nodes in KSHV(+) Castleman's disease, whereas the human IL-6 expression was detected predominantly in the germinal centers and rare in surrounding cells *(61)*. Mori et al. reported the possible existence of paracrine mechanism how vIL-6 stimulates human IL-6 production in the lymph node and the enhanced human IL-6 may be responsible for the systemic manifestations of the disease *(62)*.

Despite the fact that KSHV/HHV-8 is etiologically associated with multicentric Castleman's disease, there are some patients without KSHV/HHV-8 infection. This suggests another etiological agent likely exists for Castleman's disease.

4. IL-6 TARGETING THERAPY FOR CASTLEMAN'S DISEASE WITH THERAPEUTIC INTENT

4.1. IL-6 Receptor System

The IL-6 receptor (IL-6R) system consists of two functional membrane proteins: an 80 kDa ligand-binding chain (IL-6R, IL-6R α-chain, CD126) *(63)* and a 130 kDa non-ligand-binding but signal-transducing chain (gp130, IL-6R β-chain, CD130) *(64,65)*. When IL-6 binds to cell surface IL-6R, IL-6/IL-6R complex induces the homodimerization of gp130, and forms a high-affinity functional receptor complex of IL-6, IL-6R, and gp130. The soluble form of IL-6R (sIL-6R), lacking the intracytoplasmic portion of IL-6R, also exists in the blood and is capable of signal transduction as a ligand-binding receptor *(66)*. Thus, IL-6 binding to either a membrane-anchored IL-6R or sIL-6R introduces the signal into target cells as long as they express gp130 (Fig. 2). Based on an understanding of this unique IL-6 receptor system, a strategy has been established to inhibit IL-6 functions. Several therapeutic approaches have been proposed to block the IL-6 signal: (1) suppression of IL-6 production; (2) neutralization of IL-6; (3) blockade of IL-6 binding onto IL-6R; (4) blockade of IL-6/IL-6R complex binding to gp130; (5) suppression of IL-6R and gp130 expression; and (6) blockade of the intracytoplasmic signal from gp130. Corticosteroids are frequently used for the treatment of multicentric Castleman's disease and suppress IL-6 production. However, they also up regulate the expression of membrane-anchored IL-6R on plasma cells *(67)*. Below we discuss limited experiences with neutralization of IL-6 and interruption of IL-6 binding to IL-6R.

4.2. Monoclonal Antibody Approaches

The therapeutic value of mouse antibodies in human chronic diseases remains limited because these conditions like Castleman's disease require repetitive administrations of the antibodies. Since mouse antibodies are highly immunogenic in humans, repetitive administrations of mouse antibodies to human often results in the emergence of neutralizing human antibodies against the mouse antibodies. Such neutralizing antibodies not only

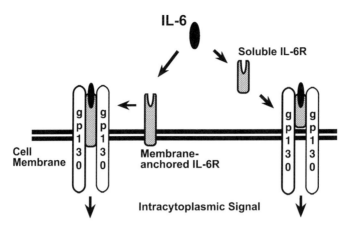

Fig. 2. IL-6 receptor system. The IL-6 receptor (IL-6R) system consists of two functional membrane proteins: a ligand-binding IL-6R and a nonligand-binding but signal-transducing gp130. When IL-6 binds to IL-6R, IL-6/IL-6R complex induces the homodimerization of gp130, which in turn forms a high-affinity functional receptor complex of IL-6, IL-6R, and gp130.

reduce the efficacy but also cause an allergic reaction to the mouse antibodies. A humanized version of an anti-human IL-6R monoclonal antibody was engineered by grafting the complimentarity determining regions from the mouse anti-IL-6R antibody into human IgG, thereby creating a functioning antigen-binding site in a reshaped human antibody *(68)*. It is nonimmunogenic and recognizes both the membrane-anchored and the soluble form of IL-6R and inhibits IL-6 actions both *in vitro (68,69)* and *in vivo (70,71)*.

Beck et al. reported that the *in vivo* administration of murine anti-IL-6 monoclonal antibody (BE-8) to a man with localized Castleman's disease of PC type showed a therapeutic benefit *(11)*. BE-8 monoclonal antibody was administered in a dose of 40 mg daily for 2 days followed by daily doses of 10 mg for 82 days. His fever and constitutional symptoms improved within 24 hours. His hemoglobin levels increased and platelet count decreased within 2 weeks after starting the therapy, although the abnormalities returned after cessation of the therapy *(11)*. The finding confirmed that IL-6 is a key cytokine in this disease.

We have employed the humanized anti-human IL-6 receptor monoclonal antibody to block the IL-6 actions for the treatment of multicentric Castleman's disease *(70)*. We treated 7 patients with multicentric Castleman's disease with either 50 mg of humanized anti-IL-6R antibody twice a week or 100 mg once a week and immediately noted improved systemic symptoms such as fever and malaise. It also normalized the CRP, fibrinogen, albumin and hemoglobin levels. After 3 mo of treatment, hypergammaglobulinemia and lymphadenopathy were remarkably alleviated *(70)*. Treatment was well tolerated, with only a transient leukopenia. Of particular interest, histopathological examination revealed that the treatment reduced both the follicular hyperplasia and vascularity. Therefore, the blockade of the IL-6 signal utilizing humanized anti-IL-6R antibody appears to have potential as a therapeutic agent in this disease.

5. CONCLUSION

On the basis of our study, clinical trials of humanized anti-IL-6R antibody for multicentric Castleman's disease are being conducted both in Japan *(72)* and in the United States. It was approved as an orphan drug for Castleman's disease in Japan in 2005. This therapy is not a nonspecific immunosuppressive therapy like corticosteroids or cytotoxic agents but rather a specific therapy that targets the IL-6 molecule that is key in the pathogenesis of this disease. However, there is still a need for studies to elucidate the exact cause(s) of Castleman's disease. KSHV/HHV-8 can be an etiological agent for Castleman's disease, but there may be others. We also need to elucidate the molecular basis for IL-6 overproduction in Castleman's disease so that additional therapeutic targets can be identified.

REFERENCES

1. Castleman B, Iverson L, Menendez VP. Localized mediastinal lymph node hyperplasia resembling thymoma. Cancer 1956;9:822–830.
2. Flendrig JA, Schillings PHM. Benign giant lymphoma: The clinical signs and symptoms. Folia Med Neerl 1969;12:119–120.
3. Keller AR, Hochholzer L, Castleman B. Hyalin-vascular and plasma-cell types of giant lymph node hyperplasia of the mediastinum and other locations. Cancer 1972;29:670–683.
4. Gaba AR, Stein RS, Sweet DL, et al. Multicentric giant lymph node hyperplasia. Am J Clin Pathol 1978;69:86–90.
5. Bartoli E, Massarelli G, Soggia G, et al. Multicentric giant lymph node hyperplasia. A hyperimmune syndrome with a rapidly progressive course. Am J Clin Pathol 1980;73:423–426.
6. Weisenburger DD, Nathwani BN, Winberg CD, et al. Multicentric angiofollicular lymph node hyperplasia: A clinicopathologic study of 16 cases. Hum Pathol. 1985;156:162–172.
7. Diebold J, Tulliez M, Bernadou A, et al. Angiofollicular and plasmacytic polyadenopathy: A pseudo-tumourous syndrome with dysimmunity. J Clin Pathol 1980;33:1068–1070.
8. Akira S, Taga T, Kishimoto T. interleukin-6 in biology and medicine. Adv Immunol 1993;54:1–78.
9. Yoshizaki K, Matsuda T, Nishimoto N, et al. Pathogenic significance of interleukin-6 (IL-6/BSF-2) in Castleman's disease. Blood 1989;74:1360–1367.
10. Hsu SM, Waldron JA, Xie SS, et al. Expression of interleukin-6 in Castleman's disease. Hum Pathol 1993;24:833–839.
11. Beck JT, Hsu SM, Wijdenes J, et al. Alleviation of systemic manifestations of Castleman's disease by monoclonal anti-interleukin-6 antibody. N Engl J Med. 1994;330:602–605.
12. Frizzera G. Castleman's disease: More questions than answers. Hum Pathol 1985;16:202–205.
13. Frizzera G, Peterson BA, Bayrd ED, Goldman A: A systemic lymphoproliferative disorder with morphologic features of Castleman's disease: Clinical findings and clinicopathologic correlations in 15 patients. J Clin Oncol 1985;3:1202–1216.
14. Kessier E: Multicentric giant lymph node hyperplasia. A report of seven cases. Cancer 1985:56; 2446–2451.
15. Johkoh T, Muller LN, Ichikado K, et al. Intrathoracic multicentric Castleman disease; CT findings in 12 patients. Radiology 1998;209:477–481.
16. Bardwick PA, Zvaifler NJ, Gill GN, et al. Plasma cell dyscrasia with polyneuropathy, organomegaly, endocrinopathy, M protein, and skin changes: The POEMS syndrome. Report on two cases and a review of the literature. Medicine 1980;59:311–322.
17. Hanson CA, Frizzera G, Patton DF et al. Clonal rearrangement for immunoglobulin and T-cell receptor genes in systemic Castleman's disease. Association with Epstein-Barr virus. Am J Pathol 1988;131:84–91.
18. Nagai M, Irino S, Uda H, et al. Molecular genetic and immunohistochemical analyses of a case of multicentric Castleman disease. Jpn J Clin Oncol 1988;18:149–157.
19. Peterson BA, Frizzera G. Multicentric Castleman's disease. Semin Oncol. 1993;20:636–647.
20. Pavlidis NA, Skopouli FN, Bai MC, et al. A successfully treated case of multicentric angiofollicular hyperlasia with oral chemotherapy (Castleman's desease). Med Pediatr Oncol 1990;18:333–335.
21. Feigert JM, Sweet DL, Coleman M, et al. Multicentric angiogollicular lymph node hyperplasia with peripheral neuropathy, pseudotumor ceebri, IgA dysproteinemia, and thrombocytosis in women. A distinct syndrome. Ann Intern Med 1990;113:362–367.
22. Muraguchi A, KishimotoT, Miki T, et al. T cell-replacing factor (TRF)-induced IgG secretion in human B blastoid cell line and demonstration of acceptors for TRF. J Immunol 1981;127:412–416.

23. Yoshizaki K, Nakagawa T, Kaieda T, et al. Induction of proliferation and Igs-production in human B leukemic cells by anti-immunoglobulins and T cell factors. J Immunol 1982;128:1296–1301.

24. Hirano T, Yasukawa K, Harada H, et al. Complementary DNA for a novel human interleukin(BSF-2) that induces B cell lymphocytes to produce immunoglobulin. Nature 1986;324:73–76.

25. Zilberatein A, Ruggieri R, Korn JH, et al. Structure and expression of cDNA and genes for human interferon-β2, a distinct species inducible by growth-stimulatory cytokines. EMBO J1986;5:2529–2537.

26. Sehgal PB, Walther Z, and Tamm I. Rapid enhancement of β2-interferon/ B-cell differntiation factor BSF-2 gene expression in human fibroblasts by diacylglycerols and calcium ionophore A23187. Proc Natl Acad Sci USA 1987;84:3633–3667.

27. Haegeman G, Content J, Volckaert G, et al. Structural analysis of the sequence encoding for an inducible 26-kDa protein in human fibroblasts. Eur J Biochem 1986;159:625–632.

28. Van Damme J, Opdenakker G, Simpson RJ, et al. Identification of the human 26-kDa protein, interferon β2 (IFNβ2), as a B cell hybridoma/ plasmacytoma growth factor induced by interleukin-1 and tumor necrosis factor. J Exp Med 1987;165:914–919.

29. Nordan RP, Pumphrey JG, Rudikoff S. Purification and NH2-terminal sequence of a plasmacytoma growth factor derived from the murine macrophage cell line P388D1. J Immunol 1987;139:813–817.

30. Andus T, Geiger T, Hirano T, et al. Recombinant human B cell stimulatory factor 2 (BSF-2/IFNβ2) regulates β-fibrinogen and albumin mRNA levels in Fao-9 cells. FEBS Lett 1987;221:18–22.

31. Gauldie J, Richards C, Harnish D, et al. Interferon-β2/ B cell-stimulatory factor type 2 shares identity with monocyte-derived hepatocyte-stimulating factor and regulates the major acute phase protein response in liver cells. Proc Natl Acad Sci USA 1987;84:7251–7255.

32. Castell JV, Gomez-Lechon MJ, David M, et al. Recombinant human interleukin-6 (IL-6/ BSF-2/ HSF) regurates the synthesis of acute phase proteins in human hepatocytes. FEBS Lett 1988;232:347–350.

33. Noma T, Mizuta T, Rosen A, et al. Enhancement of the interleukin-2 receptor expression on T cells by multiple B-lymphotropic lymphokines. Immunol Lett 1987;15:249–253.

34. Miyaura C, Onozaki K, Akiyama Y, et al. Recombinant human interleukin 6 (B-cell stimulatory factor 2) is a potent inducer of differentiation of mouse myeloid leukemia cells (M1). FEBS Lett 1988;234:17–21.

35. Ishibashi T, Kimura H, Shikama Y, et al. Interleukin-6 is a potent thrombopoietic factor in vivo in mice. Blood 1989;74:1241–1244.

36. Ikebuchi K, Wong GG, Clark SC, et al. Interleukin-6 enhancement of interleukin-3-dependent proliferation of multipotential hemopoietic progenitors. Proc Natl Acad Sci USA 1987;84:9035-9039.

37. Koike K, Nakahata T, Takagi M, et al. Synergism of BSF2/ interleukin–6 and interleukin-3 on development of multipotential hemopoietic progenitors in serum free culture. J Exp Med 1988; 168:879–890.

38. Ulich TR, del Castillo J, Guo KZ. In vivo hematologic effects of recombinant interleukin-6 on hematopoiesis and circulating numbers of RBCs and WBCs. Blood 1989;73:108–110.

39. Horii Y, Muraguchi A, Iwano M, et al. Involvement of interleukin-6 in mesangial proliferative of glomerulonephritis. J Immunol 1989;143:3949–3955.

40. Yee C, Biondi A, Wang XH, et al. A possible autocrine role for interleukin-6 in two lymphoma cell lines. Blood 1989;74:798–804.

41. Kawano M, Hirano T, Matsuda T, et al. Autocrine generation and requirement of BSF-2/IL-6 for human multiple myelomas. Nature 1988;332:83–85.

42. Miles SA, Rezai AR, Salazar-Gonzales JF, et al. AIDS Kaposi sarcoma-derived cells produce and respond to interleukin 6. Proc Natl Acad Sci USA 1990;87:4068–4072.

43. Suematsu S, Matsuda T, Aozasa K, et al. IgG1 plasmacytosis in interleukin-6 transgenic mice. Proc Natl Acad Sci USA 1989;86:7547–7551.

44. Suematsu S, Matsusaka T, Matsuda T, et al. Generation of plasmacytomas with the chromosomal translocation t(12;15) in interleukin-6 transgenic mice. Proc Natl Acad Sci USA 1992;89: 232–235.

45. Katsume A, Saito H, Yamada Y, et al. Anti-interleukin 6 (IL-6) receptor antibody suppresses Castleman's disease like symptoms emerged in IL-6 transgenic mice. Cytokine 2002;20:304–311.

46. Akira S, Isshiki H, Sugita T, et al. A nuclear factor for IL-6 expression (NF-IL6) is a member of a C/EBP family. EMBO J 1990;9:1897–1906.

47. Screpanti I, Romani L, Musiani P, et al. Lymphoproliferative disorder and imbalanced T-helper response in C/EBP beta-deficient mice. EMBO J 1995;14:1932–1941.

48. Chang Y, Cesarman E, Pessin MS, et al. Identification of herpesvirus-like DNA sequences in AIDS-associated Kaposi's sarcoma. Science 1994;266:1865–1869.

49. Soulier J, Grollet L, Oksenhendler E, et al. Kaposi's sarcoma-associated herpesvirus-like DNA sequences in multicentric Castleman's disease. Blood 1995;86:1276–1280.

50. Dupin N, Gorin I, Deleuze J, et al. Herpes-like DNA sequences, AIDS-related tumors, and Castleman's disease. N Engl J Med 1995;333:798–799.

51. Gessain A, Sudaka A, Briere J, et al. Kaposi's sarcoma-associated herpesvirus-like Virus (Human Herpesvirus Type 8) DNA sequences in multicentric Castleman's disease: Is there any relevant association in nonhuman immunodeficiency virus-infected patients? Blood 1996;87:414–416.

52. Russo JJ, Bohenzky RA, Chien MC, et al. Nucleotide sequence of the Kaposi sarcoma-associated herpesvirus (HHV8). Proc Natl Acad Sci USA. 1996;93:14862-14867.

53. Moor P S, Boshoff C, Weiss RA, et al. Molecular mimicry of human cytokine and cytokine response pathway genes by KSHV. Science 1996;274:1739–1744.

54. Nicholas J, Ruvolo VR, Burns WH, et al. Kaposi's sarcoma-associated human herpesvirus-8 encodes homologues of macrophage inflammatory protein-1 and interleukin-6. Nature Med 1997;3:287–292.

55. Neipel F, Albrecht JC, Ensser A, et al. Human herpesvirus 8 encodes a homolog of interleukin-6. J Virol 1997;71:839–842.

56. Chen KT. Multicentric Castleman's disease and Kaposi's sarcoma. Am J Surg Pathol 1984; 8:287–293.

57. Dickson D, Ben-Ezra JM, Reed J, et al. Multicentric giant lymph node hyperplasia, Kaposi's sarcoma, and lymphoma. Arch Pathol Lab Med 1985;109:1013–1018.

58. De Rosa G, Barra E, Guarino M, et al. Multicentric Castleman's disease in association with Kaposi's sarcoma. Appl Pathol 1989;7:105–110.

59. Aoki Y, Jaffe ES, Chang Y, et al. Angiogenesis and hematopoiesis induced by Kaposi's sarcoma-associated herpesvirus-encoded interleukin-6. Blood 1999;93:4034–4043.

60. Aoki Y, Tosato G. Role of vascular endothelial growth factor/vascular permeability factor in the pathogenesis of Kaposi's sarcoma-associated herpesvirus-infected primary effusion lymphomas. Blood 1999;94:4247–4254.

61. Parravicini C, Corbellino M, Paulli M, et al. Expression of a virus-derived cytokine, KSHV vIL-6, in HIV-seronegative Castleman's disease. Am J Pathol 1997;151:1517–1522.

62. Mori Y, Nishimoto N, Ohno M, et al. Human herpesvirus 8-encoded interleukin-6 homologue (viral IL-6) induces endogenous human IL-6 secretion. J Med Virol 2000;61:332–335.

63. Yamasaki K, Taga T, Hirata Y, et al. Cloning and expression of the human interleukin-6 (BSF-2/INF b2) receptor. Science 1988;241:825–828.

64. Taga T, Hibi M, Hirata Y, et al. Interleukin-6 triggers the association of its receptor with a possible signal transducer, gp130. Cell 1989;58:573–581.

65. Hibi M, Murakami M, Saito M, et al. Molecular cloning and expression of an IL-6 signal transducer, gp130. Cell 1990;63:1149–1157.

66. Heinrich PC, Graeve L, Rose-John S, et al. Membrane-bound and soluble interleukin-6 receptor: studies on structure, regulation of expression, and signal transduction. Ann N Y Acad Sci 1995;762: 222–366.

67. Ogata A, Nishimoto N, Shima Y, et al. Inhibitory effect of all-trans retinoic acid on the growth of freshly isolated myeloma cells via interference with interleukin-6 signal transduction. Blood 1994;84:3040–3046.

68. Sato K, Tsuchiya M, Saldanha J, et al. Reshaping a human antibody to inhibit the interleukin 6-dependent tumor cell growth. Cancer Res 1993;53:851–856.

69. Nishimoto N, Ogata A, Shima Y, et al. Oncostatin M, leukemia inhibitory factor, and interleukin 6 induce the proliferation of human plasmacytoma cells via the common signal transducer, gp130. J Exp Med 1994;179:1343–1347.

70. Nishimoto N, Sasai M, Shima Y, et al. Improvement in Castleman's disease by humanized anti-IL-6 receptor antibody therapy. Blood 2000;95:56–61.

71. Nishimoto N, Yoshizaki K, Maeda K, et al. Toxicity, pharmacokinetics, and dose-finding study of repetitive treatment with the humanized anti-interleukin 6 receptor antibody MRA in rheumatoid arthritis. Phase I/II clinical study. J Rheumatol 2003;30:1426–1435.

72. Nishimoto N, Kanakura Y, Aozasa K, et al. Humanized anti-interteukin-6 receptor antibody treatment of multicentric Castleman disease. Blood 2005;106:2627–2632.

9 Interleukin-10 (IL-10)

Biology, Immune Regulation, and Cancer

Shin-ichiro Fujii and Michael T. Lotze

CONTENTS

1. INTRODUCTION

The Class II alpha helical family of cytokines now includes the extended Interleukin-10 family (IL-10, IL-19, IL-20, IL-22, and IL-26) as well as the closely related Interferon-α, Interferon-γ, and Interferon-τ *(1–22)*. The importance of the distaff side of this family, the interferons *(22,23)*, for cancer biology and tumor immunology has been well defined since the initial report of substances interfering with viral infection by Isaacs and Lindenmann almost 50 yr ago *(25–27)*. Less clear, evolving, and more ambiguous has been the role of the IL-10 extended family defined in the last 15 yr, many of them with more interferon-like properties *(22)*. In cancer patients with malignant melanoma *(28)*, ovarian cancer *(29),* and other hematologic malignancies such as, lymphoma *(30)* and multiple myeloma *(31)*, IL-10 itself can be identified in the serum and/or tumor. Indeed, a negative correlation between circulating levels of IL-10 and prognosis has been reported. For this reason, IL-10 was suspected to be produced by tumor cells, followed by suppression of antitumor immune responses. IL-10 may also act as a tumor growth factor. For example, exogenous IL-10 administration causes expansion in a number of melanoma cell lines owing to the expression of IL-10 receptor *(32)*. In contrast, IL-10 produced by some activated immune cells can promote antitumor activity and is indicative of a potent antitumor immune response. Thus, elevation of IL-10 levels does not always correlate with prognosis in patients with cancer, reflecting its complex biology.

From: *Cancer Drug Discovery and Development,*
Cytokines in the Genesis and Treatment of Cancer
Edited by: M. A. Caligiuri and M. T. Lotze © Humana Press Inc., Totowa, NJ

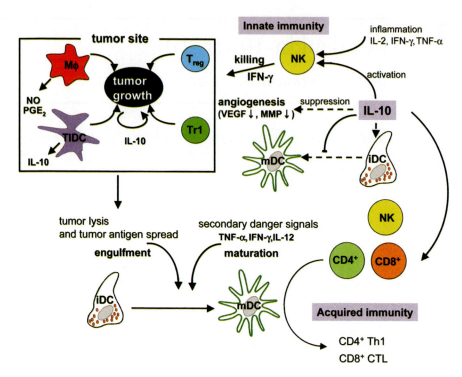

Fig. 1. Cell mediated roles of IL-10 on the link between innate immunity and acquired immunity in tumor. As shown in tumor sites, macrophages, tumor-infiltrating dendritic cells, regulatory T-cells help to grow tumors through IL-10. In innate immunity, exogenous IL-10 serves to activate NK cells and suppress the angiogenesis. After tumor cells are lysed at tumor sites by activated NK cells or IFN-γ, tumor antigens would be engulfed by immature DC. After exposure to inflammatory signals, these DCs can present tumor antigens to naïve T-cells, followed by the induction of antigen specific, Th1 cells or CTL. TIDC, tumor infiltrated dendritic cells; Mφ, macrophage; Treg, CD4$^+$CD25$^+$ regulatory T-cells; Tr1, IL-10 producing regulatory T-cells; iDC, immature DC; mDC, mature DC; NK, natural killer cell; CTL, cytotoxic T-cells; VEGF, vascular endothelial growth factor; MMP, matrix metalloproteinase.

Systemic administration of IL-10 inhibits tumor metastasis in various murine models, including melanomas, sarcomas, lymphoma and colorectal carcinomas *(33,34)*. Although the mechanisms behind these antitumor effects are still incompletely understood, the antitumor effects of IL-10 may be attributable to activation of NK cells *(6)*, CD8$^+$ T-cells *(34)*, macrophages *(35)*, and nitric oxide *(36)* (Fig. 1). In addition, IL-10 exerts a direct antitumor effect by inhibiting angiogenesis. IL-10 stimulates tissue inhibitors of metalloproteinases (TIMPs) and inhibits matrix metalloproteinase (MMP) expression, therefore affecting induction of angiogenesis in prostate and likely other cancers *(37,38)*.

More convincing data come from studies of IL-10-gene therapy in animal tumor models. IL-10 transfected cell lines derived from mouse mammary adenocarcinoma *(39)*, ovarian carcinoma *(40)*, malignant melanoma *(41)*, Burkitt lymphoma *(42)*, prostate and colon cancers *(43)* show significant inhibition of tumor growth irrespective of the induction of a predominant Th2-mediated tumor rejection response. Also, IL-10 gene transfection of melanomas inhibits tumor growth by abrogating angiogenesis, accompanied by downregulation of synthesis of vascular endothelial growth factor (VEGF) along with IL-1β, TNF-α, IL-6, MMP-9 (all known to have angiogenic properties) in tumor-surrounding macrophages *(44)*. In Burkitt lymphoma, introduction of human or viral IL-10 genes into tumors in SCID mice inhibits VEGF-induced neovascularisation of the tumors *(42)*. In human studies, only a few reports are focused on the role of IL-10 in tumor immunology. Some melanomas spontaneously regress in patients and are associated with a high level of IL-10. In advanced stages, a negative correlation between circulating levels of IL-10 and prognosis was also observed in patients with solid or hematologic malignancies, because this is possibly associated with IL-10-producing tumor cells.

2. IL-10 EFFECTS ON THE IMMUNE CELLS

IL-10 can be produced by numerous cell types, including $CD4^+$ and $CD8^+$ T-cells, macrophages, B-cells and dendritic cells (DCs). IL-10 initiates a wide variety of activities when it binds to its heterodimeric cellular receptor. The major mechanism of IL-10 inhibition of cytokine production is to suppress antigen presentation as described below. IL-10 can directly mediate effects in innate and adaptive immunity. IL-10 suppresses the inflammatory cytokine production by DCs or macrophages (Mϕ), and thereby subsequently alters the Th1/Th2 balance. The relative levels of IL-10 and IFN-γ produced by Th1cells are important for determination of immunity in tumor bearing hosts.

2.1. Stimulatory Effects of IL-10 on NK Cells

IL-10 is a potent stimulator of NK cells in vivo *(33)* although it inhibits the production of IFN-γ as well as TNF-α release from NK cells in vitro *(45)*. A link between innate and adaptive immunity has been a role increasingly posited for the NK cell. The early participation of NK cells in response to pathogen/cancer invasion may influence the subsequent development of an adaptive immune response, perhaps providing cues to indicate a "nonself or dangerous" encounter. An aberrant innate reaction to self tissue may promote autoimmunity, as demonstrated by the fact that NK cells are required for the development of an experimental autoimmune mouse model of myasthenia gravis *(46)*. Antigen-specific T-cell activity in an adaptive immunity has to be studied in relation with innate immunity mediators. IL-10 negatively affects the production of IFN-γ and TNF-α release from NK cells in vitro, however it has strong effects on NK cells in vivo *(47,48)*, i.e., it enhances the susceptibility of target cell lysis by NK cells by reducing cell surface MHC expression on tumor cells by IL-10 (Fig. 1). In fact, administration of IL-10 can also induce NK-cell activation and facilitate target-cell destruction in a dose-dependent manner. Moreover, NK cells pretreated with IL-10, either alone or in combination with other cytokines including IL-2, IL-18, and IL-12 are more efficient in enhancing the lysis of tumor cell as well activating NK cells *(47)*. It amplifies the production of IL-2-induced cytokines, such as TNF-α, GM-CSF, and IFN-γ *(48)*. Activated NK cells facilitate antigen acquisition from necrotic/apoptotic tumor cells to activated antigen-presenting cells (APCs) for cross-priming, providing a link between innate immunity and the adaptive immune response.

NKT cells activation by the CD1-ligand mimic, α-galactosylceramide (αGalCer) is dictated by its expression on various types of APCs. DCs presenting this molecule skew the subsequent immune response to one with a Th1 phenotype whereas non-DC as APC induce anergy *(49)*. However, activation of NKT cells can prime naïve $CD4^+$ T-cells and $CD8^+$ T-cells toward Th1 type T-cells by adjuvant effects of αGalCer for in vivo matured DC. In contrast, repeated injection of αGalCer induces anergy and rescued NOD SCID mice from diabetes mellitus, possibly owing to IL-4 and IL-10 production *(50)*.

2.2. Interaction Between IL-10 and Antigen Presenting Cells

APCs can directly produce many cytokines and chemokines during the innate immune response as well as promote effective antigen presentation in acquired adaptive immunity. IL-10 inhibits the differentiation of monocytes to DCs, which are the most important APCs for primary immune responses, as well as the expression of cytokines, soluble mediators and cell surface molecules by monocytes, macrophages, and myeloid DC *(51)*. Thus, IL-10 regulates the balance between the cellular immune response and tolerance in the adaptive immunity through modifying the function of antigen presenting cells.

2.2.1. EFFECTS OF IL-10 ON MONOCYTES, MACROPHAGES (Mφ) AND DCs

Monocytes in the peripheral blood are very sensitive to IL-10. There, they are not in a differentiated state, but rather reside in the circulation for 24- to 48-h before migrating into the tissues where they develop into more specialized cell populations, either Mφ or myeloid DC. As the result of the influence of IL-10 for preventing monocyte differentiation to DC, IL-10 supports monocyte maturation to Mφ, and up-regulates the sensitivity of Mφ to IL-10, owing to the induction of expression of several chemokine receptors *(51)*. IL-10 inhibits the production of proinflammatory mediators by monocytes or Mφ, including release of IL-1β, IL-6, IL-8, G-CSF, GM-CSF and TNF-α *(51)*. It also enhances the production of anti-inflammatory mediators such as IL-1RA and soluble TNF-α. Pretreatment of monocytes with chemokines, such as MCP1-4 leads to endogenous IL-10 production, followed by the suppression of the production of IL-12p70 *(52)*. IL-10 up-regulates the phagocytic activity of monocytes, macrophages, and immature DC via up-regulation of expression of IgG-Fc receptors as well as scavenger receptors *(53)*.

DCs prime naïve T-cells in the initial immune response as the professional antigen presenting cells. When IL-10 is added to immature DC, it inhibits cytokine production, such as IL-12 family members, and suppresses costimulatory molecule expression, MHC class II expression, and chemokine secretion *(51)*, in addition to modulating primary antigen-specific T-cell responses that are abrogated. IL-10 treatment of DC induces or contributes to a state of anergy in allo-antigen- or peptide-antigen-activated CD4$^+$ and CD8$^+$ T-cells *(45,54,55)*. IL-10 promotes the differentiation of CD11c^{low}CD45RB^{high} DCs that lead to the differentiation of regulatory T-cells *(56)*. IL-10 also induces the apoptosis of both freshly isolated and cultured CD4$^+$CD11c$^-$IL-3R$^+$ plasmacytoid DC. Generally, viral-induced plasmacytoid DCs promote naïve T-cells to produce both IFN-γ and IL-10 *(57)*.

In tumor models, tumor-infiltrating DCs are important, because IL-10 can promote the generation of nominally tolerogenic regulatory T-cells *(58,59)*. In this setting, tumor-infiltrating DCs (TIDCs) are largely immature, and can present tumor antigen, but are refractory to stimulation with a combination of LPS, IFN-γ, and anti-CD40 antibody. DC paralysis in this setting can be reversed by CpG plus anti-IL-10 receptor antibody treatment where it has potent therapeutic antitumor effect and induces immune memory *(59)*.

At an early stage of the immune responses, IL-10 may induce destruction of tumor cells by either directly or indirectly stimulating the innate cells of the immune response (Fig. 1). Cytokine- or NK cell-mediated cytolysis of target cells provides DC with adequate amounts of relevant tumor antigens, chemotactic peptides, and danger signal molecules (such as heat shock proteins, double-stranded DNA, HMGB1, S100 molecules, or purine metabolites such as uric acid), which initiate the process of DC maturation. Of note, in augmenting the signalling for toll-like receptors on immature DCs, IL-10 may enhance their sensibility to danger signal molecular mediators. Upon demonstration of a secondary stimulus (IL-2 and IL-12) in secondary lymphatic organs for DC maturation, CD4$^+$T-cells and CD8$^+$ T-cells promote proliferation and activating effects, thereby inducing an adaptive immune response.

During early phases of the immune response when antigen uptake by immature DCs is promoted by IL-10, combined with the inhibition of DC migration, immature DCs accumulate and are loaded with antigens from damaged tissues. This possibly could promote tolerance. In contrast, in several tumor models, IL-10 expressed within the tumors could drive rejection and elimination of the tumor. Interestingly under such conditions, the EBV expressed homologue, vIL-10 promoted tumor growth *(60)*.

2.3. Divergent Effects of IL-10 on CD4$^+$T-Cells and CD8$^+$T-Cells

2.3.1. IL-10 ACTS TO ENHANCE MAINTENANCE OF ANTITUMOR CD8$^+$T-CELLS

Besides the dominant indirect impact mediated via the APCs, IL-10 exerts direct suppressive effects on naïve T-cells *(51)*. However, IL-10 often shows stimulatory effects on CD8$^+$ T-lymphocytes (CTLs), including their recruitment, cytotoxic activity, and proliferation. IL-10 enhances the proliferative responses of murine IL-2- and IL-4-activated CD8$^+$T-cells and rescues T-cells from apoptotic cell death *(62,63)*. As such, IL-10 enhances the effects of antitumor CD8$^+$T-cells in vivo, leading to reduced growth of immunogenic tumors *(51,63)* (Fig. 1). Administration of high doses of IL-10 injections mediates rejection of tumors with contrasting effects on CD4$^+$ and CD8$^+$ T-cells that result in either immune dampening or immune potentiation of these individual cell types *in situ*, respectively *(34,63)*. IL-10 has negative effects on CD8$^+$T-cells through its effects by DCs i.e., DCs that have already been treated with IL-10, mediating its suppressive effects in vitro and in vivo.

2.3.2. IL-10 INDUCES SUPPRESSIVE EFFECTS ON CD4$^+$ T-CELLS

IL-10 positively stimulates CD8$^+$ T-cells under some conditions. In contrast, IL-10 inhibits both the Th1-type and the Th2-type responses of CD4$^+$T-cells strongly via regulatory effects on APC function. Naïve CD4$^+$T-cells are the major targets of IL-10; whereas activated and memory T-cells seem to be rather insensitive *(45)*. CD4$^+$ T-cells cultured in the presence of IL-10, or IL-10-treated APCs become nonresponsive and fail to proliferate or produce inflammatory cytokines *(64–66)*. IL-10-mediated anergy may be associated with induction of regulatory T-cells (Tr1 cells) that produce high levels of IL-10 and can suppress antigen-specific responses in vivo and in vitro *(64–66)* (Fig. 1). In contrast, natural occurring CD4$^+$CD25$^+$ regulatory T-cells (T reg) also mediate inhibition through IL-10 or TGF-β secretion in vivo but not in vitro *(67,68)*.

2.3.3. BIOLOGIC EFFECTS OF REGULATORY T-CELLS TO CONTROL IMMUNE RESPONSES

IL-10 producing regulatory T-cells (IL-10 Treg), containing Tr1 cells and CD4$^+$CD25$^+$ regulatory T-cells (CD4$^+$CD25$^+$ Treg) are independent *(69)*. In the resting state, regulatory T-cells constitutively express high levels of IL-2/IL-15Rβ and γ common chains, as well as a vast repertoire of chemokine receptors, and the homing receptor to lymph nodes, CCR7 *(70)*. CD4$^+$CD25$^+$ T-cells are generated in the thymus, and are thought to arise via "altered negative selection" by self-peptides *(71,72)*. The suppressive activity of CD4$^+$CD25$^+$ T-cells is related to their ability to inhibit IL-2 production and promote cell cycle arrest in both CD4$^+$ and CD8$^+$ T-cells. This finding suggests that direct cell–cell contact may be required. Tregs express CTLA-4 and GITR and can produce TGF-β and IL-10, which are important mediators of Treg-mediated suppression, but they are not specific markers *(69)*. The forkhead/winged helix transcription factor 3 (Foxp3) has been suggested to be a specific marker *(73)* but some CD25$^-$ cells with regulatory activity also express this molecule. In fact, Foxp3-transduced CD4$^+$CD25$^-$T-cells express enhanced amounts of mRNA of IL-10, comparable to that of naturally occurring CD4$^+$CD25$^+$T-cells, suggesting that Foxp3 directly upregulates IL-10 production, although this issue remains controversial *(74)*. In the interaction between Treg and DCs, Pasare et al showed that activation, through Toll-like receptor (TLR)-4 or TLR-9, of BM-derived DCs overcomes the inhibition of naïve T-cell proliferation mediated byCD4$^+$CD25$^+$Treg cells partly owing to the secretion of IL-6 *(75)*.

IL-10 producing T-regulatory cells, including Tr1 cells can regulate the responses of naïve and memory T-cells in vitro and in vivo as well as suppress both Th1 and Th2 cell-mediated pathology through the production of IL-10 and TGF-β *(76)*. The production of these two cytokines is interrelated where IL-10 and TGF-β stimulates each other, however lymphocytes from IL-10 deficient mice produce less TGF-β. The protective effect of IL-10 in a colitis model is also owing to its ability to produce TGF-β, mediating suppressive effects whereas IL-10 enhances production of TGF-β and also controls the ability of target cells to respond to TGF-β through up-regulation of the expression of TGF-βR2 on recently activated T-cells *(77)*. In vivo, CD4$^+$CD25$^+$Treg and IL-10Treg inhibit inflammation mainly through IL-10 and TGF-β dependent mechanism *(69,76,77)*. These two types of regulatory T-cells can promote tumor growth by suppressing immune reactions to tumor-associated antigens .

3. IMMUNOLOGIC REGULATION BY IL-10 ON TUMOR PROGRESSION AND ANTITUMOR RESPONSES

3.1. A Biologic Role of IL-10 in Tumorigenesis

Several animal experiments have focused on the role of IL-10 on tumor development, whereby diverse effects regarding the influence of IL-10 on cancer are shown. IL-10 sometimes seems to favor the existence and progression of tumors. IL-10 can also convert tumor cells to a CTL-resistant phenotype. For example, approx 50% reduction in MHC class I expression in human melanoma cells is noted after IL-10 treatment in a dose-dependent fashion. This effect may be mediated by reduced expression of the transporter associated with antigen processing (TAP)-1 and -2 that results in reduced translocation of peptides to the endoplasmic reticulum followed by the diminished MHC class I peptide loading and cell surface levels *(51)*. However, such downregulation of MHC class I expression may bring about a higher sensitivity toward NK cell activity. In in vitro and in vivo experiments, when antigen-pulsed DCs were exposed to IL-10, active CTL cannot be easily generated. In contrast, we have some evidences concerning antitumor effects that after complete establishment of CTL, IL-10 can maintain and support their functions, such as antigen specific IFN-γ production and cytolysis against tumor cells *(34,63)* (Fig. 1). In addition, when IL-10-transfected tumor is injected, the increased expression of isoforms of nitric-oxide synthase (iNOS), which demonstrates potent antitumor ability, emerges *(36)*. IL-10 also can inhibit the generation of new vessels within the tumor both directly by acting on the tumor cells and indirectly by influencing infiltrating immune cells. When IL-10 inhibited microvessel formation, IL-10 induced the tissue inhibitor of metalloproteinase-2 (TIMP-2) in primary cancer cells, such as prostate cancer cells *(37,38)*. Simultaneously, it reduced the secretion of matrix metalloproteinase (MMP)-2 and MMP-9 from these cells *(37,38)*. IL-10 can also inhibit the angiogenesis by inhibiting tumor-resident macrophages.

3.2. IL-10 Gene Polymorphisms in Cancer

The human IL-10 gene is comprised of 5 exons, spans approx 5.2 kb and is located on chromosome 1, at 1q31-1q32 *(78)*. The IL-10 promoter is highly polymorphic with two informative microsatellites, IL-10.G and IL-10.R, 1.2 kb and 4 kb upstream of the transcription start site *(78)*. A number of genetic polymorphisms have been identified within the IL-10 gene, particularly in the promoter region gene, which is associated with enhanced production of this cytokine in response to stimulation of immune cells. Certain of these polymorphisms may be associated with differential levels of IL-10 expression. Therefore, IL-10 polymorphisms by single nucleotide polymorphism (SNP) are analyzed and shown in the association with the susceptibility to cancers; some solid tumors (i.e., malignant melanoma, prostate cancer, and breast cancer) *(79)* and especially hematologic malignancies (i.e., multiple myeloma, non-Hodgkins lymphoma, AML, and ALL) *(80–82)*. In the studies demonstrating IL-10 polymorphisms and markers of disease progression, a polymorphism in the promoter region of IL-10 can be found associated with a higher incidence of melanoma, prostate, breast, and gastric cancers. Genetic predisposition to these tumors may modulate tumor growth by immune mechanisms, however it might have relatively little impact on the levels of IL-10 produced by tumor cells *(80–82)*. The first steps of angiogenesis are crucial for the development, metastasis and prognosis in many types of cancers. Therefore, in the initial tumor development, such genetic polymorphisms of IL-10 would be associated with angiogenesis, especially the production of the angiogenic cytokines, VEGF and bFGF.

3.3. IL-10 Effects on Immune Responses in Mouse Tumor Models

IL-10 can initiate and terminate inflammatory responses as well as the regulate differentiation and proliferation of T- and B-lymphocytes, NK cells, APC, mast cells, and granulocytes. IL-10 also plays a role in simultaneously enhancing tumor progression or facilitating tumor destruction in mouse models (Fig. 1). As previously described, anti-inflammatory properties mediated by IL-10 have been ascribed mainly to inhibition of macrophages or DC immune function and induction of regulatory T-cells. In IL-10 transgenic models, IL-10 reduces T- or B-cell responses to Listeria monocytogenes and Leishmania *(83)*, and in contrast they increase T-cell-mediated rejection of cancer.

In contrast, in the models for abrogating effects of IL-10 on tumors by IL-10, local administration in IL-10-transfected tumor cells prevents tumor cells from growing. In addition, systemic IL-10 administration has protective and curative effects through enhancement of tumor cell killing by NK and CD8[+] T-cells *(33–37,39–43,63,84)* (Fig. 1). In innate immunity, activated NK cells may mediate tumor destruction and enhance antigen availability. IL-10 sustains NK cell or CTL cytolytic function in vivo probably together with the release of IFN-γ, IFN-γ inducible protein-10 (IP-10) or increased granzyme levels. These effectors induced by IL-10 can destroy abnormal tumor cells.

Upon addition of a secondary pro-inflammatory cytokine, immature DCs will mature, producing chemoattractants and cytokines and upregulating costimulatory molecules. In addition, as a secondary inflammatory response, CXC chemokines inducible protein and monokine *(85)*, enhanced by IFN-γ, can mediate the local and systemic antitumor effects of IL-10. Thus, mature DC captured tumor antigen may act as potent immune cells to present naïve T-cells for establishing and maintaining tumor-specific CTLs following IL-10 responses. This pro-inflammatory activity not only comes from IL-2, but when combined with other cytokines (such as IL-2, IL-12, or IL-18), IL-10 may serve as a link between innate and adaptive antitumor immunity.

3.4. Efficacy and Vulnerability of IL-10 Effects on Immune Responses in Human Cancer Diseases

Several human cancer cell lines constitutively produce IL-10 in vitro, indicating that a large amount of the IL-10 may be produced in vivo at the site of tumor lesions. Otherwise, autocrine and paracrine IL-10 effects could be produced by the immune cells, such as macrophages or Tr1 cells around the tumor sites. Actually, an inverse correlation between circulating levels of IL-10 and prognosis was reported in patients with solid or hematologic malignancies in advanced stages. In B-cell lymphoma or some other solid tumors (especially colon cancer, gastric cancer, and renal cell cancer) *(84,86,87)*, the increased circulating IL-10 serum level has been reported as a negative prognostic factor for responsiveness to conventional therapy, such as surgery and chemotherapy, presumably owing to the impaired function of APC in tumors. Significant IL-10 mRNA expression is shown in patients with melanoma but not in healthy individuals. The proliferative rate of human melanoma cell lines is enhanced by exogenous IL-10, suggesting that this cytokine might serve as a tumor growth factor. Over-expression of IL-10 in basal cell and squamous cell carcinoma in primary tissues has also been demonstrated *(86)*. IL-10 immune suppressive effects may help tumors escape from immune recognition. Actually, lymphoma patients had significantly higher serum levels of IL-10 than healthy volunteers *(87)*. In the tissues, an elevated local expression of IL-10 was detected particularly in cutaneous T-cell lymphoma entities (CTCL) *(88)*. Increasing IL-10 gene expression was found to be correlated with the tumor progression in lymphoma. In humans, IL-10 may perform as a tumor promoting angiogenic factor, as correlations between IL-10 and VEGF expression have been reported in esophageal cancer patients *(84)*.

The role that IL-10 plays in tumor escape has not been established; high levels of IL-10 are observed in the areas of spontaneous regression of primary melanoma as an inhibitor of cancer growth. In the context of human papilloma virus-related cervical carcinoma, IL-10 also enhances synergistically with the IL-2 tumor-specific T-cell expansion as shown in murine models and cytotoxicity by increasing intracellular accumulation of perforin *(89)*. Again, IL-10 sometimes enhances the immunity against tumor cells and sometimes leads to progression.

3.5. IL-10 Release in the Local Tumor Microenvironment

When IL-10 is constitutively released in the tumor sites, microenvironment during tumor progression, biologic responses will be revealed as either an immune activation or an immune suppression. Although normal bronchial epithelial cells constitutively produce IL-10, secretion of IL-10 may be retained, or abolished in primary lung cancer *(90,91)*. Lack of IL-10 secretion predicts poor outcome of early stage nonsmall cell lung cancer. Secondary local immune responses by IL-10 release may bring about antitumor effects without tumor progression. It would be more important to understand what kinds of immune cells can play a role by secreting IL-10 in growing tumor (infiltrating macrophages, monocytes, NK cells, eosinophils, or T-cells). Inhibition of tumor growth by IL-10 could be attained through up-regulation of TIMP-2 expression or downregulation of MMP-2 and MMP-9 *(37,38)*, which will consequently inhibit micro-vessel formation. In addition, elevated levels of nitric oxide by IL-10 may be related to their toxic effects on tumor cells *(36)*.

4. AGONISTIC OR ANTAGONISTIC INTERACTION BETWEEN IL-10 AND OTHER CYTOKINES

IL-10 inhibits production of Th1 cytokines. IL-10 may inhibit cancer growth through activation of IFN-γ and IFN-γ-inducible gene Gbp-1/Mig-1 which could exert a direct antitumor effect or enhance alternations in the immune microenvironment such as limiting macrophage ingress thereby limiting tumor growth *(92)*. Among suppressive effects, IL-10 inhibits IFN-induced gene transcription, such as IP-10, which correlates with IL-10-mediated inhibition of IFN-induced STAT1 phosphorylation *(92)*. Moreover, IL-10 inhibition can be overcome by increasing IFN concentrations, suggesting competition of these cytokines. The most marked effect of IL-10 is its capability to enhance tumor growth as an inducer of expression of the suppressor of cytokine synthesis (SOCS)-3 which plays a critical role in inhibition of macrophage activation *(93)*.

IL-10 plays an important role in immune regulation by interacting with other cytokines. IL-10 is regulated together with other cytokines, especially class II cytokines, such as IFN-γ (class II cytokines; IFNs, IL-10, 19, 20, 22, 24, 26, 28, and 29) *(94)*. Class II cytokine receptors were originally defined on the basis of sequence homologies in the extracellular domains of receptors for IFNs and IL-10, and ligands known as class II cytokines, also have a common structure. IFNs exert their activities through heterodimeric receptors composed of transmembrane proteins that belong to class II cytokine receptor family. Despite the quite different functions between IFN-γ and IL-10, the IL-10 receptor (IL-10R) indeed belongs to this family of receptors. Although the homology between the sequences of IL-10 and IFNs is quite limited, the elucidation of their three-dimensional structure indicated a shared a-helical pattern, confirming that these factors are structurally related *(95)*. The IL-10Rβ chain is used by several types of cytokines, such as IL-10, 22, 26, 28, and 29. A single receptor can bind several cytokines, potentially transducing distinct signals, as indicated for type-I IFNs that have different activities mediated through a single common receptor. Despite the structural similarities and the sharing of common receptor chains used by several cytokines, the physiologic roles of class II cytokines are divergent and the homology is limited. This may reflect that IL-10 has both negative and positive effects on immune responses, especially together with the other class II cytokines. IFN-γ is a major pro-inflammatory cytokine which can activate macrophages and endothelial cells. In contrast, IL-10 downregulates the expression of activating and costimulatory molecules of APCs as well as inhibits the production of pro-inflammatory cytokines by macrophages and DCs. With regards to biologic functions, IL-10- and IFN-related cytokines seem to be antagonists to each other in in vitro models. To understand the opposing effects of these two cytokines, we can compare the lipopolysaccharide (LPS)-endotoxin shock models. Administration of LPS in an experimental model is associated with release of a number of systemic inflammatory cytokines, suggesting that TNF-α and IL-1β are crucial pro-inflammatory factors. Administration of IL-10 following LPS rescued mice from LPS-induced toxic shock by inhibiting the production of these factors *(96,97)*. In contrast, endogenous IL-10 release by LPS injection confers protection from the harmful effects of endotoxin challenge; blocking IL-10 markedly increased the sensitivity of mice to LPS *(98)*. Expression of IFNs is also upregulated by LPS with IFN-γ serving as a potent activator of macrophage/monocytes. Therefore, blocking IFN-γ increases resistance to endotoxin challenge *(99)*. Interestingly, whereas IL-10 and IFN-γ may at times be antagonistic, they may also play roles as agonistic factors for each other. A balance in the production of these factors is required to maintain the homeostasis of inflammatory process. As shown in the cases of differential effects on NK cells and CTLs, when we consider the class II family, it is no wonder that IL-10 mediates different effects on immune responses together with IFN-γ, perhaps involving other novel cytokines such as HMGB1, released from intranuclear stores *(100–102)*.

CD4+ regulatory T-cell populations that could produce high levels of IL-10 have been indicated to have an essential role in tolerance to self-antigens. The relative contribution of IL-10 in the anti-inflammatory function mediated by such regulatory T-cells may depend on the types of experimental models used.

5. CLINICAL USE OF IL-10

In humans, systemic administration of IL-10 to normal volunteers is associated with very little toxicity and pro-inflammatory properties are mediated through activation of effector cells of the innate immune response. Indeed, clinical trials were performed in healthy volunteers and consistently demonstrated the safety of IL-10 administration at doses up to 25 μg/kg *(103,104)*. Single iv or sc doses of IL-10 resulted in transient dose-dependent increases of white blood cell populations, together with neutrophilia, CD4+ and CD8+ T-lymphocytopenia, monocytosis, and reversible decline in platelet counts and hemoglobin levels. However, no significant change was observed in the bone marrow cellularity or myeloid:erythroid ratio or in the number of megakaryocytes. Intravenous administration of human recombinant IL-10 could have potential anticancer activity with production of the IFN-γ-inducible protein and inducing activation of cytotoxic T-cell and NK cells as reflected by increased levels of granzyme-β. When administered IL-10, PBMC from treated subjects resisted the LPS-induced cytokine producing responses (IL-6, IL-1, and TNF-α) *(105)*, and showed decreased proliferative responses and IFN-γ production induced by PHA (phytohemagglutinin) stimulation, indicating that IL-10 retains immunomodulatory activity when administered in vivo. In some clinical trials, the effects have been heterogenous; that is almost no effects were observed in rheumatoid arthritis, but significant effects were observed in psoriasis *(106)*.

6. CONCLUSIONS

IL-10 is the prototypic member of a regulatory cytokine family which regulates immunity. When considering IL-10, we need to focus on two aspects: one is the initiation of local responses surrounding tumor cells and the other is its role in regulating systemic responses. In innate immunity, local production and secretion of IL-10 by tumor cells or immune cells (such as infiltrating macrophages, monocytes, NK cells, eosinophils, or T-cells) can be helpful in limiting the progression of tumor growth, as well as impairment of macrophage or DC function and induction of both types of regulatory T-cells. This effect may depend upon the concentration of IL-10 within the tumor microenvironment, the density of IL-10 receptor expressed on tumor cells, or the presence of other regulatory circuits affecting signaling within the cells.

Situations associated with inadequate IL-10 expression have to be considered (inflammatory bowel disease, and psoriasis), as well as situations in which there is IL-10 overexpression (lymphoma, SLE, and intensive care unit patients). Under conditions by which high levels of IL-10 are released, such as IL 10-transfection of tumor cells, or when NK cells and anti-angiogenic cytokines are secreted, tumor growth is inhibited. Systemically, IL-10 enhances the activation of NK cells and maintains the survival of CD9[+] T-cells. However, the roles of IL-10, as is true of virtually all other cytokines, are currently incompletely understood and will require intense additional study in a multitude of model systems.

ACKNOWLEDGMENTS

We would like to thank Drs. Caroline Smith, Kanako Shimizu, Koji Fujimoto, Shohei Hori, and Michael Caligiuri for peer-reviewing.

REFERENCES

1. Bartlett NW, Dumoutier L, Renauld JC, et al. A new member of the interleukin 10-related cytokine family encoded by a poxvirus. J Gen Virol 2004;85,1401–1412.
2. Chang C, Magracheva E, Kozlov S, et al. Crystal structure of interleukin-19 defines a new subfamily of helical cytokines. J Biol Chem 2003;278,3308–3313.
3. Conti P, Kempuraj D, Frydas S, et al. IL-10 subfamily members: IL-19, IL-20, IL-22, IL-24 and IL-26. Immunol Lett 2003;88,171–174.
4. Dumoutier L, Leemans C, Lejeune D, Kotenko SV, Renauld JC. Cutting edge: STAT activation by IL-19, IL-20 and mda-7 through IL-20 receptor complexes of two types. J Immunol 201;167:3545–3549.
5. Dumoutier L, Renauld JC. Viral and cellular interleukin-10 (IL-10)-related cytokines: From structures to functions. Eur Cytokine Netw 2002;13:5–15.
6. Fickenscher H, Hor S, Kupers H, Knappe A, Wittmann S, Sticht H. The interleukin-10 family of cytokines. Trends Immunol 2002;23:89–96.
7. Gallagher G, Dickensheets H, Eskdale J, et al. Cloning, expression and initial characterization of interleukin-19 (IL-19), a novel homologue of human interleukin-10 (IL-10). Genes Immun 200;1:442–450.
8. Gallagher G, Eskdale J, Jordan W, et al. Human interleukin-19 and its receptor: A potential role in the induction of Th2 responses. Int Immunopharmacol 2004;4:615–626.
9. Kempuraj D, Frydas S, Kandere K, et al. Interleukin-19 (IL-19) network revisited. Int J Immunopathol Pharmacol 2003;16:95–97.
10. Koks S, Kingo K, Ratsep R, et al. Combined haplotype analysis of the interleukin-19 and -20 genes: Relationship to plaque-type psoriasis. Genes Immun. 2004;5(8):662–667.
11. Kotenko SV. The family of IL-10-related cytokines and their receptors: Related, but to what extent? Cytokine Growth Factor Rev 2002;13:223–240.
12. Langer JA, Cutrone EC, Kotenko S. The Class II cytokine receptor (CRF2) family: overview and patterns of receptor-ligand interactions. Cytokine Growth Factor Rev 2004;15:33–48.
13. Li MC, He SH. IL-10 and its related cytokines for treatment of inflammatory bowel disease. World J Gastroenterol 2004;10:620–625.
14. Liao YC, Liang WG, Chen FW, et al. IL-19 induces production of IL-6 and TNF-alpha and results in cell apoptosis through TNF-alpha. J Immunol 2002;169:4288–4297.

15. Nagalakshmi ML, Murphy E, McClanahan T, de Waal Malefyt R. Expression patterns of IL-10 lig-
    and and receptor gene families provide leads for biological characterization. Int Immunopharmacol
    2004;4:577–592.
16. Parrish-Novak J, Xu W, Brender T, et al. Interleukins 19, 20, and 24 signal through two distinct recep-
    tor complexes. Differences in receptor-ligand interactions mediate unique biological functions. J Biol
    Chem 2002;277:47,517–47,523.
17. Pletnev S., Magracheva E, Kozlov S, et al. Characterization of the recombinant extracellular domains
    of human interleukin-20 receptors and their complexes with interleukin-19 and interleukin-20.
    Biochemistry 2003;42:12,617–12,624.
18. Preimel D, Sticht H. Molecular modeling of the interleukin-19 receptor complexNovel aspects
    of receptor recognition in the interleukin-10 cytokine family. J Mol Model (Online) 2004;10:
    290–296.
19. Sheikh F, Baurin VV, Lewis-Antes A, et al. Cutting edge: IL-26 signals through a novel receptor com-
    plex composed of IL-20 receptor 1 and IL-10 receptor 2. J Immunol 2004:172:2006–2010.
20. Vandenbroeck K, Alloza I, Brehmer D, et al. The conserved helix C region in the superfamily of inter-
    feron-gamma /interleukin-10-related cytokines corresponds to a high-affinity binding site for the
    HSP70 chaperone DnaK. J Biol Chem 2002:277:25,668–25,676.
21. Olk K, Kunz S, Asadullah K, Sabat R. Cutting edge: Immune cells as sources and targets of the IL-10
    family members? J Immunol 2002;168:5397–5402.
22. Pestka S, Krause CD, Sarkar D, et al. Interleukin-10 and related cytokines and receptors. Annu Rev
    Immunol 2004;22:929–979.
23. Colonna M., Trinchieri G. and Liu Y. J. Plasmacytoid dendritic cells in immunity. Nat Immunol
    2004;5:1219–1226.
24. Picard C, Casanova JL. Inherited disorders of cytokines. Curr Opin Pediatr 2004;16: 648–658.
25. Isaacs A, Burke DC. Mode of action of interferon. Nature 1958;182:1073, 1074.
26. Isaacs A, Lindenmann J. Virus interference. I. The interferon. Proc R Soc Lond B Biol Sci 1957;147:
    258–267.
27. Isaacs A, Lindenmann J, Valentine R. C. Virus interference. II. Some properties of interferon. Proc R
    Soc Lond B Biol Sci 1957;147:268–273.
28. Dummer W, Becker JC, Schwaaf A, et al. Elevated serum levels of Interleukin-10 in patients with
    metastatic malignant melanoma. Melanoma Res 1995;5:67, 68.
29. Gotlieb WH, Abrams JS, Watson JM, et al. Presence of Interleukin-10(IL-10) in the ascites of patients
    with ovarian and other intra-abdominal cancers. Cytokine 1992;4:385–390.
30. Khatri VP, Caligiuri MA. A review of the association between Interleukin-10 and human B-cell
    malignancies. Cancer Immunol Immunother 1998;46:239–244.
31. Klein B, Lu ZY, Gu ZJ, et al. Interleukin-10 and Gp130 cytokines in human multiple myeloma. Leuk
    Lymphoma 1999;34:63–70.
32. Yue FY, Dummer R, Geersten R, et al. Interleukin-10 is a growth factor for human melanoma cells
    and down-regulates HLA class-1, HLA class-2 and ICAM-1 molecules. Int J Cancer 1997;71:
    630–637.
33. Zheng LM, Ojcus DM, Garaud F, et al. Interleukin-10 inhibits tumor metastasis through an NK cell-
    dependent mechanism. J Exp Med 1996;184:579–584.
34. Berman RM, Suzuki T, Tahara H, et al. Systemic administration of cellular IL-10 induces an effec-
    tive, specific, and long-lived immune response against established tumors in mice. J Immunol
    1996;157:231–238.
35. Di Carlo E, Coletti A, Modesti A, et al. Local release on Interleukin-10 by transfected mouse adeno-
    carcinoma cells exhibit pro- and anti-inflammatory activity and results in a delayed tumor rejection.
    Eur Cytokine Netw 1998;9:61–68.
36. Kundu D, Dorsey R, Jackson MJ, et al. Interleukin-10 gene transfer inhibits murine mammary tumors
    and elevates nitric oxide. Int J Cancer 1998;76:713–739.
37. Stearns ME, Fudge K, Garcia F, et al. IL-10 inhibition of human prostate PC-3 ML cell metastases in
    SCID mice: IL-10 stimulation of TIMP-1 and inhibition of MMP-2/MMP-9 expression. Invasion
    Metastasis 1997;17:62–74.
38. Stearns ME, Rhim J, Wang M. Interleukin-10(IL-10) inhibition of primary human prostate cell-
    induced angiogenesis: IL-10 stimulation of tissue inhibitor of metalloproteinase-1 and inhibition of
    matrix metalloproteinase(MMP)2/MMP-9 secretion. Clin Cancer Res 1999;5:189–196.

39. Giovarelli M, Musiani P, Modesti A, et al. Local release of IL-10 by transfected mouse mammary adenocarcinoma cells does not suppress but enhances antitumor reaction and elicits a strong cytotoxic lymphocyte and antibody-dependent immune memory. J Immunol 1995;155:3112–3123.
40. Richter G, Kruger-Krasagakes S, Hein G, et al. Interleukin-10 transfected into Chinese hamster ovary cells prevents tumor growth and macrophage infiltration. Cancer Res 1993;53:4134–4137.
41. Gerard CM, Bruyns C, Delvaux A, et al. Loss of tumorigenicity and increased immunogenicity induced by interleukin-10 gene transfer in B16 melanoma cells. Hum Gene Ther 1996;7:23–31.
42. Cervenak L, Morbidelli L, Donati D, et al. Abolished angiogenicity and tumorigenicity of Burkitt lymphoma by Interleukin-10. Blood 2000;96:2568–1273.
43. Adris S, Klein S, Jasnis M, et al. IL-10 expression by CT26 colon carcinoma cells inhibits their malignant phenotype and induces a T cell-mediated tumor rejection in the context of a systemic Th2 response. Gene Ther 1999;6:1705–1712.
44. Huang S, Ullrich SE, Bar-Eli M. Regulation of tumor growth and metastasis by interleukin-10: The melanoma experience. J Interferon Cytokine Res 1999;19:697–703.
45. Moore KW, de Waal Malefyt, R, Coffman, RL et al. Interleukin-10 and the interleukin-10 receptor. Annu Rev Immunol 2001;19:683–765.
46. Shi FD, Wang NB, Li H, et al. Natural killer cells determine the outcome of B cell-mediated autoimmunity. Nat Immunol 2000;1:245–251.
47. Shibata Y, Foster LA, Kurimoto M, Okamura H, et al. Immunoregulatory roles of IL-10 in innate immunity: IL-10 inhibits macrophages production of IFN-γ-inducing factors but enhances NK cell production of IFN-γ. J Immunol 1998;161:4283–4288.
48. Mocellin S, Panelli MC, Wang E, et al. The dual role of IL-10. Trends Immunol 2003;24:36–43.
49. Fujii S, Shimizu K, Kronenberg M, et al. Prolonged IFN-γ-producing NKT response induced with α-galactosylceramide-loaded DCs. Nat Immunol 2002;3:867–874.
50. Hong S, Wilson MT, Serizawa I, et al. The natural killer T-cell ligand α-galactosylceramide prevents autoimmune diabetes in non-obese diabetic mice. Nat Med 2001;7:1052–1056.
51. Fujii S, Lotze MT. IL-10 effects on innate immunity. In: Marincola F, ed. Interleukin-10. Landes Bioscience 2006; pp. 11–23.
52. Braun MC, Lahey E, Kelsall BL. Selective suppression of IL-12 production by chemoattractants. J Immunol. 2000;164:3009–3017.
53. Muzio M, Bosisio D, Polentarutti N, et al. Differential expression and regulation of toll-like receptors (TLR) in human leukocytes: Selective expression of TLR3 in dendritic cells. J Immunol. 2000;164:5998–6004.
54. Steinbrink K, Jonuleit H, Muller G, et al. Interleukin-10-treated human dendritic cells induce a melanoma-antigen-specific anergy in CD8+ T cells resulting in a failure to lyse tumor cells. Blood. 1999;93:1634–1642.
55. Steinbrink, K, Granulich, E, Kubsch, S, et al. CD4+ and CD8+ anergic T cells induced by interleukin-10-treated human dendritic cells display antigen-specific suppressor activity. Blood. 2002;99:2468–2476.
56. Wakkach A, Fournier N, Brun V, et al. Characterization of dendritic cells that induce tolerance and T regulatory 1 cell differentiation in vivo. Immunity 2003;18:605–617.
57. Liu YJ. Dendritic cell subsets and lineages, and their functions in innate and adaptive immunity. Cell. 2001;106:259–262.
58. Castro AG, Neighbors M, Hurst SD, et al. Anti-interleukin-10 receptor monoclonal antibody is an adjuvant for T helper cell type 1 responses to soluble antigen only in the presence of lipopolysaccharide. J Exp Med. 2000;192:1529–1534.
59. Vicari AP, Chiodoni C, Vaure C, et al. Reversal of tumor-induced dendritic cell paralysis by CpG immunostimulatory oligonucleotide and anti-interleukin-10 receptor antibody. J Exp Med. 2002;196:541–549.
60. Suzuki T, Tahara H, Narula S, et al. Viral interleukin-10 (vIL-10), the human herpes virus 4 cellular IL-10 homologue, induces local anergy to allogeneic and syngeneic tumors. J Exp Med. 1995;182:477–486.
61. Taga K, Cherney B, Tosato G. Interleukin-10 inhibits apoptotic cell death in human T cells starved of IL-2. Int Immunol 1993;5:1599–1608.
62. Cohen SB, Crawley JB, Kahan MC, et al. Interleukin-10 rescues T cells from apoptotic cell death: Association with an up-regulation of bcl-2. Immunology 1997;92:1–5.

63. Fujii S, Shimizu K, Shimizu T, et al. Interleukin-10 promotes the maintenance of antitumor CD8[+] T-cell effector function in situ. Blood 2001;98:2143–2151.

64. Levings MK, Sangregorio R, Galbiati F, et al. IFN-α and IL-10 induce the differentiation of human type 1 T regulatory cells. J Immunol 2001;166:5530–5539.

65. Asseman C, Mauze S, Leach MW, et al. An essential role for interleukin 10 in the function of regulatory T cells that inhibit intestinal inflammation. J Exp Med 1999;190:995–1004.

66. Groux H, O'Garra A, Bingler M, et al. A CD4[+] T-cell subset inhibits antigen-specific T-cell responses and prevents colitis. Nature 1997;389:737–742.

67. Annacker, O et al. CD25+CD4+ T cells regulate the expansion of peripheral CD4 T cells through the production of IL-10. J Immunol 2001;166:737–742.

68. Nakamura K, Kitani A, Strober W. Cell contact-dependent immunosuppression by CD4+CD25+ regulatory T cells is mediated by cell surface-bound transforming growth factor β. J Exp Med 2001;194: 629–644.

69. O'Garra A, Vieira P. Regulatory T cells and mechanisms of immune system control. Nat Med 2004;10:801–805.

70. Roncarolo MG, Bacchetta R, Bordignon C, et al. Type 1 T regulatory cells. Immunol Rev 2001;182: 68–79.

71. Sakaguchi S, Sakaguchi N, Shimizu J, et al. Immunologic tolerance maintained by CD25[+] CD4[+] regulatory T cells: Their common role in controlling autoimmunity, tumor immunity, and transplantation tolerance. Immunol Rev 2001;182:18–32.

72. Shevach EM. CD4[+] CD25[+] suppressor T cells: More questions than answers. Nat Rev Immunol 2002;2:389–400.

73. Hori S, Nomura T, Sakaguchi S. Control of regulatory T cell development by the transcription factor Foxp3. Science 2003;299:1057–1061.

74. Chen W, Jin W, Hardegen N, et al. Conversion of peripheral CD4+CD25- naive T cells to CD4+CD25+ regulatory T cells by TGF-β induction of transcription factor Foxp3. J Exp Med 2003;198:1875–1886.

75. Pasare C, Medzhitov R. Toll pathway-dependent blockade of CD4+CD25+ T cell-mediated suppression by dendritic cells. Science 2003;299:1033–1036.

76. Levings MK, Bacchetta R, Schulz U, et al. The role of IL-10 and TGF-β in the differentiation and effector function of T regulatory cells. Int Arch Allergy Immunol 2002;129:263–276.

77. Cottre F, Groux H. Regulation of TGF-β response during T cell activation is modulated by IL-10. J Immunol 2001;167:773–778.

78. Eskdale J, Kube D, Tesch H et al. Mapping of the human IL-10 gene and further characterization of the 5′ flanking sequence. Immunogenetics 1997;46:120–128.

79. Folkman J. Angiogenesis in cancer, vascular, rheumatoid and other diseases. Nat Med 1995;1:27–31.

80. Lauten M, Matthias T, Stanulla M et al. Association of initial response to predonisone treatment in childhood acute leukemia and polymorphism within the tumor necrosis factor and the interleukin-10 gene. Leukemia 2002;16:1437–1442.

81. Cunningham LM, Chapman C, Dunstan R et al. Plymorphisms in interleukin-10 gene promoter are associated with susceptibility to aggressive non-Hodgkin's lymphoma. Leuk Lymph 2003;44:251–255.

82. Zheng C, Huang D, Liu L et al. Interleukin-10 gene promoter polymorphisms in multiple myeloma. Int J Cancer 2001;95:184–188.

83. Groux H, Cottrez F, Rouleau M et al. A transgenic model to analyze the immunoregulatory role of IL-10 secreted by antigen-presenting cells. J Immunol 1999;162:1723–1729.

84. Asadullah K, Sterry W, Volk HD. Interleukin-10 therapy-review of a new approach. Pharmacol Rev 2003;55:241–269.

85. Dorsey R, Kundu N, Yang Q et al. Immunotherapy with interleukin-10 depends on the CXC chemokines inducible protein-10 and monokine induced by IFN-γ. Cancer Res 2002;62:2606–2610.

86. Ordemann J, Jacobi CA, Braumann, C et al. Immunomodulatory changes in patients with colorectal cancer. Int J Colorectal Dis 2002;17:37–41.

87. Blay JY, Burdin N, Rousset F et al. Serum interleukin-10 in non-Hodgkin's lymphoma: A prognostic factor. Blood 1993;82:2169–2174.

88. Asadullah K, Docke WD, Volk HD, et al. Cytokines and cutaneous T-cell lymphomas. Exp Dermatol 1998;7:314–320.

89. Santin AD, Hermonat PL, Ravaggi A, et al. Interleukin-10 increases Th1 cytokine production and cytotoxic potential in human papillomavirus-specific CD8[+] cytotoxic T lymphocyts. J Virol 2000 74: 4729–4737.

90. Soria JC, Moon C, Kemp BL et al. Lack of interleukin-10 expression is closely correlated with the expression of granulocyte-macrophage colony-stimulating factor in nonsmall cell lung cancer. Clin Cancer Res 2003;9:1785–1791.

91. Mocellin S, Marincola FM, Rossi CR, et al. The multifaced relationship between IL-10 and adaptive immunity: Putting together the pieces of a puzzle. Cytokine Growth Factor Rev 2004;61–76.

92. Sun H, Jackson MJ, Kundu N, et al. Interleukin-10 gene transfer activates interferon-gamma and the interferon-gamma-inducible genes Gbp-1/Map-1 and Mig-1 in mammary tumors. Int J Cancer 1999; 80:624–629.

93. Berlato C, Cassatella MA, Kinjiyo I, et al. Involvement of suppressor of cytokine signaling-3 as a mediator of the inhibitory effects of IL-10 on LPS induced macrophage activation. J Immunol 2002;168:6404–6411.

94. Renauld JC. Class II cytokine receptors and their ligands: Key antiviral and inflammatory modulators. Nat Rev 2003;3:667–675.

95. Walter MR. Crystal structures of α-helical cytokine receptor complexes: We've only scratched the surface. Biotechniques Suppl, 2002;S50–S57.

96. Howard M, Muchamuel T, Andrade S, Menon, S. Interleukin 10 protects mice from lethal endotoxemia. J Exp Med 1993;177, 1205–1208.

97. Gerard C, Bruyns C, Marchant A, et al.. Interleukin 10 reduces the release of tumor necrosis factor and prevents lethality in experimental endotoxemia. J Exp Med 1993;177:547–550.

98. Ishida H, Hastlngs R, Thompson-Snipes L, Howard M. Modified immunological status of anti-IL-10 treated mice. Cell Immunol 1993;148, 371–384.

99. Lotze MT, Tracey KJ. HMGB1: Nuclear Weapon in the Immune Arsenal. 2005;Nature Reviews Immunology 2005;5:331–342.

100. Rendon-Mitchell B, Ochani M, Li J, et al. IFN-γ induces high mobility group box 1 protein release partly through a TNF-dependent mechanism. J Immunol 2003;170, 3890–3897.

101. Wang H, Bloom O, Zhang M, et al. HMG-1 as a late mediator of endotoxin lethality in mice. Science 1999;285, 248–251.

102. Heremans H, Van Damme J, Dillen C, Dijkmans R, Billau A. Interferon-γ, a mediator of lethal lipopolysaccharide-induced Shwartzman-like shock reactions in mice. J Exp Med 1990;171: 1853–1869.

103. Hall GL, Compston A, Scolding NJ. β-interferon and multiple sclerosis. Trends Neurosci 1997;20: 63–67.

104. Chernoff AE, Granowitz EV, Shapiro L, et al. A randomized, controlled trial of IL-10 in humans. Inhibition of inflammatory cytokine production and immune responses. J Immunol 1995;154: 5492–5499.

105. Huhn RD, Radwanski E, O'Connell SM, et al. Pharmacokinetics and immunomodulatory properties of intravenously administered recombinant human interleukin-10 in healthy volunteers. Blood 1996;87:699-705.

106. Radwanski E, Chakraborty A, Van Wart S, et al. Pharmacokinetics and leukocyte responses of recombinant human interleukin-10. Pharm Res 1998;15:1895–1901.

10 Cytokines in Multiple Myeloma

Therapeutic Implications

Dharminder Chauhan, Teru Hideshima, and Kenneth C. Anderson

CONTENTS

1. INTRODUCTION

Multiple myeloma (MM) is a clonal plasma cell neoplasm which remains incurable despite conventional therapy; and new treatment strategies are therefore urgently required *(1,2)*. MM cells predominantly localize in bone marrow (BM), and their interaction with BM stromal cells (BMSCs) stimulates transcription and secretion of cytokines from BMSCs. Cytokines in turn not only promote the growth and survival of MM cells, but also reduce efficacy of conventional drugs *(2)*. For example, adherence of MM cells to BMSCs triggers interleukin-6 (IL-6) and insulin-like growth factor-I (IGF-I), and vascular endothelial growth factor (VEGF) production from BMSCs, which induces MM cell growth and protect against dexamethasone (Dex)-induced MM apoptosis *(3–8)*. High serum levels of IL-6 and IGF-I in MM patients *(9,10)* also correlate with clinical drug-resistance in MM. Cytokines trigger three signaling cascades in

From: *Cancer Drug Discovery and Development,*
Cytokines in the Genesis and Treatment of Cancer
Edited by: M. A. Caligiuri and M. T. Lotze © Humana Press Inc., Totowa, NJ

MM cells: mitogen-activated extracellular kinase 2(MEK)/extracellular signal-regulated kinase (ERK); phosphatidylinositol-3 kinase (PI3-kinase)/AKT; and Janus kinases (JAK)-signal transducer and activator of transcription (STAT) pathways. Novel treatment strategies based on targeting these signaling pathways are now being designed to block cytokine-mediated growth/survival and drug-resistance. In this chapter, we review the role of various cytokines in the biology of MM, as well as novel therapies that overcome cytokine-mediated growth, survival, migration and chemoresistance.

2. INTERLEUKIN-6 (IL-6) AND MM

Multiple lines of evidence support the role of IL-6 in the biology of MM: 1) IL-6 induces proliferation of MM cells *(3,11–13)*; 2) in vitro studies using antibodies to IL-6 receptor show marked inhibition of MM cell proliferation *(14–16)*; 3) IL-6 transgenic mice develop plasmacytosis *(17)*; 4) deletion of IL-6 gene blocks the generation of pristine-induced plasmacytomas in BALB/c mice *(18)*; 5) elevated IL-6 serum levels correlate with poor prognosis and high tumor mass *(9)*; 6) IL-6 serve as an osteoclast activating factor in MM bone disease *(19)*; 7) IL-6 induces X-box binding protein (XBP)-1 *(20,21)*, a transcription factor essential for differentiation of normal B-cells to plasma cells *(22,23)*, which is highly upregulated in patient MM cells *(21,24)*; and finally, 7) high IL-6 levels correlate with high telomerase activity and short telomerase length in patients with poor prognosis *(25)*.

The major signaling cascades triggered by IL-6 in MM cells are MAPK, PI3K/Akt, and JAK-STAT pathways *(24,26,27)*. The following events are triggered upon binding of soluble IL-6 to IL-6R cells: Oligomerization of signal transducer glycoprotein gp130 cross-phosphorylation on tyrosine residues and activation of JAK family members JAKs then phosphorylate tyrosine motifs in the cytoplasmic tail of gp130 creating recognition sites for signaling proteins with Src-homology-2 (SH2) domains or other tyrosine domains. The SH2-domain containing proteins, such as members of the signal transducers and activators of transcription (STATs) family or tyrosine phospahatase SHP2, are phosphorylated by JAKs upon binding to the gp130, thereby enabling them to dimerize and translocate to nucleus where they bind to IL-6 response elements (ILRE) within the promoter region of IL-6-responsive genes and trigger their transcription *(26,28–32)*. Upon activation, STAT3 homodimers or hetrodimers migrate to the nucleus, where they bind to the promoter regions of several anti-apoptotic proteins, including Bcl2, Bcl-x, *(33)* or Mcl-1 *(34,35)*, and initiate their transcription. Besides triggering JAK-STAT signaling, IL-6 also induces the growth via the conventional Ras-dependent MAPK cascade, which involves sequential activation of SHP2-Grb2-Sos1-Ras-Raf-MEK-MAPK and results in activation of transcription factors mediating growth and survival, such as nuclear factor-κB (NF-κB), nuclear factor-IL-6 (NF-IL6), and activating protein-1 (AP-1) complex (Jun/Fos) *(28,29,36)*. IL-6 also triggers growth of MM cells via activating PI3-K/Akt signaling pathway *(37,38)*. Finally, our recent study showed that IL-6 induced growth requires phosphorylation of caveolin-1, a component of lipid rafts on cell surface *(39)*.

The above findings confirm that the signaling transduction pathways triggered by IL-6 in MM cells involve several protein kinases and phosphatases, which may be targeted for therapy (Fig. 1). Drugs designed to specifically inhibit growth pathways fall into two categories: 1) modified protein ligands or small synthetic molecules; and 2) monoclonal

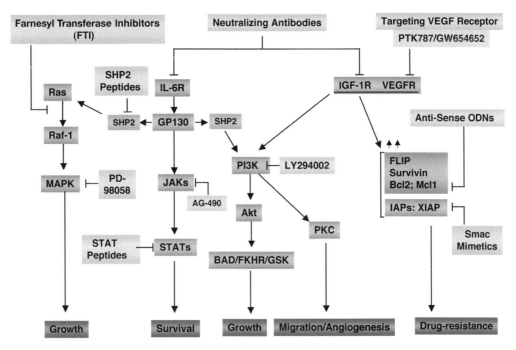

Fig. 1. Therapeutic strategies to abrogate signaling pathways mediating growth, survival, and drug-resistance in MM cell. IL-6, IGF-1 and VEGF induce growth and survival by activating MAPK, PI3K/Akt, and JAK/STAT pathways. These pathways can be interrupted at various potential sites by using specific biochemical inhibitors, neutralizing antibodies, small peptides, or antisense oligonucleotides (ODNs) against the molecules mediating growth and survival. *See* text for details. MAPK, mitogen-activated protein kinase; STAT, signal transducer and activator of transcription; IL, interleukin; JAKs, Janus kinases; VEGFR, vascular endothelial growth factor receptor; PTK, VEGF receptor tyrosine kinase inhibitor.

antibodies. Examples of biochemical inhibitors of these pathways include, antisense-oligonucleotides (ODNs) against MAPK (30), MEK1 inhibitors PD98059, or MEK1/2 inhibitor U0126 *(40)*; piceatannol (JAK1/STAT3 inhibitor) and tyrphostin AG490 (JAK2/STAT3 inhibitor) *(41)*; and PI3K inhibitor LY294002 and wortmannin *(37,42)*. Importantly, the sensitization induced by these inhibitors correlated with attenuation of anti-apoptotic proteins including, Bcl-2, Bcl-xL, and inhibitors of apoptosis proteins (IAPs). A recent study demonstrated that a fusion protein of gp130 and interleukin-6R-alpha ligand-binding domains acts as a potent IL-6 inhibitor *(43)*.

Because IL-6 activates Ras-Raf-MAPK signaling to induce growth in MM cells, mutations in Ras may result in loss of proliferation in these cells; however, a recent report showed that ectopic expression of mutated K-ras or N-ras in the IL-6-dependent MM cells induces cytokine-independent growth, which associated with constitutive activation of ERK, PI3 kinase/AKT, mammalian target of rapamycin (mTOR)/p70S6-kinase, and NF-κB) pathways *(42)*. In contrast, no STAT-3 activation was noted in ras-mutant cells. The mTOR inhibitors rapamycin and CCI-779, the PI3 kinase inhibitor LY294002, and the MEK inhibitor PD98059, all markedly inhibit growth of ras-mutant MM cells. Growth of N-ras-mutant MM cells was blocked by overexpression of the IκB super-repressor gene, which abrogated NF-κB activation. These findings suggest that several pathways mediating cytokine-independent growth are activated downstream of oncogenic ras, and that therapeutic strategies targeting these pathways may be specifically beneficial for MM patients with ras mutations.

Although various studies have provided evidence for the role of IL-6 in the growth and survival of MM cells, some cells grow in an IL-6-independent fashion. Genetic abnormalities *(44)* underlying this growth mechanism include the following: K-ras and N-ras mutations *(45,46)*; H-Ras mutant isolated from a MM cell line led to factor-independent cell growth *(47)*; the t(4;14)(p16.3;q32) translocation, which occurs uniquely in a subset of MM tumors, results in ectopic expression of wild-type fibroblast growth factor receptor-3 (FGFR3), and enhanced expression of MMSET, which may have a role in MM progression *(48,49)*; alterations in cyclin D1 (11q13), c-Myc *(50)*, c-Maf (16q23) *(51)* maf-B (20q11), and cyclin D3 (6p21) *(52,53)* oncogenes *(54)*; abnormalities of cell cycle regulatory protein Retinoblastoma (Rb), p16, and p21 *(55,56)*; and intrinsic activation of signaling cascades *(57)*. For example, a lack of Sos-1 activation is associated with the loss of IL-6 responsiveness in MM cells, and growth independent of IL-6 *(58)*.

3. INTERLEUKIN-6 AS AN ANTI-APOPTOTIC FACTOR

We and others have shown that IL-6 also functions as an anti-apoptotic agent in MM cells *(6,59–61)*. Apoptosis induced by Fas and γ-irradiation (IR) is associated with activation of various serine/threonine kinases, such as stress activated protein kinase (SAPK) or c-Jun-N-terminal kinase (JNK) and p38 kinase. Although IL-6 does not rescue MM cells from IR-induced apoptosis, it protects them against FAS-induced apoptosis via inhibition of the JNK/SAPK pathway *(62,63)*. Dex-induced apoptosis, in contrast, is associated with a significant decrease in the activities of growth related kinases, such as MAPK and p70^{RSK}, without activation of JNK/SAPK and p38 stress kinases *(60)*. Importantly, IL-6 inhibits both Dex-induced apoptosis and the associated downregulation of MAPK *(60)*. The mechanism whereby IL-6 functions as an anti-apoptoic factor is unclear. Our previous study also demonstrated the role of protein tyrosine phosphatase SHP2 in mediating the protective effects of IL-6 against Dex-induced apoptosis. Specifically, IL-6 activates SHP2 in MM cells, and treatment of MM cells with IL-6 and Dex induces binding of activated SHP2 with RAFTK, resulting in dephosphorylation of related adhesion focal tyrosine kinase (RAFTK). Importantly, we showed that RAFTK is a substrate of SHP2, both in vitro and in vivo. Overexpression of dominant negative (DN)-SHP2 abrogates the protective function of IL-6 against Dex-induced apoptosis. In concert with our findings, fibroblasts from SHP2 mutant mice show impaired MAPK activation in response to other growth factors, such as fibroblast growth factor, epidermal growth factor, and insulin growth factor *(64)*, suggesting a role of SHP2 during growth and survival signaling. Together, these findings demonstrate that SHP2 mediates the protective effect of IL-6 against Dex-induced apoptosis, and both RAFTK and SHP2 are novel therapeutic targets in MM *(65)*.

Besides affecting the cytoplasmic apoptotic signaling cascades, IL-6 also negatively regulates mitochondria-mediated cell death pathways. It is well established that mitochondria play an important role during apoptosis, because various cell death inducers cause a disruption in mitochondrial membrane potential, which precedes either apoptosis or cytolysis *(66)*. Mitochondria harbor two key enzymes, cytochrome-c (cyto-c) and second mitochondrial activator of caspases (Smac), which are released to the cytoplasm during apoptosis, thereby triggering activation of caspase-9 and caspase-3 (67). In the context of MM, our studies have shown that Dex-induced apoptosis in MM cells is associated with release of Smac from mitochondria to cytosol (61,68). Importantly, IL-6 blocks the Dex-induced Smac release, thereby preventing Dex-induced caspase-9/3 activation and apoptosis (68). Furthermore, IL-6 inhibits Dex-induced decreases in mitochondrial membrane potential (69). Together, these data suggest that IL-6 prevents Dex-induced cytotoxicity in MM cells by blocking mitochondrial alterations.

4. INSULIN-LIKE GROWTH FACTOR (IGF)-1

IGF-I, like IL-6, is a potent growth and survival factor for myeloma and triggers growth via activation of MEK/ERK and PI3-K/Akt signaling cascades (7,70–72). Importantly, IGF-1 confers protection against Dex-induced apoptosis (73,74). Besides MEK/PI3 kinase, IGF-1 also stimulates phosphorylation of forkhead transcription factor (FHKR); causes accumulation of intracellular anti-apoptotic proteins including, FLIP, survivin, cIAP-2, A1/Bfl-1, and XIAP (8); and increases telomerase activity via PI3-K/Akt/NF-κB pathway (75). IGF-1-triggered MM cell growth is inhibited by inhibition of PI3 kinase, but not by inhibition of MAPK (76). Another study demonstrates that IGF-I promotes MM cell migration via PI3 kinase/PKC and PI3 Kinase/RhoA pathways independent of Akt (77). Although IGF-1, like IL-6, triggers growth in MM cells, it triggers a differential pathophysiologic sequelae in MM cells compared to IL-6 (8). For example, IGF-1 induces a sustained activation of NF-κB and Akt, whereas IL-6 induces transient activity of these molecules. Interestingly, IL-6 induces IGF-1R phosphorylation independent of JAKs via complex formation between IL6R and IGF-1R in an IL-6R-α-transfected MM cell line, suggesting a cross-talk between IL-6R and IGF-1R in a synergistic manner (78). Finally, inhibition of IGF-1R activity with neutralizing antibodies (Fig. 1), antagonistic peptide, or the selected kinase inhibitor NVP-ADW742 induced remarkable antitumor activity even in MM cells resistant to various conventional therapies (72). Moreover, NVP-ADW742 as a single agent or in combination with other chemotherapy triggered significant antitumor activity in an orthotopic xenograft MM model. Together, these studies suggest potential clinical use of IGF-1R inhibitors in MM.

5. TRANSFORMING GROWTH FACTOR-β (TGF-β)

Our previous study showed that MM cells produce TGF-β which in turn, triggers IL-6 production from BMSCs (79). Inhibition of TGF-β receptor blocks IL-6 secretion from BMSCs and related MM cell growth. Serum TGF-β is associated with the degree of immunoparesis in MM patients (80). A recent study on 162 MM patient samples showed significant serum levels of TGF-β, VEGF, and FGF. Importantly all three are angiogenic cytokines and facilitate angiogenesis in MM (81). Interestingly, another member of the TGF-β superfamily, bone morphogenetic protein-2 (BMP-2), induces apoptosis in MM cell lines and patient's MM cells (82). The mechanism of BMP-2-induced apoptosis is blockade of IL-6 autocrine loop, associated with: down-regulation of Bcl-xL, up-regulation of p21 (WAF1)/p27(KIP1), hypo-phosphorylation of Rb, and inactivation of STAT3. These data suggest potential therapeutic use of BMP-2 in MM patients with frequent bone lesions.

6. HEPARIN BINDING EGF-LIKE GROWTH FACTORS

Syndecan-1, a heparan sulfate proteoglycan is expressed on the MM cell surface and functions by integrating extracellular signals to cytoplasmic domains of other growth factor receptors *(83)*. Specifically, it binds to various heparin-binding growth factors (HB-EGF) and mediates their signaling. Gene microarray studies showed high expression of HB-EGF transcripts in MM cells *(84)*. Importantly, HB-EGF cooperates with IL-6 to induce optimal survival of MM cells both via interaction of gp130 and EGF receptors and through PI3 kinase/Akt pathway *(85)*. Eleven members of the EGF receptor family are coexpressed in MM cells, suggesting their involvement in MM pathogenesis, and confirming their use as potential novel therapeutic targets in MM.

Hepatocyte growth factor (HGF) is also a heparin-binding MM growth factor, which increases bone resorption in MM patients *(86)*. HGF serum levels are high in MM patients and considered as a prognostic marker *(87)*. Recent studies have also shown that FGF, like HB-EGF or HGF, binds to syndecan-1 and may play a role in MM biology *(88)*; however, more comprehensive studies in MM are ongoing.

7. VASCULAR ENDOTHELIAL GROWTH FACTOR (VEGF)

VEGF is an angiogenic factor for MM cells *(89–91)*. A marked increase in VEGF secretion occurred in response to either adhesion of MM cells to BMSCs or upon treatment of MM cell with recombinant IL-6 *(92–94)*. Conversely, exposure of BMSCs to rVEGF triggered IL-6 secretion *(92)*. These findings suggest paracrine interactions between MM cells and BMSCs triggered by VEGF and IL-6 *(92)*. VEGF induces MM cell growth via phosphorylation of Flt-1 and activation of MAPK, whereas VEGF-triggered MM cell migration occurs in a PKC-dependent manner *(93)* (Fig. 1). Blocking MAPK pathway with the specific inhibitor PD184352 significantly reduced basal, as well as IL-6-induced, VEGF secretion from MM cells *(95)*. Moreover, PI3K kinase inhibitors, but not p38 MAPK inhibitors, reduced VEGF secretion by MM cells and increased the inhibitory effect of MEK1 inhibitors. A recent study shows that oncogene c-*maf* is overexpressed in MM and the c-*maf*-driven expression of integrin-β7 enhanced MM adhesion to BMSCs and secretion of VEGF *(96)*. Importantly, VEGF triggers PI3 kinase-dependent MM cell migration *(97)*. Taken together, these data indicate that VEGF not only triggers angiogenesis, but also proliferation and migration of the MM cells in the BM milieu *(93)*. They support the development of novel therapies based upon targeting VEGF and/or its receptor. In this context, our study showed that the VEGF receptor tyrosine kinase inhibitor PTK787 blocked MM growth and migration *(98)*. Finally, the pan-VEGF receptor inhibitor GW654652 demonstrated significant activity against MM cells in the BM milieu, without major toxicity in preclinical mouse models *(99)*. These data provide the framework for clinical trials of this drug-class to improve patient outcome in MM.

8. INTERLEUKIN-1

An earlier study demonstrated that recombinant IL-1α stimulates secretion of MM cell growth factor IL-6 *(100)*. IL-1β was later shown to mediate bone-resorbing activity in MM *(101)*. Other studies confirmed both the presence of IL-1β transcripts in MM cells and its role as an osteoclast activating factor (OAF) *(102–104)*. Moreover, IL-1β was reported as a marker whose presence in MGUS cells may identify patients likely to progress to MM *(105)*. Based on these observations, blocking IL-1β activity may be useful in preventing MM bone disease. In contrast, a recent study using murine MM cell line MPC-11 to evaluate use of IL-1β receptor antagonist to prevent bone disease showed that IL-1β is not a primary factor mediating in vivo bone destruction by the MPC-11 cell line *(106)*. Because bone destruction is a hallmark of MM in the majority of patients, the therapeutic strategies based upon inhibiting the production or function of OAFs may be useful, but more extensive preclinical studies are needed.

9. TUMOR NECROSIS FACTOR FAMILY

Previous studies have shown that 1) MM patients with bone disease have high TNFα levels *(107,108)*, and that 2) TNFα triggers a modest (< twofold) proliferation of MM cells associated with activation of MAPK but not STAT-3 *(109,110)*. Inhibitors of TNFα (pentoxyphylline and roloxifen) blocked TNFα-induced proliferation of MM cells. Importantly, TNFα triggers NF-κB-dependent upregulation of ICAM-1, VCAM-1, or MUC-1 on human MM cells, thereby promoting not only interaction between MM and BMSCs, but also adhesion-related cytokine (IL-6/IGF-1/TGF-β) secretion and MM cell growth *(111)*. In addition to providing evidence for TNF-α as a growth/survival factor for MM *(112)*, these findings confirm the involvement of NF-κB during interaction of MM and BMSCs *(5)*. Furthermore, oligonucleotide array analyses showed significantly increased NF-κB binding activity in MM cells adherent to fibronectin compared to cells in suspension *(113)*. Together, these observations suggest that TNF-α in the BM microenvironment triggers NF-κB activation and thereby promotes growth/survival of MM cells.

10. OTHER TNF FAMILY MEMBERS

CD40 is a 48 kDa glycosylated phosphoprotein that is a member of the TNF-receptor superfamily. CD40 was originally identified in B-lymphocytes, and is also found on monocytes, dendritic cells, some carcinoma cell lines, and the thymic epithelium. CD40 is also expressed on freshly isolated myeloma cells: CD40 specific MoAb G28-5 induces proliferation in these cells, which can be inhibited by IL-6-neutralizing mAb. *(114)*. Furthermore, CV-1/EBNA cells expressing the human CD40 ligand also induced the proliferation of the MM cells *(114,115)*. CD40 ligand is a TNFα family member, which affects MM cell biology both directly and indirectly through its effects on the BM microenvironment. For example, CD40 ligation induces VEGF secretion in BMSCs, which in turn mediates MM-cell homing and migration, as well as angiogenesis *(116)*. Treatment of MM cells with either sCD40L or anti-CD40 Ab induces MM cell migration *via* activation of PI3/Akt NF-κB (116). Interestingly, presence or absence of p53 may determine CD40-triggered biologic sequelae in MM cells *(117)*. Finally, a recent study also showed that rhuCD40 mAb triggers autologous antibody-dependent cellular cytotoxicity against patient MM cells *(118)*, which is providing the framework for clinical evaluation of rhuCD40 mAb immunotherapy to improve patient outcome in MM.

11. BAFF AND APRIL

BAFF/BlyS (B-cell activating factor/B-lymphocyte stimulator), a member of TNF family, is a survival factor for B-cells *(119)*. BAFF has been identified as a potential therapeutic target on autoreactive B-cells *(120)*. APRIL is a related factor that shares receptors with BAFF and yet plays a distinct biologic role *(119)*. The mechanism whereby BAFF exerts its effect involves binding to three receptors: transmembrane activator and CAML interactor (TACI); B-cell maturation antigen (BCMA); and BAFF receptor (BAFF-R). Recent studies showed that BAFF and APRIL as well as their receptors, are expressed on MM cells and modulate growth in an autocrine manner *(121,122)*. Importantly, both BAFF and APRIL triggered activation of NF-κB, PI3 kinase/AKT, and MAPK kinase pathways, as well as inducing upregulation of Mcl-1 and Bcl-2 anti-apoptotic proteins in MM cells. Additionally, BAFF or APRIL augments survival of patient MM cells in BM microenvironment and protect against Dex-induced apoptosis. Finally, MM patient serum contains higher BAFF and APRIL levels compared to healthy donors. Together, these findings suggest that inhibitors of BAFF or APRIL, such as anti-BAFF/APRIL antibody or receptor-Fc fusion proteins, may have clinical utility in MM, both either alone or in combination with Dex.

12. OSTEOCLAST ACTIVATING FACTORS (OAFs): RANKL AND MIP-1α

MM is associated with the development of bone disease owing to the increased activity of osteoclasts (OCLs) present within the BM milieu *(123)*. The secretion of OAFs from MM cells *(124)* and BMSCs activate OCLs *(125,126)*. Besides TNF-β and IL-6, receptor activator of NF-κB (RANKL) and macrophage inflammatory protein-1α (MIP-1α) are other OAFs implicated in MM bone disease. Osteoprotegerin (OPG), a member of the TNF receptor family, binds to the receptor RANKL and thereby inhibits bone resorption in the normal marrow milieu; in contrast, in MM BM microenvironment the balance between OPG and RANKL is disrupted: increased RANKL and decreased OPG results in bone loss. OPG blocks TRAIL/Apo2L-induced apoptosis in MM cells, which can be prevented by soluble RANKL. These studies suggest that OPG may function as a paracrine survival factor for MM. Transgenic animals that overexpressed OPG developed osteopetrosis, providing a rationale for using OPG to inhibit the imbalance in bone formation/resorption seen in MM. Indeed, study in the 5T33MM murine model of MM showed that inhibiting the interaction between RANKL and RANK with Fc-OPG inhibits the development of MM bone disease *(127)*. RANK-L antagonist RANK-Fc also reduces MM-induced osteoclastogenesis, development of bone disease, and MM progression *(125,128)*.

MIP-1α is a chemokine and an OAF in MM *(129,130)*. Increased IL-3 mRNA levels in the BM milieu, together with MIP-1α and RANKL, enhanced osteolytic activity and bone resorption, suggesting a coordinated activity of OAFs contributing to bone destruction in MM *(131)*. However, another in vivo study using RANK knock-out mice showed that MIP-1α alone is sufficient to induce MM-like destructive lesions in bone *(132)*. Finally, examination of gene expression profiles on 92 primary MM cells demonstrated a strong correlation between kappa-positive MM patient subgroup with high levels of MIP-1α transcripts and active MM bone disease *(133)*.

13. ADDITIONAL GROWTH FACTORS AND CHEMOKINE-RELATED CYTOKINES

Oncostatin M (OSM), leukemia inhibitory factor, and ciliary neurotropic factor induce growth in MM cells using the common gp130 receptor *(134,135)*. OSM triggers tyrosine phosphorylation and activation of JAK2, but not JAK1 or Tyk2, kinases and direct interaction of JAK2 kinase with Grb2 *(135)*. IL-10 affects MM cells by stimulating secondary signals for MM cell growth through OSM and IL-11 *(136)*. In addition, IL-10 prevents all trans retinoic acid (ATRA)-induced growth inhibition of MM cells *(136)*. A close relationship between OSM and IL-6 has also been demonstrated *(137)*.

Granulocyte/macrophage-colony stimulating factor (GM-CSF) has been reported to enhance the IL-6 responsiveness of MM cells *(138)*. GM-CSF has acceptable toxicity in patients with MM, but increased PCLI in selected MM patients *(139)*. Interleukin-11 can support the growth of IL-6 dependent cell lines and promote B-cell differentiation, but does not augment DNA synthesis by purified MM cells *(140,141)*. Autocrine growth mediated by IL-15 has been demonstrated in both MM cell lines and patient cells *(142)*. IL-21 is a recently cloned cytokine with homology to IL-2, IL-4, and IL-15, which triggers growth/survival in MM *via* phosphorylation of Jak1, STAT3, and ERK *(143)*.

Finally, the chemokine stromal cell-derived factor-1α (SDF-1α) rapidly and transiently up-regulated VLA-4-mediated MM cell adhesion to both CS-1/fibronectin and VCAM-1, suggesting its contribution to the trafficking and localization of these cells in the BM microenvironment *(144)*. SDF-1α induces proliferation, migration, and protection against Dex-induced apoptosis via MAPK, PI3 Kinase/Akt, and NF-κB signaling cascades, respectively. Importantly, SDF-1α also triggers secretion of IL-6 and VEGF from BMSCs, thereby further promoting MM cell growth, survival, drug-resistance, and migration in a paracrine manner *(111)*. Recent studies further established the role of chemokines in the homing of MM cells to BM: MM cell lines express functional CCR1, CXCR3 and CXCR4 receptors; and MM cells migrated in response to CCR1 ligands RANTES and MIP-1α as well as CXCR4 ligand SDF-1 *(145)*. Thus, binding of chemokine receptors to ligands localizes MM cells in the BM. Long-term engraftment of both MM cell lines and freshly isolated cells from MM BM has been reported in severe combined immunodeficient (SCID) mice and in SCID-hu mice, providing additional models for growth of MM in vivo *(146,147)*.

14. THERAPIES TARGETING MM AND BM MICROENVIRONMENT

The above studies define the role of multiple cytokines and the mechanisms whereby they mediate growth and survival of MM cells. Various biochemical inhibitors of these growth/survival signaling cascades trigger or enhance chemotherapy-induced apoptosis in MM cells and have therapeutic use *(148)* (Fig. 1): farnesyl transferase inhibitor (FTI) to block Ras/MAPK; 7-hydroxystarosporine (UCN-01) and MEK/2 inhibitor *(149)*; JAK/STAT pathway inhibitor piceatannol (JAK1/STAT3 inhibitor) and tryphostin AG490 (JAK/STAT3 inhibitor) *(41)*; STAT peptides; protein tyrosine phosphatase SHP2 peptides; and small inducible RNA (siRNA) against anti-apoptotic proteins such as, Bcl2, Mcl-1, cIAPs, and XIAP, and finally, inhibitors of NF-κB pathway including PS-1145, Bay 11-7082, UCN-01, or curcumin.

Delineation of the cytokine network in MM has also provided the framework to evaluate, validate, and define mechanisms of many novel drugs *(2,27,111)*. For example, the following drugs modulate interaction between MM to BMSCs and related growth/survival cytokine signaling, and have demonstrated remarkable anti-MM activity: PS-341 (Velcade) *(150,151)*; triterpinoid CDDO-Im *(74)*; thalidomide/Relvimid *(152,153)*; IGF-1R inhibitor *(72)*; VEGF receptor kinase inhibitor PTK787 *(98)*; HDAC inhibitor

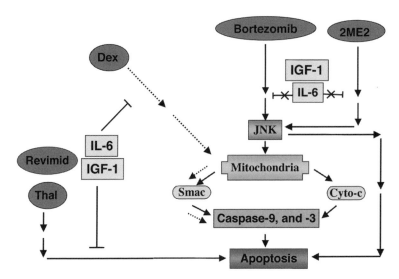

Fig. 2. Delineation of conventional and novel apoptosis-inducing agents within the signaling cascades of MM cells. Bortezomib, 2ME2, or Triterpenoid CDDO-Im induce activation of JNK, which translocates to mitochondria and triggers the release of cyto-c and Smac. Dex-induced apoptotic signaling proceeds without concurrent JNK activation and cyto-c release; however, Dex triggers Smac release and downstream activation of caspase-9 and -3. Both IL-6 and IGF-1 block Dex-triggered apoptotic signaling. Bortezomib, 2ME2 or CDDO-Im induce MM cell apoptosis even in the presence of IL-6 and/or IGF-1, suggesting that these novel anti-MM agents overcome the protective effects of cytokines. *See* text for details. Dex, dexamethasone; IL, interleukin; IGF, insulin-like growth factor; ME, methoxyestradiol; JNK, c-Jun-N-terminal kinase; Smac, second mitochondrial activator of caspases.

SAHA *(154)*; LAQ-824 *(155)*; 2-Methoxyestradiol (2-ME2) *(156)*; arsenic trioxide *(157)*; LPAAT-beta inhibitor *(158)*; HSP-90 inhibitor *(159)*; or TRAIL *(160)*. Importantly, many of the novel drugs overcome the anti-apoptotic effects of cytokines present in the BM milieu, such as IL-6 or IGF-1 against conventional therapies (Fig. 2). Based on preclinical and clinical studies, the FDA recently approved Bortezomib/Velcade for the treatment of relapsed/refractory MM *(150,151)*. In addition, both thalidomide and Relvimid are effective therapies for refractory MM *(152,153)*.

Ongoing and future studies using genomics and proteomics will identify and characterize not only new signaling molecules, but also unveil the complex crosstalk between growth and apoptotic signaling cascades. These studies will establish the framework for validating novel drugs to target both the tumor cell and the microenvironment, overcome drug resistance, and improve patient outcome in MM.

REFERENCES

1. Greenlee RT, Murray T, Bolden S, Wingo PA. Cancer statistics, 2000. CA Cancer J Clin 2000; 50(1):7–33.
2. Anderson KC. Moving disease biology from the lab to the clinic. Cancer 2003;97(3 Suppl):796–801.
3. Klein B, Zhang XG, Jourdan M, et al. Paracrine rather than autocrine regulation of myeloma-cell growth and differentiation by interleukin-6. Blood 1989;73(2):517–526.
4. Uchiyama H, Barut BA, Mohrbacher AF, Chauhan D, Anderson KC. Adhesion of human myeloma-derived cell lines to bone marrow stromal cells stimulates IL-6 secretion. Blood 1993;82:3712–3720.

5. Chauhan D, Uchiyama H, Akbarali Y, et al. Multiple myeloma cell adhesion-induced interleukin-6 expression in bone marrow stromal cells involves activation of NF-kappa B. Blood 1996; 87(3): 1104–1112.
6. Lichtenstein A, Tu Y, Fady C, Vescio R, Berenson J. Interleukin-6 inhibits apoptosis of malignant plasma cells. Cell Immunol 1995;162:248–255.
7. Freund GG, Kulas DT, Mooney RA. Insulin and IGF-1 increase mitogenesis and glucose metabolism in the multiple myeloma cell line, RPMI 8226. J Immunol 1993;151(4):1811–1820.
8. Mitsiades CS, Mitsiades N, Poulaki V, et al. Activation of NF-kappaB and upregulation of intracellular anti-apoptotic proteins via the IGF-1/Akt signaling in human multiple myeloma cells: Therapeutic implications. Oncogene 2002;21(37):5673–5683.
9. Bataille R, Jourdan M, Zhang XG, et al. Serum levels of interleukin-6, a potent myeloma cell growth factor, as a reflection of disease severity in plasma cell dyscrasias. J Clin Invest 1989;84:2008–2011.
10. Tucci A, Bonadonna S, Cattaneo C, Ungari M, Giustina A, Guiseppe R. Transformation of a MGUS to overt multiple myeloma: The possible role of a pituitary macroadenoma secreting high levels of insulin-like growth factor 1 (IGF-1). Leuk Lymphoma 2003;44(3):543–545.
11. Kawano MM, Hirano T, Matsuda T, et al. Autocrine generation and requirement of BSF-2/IL-6 for human multiple myeloma. Nature 1988;332:83–85.
12. Anderson KC, Jones RM, Morimoto C, Leavitt P, Barut BA. Response patterns of purified myeloma cells to hematopoietic growth factors. Blood 1989;73(7):1915–1924.
13. Barut BA, Zon LI, Cochran MK, et al. Role of interleukin 6 in the growth of myeloma-derived cell lines. Leuk Res 1992;16(10):951–959.
14. Klein B, Wijdenes J, Zhang XG, et al. Murine anti-interleukin-6 monoclonal antibody therapy for a patient with plasma cell leukemia. Blood 1991;78(5):1198–1204.
15. Bataille R, Barlogie B, Lu ZY, et al. Biologic effects of anti-interleukin-6 murine monoclonal antibody in advanced multiple myeloma. Blood 1995;86(2):685–691.
16. Sporeno E, Savino R, Ciapponi L, et al. Human interleukin-6 receptor super-antagonists with high potency and wide spectrum on multiple myeloma cells. Blood 1996;87(11):4510–4519.
17. Suematsu S, Matsuda T, Aozasa K, et al. IgG1 plasmacytosis in interleukin 6 transgenic mice. Proc Natl Acad Sci U S A 1989;86(19):7547–7551.
18. Lattanzio G, Libert C, Aquilina M, et al. Defective development of pristane-oil-induced plasmacytomas in interleukin-6-deficient BALB/c mice. Am J Pathol 1997;151(3):689–696.
19. Barille S, Collette M, Bataille R, et al. Myeloma cells upregulate IL-6 but downregulate osteocalcin production by osteoblastic cells through cell to cell contact. Blood 1995;86:3151–3159.
20. Wen XY, Stewart AK, Sooknanan RR, et al. Identification of c-myc promoter-binding protein and X-box binding protein 1 as interleukin-6 target genes in human multiple myeloma cells. Int J Oncol 1999;15(1):173–178.
21. Chauhan D, Li G, Auclair D, et al. Identification of genes regulated by 2-methoxyestradiol (2ME2) in multiple myeloma cells using oligonucleotide arrays. Blood 2003;101(9):3606–3614.
22. Reimold AM, Iwakoshi NN, Manis J, et al. Plasma cell differentiation requires the transcription factor XBP-1. Nature 2001;412(6844):300–307.
23. Iwakoshi NN, Lee AH, Vallabhajosyula P, Otipoby KL, Rajewsky K, Glimcher LH. Plasma cell differentiation and the unfolded protein response intersect at the transcription factor XBP-1. Nat Immunol 2003;4(4):321–329.
24. Klein B, Tarte K, Jourdan M, et al. Survival and proliferation factors of normal and malignant plasma cells. Int J Hematol 2003;78(2):106–113.
25. Wu KD, Orme LM, Shaughnessy J, Jr., Jacobson J, Barlogie B, Moore MA. Telomerase and telomere length in multiple myeloma: Correlations with disease heterogeneity, cytogenetic status, and overall survival. Blood 2003;101(12):4982–4989.
26. Heinrich PC, Behrmann I, Haan S, Hermanns HM, Muller-Newen G, Schaper F. Principles of interleukin (IL)-6-type cytokine signalling and its regulation. Biochem J 2003;374(Pt 1):1–20.
27. Chauhan D, Anderson KC. Mechanisms of cell death and survival in multiple myeloma (MM): Therapeutic implications. Apoptosis 2003;8(4):337–343.
28. Kishimoto T, Taga T, Akira S. Cytokine signal transduction. Cell 1994;76:253.
29. Kishimoto T, Akira S, Narazaki M, Taga T. Interleukin-6 family of cytokines and gp130. Blood 1995;86:1243.
30. Ogata A, Chauhan D, Teoh G, et al. Interleukin-6 triggers cell growth via the *ras*-dependent mitogen-activated protein kinase cascade. J Immunology 1997(159):2212–2221.

31. Feng GS, Hui CC, Pawson T. SH2-containing phosphotyrosine phosphatase as a target of protein-tyrosine kinases. Science 1993;259(5101):1607–1611.
32. Vogel W, Lammers R, Huang J, Ullrich A. Activation of a phosphotyrosine phosphatase by tyrosine phosphorylation. Science 1993;259(5101):1611–1614.
33. Catlett-Falcone R, Landowski TH, Oshiro MM, et al. Constitutive activation of STAT3 signaling confers resistance to apoptosis in human U266 myeloma cells. Immunity 1999;10:105–115.
34. Puthier D, Bataille R, Amiot M. IL-6 up-regulates mcl-1 in human myeloma cells through JAK/STAT rather than ras / MAP kinase pathway. Eur J Immunol 1999;29(12):3945–3950.
35. Derenne S, Monia B, Dean NM, et al. Antisense strategy shows that Mcl-1 rather than Bcl-2 or Bcl-x(L) is an essential survival protein of human myeloma cells. Blood 2002;100(1):194–199.
36. Neumann C, Zehentmaier G, Danhauser-Riedl S, Emmerich B, Hallek M. Interleukin-6 induces tyrosine phosphorylation of the Ras activating protein Shc, and its complex formation with Grb2 in the human multiple myeloma cell line LP-1. Eur J Immunol 1996;26(2):379–384.
37. Hideshima T, Nakamura N, Chauhan D, Anderson KC. Biologic sequelae of interleukin-6 induced PI3-K/Akt signaling in multiple myeloma. Oncogene 2001;20(42):5991–6000.
38. Hsu JH, Shi Y, Hu L, Fisher M, Franke TF, Lichtenstein A. Role of the AKT kinase in expansion of multiple myeloma clones: Effects on cytokine-dependent proliferative and survival responses. Oncogene 2002;21(9):1391–1400.
39. Podar K, Tai YT, Cole CE, et al. Essential role of caveolae in interleukin-6- and insulin-like growth factor I-triggered Akt-1-mediated survival of multiple myeloma cells. J Biol Chem 2003;278(8):5794–5801.
40. Dai Y, Pei XY, Rahmani M, Conrad DH, Dent P, Grant S. Interruption of the NF-{kappa}b pathway by Bay 11-7082 promotes UCN-01-mediated mitochondrial dysfunction and apoptosis in human multiple myeloma cells. Blood 2004;103(7):2761–2770.
41. Alas S, Bonavida B. Inhibition of constitutive STAT3 activity sensitizes Resistant non-Hodgkin's lymphoma and multiple myeloma to chemotherapeutic drug-mediated apoptosis. Clin Cancer Res 2003;9(1):316–326.
42. Hu L, Shi Y, Hsu JH, Gera J, Van Ness B, Lichtenstein A. Downstream effectors of oncogenic ras in multiple myeloma cells. Blood 2003;101(8):3126–3135.
43. Ancey C, Kuster A, Haan S, Herrmann A, Heinrich PC, Muller-Newen G. A fusion protein of the gp130 and interleukin-6Ralpha ligand-binding domains acts as a potent interleukin-6 inhibitor. J Biol Chem 2003;278(19):16,968–16,972.
44. Fonseca R, Barlogie B, Bataille R, et al. Genetics and cytogenetics of multiple myeloma: A workshop report. Cancer Res 2004;64(4):1546–1558.
45. Billadeau D, Liu PC, Jelinek D, Shah N, Lebien TW, Vanness B. Activating mutations in the N- and K-ras oncogenes differentially affect the growth properties of the IL-6 dependent myeloma cell line. Cancer Res 1997;57(11):2268–2275.
46. Bezieau S, Devilder MC, Avet-Loiseau H, et al. High incidence of N and K-Ras activating mutations in multiple myeloma and primary plasma cell leukemia at diagnosis. Hum Mutat 2001;18(3):212–224.
47. Crowder C, Kopantzev E, Williams K, Lengel C, Miki T, Rudikoff S. An unusual H-Ras mutant isolated from a human multiple myeloma line leads to transformation and factor-independent cell growth. Oncogene 2003;22(5):649–659.
48. Chesi M, Bergsagel PL, Kuehl WM. The enigma of ectopic expression of FGFR3 in multiple myeloma: A critical initiating event or just a target for mutational activation during tumor progression. Curr Opin Hematol 2002;9(4):288–293.
49. Winkler JM, Greipp P, Fonseca R. t(4;14)(p16.3;q32) is strongly associated with a shorter survival in myeloma patients. Br J Haematol 2003;120(1):170–171.
50. Kuehl WM, Brents LA, Chesi M, Huppi K, Bergsagel PL. Dysregulation of c-myc in multiple myeloma. Curr Top Microbiol Immunol 1997;224:277–282.
51. Chesi M, Bergsagel PL, Shonukan OO, et al. Frequent dysregulation of the c-maf proto-oncogene at 16q23 by translocation to an Ig locus in multiple myeloma. Blood 1998;91(12):4457–4463.
52. Bergsagel PL, Kuehl WM. Chromosome translocations in multiple myeloma. Oncogene 2001; 20(40):5611–5622.
53. Shaughnessy J, Jr., Gabrea A, Qi Y, et al. Cyclin D3 at 6p21 is dysregulated by recurrent chromosomal translocations to immunoglobulin loci in multiple myeloma. Blood 2001;98(1):217–223.
54. Rasmussen T, Theilgaard-Monch K, Hudlebusch HR, Lodahl M, Johnsen HE, Dahl IM. Occurrence of dysregulated oncogenes in primary plasma cells representing consecutive stages of myeloma pathogenesis: Indications for different disease entities. Br J Haematol 2003;123(2):253–262.

55. Urashima M, Ogata A, Chauhan D, et al. Interleukin-6 promotes multiple myeloma cell growth via phosphorylation of retinoblastoma protein. Blood 1996;88(6):2219–2227.
56. Urashima M, Teoh G, Ogata A, et al. Role of CDK4 and p16[INK4A] in interleukin-6-mediated growth of multiple myeloma. Leukemia 1997;11:1957–1963.
57. Chauhan D, Hideshima T, Anderson KC. Apoptotic signaling in multiple myeloma: Therapeutic implications. Int J Hematol 2003;78(2):114–120.
58. Ogata A, Chauhan D, Urashima M, Teoh G, Treon SP, Anderson KC. Blockade of mitogen-activated protein kinase cascade signaling in interleukin-6 independent multiple myeloma cells. Clinical Cancer Research 1997;3:1017–1022.
59. Hardin J, MacLeod S, Grigorieva I, et al. Interleukin-6 prevents dexamethasone-induced myeloma cell death. Blood 1994;84(9):3063–3070.
60. Chauhan D, Pandey P, Ogata A, et al. Dexamethasone induces apoptosis of multiple myeloma cells in a JNK/SAP kinase independent mechanism. Oncogene 1997;15:837–843.
61. Chauhan D, Pandey P, Ogata A, et al. Cytochrome-c dependent and independent induction of apoptosis in multiple myeloma cells. J Biol Chem 1997;272:29,995–29,997.
62. Chauhan D, Kharbanda S, Ogata A, et al. Interleukin-6 inhibits Fas-induced apoptosis and stress-activated protein kinase activation in multiple myeloma cells. Blood 1997;89:227–234.
63. Xu FH, Sharma S, Gardner A, et al. Interleukin-6-induced inhibition of multiple myeloma cell apoptosis: Support for the hypothesis that protection is mediated via inhibition of the JNK/SAPK pathway. Blood 1998;92(1):241–251.
64. Saxton TM, Pawson T. Morophogenetic movements at gastrulation require the SH2 tyrosine phosphatase Shp2. Proc Natl Acad Sci USA 1999;96(7):3790–3795.
65. Chauhan D, Pandey P, Hideshima T, et al. SHP2 mediates the protective effect of interleukin-6 against dexamethasone-induced apoptosis in multiple myeloma cells. J Biol Chem 2000;275(36): 27,845–27,850.
66. Bossy-Wetzel E, Green DR. Apoptosis: Checkpoint at the mitochondrial frontier. Mutat Res 1999; 434(3):243–251.
67. Ferri KF, Kroemer G. Mitochondria—the suicide organelles. Bioessays 2001;23(2):111–115.
68. Chauhan D, Hideshima T, Rosen S, Reed JC, Kharbanda S, Anderson KC. Apaf-1/cytochrome c-independent and Smac-dependent induction of apoptosis in multiple myeloma (MM) cells. J Biol Chem 2001;276(27):24,453–24,456.
69. Chauhan D, Li G, Sattler M, et al. Superoxide-dependent and -independent mitochondrial signaling during apoptosis in multiple myeloma cells. Oncogene 2003;22(40):6296–6300.
70. Georgii-Hemming P, Wiklund HJ, Ljunggren O, Nilsson K. Insulin-like growth factor I is a growth and survival factor in human multiple myeloma cell lines. Blood 1996;88:2250.
71. Jelinek DF, Witzig TE, Arendt BK. A role for insulin-like growth factor in the regulation of IL-6-responsive human myeloma cell line growth. J Immunol 1997;159(1):487–496.
72. Mitsiades C, Mitsiades N, McMullan C, et al. Inhibition of the insulin-like growth factor-1 tyrosine kinase activity as a therapeutic strategy for multiple myeloma, other hematologic malignancies, and solid tumors. Cancer cell 2004;5:221–230.
73. Tu Y, Gardner A, Lichtenstein A. The phosphatidylinositol 3-kinase/AKT kinase pathway in multiple myeloma plasma cells: Roles in cytokine-dependent survival and proliferative responses. Cancer Res 2000;60(23):6763–6770.
74. Chauhan D, Li G, Podar K, et al. The bortezomib/proteasome inhibitor PS-341 and triterpenoid CDDO-Im induce synergistic anti-multiple myeloma (MM) activity and overcome bortezomib resistance. Blood 2004;103(8):3158–3166.
75. Akiyama M, Hideshima T, Hayashi T, et al. Cytokines modulate telomerase activity in a human multiple myeloma cell line. Cancer Res 2002;62(13):3876–3882.
76. Qiang YW, Kopantzev E, Rudikoff S. Insulinlike growth factor-I signaling in multiple myeloma: Downstream elements, functional correlates, and pathway cross-talk. Blood 2002;99(11):4138–4146.
77. Qiang YW, Yao L, Tosato G, Rudikoff S. Insulin-like growth factor I induces migration and invasion of human multiple myeloma cells. Blood 2004;103(1):301–308.
78. Abroun S, Ishikawa H, Tsuyama N, et al. Receptor synergy of interleukin-6 (IL-6) and insulin-like growth factor-I in myeloma cells that highly express the IL-6 receptor {alpha}. Blood 2004;103(6): 2291–2298.
79. Urashima M, Ogata A, Chauhan D, et al. Transforming growth factor-beta1: Differential effects on multiple myeloma vs normal B cells. Blood 1996;87(5):1928–1938.

80. Kyrtsonis MC, Repa C, Dedoussis GV, et al. Serum transforming growth factor-beta 1 is related to the degree of immunoparesis in patients with multiple myeloma. Med Oncol 1998;15(2):124–128.

81. Urba ska-Rys H, Wierzbowska A, Robak T. Circulating angiogenic cytokines in multiple myeloma and related disorders. Eur Cytokine Netw 2003;14(1):40–51.

82. Kawamura C, Kizaki M, Yamato K, et al. Bone morphogenetic protein-2 induces apoptosis in human myeloma cells with modulation of STAT3. Blood 2000;96(6):2005–2011.

83. Zimmermann P, David G. The syndecans, tuners of transmembrane signaling. FASEB J 1999;13 Suppl:S91–S100.

84. De Vos J, Couderc G, Tarte K, et al. Identifying intercellular signaling genes expressed in malignant plasma cells by using complementary DNA arrays. Blood 2001;98(3):771–780.

85. Wang YD, De Vos J, Jourdan M, et al. Cooperation between heparin-binding EGF-like growth factor and interleukin-6 in promoting the growth of human myeloma cells. Oncogene 2002;21(16): 2584–2592.

86. Derksen PW, Keehnen RM, Evers LM, van Oers MH, Spaargaren M, Pals ST. Cell surface proteoglycan syndecan-1 mediates hepatocyte growth factor binding and promotes Met signaling in multiple myeloma. Blood 2002;99(4):1405–1410.

87. Seidel C, Borset M, Turesson I, et al. Elevated serum concentrations of Hepatocyte growth factor in patients with multiple myeloma. Blood 1998;91:806–812.

88. Sato N, Hattori Y, Wenlin D, et al. Elevated level of plasma basic fibroblast growth factor in multiple myeloma correlates with increased disease activity. Jpn J Cancer Res 2002;93(4):459–466.

89. Di Raimondo F, Azzaro MP, Palumbo G, et al. Angiogenic factors in multiple myeloma: Higher levels in bone marrow than in peripheral blood. Haematologica 2000;85(8):800–805.

90. Rajkumar SV, Witzig TE. A review of angiogenesis and antiangiogenic therapy with thalidomide in multiple myeloma. Cancer Treat Rev 2000;26(5):351–362.

91. Xu JL, Lai R, Kinoshita T, Nakashima N, Nagasaka T. Proliferation, apoptosis, and intratumoral vascularity in multiple myeloma: Correlation with the clinical stage and cytological grade. J Clin Pathol 2002;55(7):530–534.

92. Dankar B, Padro T, Leo R, et al. Vascular endothelial growth factor and interleukin-6 in paracrine tumor-stromal cell interactions in multiple myeloma. Blood 2000;95(8):2630–2336.

93. Podar K, Tai YT, Davies FE, et al. Vascular endothelial growth factor triggers signaling cascades mediating multiple myeloma cell growth and migration. Blood 2001;98(2):428–435.

94. Gupta D, Treon SP, Shima Y, et al. Adherence of multiple myeloma cells to bone marrow stromal cells upregulates vascular endothelial growth factor secretion: Therapeutic applications. Leukemia 2001;15(12):1950–1961.

95. Giuliani N, Lunghi P, Morandi F, et al. Downmodulation of ERK protein kinase activity inhibits VEGF secretion by human myeloma cells and myeloma-induced angiogenesis. Leukemia 2004; 18(3):628–635.

96. Hurt EM, Wiestner A, Rosenwald A, et al. Overexpression of c-maf is a frequent oncogenic event in multiple myeloma that promotes proliferation and pathological interactions with bone marrow stroma. Cancer Cell 2004;5(2):191–199.

97. Podar K, Tai YT, Lin BK, et al. Vascular endothelial growth factor-induced migration of multiple myeloma cells is associated with beta 1 integrin- and phosphatidylinositol 3-kinase-dependent PKCalpha activation. J Biol Chem 2002;277(10):7875–7881.

98. Lin B, Podar K, Gupta D, et al. The vascular endothelial growth factor receptor tyrosine kinase inhibitor PTK787/ZK222584 inhibits growth and migration of multiple myeloma cells in the bone marrow microenvironment. Cancer Res 2002;62(17):5019–5026.

99. Podar K, Catley LP, Tai YT, et al. GW654652, the pan-inhibitor of VEGF receptors, blocks the growth and migration of multiple myeloma cells in the bone marrow microenvironment. Blood 2004; 103(9):3474–3479.

100. Kawano M, Tanaka H, Ishikawa H, al. e. Interleukin-1 accelerates autocrine growth of myeloma cells through interleukin-6 in human myeloma. Blood 1989;73:2145–2148.

101. Cozzolino F, Torcia M, Aldinucci D, et al. Production of interleukin-1 by bone marrow myeloma cells: Its role in the pathogenesis of lytic bone lesions. Blood 1989;74:380–387.

102. Costes V, Portier M, Lu ZY, Rossi JF, Bataille R, Klein B. Interleukin-1 in multiple myeloma: Producer cells and their role in the control of IL-6 production. Br J Haematol 1998;103(4): 1152–1160.

103. Lust JA, Donovan KA. The role of interleukin-1 beta in the pathogenesis of multiple myeloma. Hematol Oncol Clin North Am 1999;13(6):1117–1125.

104. Donovan KA, Lacy MQ, Gertz MA, Lust JA. IL-1beta expression in IgM monoclonal gammopathy and its relationship to multiple myeloma. Leukemia 2002;16(3):382–385.
105. Lacy MQ, Donovan DA, Heimbach JH, et al. Comparison of interleukin-1b expression by in situ hybridization in monoclonal gammopathy of undetermined significance and multiple myeloma. Blood 1999;93:300–305.
106. Ferguson VL, Simske SJ, Ayers RA, et al. Effect of MPC-11 myeloma and MPC-11 + IL-1 receptor antagonist treatment on mouse bone properties. Bone 2002;30(1):109–116.
107. Thompson MA, Witzig TE, Kumar S, et al. Plasma levels of tumour necrosis factor alpha and interleukin-6 predict progression-free survival following thalidomide therapy in patients with previously untreated multiple myeloma. Br J Haematol 2003;123(2):305–308.
108. Alexandrakis MG, Passam FH, Sfiridaki K, et al. Interleukin-18 in multiple myeloma patients: Serum levels in relation to response to treatment and survival. Leuk Res 2004;28(3):259–266.
109. Hideshima T, Chauhan D, Schlossman R, Richardson P, Anderson KC. The role of tumor necrosis factor alpha in the pathophysiology of human multiple myeloma: Therapeutic applications. Oncogene 2001;20(33):4519–4527.
110. Bharti AC, Donato N, Singh S, Aggarwal BB. Curcumin (diferuloylmethane) down-regulates the constitutive activation of nuclear factor-kappa B and Ikappa Balpha kinase in human multiple myeloma cells, leading to suppression of proliferation and induction of apoptosis. Blood 2003;101(3):1053–1062.
111. Hideshima T, Anderson KC. Molecular mechanisms of novel therapeutic approaches for multiple myeloma. Nat Rev Cancer 2002;2(12):927–937.
112. Hideshima T, Chauhan D, Richardson P, et al. NF-kappa B as a therapeutic target in multiple myeloma. J Biol Chem 2002;28:28.
113. Landowski TH, Olashaw NE, Agrawal D, Dalton WS. Cell adhesion-mediated drug resistance (CAM-DR) is associated with activation of NF-kappa B (RelB/p50) in myeloma cells. Oncogene 2003;22(16):2417–2421.
114. Westendorf JJ, Ahmann GJ, Armitage RJ, et al. CD40 expression in malignant plasma cells. Role in stimulation of autocrine IL-6 secretion by a human myeloma cell line. J Immunol 1994;152(1):117–128.
115. Tong AW, Stone MJ. CD40 and the effect of anti-CD40-binding on human multiple myeloma clonogenicity. Leuk Lymphoma 1996;21(1-2):1–8.
116. Tai YT, Podar K, Mitsiades N, et al. CD40 induces human multiple myeloma cell migration via phosphatidylinositol 3-kinase/AKT/NF-kappa B signaling. Blood 2003;101(7):2762–2769.
117. Teoh G, Tai YT, Urashima M, et al. CD40 activation mediates p53-dependent cell cycle regulation in human multiple myeloma cell lines. Blood 2000;95(3):1039–1046.
118. Hayashi T, Hideshima T, Akiyama M, et al. Ex vivo induction of multiple myeloma-specific cytotoxic T lymphocytes. Blood 2003;102(4):1435–1442.
119. Mackay F, Schneider P, Rennert P, Browning J. BAFF and APRIL: A tutorial on B cell survival. Annu Rev Immunol 2003;21:231–264.
120. Kalled SL, Ambrose C, Hsu YM. BAFF: B cell survival factor and emerging therapeutic target for autoimmune disorders. Expert Opin Ther Targets 2003;7(1):115–123.
121. Moreaux J, Legouffe E, Jourdan E, et al. BAFF and APRIL protect myeloma cells from apoptosis induced by interleukin-6 deprivation and dexamethasone. Blood 2004;103(8):3148–3157.
122. Novak AJ, Darce JR, Arendt BK, et al. Expression of BCMA, TACI, and BAFF-R in multiple myeloma: A mechanism for growth and survival. Blood 2004;103(2):689–694.
123. Callander NS, Roodman GD. Myeloma bone disease. Semin Hematol 2001;38(3):276–285.
124. Mundy GR, Raisz L, G,, Cooper RA, Schecter GP, Salmon SE. Evidence for the secretion of an osteoclast stimulating factor in myeloma. N Engl J Med 1974;291:1041–1046.
125. Sordillo EM, Pearse RN. RANK-Fc: A therapeutic antagonist for RANK-L in myeloma. Cancer 2003;97(3 Suppl):802–812.
126. Lacey DL, Timms E, Tan H-L, et al. Osteoprotegerin ligand is a cytokine that regulates osteoclast differentiation and activation. Cell 1998;93:165-76.
127. Vanderkerken K, De Leenheer E, Shipman C, et al. Recombinant osteoprotegerin decreases tumor burden and increases survival in a murine model of multiple myeloma. Cancer Res 2003;63(2):287–289.
128. Barille-Nion S, Barlogie B, Bataille R, et al. Advances in biology and therapy of multiple myeloma. Hematology (Am Soc Hematol Educ Program) 2003:248–278.

129. Choi SJ, Cruz JC, Craig F, et al. Macrophage inflammatory protein 1-alpha is a potential osteoclast stimulatory factor in multiple myeloma. Blood 2000;96(2):671–675.
130. Abe M, Hiura K, Wilde J, et al. Role for macrophage inflammatory protein (MIP)-1alpha and MIP-1beta in the development of osteolytic lesions in multiple myeloma. Blood 2002;100(6):2195–2202.
131. Lee JW, Chung HY, Ehrlich LA, et al. IL-3 expression by myeloma cells increases both osteoclast formation and growth of myeloma cells. Blood 2004;103(6):2308–2315.
132. Oyajobi BO, Franchin G, Williams PJ, et al. Dual effects of macrophage inflammatory protein-1alpha on osteolysis and tumor burden in the murine 5TGM1 model of myeloma bone disease. Blood 2003; 102(1):311–319.
133. Magrangeas F, Nasser V, Avet-Loiseau H, et al. Gene expression profiling of multiple myeloma reveals molecular portraits in relation to the pathogenesis of the disease. Blood 2003;101(12): 4998–5006.
134. Zhang XG, Gu JJ, Lu ZY, et al. Ciliary neurotropic factor, interleukin 11, leukemia inhibitory factor, and oncostatin M are growth factors for human myeloma cell lines using the interleukin 6 signal transducer gp130. J Exp Med 1994;179(4):1337–1342.
135. Chauhan D, Kharbanda SM, Ogata A, et al. Oncostatin M induces association of Grb2 with Janus kinase JAK2 in multiple myeloma cells. J Exp Med 1995;182(6):1801–1806.
136. Otsuki T, Yata K, Sakaguchi H, et al. IL-10 in myeloma cells. Leuk Lymphoma 2002;43(5):969–974.
137. Koskela K, Pelliniemi TT, Pelliniemi LJ, et al. Autocrine production and synergistic growth-promoting activity of interleukin-6 and oncostatin M in a new human myeloma cell line TU-1. Acta Haematol 2002;107(1):23–28.
138. Zhang XG, Bataille R, Jourdan M, et al. Granulocyte-macrophage colony-stimulating factor synergizes with interleukin-6 in supporting the proliferation of human myeloma cells. Blood 1990;76:2599.
139. Hussein MA, Sandstrom K, Elson P, et al. GM-CSF safety and effects in the management of advanced/refractory multiple myeloma patients: A phase I trial. J Cancer Res Clin Oncol 2001; 127(10):619–624.
140. Anderson KC, Morimoto C, Paul SR, et al. Interleukin-11 promotes accessory cell dependent B cell differentiation in man. Blood 1992;80:2797–2804.
141. Paul SD, Barut BA, Cochran MA, Anderson KC. Lack of a role of interleukin-11 in the growth of multiple myeloma. Leukemia Research 1992;16:247–252.
142. Tinhofer I, Marschitz I, Henn T, Egle A, Greil R. Expression of functional interleukin-15 receptor and autocrine production of interleukin-15 as mechanisms of tumor propagation in multiple myeloma. Blood 2000;95(2):610–618.
143. Brenne AT, Baade Ro T, Waage A, Sundan A, Borset M, Hjorth-Hansen H. Interleukin-21 is a growth and survival factor for human myeloma cells. Blood 2002;99(10):3756–3762.
144. Sanz-Rodriguez F, Hidalgo A, Teixido J. Chemokine stromal cell-derived factor-1alpha modulates VLA-4 integrin-mediated multiple myeloma cell adhesion to CS-1/fibronectin and VCAM-1. Blood 2001;97(2):346–351.
145. Moller C, Stromberg T, Juremalm M, Nilsson K, Nilsson G. Expression and function of chemokine receptors in human multiple myeloma. Leukemia 2003;17(1):203–210.
146. Urashima M, Chen BP, Chen S, et al. The development of a model for the homing of multiple myeloma cells to human bone marrow. Blood 1997;90(2):754–765.
147. Yaccoby S, Barlogie B, Epstein J. Primary myeloma cells growting in SCID-hu mice: A model for studying the biology and treatment of myeloma and its manifestations. Blood 1998;92:2908–2913.
148. Raje N, Hideshima T, Anderson KC. Plasma Cell Tumors. In: Holland JF, Frei III E, Bast RC, Kufe DW, Norton DL, Weichselbaum RR, eds. Cancer Medicine. 4th ed. Baltimore: Williams and Wilkins; 2002:2066–2085.
149. Dai Y, Landowski TH, Rosen ST, Dent P, Grant S. Combined treatment with the checkpoint abrogator UCN-01 and MEK1/2 inhibitors potently induces apoptosis in drug-sensitive and -resistant myeloma cells through an IL-6-independent mechanism. Blood 2002;100(9):3333–3343.
150. Hideshima T, Richardson P, Chauhan D, et al. The proteasome inhibitor PS-341 inhibits growth, induces apoptosis, and overcomes drug resistance in human multiple myeloma cells. Cancer Res 2001;61(7):3071–3076.
151. Richardson PG, Barlogie B, Berenson J, et al. A phase 2 study of bortezomib in relapsed, refractory myeloma. N Engl J Med 2003;348(26):2609–2617.

152. Hideshima T, Chauhan D, Shima Y, et al. Thalidomide and its analogs overcome drug resistance of human multiple myeloma cells to conventional therapy. Blood 2000;96(9):2943–2950.
153. Richardson PG, Schlossman RL, Weller E, et al. Immunomodulatory drug CC-5013 overcomes drug resistance and is well tolerated in patients with relapsed multiple myeloma. Blood 2002;100(9): 3063–3067.
154. Mitsiades N, Mitsiades CS, Richardson PG, et al. Molecular sequelae of histone deacetylase inhibition in human malignant B cells. Blood 2003;101(10):4055–4062.
155. Catley L, Weisberg E, Tai YT, et al. NVP-LAQ824 is a potent novel histone deacetylase inhibitor with significant activity against multiple myeloma. Blood 2003;102(7):2615–2622.
156. Chauhan D, Catley L, Hideshima T, et al. 2-Methoxyestradiol overcomes drug resistance in multiple myeloma cells. Blood 2002;100(6):2187–2194.
157. Hayashi T, Hideshima T, Akiyama M, et al. Arsenic trioxide inhibits growth of human multiple myeloma cells in the bone marrow microenvironment. Mol Cancer Ther 2002;1(10):851–860.
158. Hideshima T, Chauhan D, Hayashi T, et al. Antitumor activity of lysophosphatidic acid acyltransferase-beta inhibitors, a novel class of agents, in multiple myeloma. Cancer Res 2003;63(23): 8428–8436.
159. Mitsiades N, Mitsiades CS, Poulaki V, et al. Molecular sequelae of proteasome inhibition in human multiple myeloma cells. Proc Natl Acad Sci U S A 2002;99(22):14,374–14,379.
160. Mitsiades CS, Treon SP, Mitsiades N, et al. TRAIL/Apo2L ligand selectively induces apoptosis and overcomes drug resistance in multiple myeloma: Therapeutic applications. Blood 2001;98(3): 795–804.

11

In Vivo Murine Cytokine Models and the Genesis of Cancer

Todd A. Fehniger, Megan A. Cooper, and Michael A. Caligiuri

CONTENTS

1. INTRODUCTION

Cytokines and their receptors comprise a critical communication pathway among the various cell types of the immune system that regulate cell growth, survival, differentiation, activation, and trafficking. As such, dysregulation of cytokine expression or secretion, cytokine-receptor expression, and their linked intracellular signaling pathways can result in undesired cell growth, survival, and ultimately malignant transformation. Use of transgenic mouse technology provides a powerful tool to better understand the physiologic sequelae resulting from unregulated activation of a cytokine/receptor pair at the level of the whole organism. In addition to altered expression of cytokine/receptor pairs leading directly to malignancy, indirect effects may also be elucidated using carcinogen models. Although other chapters in this book provide in depth review of individual cytokines' role in the genesis or therapy of cancer, here we generally discuss transgenic and knock-out mouse models that lead to malignant transformation. When relevant, studies from patients with cancer are also mentioned to provide some correlation with human disease, in addition to other chapters in this volume. One common theme that emerges from these models is the importance of chronic cytokine-induced growth, survival, or

From: *Cancer Drug Discovery and Development,*
Cytokines in the Genesis and Treatment of Cancer
Edited by: M. A. Caligiuri and M. T. Lotze © Humana Press Inc., Totowa, NJ

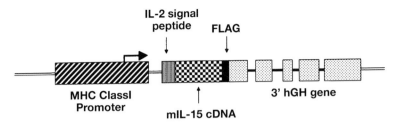

Fig. 1. An example transgene: the IL-15 transgene schematic. This transgene was engineered to be globally overexpressed via an MHC class I promoter. The poorly translated and secreted IL-15 signal peptide was replaced with the murine IL-2 signal peptide, cloned in frame with the murine IL-15 cDNA, and a FLAG epitope tag. The 3′ region of the human growth hormone gene was cloned out of frame, providing an easy method of measuring transgene transcript expression and optimizing expression in vivo.

inflammatory signals as a background leading to malignant transformation. Ultimately, better understanding of the cellular and molecular events that lead to the development of cancer will help provide novel targets for therapeutic intervention.

2. OVERVIEW OF TRANSGENIC AND "KNOCK-OUT" MOUSE TECHNOLOGY

Transgenic mouse technology was developed in the early 1980s (1) and provides powerful tools to elucidate the function of individual genes at the organism level. "Transgenic" commonly refers to insertion of a gene randomly into the mouse genome resulting in a gain-of-function genotype, and thereby allows the evaluation of the consequent phenotype in vivo. By using different promoter and regulatory elements the expression of the transgene can be global (i.e., in all tissues) or targeted to a specific tissue or cell type. In addition, strategies to include 3′ genomic DNA and a polyadenosine tail maximize transgene expression in vivo. For example, IL-15 transgenic mice were engineered using an MHC class I promoter to achieve global over expression, and the 3′ genomic region of the human growth hormone gene to optimize in vivo expression (Fig. 1; Section 7). Most of the murine transgenic models described in this chapter were engineered with transgenes randomly inserted into the mouse genome by the common methodology of pronuclear injection. Transgenic technologies continue to progress, and more sophisticated transgene expression can be achieved using tissue specific and conditionally expressed regulatory elements (2). Furthermore, by utilizing homologous recombination to insert a transgene at a specific regulatory site in the mouse genome, one can provide endogenous control of the transgene creating a "knock-in" model.

Although transgenic mice provide useful models for gain-of-function genotypes, targeted disruption of a single gene using homologous recombination ("knockout") allows for loss-of-function genotypes and investigation of the resultant phenotypes. This typically involves engineering a targeting vector with flanking arms of genomic DNA surrounding a mutated exon(s) containing a selectable marker gene cassette, such as neomycin. Following electroporation into mouse ES cells, homologous recombination of the targeting vector and the endogenous gene locus will in the end result in founders with one disrupted copy of the gene. Heterozygotes may then be bred to generate homozygous gene targeted mice *(2)*. For example, the strategy to generate TNF$^{-/-}$ mice used a targeting vector that replaced 438 bp of the 5′ UTR and exon 1 of the murine TNF-α gene with a neomycin expression cassette *(3)*. Although loss-of-function gene targeted mouse models have less commonly resulted in a carcinogenic phenotype, the example of TNF$^{-/-}$ mice is discussed below (Section 8).

The strategies to generate cytokine transgenic mice employ different patterns of gene expression (e.g., promoter specificity), human or murine genes, inbred mouse strains, random insertion sites, copy number, and levels of gene expression. It is important to keep such pivotal variables in mind when comparing various mouse models, and their relationship to human disease.

3. IL-6

3.1. IL-6 and B-Cell Neoplasms

IL-6 is a multifunctional cytokine originally identified as a B-cell differentiation factor, but was later found to also effect T-cells, hematopoietic stem cells, hepatocytes, and neuronal cells *(4,5)*. In humans, IL-6 has been associated with several hematologic malignancies, including multiple myeloma *(6–8)*, B-cell lymphoma *(9)*, and Castleman disease *(10)*. A group from Osaka, Japan first created human IL-6 transgenic mice driven by a murine MHC Class I promoter within FVB *(11)* and C57bl/6 (B6) *(12)* inbred mice. The phenotype of these FVB and B6 mice included marked plasmacytosis, elevations in serum IgG1, and fatal infiltration of multiple organs by an expanded population of polyclonal plasma cells. However, these hIL-6tg mice did not develop a transplantable, monoclonal plasmacytoma. Subsequently, B6 hIL-6tg mice were crossed the BALB/c background where transplantable, monoclonal plasmactyomas exhibiting the t(12;15) chromosomal translocation and abnormal *c-myc* expression developed *(12)*. This suggested certain genetic factors in the BALB/c inbred mouse strain contributed to plasmacytoma development in the setting of IL-6 overexpression, and agreed with known differences in mouse strain susceptibilities to induced plasmacytoma growth. Kovulcheck and colleagues backcrossed the MHC-Class I driven human IL-6 transgene onto the BALB/c background for 20 generations, creating a complete congenic BALB/c hIL-6tg line *(13)*. The majority of these congenic BALB/c hIL-6tg mice developed spontaneous plasmacytomas (25/45 mice) in the lymph nodes, peyers patches, and spleen that contained t(12;15) translocation, abnormal c-myc expression, and were transplantable. Interestingly, these BALB/c hIL-6tg mice were also found to produce follicular (13/45 mice) and diffuse large B-cell (4/45 mice) lymphomas. Woodroofe et al. developed murine IL-6 transgenic mice that had an increased incidence of lymphoma in elderly mice, further supporting the link between IL-6 and lymphoma *(14)*.

The soluble (s)IL-6R binds to IL-6 and acts in an agonist fashion, allowing the IL-6/sIL-6R to act on cell types not responsive to IL-6 alone. Schirmacher et al. bred hIL-6tg mice *(15)* controlled by a metallothionein (MT)-1 promoter and hsIL-6Rtg mice expressed via a liver and kidney specific phosphoenolpyruvate carboxykinase (PEPCK) promoter to yield double hIL-6/hsIL-6Rtg mice *(16)*. The double hIL-6/hsIL-6Rtg mice showed accelerated spontaneous development of plasmacytomas compared with hIL-6tg mice *(17)*. Pristane oil, when injected into the peritoneal cavity of BALB/C mice, results in the development of plasmacytomas, and is a commonly used to model plasmacytoma in vivo. Further evidence of the important in vivo role of IL-6 in the genesis of B-cell tumors is the observation that mice with targeted disruption of the IL-6 gene (IL-6$^{-/-}$) fail to develop pristane-induced plasmactyomas *(18)*.

3.2. IL-6 and Hepatic Adenoma

hIL-6/shIL-6Rtg mice also demonstrated marked hepatocellular proliferation, without the development of frank hepatoma *(17)*. Maione and colleagues crossed the hIL-6tg mice with BALB/C × C57Bl/6 F1 mice, and then bred double hIL-6/hsIL-6Rtg mice. On this inbred background, high transgene expressing hIL-6/hsIL-6Rtg mice developed both hepatocellular proliferation and frank hepatocellular carcinoma *(19)*. These data suggest that in addition to B-cell neoplasms, IL-6/sIL-6R driven proliferation of hepatocytes may also contribute to the development of hepatocellular carcinoma. These studies also highlight the importance of inbred strain specificity and the ultimate phenotype of transgenic mice.

4. IL-7 AND LYMPHOMA

IL-7 is a critical cytokine for B- and T-cell development, differentiation, and homeostasis as well as peripheral lymphocyte function *(20)*. IL-7 has been implicated as a growth factor in cutaneous T-cell lymphoma patients *(21)*. Rich and colleagues engineered a murine IL-7 transgene expressed via a human immunoglobulin heavy chain promoter. These mice develop a prolonged preneoplastic polyclonal lymphoproliferative syndrome, which eventually transforms into monoclonal B- and T-cell lymphomas *(22)*. Notably, 42/42 IL-7tg mice evaluated after 130 d of age had histologic evidence of lymphoma. As the lymphomas appear to arise after chronic polyclonal expansion, the authors hypothesize that additional genetic hits are necessary to transform the benign lymphoproliferation into lymphoma. Fisher et al. *(23)* and Valenzona et al. (24) also documented immature B-cell expansion in IL-7 transgenic mice. Valenzona et al. examined the B-cell compartments in MHC Class II-driven IL-7tg mice in the prelymphoma phase, and noted a marked increase in the proliferation of pro-B and pre-B-cells *(24)*. This study provides additional support for the hypothesis that uncontrolled proliferation in a broad array of immature B-cells susceptible to additional genetic mutations may lead to lymphoma.

5. IL-9 AND THYMIC LYMPHOMA

IL-9 is a multifunctional cytokine produced by Th2 cells that acts on B-cells and mast cells *(25)*, and has been implicated in Hodgkin's disease and anaplastic large cell lymphoma *(26,27)*. Renauld et al. engineered mIL-9tg mice driven by the pim-1 promoter and murine immunoglobulin heavy chain enhancer, resulting in global overexpression of IL-9 *(28)*. Small percentages (7%) of these mice spontaneously develop clonal CD4$^+$CD8$^+$ thymic lymphomas at 3–9 mo of age. Suspecting that additional genetic hits contributed to lymphoma development, the authors noted a very high susceptibility of IL-9tg mice to the thymus-tropic *N*-methyl-*N*-nitrosourea (MNU) carcinogen. Explanted tumors demonstrated an autocrine IL-9 growth pattern. Further, IL-9 has been shown to stimulate proliferation and inhibit apoptosis of murine thymic lymphoma in vitro *(29)*. The authors concluded that IL-9 driven chronic proliferation and survival may predispose to additional genetic mutations, and explain the low but consistent frequency of thymic lymphomas.

Anaplastic large cell lymphoma (ALCL) is a T-cell lymphoma that typically over expresses the anaplastic lymphoma kinase (ALK), usually via a t(2;5) chromosomal translocation resulting in a fusion between the nucleophosmin (NPM) and ALK genes *(30,31)*. Lange and colleagues used a retrovirus to transduce murine bone marrow progenitor cells with the NPM-ALK fusion gene, and reconstituted IL-9tg and wild-type mice *(32)*. The authors observed an increase in the spontaneous development of thymic lymphoma in the IL-9tg/NPM-ALK mice, compared to both IL-9tg and WT/NPM-ALK mice. Although suggestive that IL-9 over expression may be an early factor that contributes to T-cell lymphoma, one must be cautious in drawing definitive conclusions from a model system that employs concurrent cytokine transgene and retroviral reconstitution with a known fusion oncogene that causes lymphoma.

6. IL-10 AND LEWIS LUNG CANCER MODEL

IL-10 is cytokine that limits immune activation, including inflammation, antigen presentation, T-cell activation, and cytokine and chemokine release, as well as adhesion and costimulatory molecule expression *(33)*. Transgenic mice expressing mIL-10 were engineered under the control of the human IL-2 promoter, and were more susceptible to injection of the immunogenic murine 3LL Lewis lung carcinoma line *(34)*. The 3LL lung cancer line has well characterized immunodominant epitopes and is normally controlled via a CD8+ CTL response by immunocompetent mice in vivo. Corroborating evidence from patients shows that nonsmall-cell lung cancer induced 10–100-fold elevations in the T-cell-derived IL-10, postulated as one method to avoid CTL responses *(35)*. In follow-up studies, Sharma et al. demonstrated that the tumor-promoting IL-10 effect was transferable, in that IL-10tg T-cells transferred to wild-type mice conferred increased susceptibility to 3LL tumor cell challenge. Further, they documented defects in both T-cells and antigen-presenting cells suggesting that overproduction of IL-10 results in multiple immune defects preventing the recognition and control of the 3LL lung cancer *(36)*. Thus, over expression of a cytokine that suppresses type 1 CTL responses increased susceptibility to transplanted tumors in vivo.

7. IL-15 AND T, NK, T/NK MALIGNANCIES

IL-15 is a pleiotropic cytokine produced by a variety of cell types including monocyte/ macrophages, dendritic cells, and bone marrow stromal cells that acts primarily on lymphocytes *(37)*. IL-15 appears central to NK cell differentiation and survival, and also affects memory CD8+ T-cell homeostasis. As a central cytokine in lymphocyte growth, differentiation, and homeostasis it follows that IL-15 dysregulation leads to neoplastic disease. Indeed, IL-15 has been implicated in cutaneous T-cell lymphoma *(38,39)*, large granular lymphocytic leukemia *(40)*, and multiple myeloma *(41)*.

7.1. IL-15 and T, NK, T/NK Cell Leukemia/Lymphoma

Fehniger and colleagues generated FVB transgenic mice that over express murine IL-15 protein via an MHC class I promoter by eliminating several post-transcriptional checkpoints that limit endogenous IL-15 expression (Fig. 1) *(42)*. Early in life, IL-15tg mice develop a benign lymphocytosis consisting of NK cells and CD8+ T-cells with a memory phenotype. Later in life, the majority of these mice develop a spontaneous, fatal, clonal lymphocytic leukemia/lymphoma. The phenotype of the malignant clones is heterogeneous: either T-cell large granular leukemia (T-LGL and TCRβ+DX5+) with monoclonal TCR rearrangements, NK-LGL (TCRβ-DX5+) with monoclonal NK receptor expression, or rarely T-cell leukemia (CD8+TCRβ+DX5-) with monoclonal TCR rearrangements *(42,43)*. The neoplastic cells invade secondary lymphoid organs (spleen and lymph nodes), liver, lung, and skin, ultimately leading to death by 3–6 mo-of-age. Clonal malignancy was documented in 3 separate IL-15 transgenic lines. As the IL-15tg mice show a period of benign NK and T-cell growth and prolonged survival, followed by the development of heterogeneous leukemia/lymphomas, it follows that the initial phase of extended proliferation and survival may create an environment favoring secondary genetic mutations that ultimately lead to malignancy. These IL-15tg mice are therefore an interesting model to study the genetic changes leading to the spontaneous malignant transformation of lymphocytes, especially NK cells, NK/T-cells, and T-cells.

7.2. Mutated HMGI-C Increases IL-15 Expression Causing T-NK Lymphoma

High mobility group (HMG) proteins enhance transcription by both binding to DNA via AT-hooks and protein–protein interactions with transcription factors, and can regulate cytokine gene expression. Mice engineered to express a truncated form of HMG1-C exhibit a giant phenotype and lipomatosis *(44)*. In addition, late in life (>12 mo) these animals were noted to develop NK and T/NK lymphoma *(45)*. This correlated with aberrant over expression of IL-15 and IL-15 receptor components. Further, follow-up experiments demonstrated that the mutated HMG1-C directly activates the IL-15 promoter in vitro. Thus, a second model where IL-15 is indirectly up regulated by expression of a mutated transcription enhancer protein also results in the late development of murine NK/T lymphomas, providing additional evidence that chronic stimulation with IL-15 leads to NK/T malignancies.

7.3. Clues to the Pathogenesis of IL-15-Associated T/NK Leukemia: Epigenetic Alterations

IL-15 can induce both enhanced proliferation and enhanced survival of CD8 memory cells and NK cells, two components that are likely requisite for the additional or secondary hits that can lead to malignant transformation. However, the nature of such secondary events leading to malignant transformation of T/NK cells, in this instance, is poorly understood. Yu et al. used a technique called restriction landmark genomic scanning (RLGS) to perform a genome-wide analysis to determine if and how aberrant promoter DNA methylation and consequent gene silencing might contribute to leukemic transformation *(46)*. Comparative samples were taken from wild-type FVB splenocytes, FVB IL-15tg splenocytes with polyclonal expansion of T- and NK-cells, and splenocytes from FVB IL-15tg mice that had developed T/NK acute lymphoblastic leukemia (ALL). Using a novel mouse *Not*I-*Eco*RV arrayed library *(47)*, a total of 2447 fragments on each RLGS profile were analyzed. Only one to two variable changes consistent with aberrant methylation were detected by RLGS in spleens from either wild-type mice or those with polyclonal T/NK expansion. In contrast, the eight T/NK ALL spleens had 45–209 changes (1.8–8.5% of total fragments) consistent with aberrant DNA methylation *(46)*. The association of RLGS fragment loss or reduced intensity with leukemic transformation versus polyclonal expansion was highly significant ($P < 0.001$). Fifty-five methylated sequences were cloned from RLGS gels and nearly 90% had sequence characteristics of CpG islands, with the majority in the 5′ region of genes. The promoter of *inhibitor of DNA binding 4* (*Id4*) was found methylated in over 85% of the mouse T/NK ALLs, and was silenced secondary to promoter methylation in all cases examined. Over expression of *Id4* induced apoptosis in mouse cell line YAC-1 and inhibited tumor growth both in vitro and in vivo. Subsequent studies in human leukemias established that *ID4* was methylated in 72 of 84 primary acute myeloid leukemias (AML) and in 100% of 61 chronic lymphocytic leukemias (CLL), and was silenced in all cases examined *(46)*. Thus, one mechanism that is likely operative in this instance of IL-15-induced T/NK ALL is aberrant, nonrandom methylation of putative tumor suppressor genes that in turn contribute towards the malignant phenotype.

8. TNF-α AND SKIN CANCER

Many mouse models implicate cytokines in cancer pathogenesis by over expressing the culprit protein via transgene and observing the development of disease. An alternative strategy to analyzing the contribution of cytokines in the early stages of neoplasia involves comparing the incidence of induced tumor formation in mice with targeted disruption of the cytokine gene in question. Using this approach, the Balkwill laboratory has shown that mice deficient in tumor necrosis factor (TNF)-α (TNF-$\alpha^{-/-}$) are resistant to chemically induced skin carcinogenesis. Moore et al. demonstrated that mice deficient in TNF-α had a significantly lower incidence of skin carcinogenesis and progression using multiple tumor-inducing regimens and two different murine genetic backgrounds *(48)*. Furthermore, animals deficient in the TNF-α-inducible chemokine monocyte chemoattractant protein 1 (MCP-1) also had a lower incidence of carcinogenesis, although not to the same extent as TNF-$\alpha^{-/-}$ mice. TNF-α was found to be important only for the early stages of chemically induced skin carcinogenesis: shortly after carcinogen treatment of wild-type mice an increase in TNF-α protein was detected in the epidermis and inflammation and proliferation of keratinocytes was evident. Moreover, in TNF-$\alpha^{-/-}$ mice there was a marked reduction in this early inflammatory process, suggesting that the proliferation of the keratinocytes may be regulated by TNF-α *(48)*. TNF-α was not involved in the later stages of the tumor and had no effect on late tumor progression. This in vivo murine model identifies TNF-α as a contributor to skin carcinogenesis and a potential target for anticytokine therapy for the prevention of this cancer or treatment of the early stages of malignant transformation.

9. CONCLUSIONS

Transgenic and gene targeting in mice are powerful tools that allow the functional analysis of an individual gene at the level of the whole organism. Using such murine models, cytokines have been shown to contribute to carcinogenesis in vivo. Many transgenic models discussed above support the idea that cytokine growth factors provide early sustained signals for cell survival and proliferation, which then sets the stage for acquiring additional mutations, ultimately leading to autonomous cell growth and malignant transformation (Fig. 2; Table 1). This includes IL-6 and plasmacytomas, IL-7 and cutaneous lymphoma, IL-9 and thymic lymphoma, and IL-15 and NK, T,

Table 1

Murine Cytokine Transgenic and Gene Targeted Models of Malignant Transformation[a]

Cytokine	Promoter	Strain	Phenotype	Ref
hIL-6	IL-6/Eμ enhancer	FVB, B6	Massive polyclonal plasmacytosis with organ infiltration	(11)
hIL-6	MHC Class I (H-2L[d])	B6->BALB/C	Monoclonal plasmacytoma	(12)
hIL-6	MHC Class I (H-2L[d])	BALB/C	Monoclonal plasmacytoma, follicular lymphoma, diffuse large B-cell lymphoma	(13)
mIL-6	MHC Class I	B6 × SJL	B-cell lymphoma later in life (>18 mo)	(14)
hIL-6/hsIL–6R	MT-1/PEPCK	B6 × DBA/B6 × NMR	Plasmacytoma, hepatocyte proliferation, liver necrosis	(17)
hIL-6/hsIL–6R	MT-1/PEPCK	BALB/C × B6/B6 × NMR	Hepatoma	(19)
IL-6 –/–	—	B6 × BALB/C	Failed to develop pristane–induced plasmacytoma	(18)
mIL-7	hPμ/mEμ	FVB/N	Cutaneous lymphoma (T and B)	(22)
mIL-7	MHC Class II (Eα)	B6 × DBA2-B6	Immature B-cell expansion	(23)
mIL-7	MHC Class II (Eα)	B6 × DBA2-B6	Pro-B and Pre-B-cell expansion and proliferation	(24)
mIL-9	Pim-1/ Eμ enhancer	FVB/N	Thymic lymphoma, enhanced susceptibility to thymus–tropic MNU carcinogen	(28)
mIL-9/npm-alk	Pim-1/Eμ enhancer >BMT w/NPM-ALK	FVB/N	Increased incidence of thymic lymphoma	(32)
mIL-10tg	hIL-2/hIL–2 enhancer	B6	Increased susceptibility to Lewis lung (3LL) tumor challenge	(34)
mIL-10tg	hIL-2/hIL2 enhancer	B6	Increased susceptibility to Lewis lung (3LL) tumor challenge	(36)
mIL-15tg	MHC Class I	FVB/N	T, NK, T/NK leukemia/lymphoma	(42)
HMG1-C–/–	—	B6	NK, T/NK lymphoma, HMG1–C deficiency increased expression of IL–15	(45)
TNFα –/–	—	129 × B6	Increased susceptibility to skin cancer	(46)

[a]Abbreviations: C57Bl/6, B6; major histocompatibility complex, MHC; phosphoenolpyruvate carboxykinase, PEPCK; metallothionein, MT; Pμ, immunoglobulin heavy chain promoter; Eμ, heavy chain immunoglobulin enhancer; N-methyl–N-nitrosourea, MNU; bone marrow transplant, BMT; anaplastic lymphoma kinase, ALK; nucleophosmin, NPM; high mobility group, HMG.

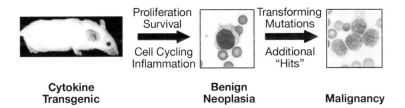

Fig. 2. Model of cytokine-induced carcinogenesis transgenic mice. Prolonged exposure to growth, cell cycle, and survival signals by cytokines on their normal physiologic target cells results in predisposition to acquiring additional genetic mutations and ultimately malignant transformation.

NK/T-cell malignancies. Transgenic models provide a framework to study the contribution of cytokines to carcinogenesis and further identify the cellular and molecular events and mechanisms critical to the development of cancer. These mouse models also provide an arena to test experimental therapeutic interventions, with the ultimate goal to improve our understanding and treatment of malignancies in our patients.

REFERENCES

1. Palmiter RD, Brinster RL, Hammer RE, et al. Dramatic growth of mice that develop from eggs microinjected with metallothionein-growth hormone fusion genes. Nature. 1982;300:611–615.
2. Hofker MH, VanDeursen J. Transgenic mouse methods and protocols. *In:* Walker JM ed. *Methods in Molecular Biology,* Vol. 209. Humana Press, Totowa, New Jersey, p. 374, 2003.
3. Pasparakis M, Alexopoulou L, Episkopou V, Kollias G. Immune and inflammatory responses in TNF alpha-deficient mice: A critical requirement for TNF alpha in the formation of primary B cell follicles, follicular dendritic cell networks and germinal centers, and in the maturation of the humoral immune response. J Exp Med. 1996;184:1397–1411.
4. Kishimoto T, Akira S, Narazaki M, Taga T. Interleukin-6 family of cytokines and gp130. Blood. 1995;86:1243–1254.
5. Naka T, Nishimoto N, Kishimoto T. The paradigm of IL-6: From basic science to medicine. Arthritis Res. 2002;4:S233–242.
6. Kawano M, Hirano T, Matsuda T, et al. Autocrine generation and requirement of BSF-2/IL-6 for human multiple myelomas. Nature. 1988;332:83–85.
7. Zhang XG, Klein B, Bataille R. Interleukin-6 is a potent myeloma-cell growth factor in patients with aggressive multiple myeloma. Blood. 1989;74:11–13.
8. Klein B, Zhang XG, Lu ZY, Bataille R. Interleukin-6 in human multiple myeloma. Blood. 1995; 85:863–872.
9. Tosato G, Jones K, Breinig MK, McWilliams HP, McKnight JL. Interleukin-6 production in post-transplant lymphoproliferative disease. J Clin Invest. 1993;91:2806–2814.
10. Yoshizaki K, Matsuda T, Nishimoto N, et al. Pathogenic significance of interleukin-6 (IL-6/BSF-2) in Castleman's disease. Blood. 1989;74:1360–1367.
11. Suematsu S, Matsuda T, Aozasa K, et al. IgG1 plasmacytosis in interleukin 6 transgenic mice. Proc Natl Acad Sci U S A. 1989;86:7547–7551.
12. Suematsu S, Matsusaka T, Matsuda T, et al. Generation of plasmacytomas with the chromosomal translocation t(12;15) in interleukin 6 transgenic mice. Proc Natl Acad Sci U S A. 1992;89:232–235.
13. Kovalchuk AL, Kim JS, Park SS, et al. IL-6 transgenic mouse model for extraosseous plasmacytoma. Proc Natl Acad Sci U S A. 2002;99:1509–1514.
14. Woodroofe C, Muller W, Ruther U. Long-term consequences of interleukin-6 overexpression in transgenic mice. DNA Cell Biol 1992;11:587–592.
15. Fattori E, Della Rocca C, Costa P, et al. Development of progressive kidney damage and myeloma kidney in interleukin-6 transgenic mice. Blood 1994;83:2570–2579.
16. Peters M, Jacobs S, Ehlers M, et al. The function of the soluble interleukin 6 (IL-6) receptor in vivo: Sensitization of human soluble IL-6 receptor transgenic mice towards IL-6 and prolongation of the plasma half-life of IL-6. J Exp Med 1996;183:1399–1406.

17. Schirmacher P, Peters M, Ciliberto G, et al. Hepatocellular hyperplasia, plasmacytoma formation, and extramedullary hematopoiesis in interleukin (IL)-6/soluble IL-6 receptor double-transgenic mice. Am J Pathol. 1998;153:639–648.

18. Hilbert DM, Kopf M, Mock BA, Kohler G, Rudikoff S. Interleukin 6 is essential for in vivo development of B lineage neoplasms. J Exp Med 1995;182:243–248.

19. Maione D, Di Carlo E, Li W, et al. Coexpression of IL-6 and soluble IL-6R causes nodular regenerative hyperplasia and adenomas of the liver. EMBO J 1998;17:5588–5597.

20. Fry TJ, Mackall CL. Interleukin-7: From bench to clinic. Blood 2002;99:3892–3904.

21. Qin, JZ, Dummer, R, Burg, G, and Dobbeling, U. Constitutive and interleukin-7/interleukin-15 stimulated DNA binding of Myc, Jun, and novel Myc-like proteins in cutaneous T-cell lymphoma cells. Blood 1999;93:260–267.

22. Rich BE, Campos-Torres J, Tepper RI, Moreadith RW, Leder P. Cutaneous lymphoproliferation and lymphomas in interleukin 7 transgenic mice. J Exp Med 1993;177:305–316.

23. Fisher AG, Burdet C, Bunce C, Merkenschlager M, Ceredig R. Lymphoproliferative disorders in IL-7 transgenic mice: Expansion of immature B cells which retain macrophage potential. Int Immunol 1995;7:415–423.

24. Valenzona HO, Pointer R, Ceredig R, Osmond DG. Prelymphomatous B cell hyperplasia in the bone marrow of interleukin-7 transgenic mice: Precursor B cell dynamics, microenvironmental organization and osteolysis. Exp Hematol 1996;24:1521–1529.

25. Demoulin JB, Renauld JC. Interleukin 9 and its receptor: An overview of structure and function. Int Rev Immunol 1998;16:345–364.

26. Merz H, Houssiau FA, Orscheschek K, et al. Interleukin-9 expression in human malignant lymphomas: Unique association with Hodgkin's disease and large cell anaplastic lymphoma. Blood 1991;78:1311–1317.

27. Fischer M, Bijman M, Molin D, et al. Increased serum levels of interleukin-9 correlate to negative prognostic factors in Hodgkin's lymphoma. Leukemia 2003;17:2513–2516.

28. Renauld JC, van der Lugt N, Vink A, et al. Thymic lymphomas in interleukin 9 transgenic mice. Oncogene 1994;9:1327–1332.

29. Renauld JC, Vink A, Louahed J, Van Snick J. Interleukin-9 is a major anti-apoptotic factor for thymic lymphomas. Blood 1995;85:1300–1305.

30. Morris SW, Kirstein MN, Valentine MB, et al. Fusion of a kinase gene, ALK, to a nucleolar protein gene, NPM, in non-Hodgkin's lymphoma. Science 1994;263:1281–1284.

31. Morris SW, Xue L, Ma Z, Kinney MC. Alk+ CD30+ lymphomas: A distinct molecular genetic subtype of non-Hodgkin's lymphoma. Br J Haematol 2001;113:275–295.

32. Lange K, Uckert W, Blankenstein T, et al. Overexpression of NPM-ALK induces different types of malignant lymphomas in IL-9 transgenic mice. Oncogene 2003;22:517–527.

33. Pestka S, Krause CD, Sarkar D, Walter MR, Shi Y, Fisher PB. Interleukin-10 and related cytokines and receptors. Annu Rev Immunol 2004;22:929–979.

34. Hagenbaugh A, Sharma S, Dubinett SM, et al. Altered immune responses in interleukin 10 transgenic mice. J Exp Med 1997;185:2101–2110.

35. Huang M, Sharma S, Mao JT, Dubinett SM. Non-small cell lung cancer-derived soluble mediators and prostaglandin E2 enhance peripheral blood lymphocyte IL-10 transcription and protein production. J Immunol 1996;157:5512–5520.

36. Sharma S, Stolina M, Lin Y, et al. T cell-derived IL-10 promotes lung cancer growth by suppressing both T cell and APC function. J Immunol 1999;163:5020–5028.

37. Fehniger TA, Caligiuri MA. Interleukin 15: Biology and relevance to human disease. Blood 2001;97:14–32.

38. Leroy S, Dubois S, Tenaud I, et al. Interleukin-15 expression in cutaneous T-cell lymphoma (mycosis fungoides and Sezary syndrome). Br J Dermatol 2001;144:1016–1023.

39. Dobbeling U, Dummer R, Laine E, Potoczna N, Qin JZ, Burg G. Interleukin-15 is an autocrine/paracrine viability factor for cutaneous T-cell lymphoma cells. Blood 1998;92:252–258.

40. Zambello R, Facco M, Trentin L, et al. Interleukin-15 triggers the proliferation and cytotoxicity of granular lymphocytes in patients with lymphoproliferative disease of granular lymphocytes. Blood 1997;89:201–211.

41. Tinhofer I, Marschitz I, Henn T, Egle A, Greil R. Expression of functional interleukin-15 receptor and autocrine production of interleukin-15 as mechanisms of tumor propagation in multiple myeloma. Blood 2000;95:610–618.

42. Fehniger TA, Suzuki K, Ponnappan A, et al. Fatal leukemia in interleukin 15 transgenic mice follows early expansions in natural killer and memory phenotype CD8+ T cells. J Exp Med 2001;193: 219–231.

43. Fehniger TA, Suzuki K, VanDeusen JB, Cooper MA, Freud AG, Caligiuri MA. Fatal leukemia in interleukin-15 transgenic mice. Blood Cells Mol Dis 2001;27:223–230.

44. Battista S, Fidanza V, Fedele M, et al. The expression of a truncated HMGI-C gene induces gigantism associated with lipomatosis. Cancer Res 1999;59:4793–4797.

45. Baldassarre G, Fedele M, Battista S, et al. Onset of natural killer cell lymphomas in transgenic mice carrying a truncated HMGI-C gene by the chronic stimulation of the IL-2 and IL-15 pathway. Proc Natl Acad Sci U S A. 2001;98:7970–7975.

46. Yu L, Liu C, Vandeusen J, et al. Global assessment of promoter methylation in a murine model of cancer identifies ID4 as a putative tumor suppressor gene in human leukemia. Nat Genet 2005; 37: 265–274.

47. Yu L, Liu C, Bennett K, et al. A NotI-EcoRV promoter library for studies of genetic and epigenetic alterations in mouse models of human malignancies. Genomics 2004;84:647–660.

48. Moore RJ, Owens DM, Stamp G, et al. Mice deficient in tumor necrosis factor-alpha are resistant to skin carcinogenesis. Nat Med 1999;5:828–831.

12 Experimental Models of Cytokines and Cancer Prevention

Mark J. Smyth, Erika Cretney,
Shayna E. A. Street, and Yoshihiro Hayakawa

Contents

1. INTRODUCTION: CYTOKINES IN CANCER IMMUNITY

Cancer immunosurveillance has been debated for well over a century, but more recent experimental data over the past 15 years has clearly been supportive for an important role for cytokines and other effector molecules in host resistance to transformation *(1,2)*. Importantly, this molecular biology era has brought with it the discovery of new hormones (cytokines such as IL-2 and interferons [IFNs]) and messengers (chemokines) that activate and direct leukocytes in a coordinated fashion. Clinical application quickly followed *(3)* and immune cell/cytokine immunotherapies now herald the promise of new forms of cancer therapy. Cytokines have pivotal effects on the carcinogenic process. On the one hand they can be involved in the activation of immune effector mechanisms that limit the growth of the tumor, but on the other they may contribute to inflammation, transformation, tumor growth, invasion, and metastasis (as discussed in earlier chapters). Cytokines are produced by host stromal and immune cells, in response to molecules secreted by the tumor cells or as part of inflammation that frequently accompanies tumor growth. Tumor cells also produce cytokines in the same environment. How a local cytokine network operates in tumors is determined by the

From: *Cancer Drug Discovery and Development,*
Cytokines in the Genesis and Treatment of Cancer
Edited by: M. A. Caligiuri and M. T. Lotze © Humana Press Inc., Totowa, NJ

array of cytokines and receptors expressed and their relative concentrations. The net cytokine environment likely varies at various stages of tumor development.

The "danger model" *(4)* postulates that dendritic cells (DC) act as sentinel cells for monitoring tissue stress, damage and/or transformation and thereby initiate the immune response. Danger signals may act on DC precursors and promote DC maturation and activity. These signals may be heat-shock proteins (HSPs), released as a result of tumor-cell damage or necrosis, and proinflammatory factors, including cytokines, released by dying tumor cells, as well as reactive host cells such as macrophages, NK cells and other cells characteristic of the innate response. Cytokines, such as interleukin-1 (IL-1), tumor necrosis factor (TNF-α), type I IFN, granulocyte–macrophage colony-stimulating factor (GM-CSF), and IL-15, can promote DC differentiation and activity by multiple mechanisms, including increased costimulation between DCs and T-cells. Tumor-associated antigens (TAAs) are captured by DCs by several mechanisms, including the uptake of tumor-cell apoptotic bodies or necrotic materials. DCs may then acquire a highly activated mature phenotype and, as a result of exposure to distinct chemokines and/or cytokines, migrate to the lymph nodes, where the processed TAA-derived peptides are presented to CD4$^+$ or CD8$^+$ T-cells in the context of MHC class-II or class-I molecules, respectively. Activation of other immune components such as B-cells also has important consequences for host immunity to tumor. The cytokine environment created at the tumor site may direct an immune response towards tolerance or immunity. Type-1 cytokines (i.e., TNF and IFN-γ) are involved in T-helper 1 (Th1) immune responses and mainly induce cell-mediated immunity; by contrast, type-2 cytokines (i.e., IL-4, IL-5, IL-6, IL-10, and IL-13) are involved in Th2 immune responses and promote humoral immunity against tumors and/or immune deviation to a state of tolerance. In the case of effective antitumor immunity, CD4$^+$ and CD8$^+$ T-cells can migrate to the tumor site, where the attack on tumor relies on both innate and adaptive cellular and humoral responses.

An important advance in the molecular biology era has been the new capability to assess the physiologic function of a particular cytokine gene by gene-targeting specific mutations in mice. This technology has had a considerable impact on our ability to study both cancer and immunity in experimental mice and has played a large part in rekindling the concept of cancer immunosurveillance (Table 1). Mice gene-targeted for cytokines and their receptor counterparts, such as members of the IFN family and members of the TNF superfamily have all proven extremely informative tools for studying tumor immunity. This review focuses on the most important developments that elucidate a role for these types of cytokines in promoting tumor immunity. Studies where cytokines have been examined in an ectopic or immunotherapy context have previously been published and reviewed extensively and will not be discussed here *(5–12)*. We will concern ourselves with studies using mice deficient in cytokines by virtue of gene-targeting or neutralizing antibodies.

2. CYTOKINES THAT PROMOTE TUMOR IMMUNITY

2.1. Type I IFNs in Tumor Immunity

The type I IFN family consists of at least 13 functional subtypes of IFN-α, IFN-β, and IFN-ω *(13)*, which share the same receptor system and exhibit similar, but not yet fully discernable, biologic activities. Type I IFN are currently used in cancer therapy *(14)*, but despite much experience in the clinical use of IFN, the primary mechanisms underlying the antitumor response are multiple, complex, and not completely understood. IFN may

Table 1
Cytokines Promoting Cancer Immunosurveillance

Mice/treatment	Deficiency	Tumor susceptibility
STAT1$^{-/-}$	IFN-γ and IFN-α/β mediated signaling	Spontaneous intestinal and mammary neoplasia (41)
STAT1$^{-/-}$	IFN-γ and IFN-α/β mediated signal	MCA-induced sarcomas Wider spectrum in p53$^{-/-}$ background Mammary carcinomas (41)
IFNGR1$^{-/-}$	IFN-γ receptor 1, IFN-γ sensitivity	MCA-induced sarcomas (33) Wider spectrum in p53$^{-/-}$ background
IFN-γ$^{-/-}$	IFN-γ production	MCA-induced sarcomas Spontaneous disseminated lymphomas (34,35) Spontaneous lung adenocarcinomas in BALB/c background (34)
GM-CSF$^{-/-}$ IFN-γ$^{-/-}$	GM-CSF and IFN-γ production	Spontaneous lymphomas Variety of non-lymphoid solid tumors (39)
Perforin$^{-/-}$ IFN-γ$^{-/-}$	Perforin-mediated cytotoxicity and IFN-γ production	MCA-induced sarcomas Spontaneous disseminated lymphomas (34)
LMP2$^{-/-}$	IFN-γ-inducible low molecular mass polypeptide-2 (LMP2) subunit	Spontaneous uterine neoplasias (40)
TRAIL$^{-/-}$	TRAIL-mediated cytotoxicity	MCA-induced sarcomas (88)
Anti-TRAIL	TRAIL-mediated cytotoxicity	MCA-induced sarcomas Spontaneous sarcomas, disseminated lymphomas in p53$^{+/-}$ background (89)
IL-12 p40$^{-/-}$	IL-12 p40 subunit, IL-12 and IL-23 production	MCA-induced sarcomas (70)

act directly on the tumor, but most often IFN appears to induce host mechanisms, including immunity, to achieve inhibition of the primary tumor and metastases.

IFN-α has a well-known antitumor activity in mouse and human malignancies (reviewed in refs. 9 and 10). It was first postulated that IFN acted primarily through host-dependent mechanisms (Fig. 1A). Locally produced IFN-α stimulates increased cytotoxic killing activity of regional NK cells (15,16) and stimulates the proliferation of NK cells (17,18). IFN-α stimulation of NK cell-mediated cytotoxicity of tumors is important in the clinical remission of chronic myelogenous leukemia (CML). IFN-α also enhances the production or secretion of other cytokines by the NK cell through the autocrine IFN-γ loop (16,19,20). IFN-α influences CD8$^+$ T-cell and B-cell adaptive-immune responses (21,22), by up-regulating class I and class II MHC expression (23,24), and increasing antigen presentation, immune surveillance, and cognate CD8$^+$ T-cell-mediated killing of neoplastic cells (23,21). The absence of CTL activity typically observed in patients with post-transplant lymphoproliferative disorders can be restored with IFN-α therapy (25). The essential role of IgG2a antibodies specific for TAAs and CD4$^+$ T-cells was revealed in IFN-α induced suppression of tumor growth in mice (reviewed in ref. 9). Other mechanisms also contribute to IFN antitumor activity. Important recent studies have demonstrated the importance of IFN in the induction of apoptosis in cancerous cells by a variety

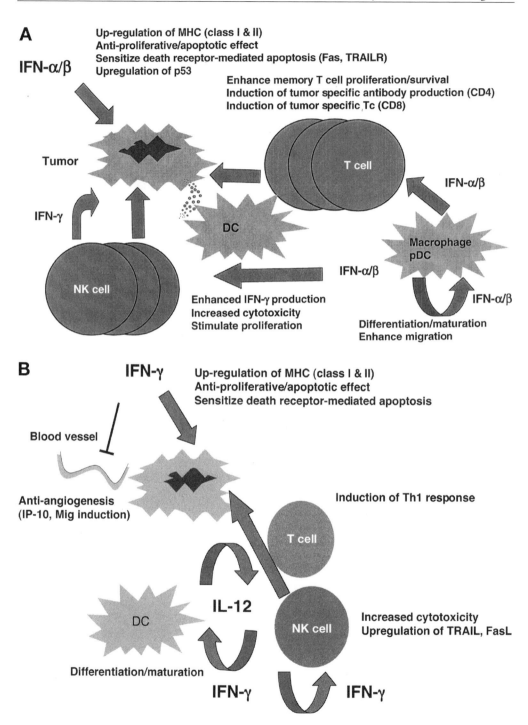

Fig. 1. (A) Mechanism of action of type I IFN.IFN-α expression occurs before the majority of the other innate-immune response cytokines, and it has been proposed that IFN is the first cytokine secreted by APC after antigen stimulation *(163)*. Plasmacytoid DC precursors (pDC) are the professional IFN-α/β secretor cells *(164)* that secrete between 200 and 1000 times more IFN-α than any other white blood cell *(165)*. In addition, type I IFN acts as an important signal for differentiation and maturation of DCs *(166,167)*. A possible sequence of events might be that IFN-α, produced by cells

(Continued next page)

of mechanisms *(26,27)*. Transcription of the p53 gene is induced by IFN, thereby boosting p53 responses to stress signals. IFN has also been shown to inhibit hepatocarcinogenesis in a rat model in a p53-independent manner *(28)*.

Few studies to date have reported tumor growth and metastasis in IFN- or IFN receptor-deficient mice. One recent study has demonstrated that IFN-β-deficient mice are more susceptible to experimental lung carcinoma growth *(29)*. An elegant series of studies using Stat-1-deficient tumors and Stat-1-deficient mice illustrated that NK cells mediated the antitumor effects of IFN-α and Stat-1 function in immune cells was key for the antitumor activity of IFN-α *(30)*. Future studies with conditional type I IFN and IFN receptor gene-targeted mice will be required to further our understanding of the primary role IFN plays in cancer immunosurveillance. Families have been described which lack the IFN-γ receptor *(31)*. These individuals appear to be highly susceptible to mycobacterial infection, but to date no increase in the frequency of malignancies has been noted. We are not aware of any reports of individuals lacking the genes for type I IFN receptor, suggesting they are essential molecules for survival. The therapeutic activity of type I IFN has been elaborated in great detail in Chapter 19 of this book.

2.2. IFN-γ/ IFN-γ Receptor Pathway in Tumor Immunity

Dighe et al. first observed that immunogenic fibrosarcomas grew avidly at higher incidence in mice treated with a neutralizing monoclonal antibody (mAb) against IFN-γ *(32)*. Furthermore, over expression of a dominant-negative mutant of IFN-γ receptor in these sarcoma cell lines abrogated tumor sensitivity to IFN-γ, and those tumors with mutant receptors showed reduced immunogenicity in syngeneic mice. Thus, the IFN-γ sensitivity of the developing tumor was critical for its immune recognition and elimination. More recently, supporting studies using both IFN-γ receptor (IFN-γR)-deficient mice *(33)* and IFN-γ-deficient mice *(34,35)* have confirmed that host IFN-γ suppresses tumor metastasis, methylcholanthrene (MCA)-induced sarcoma formation, and spontaneous tumor formation in p53 mutant mice. In the MCA model previous studies have implicated NK cell and NKT-cell IFN-γ production in the host response *(36)*, but recent work suggests that γδ+T-cells are also an important source of IFN-γ during the protective phase *(37)*. Mice either lacking IFN-γ or IFN-γ-R were considerably more

---

Fig. 1. *(Continued)* such as pDCs and macrophages, enhances innate immunity by activating NK cells and other host reactive cells. This allows destruction of tumor cells and the capture and presentation of tumor associated antigens by DCs. IFN-α then promotes the differentiation, migration and activity of DCs. Lastly, IFN-α enhances the in vivo proliferation and survival of memory T-cells, thus leading to an increase of overall humoral and cellular antitumor immunity. IFN-α may also have direct antiproliferative or sensitize tumor cells to apoptosis through the up-regulation of tumor cell-surface expression of the TRAILR and Fas *(85,168)*. IFN-α has also been shown to influence lymphocyte trafficking through autocrine effects by contributing to the mobilization and sustanance of the adaptive-immune response *(169,170)*. **(B)** Mechanism of action of type II IFN. IFN-γ has also been shown to function at many additional points in the cancer immunosurveillance process *(51,171,172)*. IFN-γ sensitivity in the tumor cells has been shown to be critical for efficient up regulation of the MHC class I and II antigen processing and presentation pathway in the tumor and recognition by tumor specific CD8+ T-cells *(41)* as well as for the induction of angiostatic chemokines [i.e., CXCL9 (MIG) and CXCL-10 (IP-10)] that inhibit angiogenesis within the developing tumor *(173)*. IFN-γ production by NK cells and T-cells in response to dendritic cell (DC) IL-12 production may result in the contribution of IFN-γ to DC maturation, and IL-12 driven lymphocyte cytotoxicity or cytokine effector function. IFN-γ secretion may also regulate the level of death ligands, TRAIL and FasL, on NK cells.

susceptible to MCA-induced sarcoma and all tumor types resulting from the loss of p53 alleles. More recently, HTLV1 Tax transgenic mice were shown to develop T-cell lymphoma earlier on an IFN-γ-deficient background *(38)*. Signal transducers and activators of transcription 1 (STAT1) is a critical transcription factor for IFN-γ R induced signal transduction and STAT1-deficient mice display a low incidence of mammary tumor development on the 129 Sv background. We have shown that a small proportion (<15%) of BALB/c IFN-γ deficient mice developed lung adenocarcinoma, but otherwise failed to develop tumors, whereas almost half the IFN-γ-deficient mice on a C57BL/6 background developed a spectrum of various T-cell lymphomas *(34)*. By contrast Enzler et al. *(39)* reported a mixture of solid and lymphoid neoplasms in C57BL/6 mice deficient for both GM-CSF and IFN-γ, but no tumors in C57BL/6 IFN-γ-deficient mice. Collectively, the findings suggest that the immune system does regulate some lymphoid and epithelial malignancies through pathways controlled by IFN-γ and the genetic background of mice appears to an important factor in spontaneous tumor development. Increased tumor formation in LMP2 (IFN-γ-inducible low molecular mass polypeptide-2 subunit)-deficient mice *(40)*, further demonstrates the diverse role IFN-γ plays in tumor immunity. Immunohistochemical studies have shown that human tumors frequently downregulate peptide transporters associated with antigen processing (TAP-1 and TAP-2), and proteasome subunits LMP-2 and LMP-7. In most cases, TAP expression can be restored by treatment with IFN-γ, suggesting a reversible inhibition of gene transcription. Thus, specifically, the data indicate that IFN-γ plays a central coordinating role leading to activation of both immune and nonimmune processes that result in destruction of developing tumors in which the tumor cell itself is a critical target of IFN-γ activities (Fig. 1B).

IFN-γ sensitivity in the tumor cells has been shown to be critical for efficient upregulation of MHC class I antigen processing and the induction of angiostatic chemokines that inhibit angiogenesis within the developing tumor. In particular, recent work has shown that immune system components such as IFN-γ may also promote the emergence of primary tumors with reduced immunogenicity that are capable of avoiding immune destruction *(41)*. Poorly immunogenic MCA-sarcoma cells derived from IFNγR1[-/-] mice became highly immunogenic after ectopic expression of wild-type IFNγR1 and restoration of IFN-γ sensitivity *(33)*. These observations prompted the development of the cancer immunoediting hypothesis by Schreiber and colleagues to more accurately reflect the sculpting of tumors by the immune system throughout tumor development *(2,42)*. Studies in the MCA model have also suggested a possible role for IFN-γ in generating a foreign body reaction to the carcinogen that limits its spread and DNA damage *(43)*, but many other roles for IFN-γ remain plausible. Constitutive activation of telomerase is a key step in the development of human cancers and recently IFN-γ has been shown to repress human teleomerase reverse transcriptase (hTERT) transcription in an IRF-1-dependent manner *(44)*. In addition, the antitumor activities of many other cytokines and immunotherapies appear to depend upon host IFN-α and/or IFN-γ (e.g., IL-27, CCL19, α-GalCer, BCG, CpG) *(45–52)*.

2.3. IL-12 in Tumor Immunity

The biology of IL-12 and its receptor subunits has been previously reviewed *(8)*. IL-12 plays an essential role in the interaction between the innate and adaptive arms of immunity *(53)*. Produced by phagocytic cells, B-cells, DC, and possibly other APC following the encounter with pathogens, IL-12 acts on NK cells and T-cells to generate cytotoxic lymphocytes. IL-12 is also responsible for Th1 cell differentiation, allowing potent production of IFN-γ. IFN-γ, in turn, has a powerful enhancing effect on the ability of phagocytes and DC to produce IL-12, thereby creating a potent positive feedback mechanism that promotes strong cell-mediated immunity. IL-12 receptors (IL-12R) are expressed on activated T- and NK-cells *(54)*, although expression of IL-12R on other cell types has also been shown. IL-12 and IFN-γ are the only cytokines that induce the activation of STAT4 *(55)*. IL-12 induces the activation of STAT4 and STAT4, through the production of IFN-γ, mediates most but not all of the biologic activities of IL-12.

It has been clear that IL-12 has potent antitumor activity since the pivotal study by Brunda et al. *(56)*. A number of different experimental mouse tumor models have been used and the behavior of IL-12 in these settings has been elegantly reviewed *(8)*. A range of papers reporting IL-12 antitumor activity against a variety of transplantable murine tumors have highlighted that IL-12 activity depends on tumor immunogenicity, cytokine dose, route of injection, production of extracellular-matrix proteins, sensitivity to IFN-γ, and dependence on neo-angiogenesis. Effector cells required for the antitumor effects of IL-12 include NK, NKT, and both CD8$^+$ and CD4$^+$ T-cells (reviewed in refs. *8,57–59*). IL-12-activated NK cells may directly cause tumor cell death or affect the integrity of the tumor vascular endothelium. IFN-γ, TNF, and other pro-inflammatory cytokines induced by IL-12, cause the production of CXCR3 ligands, such as the IP-10 and Mig chemokines; that affect the differentiation of newly formed vessels or attract activated NK and T-cells that damage endothelial cells (reviewed in ref. 8). IFN-γ and a cascade of other pro-inflammatory cytokines induced by IL-12 have a direct toxic effect on the tumor cells or may activate potent anti-angiogenic mechanisms *(60–63)*. IL-12, through IFN-γ and other pro-inflammatory cytokines, also induces the production of oxygen and nitrogen metabolites that are toxic for certain tumors. Several other cell types may also be indirect targets of IL-12, including DC, macrophages, neutrophils, and endothelial cells *(64,65)*. IL-12 can also enhance the production of antibodies able to activate the complement cascade and to opsonize tumor cells rendering them sensitive to the cytotoxic activity of myeloid and NK cells. In particular, IL-12 induction of Th1 responses augments the production of opsonizing and C′ fixing classes of IgG antibodies that have been demonstrated to have antitumor activity in vivo.

In most experimental models, the antitumor effect of IL-12 was IFN-γ-dependent and at low doses, the ability of IL-12 to induce an antigen-specific immunity relies mostly on its capacity to induce Th1 and CTL responses *(66)*. Several promising immunomodulators such as the CD1d reactive glycolipid α-galactosylceramide (α-GalCer) *(67)* stimulate IL-12-dependent antitumor immunity in mice. The ability of IL-12 to augment antigen-specific immune responses and to deviate the immune response to the effector mechanisms most active against tumors makes it a potentially efficient adjuvant for cancer vaccine. A good recent example would be the adjuvant effect of IL-12 in promoting a vaccine that prevents spontaneous mouse gastrointestinal tumors via humoral immunity *(68)*. However, the variability and the lack of general rules underlining the antitumor function of IL-12, might explain why its initial clinical use has been troublesome. New approaches such as evaluating new gene targets for IL-12 activity by microarray may prove useful in this respect *(69)*.

Endogenous IL-12 appears also to be important for host resistance to transplantable tumors and to MCA-induced fibrosarcoma *(70)*. Exogenous IL-12 treatment also has often a dramatic antitumor effect on transplantable tumors, on chemical carcinogen-induced tumors *(71,72)*, and in tumors arising spontaneously in genetically modified mice *(73,74)*. Patients with genetic deficiencies in the expression of IL-12 p40 chain or the IL-12R1 chain are susceptible to bacterial infections *(75)*, but the development of malignancies in these patients has not been reported. Reported clinical trials with IL-12 have been limited until now. IL-12 has shown to have only a modest clinical efficacy in the face of considerable toxicity (reviewed in ref. *8*). IL-23 comprising IL-12p40 and a distinct p19 subunit, is produced predominantly by macrophages and DC. The antitumor effects of IL-23 remain comparatively poorly studied, however the growth of tumors expressing IL-23 was suppressed *(76)*. The IL-12 family member, IL-27, also suppresses tumor metastases in mice in a CD8$^+$ T-cell-, T-bet- and IFN-γ-dependent manner *(45)*.

3. DEATH RECEPTOR CYTOKINE PATHWAYS IN TUMOR IMMUNITY

3.1. TRAIL

Members of the TNF superfamily that induce tumor cell apoptosis have been shown to contribute to tumor immunity. TNF-related apoptosis-inducing ligand (TRAIL), also known as Apo2 ligand, is a type II transmembrane protein belonging to the TNF super-family *(77)*. At least five receptors for TRAIL have been identified in humans (only one, DR5 [TRAIL-R2] in mice) and two of them, DR4 (TRAIL-R1) and DR5, are capable of transducing an apoptotic signal *(78)*. The other three receptors (TRAIL-R3, TRAIL-R4 and a soluble receptor called osteoprotegerin [OPG, TRAIL-R5]) lack death domains but may serve as decoy receptors to regulate TRAIL-mediated cell death. TRAIL expression is only found on a small subset of immature liver NK cells (~25–35%) *(79, 80)*, although expression can be induced on NK, T, monocytes and dendritic cells upon stimulation with cytokines such as IL-2, IFN or IL-15 *(81–85)*. IFN$^{-/-}$ and IFNR$^{-/-}$ mice have decreased TRAIL expression on NK cells *(79,86)*, suggesting that IFN is important in the in vivo regulation of TRAIL. In mice, TRAIL has been shown to contribute to NK cell suppression of primary subcutaneous or orthotopic tumor growth *(87,88)* and tumor metastasis. In experimental models, natural TRAIL-mediated antimetastatic activity was restricted to the liver *(79,80,88,89)*. Administration of a neutralizing anti-TRAIL mono-clonal antibody has also been shown to promote fibrosarcoma development in mice sub-cutaneously injected with the chemical carcinogen methylcholanthrene and TRAIL-deficient mice have an earlier onset and increased susceptibility to these tumors. The protective effect of TRAIL was at least partly mediated by NK cells and completely dependent on IFN *(88,89)*. In addition, TRAIL has also been shown to play a role in con-trol of spontaneous tumor development in p53$^{+/-}$ mice, where IFN- has also been impli-cated in surveillance *(89)*. It appears that IFN- regulates TRAIL-mediated tumor surveillance by controlling TRAIL expression on effector cells, but also by sensitizing tumor cells to TRAIL-mediated cytotoxicity *(89)*. Indeed, tumors emerging from wild-type mice appear generally TRAIL resistant, whereas those from TRAIL-deficient mice are most often TRAIL-sensitive. These data suggest that TRAIL is an important immu-noediting mechanism in tumor development. Tumor cells are inherently more resistant to TRAIL when they over express cFLIP *(90)*. In contrast to perforin that selectively pro-tected mice from disseminated lymphoma *(91)*, TRAIL, like IFN-γ, additionally sup-pressed sarcoma formation in p53 mutant mice. Recently, a role for TRAIL in

T-cell-mediated graft vs leukemia has been shown in mice *(92)*. In humans, TRAIL expression is up-regulated on CD56⁺ NK cells in hepatocarcinoma patients responding to chemotherapy *(93)* and TRAIL positive effector cells have been found in regressing primary melanomas of patients undergoing IFN therapy *(94)*. This data support the contention that TRAIL on NK cells might also be a therapeutically useful pathway in humans. Strikingly, a recent clinical study has shown that bladder carcinoma patients that responded to BCG therapy had significantly higher urine TRAIL levels vs nonresponders and TRAIL expressing neutrophils *(95)*. TRAIL is a rare example of an effector molecule that kills many types of transformed cells, but spares most normal cells *(96)*. One of the attractive features of TRAIL is its ability to kill cancers with mutations in the p53 gene. The combination of TRAIL with chemotherapeutic agents has been found to be particularly effective in killing cancers with wild-type p53, presumably through induction of DR5 expression *(97)*. Not all cancer cells are sensitive to the cytotoxic effects of TRAIL *(98)*. Bax mutation in mismatch repair-deficient tumors can cause resistance to TRAIL therapy, but pre-exposure to chemotherapy rescues tumor sensitivity *(99)*. A very recent study has highlighted the important role MYC over expression may play in tumor sensitivity to TRAIL/DR5-mediated cell death *(100)*.

3.2. FasL

Among other members of the TNF superfamily, mice and humans mutant for Fas ligand (FasL) have also been shown to develop lymphoid malignancies *(101,102)*. In addition, about 10% of multiple myeloma patients have Fas mutations that may affect function *(103)*. Together, these findings suggest a role for the Fas/FasL pathway in the inhibition of tumor development. Lpr (Fas mutant) and gld (FasL mutant) mice exhibit an increased incidence of tumor development when backcrossed to bcl-2- or E-myc-transgenic mice *(104,105)*, suggesting that a defective Fas/FasL pathway allows the accumulation of mutations that initiate tumor development, but alone are weak inducers of tumorigenesis. Fas-sensitive melanomas have been demonstrated to metastasize to the lung in gld mice but not in wild-type mice *(106)*, and IL-18-mediated suppression of tumor metastases in mice is mediated predominantly by FasL expressing NK cells *(107)*. These data demonstrate the importance of the Fas/FasL pathway in the control of tumor spread. Although high levels of Fas expression have been reported on some colon, ovary, breast, prostate, and liver tumors *(108,109)*, many tumor cells do not constitutively express Fas. NK cells have been demonstrated to stimulate Fas expression on tumor cells in vitro, and to subsequently induce Fas-dependent apoptosis in these targets *(110)*. Tumor cells that lack Fas expression have also been shown to up-regulate Fas when passaged in vivo *(110)*. Expression of FLIP or CrmA in Fas sensitive tumors has been shown to protect them from Fas mediated apoptosis, suggesting that FLIP and CrmA may function as tumor progression factors, protecting MHC class I-deficient tumors from NK-cell mediated rejection in vivo *(90,110)*. Collectively, these data indicate that FasL-mediated apoptosis might in some situations be an important means of NK cell-mediated tumor clearance. FasL/Fas interactions were also important in the therapeutic activity of adoptive immunotherapy using CTL in a mouse model of experimental tumor metastases *(111)*.

3.3. TNF

TNF binds as a homotrimer to two distinct homotrimeric receptors on the cell surface: TNFRI (p55 receptor) and TNFRII (p75 receptor) *(112)*. TNF is a vital cytokine involved in inflammation, immunity, and cellular organization *(113)*. It was first isolated from the serum of mice infected with *Bacillus Calmette-Guérin* treated with endotoxin, and was shown to replicate the ability of endotoxin to induce hemorrhagic tumor necrosis *(114)*, thus ending a long search for an important component of "Coley's mixed toxins." Although activated macrophages are a major source of TNF, TNF is also produced by other cells including fibroblasts, astrocytes, Kupffer cells, smooth-muscle cells, keratinocytes, and tumor cells.

Paradoxically, TNF-deficient mice have provided evidence both of a role in tumor immunosurveillance for TNF *(115,116)* and a role for TNF in tumor development and metastasis *(117,118)*. In preventing tumor formation, TNF may have its most significant role in promoting immune cell migration and chemotaxis *(116)*. However in some situations, promoting lymphocyte trafficking to lymphoid organs can also contribute to tumor formation. Plasmacytoid tumors that develop in FasL mutant mice were reduced in mice additionally deficient for TNF *(119)*. TNF may have induced the expression of chemokines (chemotactic cytokines), which regulate trafficking and accumulation of potentially transformed cells into lymph nodes *(119)*. TNF-deficient mice had ten times fewer skin tumors than wild-type mice after initiation with a carcinogen and repeated application of 12-O-tetradecanoylphorbol-13-acetate (TPA) *(117)*. TNF-deficient mice exposed to carcinogen had reduced levels of matrix metalloproteases and it is known that TNF promotes further tumor remodelling by stimulating fibroblast activity, tumor-cell motility, and tumor invasion via the induction of matrix metalloproteinases *(120–122)*. Similarly, TNFRI$^{-/-}$ mice, and to a lesser extent TNFRII$^{-/-}$ mice, also showed resistance to skin carcinogenesis. A tumor-promoting role of TNF has also been demonstrated in models of hepatic carcinogenesis and metastasis *(123–125)*. Expression studies have confirmed elevated concentrations of TNF in tumors and associations between single nucleotide polymorphisms (SNPs) in the TNF gene and a range of cancers exist (reviewed in ref. *126*). In summary, TNF has a paradoxical role in cancer, inducing destruction of blood vessels and cell-mediated killing of certain tumors, as well as acting as a tumor promoter. Its role in cancer progression has generated interest in the use of TNF antagonists for the prevention and treatment of cancer. This is reviewed extensively in Chapters 4 and 23.

The TNF superfamily member LIGHT (also known as TNFSF-14) is a ligand of stromal cell-expressed lymphotoxin-β receptor and T-cell-expressed herpes viral entry mediator (HVEM). Forced expression of LIGHT in the tumor environment induces a massive infiltration of naive T-lymphocytes and activation of these infiltrating T-cells, possibly through HVEM, leads to the rejection of established, highly progressive tumors at local and distal sites *(127)*. Several members of the TNFR superfamily including OX40, 4-1BB, CD27, CD30, and HVEM deliver costimulatory signals both early and late after encounter with antigen (reviewed in ref. *128*) and thus have the capacity to initiate and sustain T-cell responses to tumors.

4. GM-CSF AND FLT3 LIGAND IN TUMOR IMMUNITY

4.1. Mechanism of Action

Another group of cytokines are particularly important in their effects on APC. The ability of GM-CSF to enhance antitumor immunity was identified through an in vivo screen of a large number of immunostimulatory molecules. GM-CSF-secreting tumor cells have been revealed as powerful vaccines in a number of model systems (reviewed in ref. *7*), where GM-CSF generates mature CD8⁺CD11b⁺ DCs that effectively capture dying cancer cells and induce coordinated cellular and humoral immunity *(129,130)*. An alternative approach is to expand and activate DC in vivo using the cytokine Flt3 Ligand (FL). FL drives the expansion of both lymphoid-related DC and myeloid-related DC. Immunization of FL-treated mice with a protein antigen leads to increased production of antigen-specific antibodies and Th cell responses. FL administration leads to the generation of protective antitumor immune responses in mouse experimental tumor models, and these effects were mediated by CTL and/or NK cells *(131,132)* (reviewed in ref. *133*). When, FL has only minor or short term effects, the antitumor response can be significantly amplified by adding other cytokines, known to act at the T-cell level, such as IL-12 or CD40 ligand (CD40L) or 4-1BBL, a TNF family member.

Many new cancer immunotherapies in humans are based on the administration of DC pulsed with TAAs. Several differences between the DCs elicited by GM-CSF and FL may account for their distinct vaccination abilities. GM-CSF-generated DCs are exclusively CD8⁺CD11b⁺ and they possess a superior ability to phagocytose particulate material, thereby enabling enhanced priming. GM-CSF stimulated higher levels of the costimulatory molecule CD80 on DCs, indicative of greater maturation of the APC. Lastly, GM-CSF, but not FL, stimulates CD1d-restricted invariant NKT cells and these cells are thought to be important in the potency of the vaccine. The broad cytokine production elicited by vaccination with GM-CSF-secreting tumor cells is in concert with a requirement for CD4⁺ T-cells in priming *(129,134)*. There are many possibilities for appropriately delivering GM-CSF as a vaccine including the use of fusion-protein vaccines, gene transfection into tumor cells or DCs, and DNA immunization. Treatment with GM-CSF has been shown to promote protective and therapeutic immunity in a variety of mouse tumor models (reviewed in ref. *7*).

4.2. Therapeutic Activity of GM-CSF

The promising results of preclinical studies have prompted the testing of GM-CSF gene-transduced tumor vaccines in phase I and phase II clinical trials for cancer immunotherapy. A phase I trial investigating the biologic activity of vaccination with irradiated autologous melanoma cells engineered to secrete GM-CSF have been conducted in patients with stage IV metastatic melanoma *(135)*. No significant toxicities attributable to the treatment, but sites of immunization were intensely infiltrated with mature DCs, macrophages, and eosinophils in all evaluable patients *(136)*. Initial evaluation of GM-CSF based tumor vaccines has demonstrated the consistent induction of immunity in patients without significant toxicity. Similar favorable findings have been reported in non-small -cell cancer and pancreatic cancer *(137,138)*. Active clinical programs are under way for patients with malignant melanoma, multiple myeloma, leukemia, and carcinomas of the lung, ovary, prostate, pancreas, and kidney (reviewed in ref. *7* and in Chapter 23).

5. γ-CHAIN CYTOKINES IN TUMOR IMMUNITY

5.1. Experimental Activity

Cytokines that use receptors of the common cytokine receptor γ-chain family (CD132) cytokines are implicated in the process of memory-cell generation and maintenance. Of the γc cytokines, the antitumor activity of IL-2 is best characterized and has been reviewed extensively *(139,140)*. The ability of IL-2 to stimulate T-cells led to interest in its use to stimulate the immune response against cancer. Subsequently, systemically administered IL-2 was demonstrated to impact on established lung metastases of sarcoma in mice *(141)*. High dose IL-2 was also demonstrated to inhibit disseminated murine leukemia *(142)*. Selective depletion of lymphocyte subsets identified the mechanism responsible for tumor responses involved contributions from CD4+ and CD8+ T-cells as well as asialo-GM1+ lymphokine-activated killer (LAK) cells *(143)*. IL-2 was also used in combination with adoptively transferred lymphocytes and shown to inhibit the growth of lung and liver metastases in mice *(144,145)*.

IL-21 is structurally related to the lymphoid cytokines IL-2, IL-4, and IL-15 and has been demonstrated to be expressed by activated CD4+ T-lymphocytes *(146)*. The IL-21R is expressed in lymphoid tissues, shows homology to the β-chain of IL-2/IL-15Rs, and forms a complex with the common γ-chain. IL-21 has pleiotropic roles in the lymphoid lineages, including the promotion of CD8+ T-cell function *(147)*. Within the NK cell lineage, IL-21 enhances maturation from human multipotent bone marrow progenitors and activates peripheral NK cells in the absence of other stimuli *(148)*. Once mouse NK cells are stimulated, IL-21 has been demonstrated to increase cytotoxicity and cytokine production over that observed for IL-15 alone *(149)*. In vivo treatment with IL-21 results in a very similar activation and phenotypic maturation of NK cells as well as a potent increase in NK cell-mediated antitumor immunity that is perforin-dependent *(149)*. IL-21 stimulation of NK cell and T-cell immunosurveillance of tumors has been supported by several groups *(150,151)* and this early data and new data with promotion of CD8+ T-cell responses *(152)* suggests that IL-21 may have great promise as an adjuvant immunotherapy in humans.

5.2. Therapeutic Activity of IL-2

Promising results in mouse tumor models led to the use of IL-2 in clinical trials. IL-2 alone, or in combination with LAK cells or tumor-infiltrating lymphocytes (TIL), has been used to treat metastatic melanoma and renal cell carcinoma (reviewed in ref. *153*). Overall response rates in 15–20% of patients were observed in these trials, with 4–6% of patients achieving complete responses that were often durable *(154)*, however there was some accompanying toxicity *(155)*. Clinical studies with high- and intermediate-dose IL-2 have been comprehensively reviewed elsewhere *(153,156)*. High- and intermediate-dose regimens seek to activate immune cells against tumors. The precise mechanism of high dose IL-2 activity is not known, but presumed to be augmentation of inadequate T-cell responses against the tumor cells *(153)*. However, other possibilities may be activation of other immune cells such as macrophages and NK cells. The future of higher doses of IL-2 appears most promising when used in multiple courses of limited duration in combination with NK cell expanding and tumor-specific agents. IL-2 has also been used in combination with vaccines to enhance T-cell activation and antitumor effects in the treatment of melanoma. Response rates of up to 42% have been observed in melanoma patients receiving a modified gp100 peptide in incomplete Freunds adjuvant and 720,000 IU/kg of IL-2 intravenously to tolerance *(157)*. The inclusion of IL-2 in chemotherapeutic regimens has also been investigated using any of several agents including cisplatin, dacarbazine, and tamoxifen *(158)*. No increased survival or reductions in treatment-related toxicities were observed in these studies. The best response rates in melanoma to date using IL-2 have been achieved in combination with adoptive T-cell transfer following nonmyeloablative preconditioning *(159)*. Objective responses of approx 50% have been observed in patients undergoing this form of treatment. Low dose IL-2 has also been used to promote type 1 cytokine profiles in patients with AIDS and AIDS-associated malignancies *(160)*, although positive effects on these malignancies are yet to be reported. Epstein-Barr virus-associated lymphoproliferative disease (EBV-LPD) is a potentially life threatening complication in immune-deficient patients and effects among 2–20% of solid organ transplants performed annually in the United States. An extensive series of studies in human PBL-scid mouse models illustrated the ability of both IL-2 and GM-CSF to induce specific cellular immunity against EBV-LPD *(161,162)*. Human NK cells, CD8[+] T-cells, and monocytes were all required for the effective combination therapy. New cytokines such as IL-21 will also be interesting to test in these same settings.

6. CONCLUSIONS

The role of many cytokines in promoting tumor immunity is becoming clearer, but a significant gap in our knowledge of what the immune system contributes to each phase of tumor development seriously impedes our progress in finding more effective immunotherapies for cancer. More studies that actively examine the role of host cytokines in the best available animal models of cancer are warranted to determine when and how exactly these cytokines function in tumor/stroma/immune cell networks. The role of IFN and the death-receptor-mediated pathways they stimulate appears to be in driving both innate and adaptive arms of the immune response to suppress tumor initiation, growth, and metastasis. We now must embark on some detailed analysis of why these immune mediators often fail to prevent cancer as well as rationally designing trials that employ the antitumor potential of these pathways.

ACKNOWLEDGMENTS

This work was supported by Cancer Research Institute Post-Doctoral Fellowship to Y.H., a Medical Research Scholarship from the University of Melbourne to E.C., and National Health and Medical Research Council of Australia (NH&MRC) Research Dora Lush Scholarship to S.E.A.S and a NH&MRC Research Fellowship and Program Grant to M.J.S. The authors apologize to authors of articles we could not cite due to space constraints.

REFERENCES

1. Dunn GP, Bruce AT, Ikeda H, Old LJ, Schreiber RD. Cancer immunoediting: From immunosurveillance to tumor escape. Nat Immunol 2002;3(11):991–998.
2. Dunn GP, Old LJ, Schreiber RD. The Three Es of Cancer Immunoediting. Annu Rev Immunol 2004; 22:329–360.
3. Rosenberg SA, Lotze MT. Cancer immunotherapy using interleukin-2 and interleukin-2-activated lymphocytes. Annu Rev Immunol 1986;4:681–709.
4. Matzinger P. Tolerance, danger, and the extended family. Annu Rev Immunol 1994;12:991–1045.
5. Forni G, Fujiwara H, Martino F, et al. Helper strategy in tumor immunology: Expansion of helper lymphocytes and utilization of helper lymphokines for experimental and clinical immunotherapy. Cancer Metastasis Rev 1988;7(4):289–309.
6. Dranoff G, Mulligan RC. Gene transfer as cancer therapy. Adv Immunol 1995;58:417–54.
7. Dranoff G. GM-CSF-based cancer vaccines. Immunol Rev 2002;188:147–54.
8. Colombo MP, Trinchieri G. Interleukin-12 in anti-tumor immunity and immunotherapy. Cytokine Growth Factor Rev 2002;13(2):155–68.
9. Gresser I, Belardelli F. Endogenous type I interferons as a defense against tumors. Cytokine Growth Factor Rev 2002;13(2):111–118.
10. Belardelli F, Ferrantini M, Proietti E, Kirkwood JM. Interferon-α in tumor immunity and immunotherapy. Cytokine Growth Factor Rev 2002;13(2):119–134.

11. Apte RN, Voronov E. Interleukin-1—a major pleiotropic cytokine in tumor-host interactions. Semin Cancer Biol 2002;12(4):277–290.

12. Ferrantini M, Belardelli F. Gene therapy of cancer with interferon: Lessons from tumor models and perspectives for clinical applications. Semin Cancer Biol 2000;10(2):145–157.

13. Mogensen KE, Lewerenz M, Reboul J, Lutfalla G, Uze G. The type I interferon receptor: Structure, function, and evolution of a family business. J Interferon Cytokine Res 1999;19(10):1069–1098.

14. Pfeffer LM, Dinarello CA, Herberman RB, et al. Biological properties of recombinant α-interferons: 40th anniversary of the discovery of interferons. Cancer Res 1998;58(12):2489–2499.

15. Trinchieri G, Santoli D, Granato D, Perussia B. Antagonistic effects of interferons on the cytotoxicity mediated by natural killer cells. Fed Proc 1981;40(12):2705–2710.

16. Salazar-Mather TP, Ishikawa R, Biron CA. NK cell trafficking and cytokine expression in splenic compartments after IFN induction and viral infection. J Immunol 1996;157(7):3054–3064.

17. Biron CA, Sonnenfeld G, Welsh RM. Interferon induces natural killer cell blastogenesis in vivo. J Leukoc Biol 1984;35(1):31–37.

18. Biron CA. Interferons α and beta as immune regulators—a new look. Immunity 2001;14(6): 661–664.

19. Ortaldo JR, Phillips W, Wasserman K, Herberman RB. Effects of metabolic inhibitors on spontaneous and interferon-boosted human natural killer cell activity. J Immunol 1980;125(4):1839–1844.

20. Ortaldo JR, Mantovani A, Hobbs D, Rubinstein M, Pestka S, Herberman RB. Effects of several species of human leukocyte interferon on cytotoxic activity of NK cells and monocytes. Int J Cancer 1983;31(3):285–289.

21. Tough DF, Borrow P, Sprent J. Induction of bystander T cell proliferation by viruses and type I interferon in vivo. Science 1996;272(5270):1947–1950.

22. Finkelman FD, Svetic A, Gresser I, et al. Regulation by interferon α of immunoglobulin isotype selection and lymphokine production in mice. J Exp Med 1991;174(5):1179–1188.

23. Fellous M, Nir U, Wallach D, Merlin G, Rubinstein M, Revel M. Interferon-dependent induction of mRNA for the major histocompatibility antigens in human fibroblasts and lymphoblastoid cells. Proc Natl Acad Sci USA 1982;79(10):3082–3086.

24. Steimle V, Siegrist CA, Mottet A, Lisowska-Grospierre B, Mach B. Regulation of MHC class II expression by interferon-γ mediated by the transactivator gene CIITA. Science 1994;265(5168): 106–109.

25. Taguchi Y, Purtilo DT, Okano M. The effect of intravenous immunoglobulin and interferon-α on Epstein-Barr virus-induced lymphoproliferative disorder in a liver transplant recipient. Transplantation 1994;57(12):1813–1815.

26. Takaoka A, Hayakawa S, Yanai H, et al. Integration of interferon-α/β signalling to p53 responses in tumour suppression and antiviral defence. Nature 2003;424(6948):516–523.

27. Li C, Chi S, He N, et al. IFNα induces Fas expression and apoptosis in hedgehog pathway activated BCC cells through inhibiting Ras-Erk signaling. Oncogene 2004;23(8):1608–1617.

28. Nakaji M, Yano Y, Ninomiya T, et al. IFN-α prevents the growth of preneoplastic lesions and inhibits the development of hepatocellular carcinoma in the rat. Carcinogenesis 2004;25(3):389–397.

29. Deonarain R, Verma A, Porter AC, Gewert DR, Platanias LC, Fish EN. Critical roles for IFN-β in lymphoid development, myelopoiesis, and tumor development: Links to tumor necrosis factor α. Proc Natl Acad Sci USA 2003;100(23):13,453–13,458.

30. Lesinski GB, Anghelina M, Zimmerer J, et al. The antitumor effects of IFN-α are abrogated in a STAT1-deficient mouse. J Clin Invest 2003;112(2):170–180.

31. Newport MJ, Huxley CM, Huston S, et al. A mutation in the interferon-γ-receptor gene and susceptibility to mycobacterial infection. N Engl J Med 1996;335(26):1941–1949.

32. Dighe AS, Richards E, Old LJ, Schreiber RD. Enhanced in vivo growth and resistance to rejection of tumor cells expressing dominant negative IFN γ receptors. Immunity 1994;1(6):447–456.

33. Kaplan DH, Shankaran V, Dighe AS, et al. Demonstration of an interferon γ-dependent tumor surveillance system in immunocompetent mice. Proc Natl Acad Sci USA 1998;95(13):7556–7561.

34. Street SE, Trapani JA, MacGregor D, Smyth MJ. Suppression of lymphoma and epithelial malignancies effected by interferon γ. J Exp Med 2002;196(1):129–134.

35. Street SE, Cretney E, Smyth MJ. Perforin and interferon-γ activities independently control tumor initiation, growth, and metastasis. Blood 2001;97(1):192–197.

36. Smyth MJ, Crowe NY, Godfrey DI. NK cells and NKT cells collaborate in host protection from methylcholanthrene-induced fibrosarcoma. Int Immunol 2001;13(4):459–463.

37. Gao Y, Yang W, Pan M, et al. Gamma delta T cells provide an early source of interferon γ in tumor immunity. J Exp Med 2003;198(3):433–442.
38. Mitra-Kaushik S, Harding J, Hess J, Schreiber R, Ratner L. Enhanced tumorigenesis in HTLV-1 Tax-transgenic mice deficient in interferon-γ. Blood 2004;104(10):3305–3311.
39. Enzler T, Gillessen S, Manis JP, et al. Deficiencies of GM-CSF and interferon γ link inflammation and cancer. J Exp Med 2003;197(9):1213–1219.
40. Hayashi T, Faustman DL. Development of spontaneous uterine tumors in low molecular mass polypeptide-2 knockout mice. Cancer Res 2002;62(1):24–27.
41. Shankaran V, Ikeda H, Bruce AT, et al. IFNγ and lymphocytes prevent primary tumour development and shape tumour immunogenicity. Nature 2001;410(6832):1107–1111.
42. Dunn GP, Old LJ, Schreiber RD. The immunobiology of cancer immunosurveillance and immunoediting. Immunity 2004;21(2):137–148.
43. Qin Z, Kim HJ, Hemme J, Blankenstein T. Inhibition of methylcholanthrene-induced carcinogenesis by an interferon γ receptor-dependent foreign body reaction. J Exp Med 2002;195(11): 1479–1490.
44. Lee SH, Kim JW, Lee HW, et al. Interferon regulatory factor-1 (IRF-1) is a mediator for interferon-γ induced attenuation of telomerase activity and human telomerase reverse transcriptase (hTERT) expression. Oncogene 2003;22(3):381–391.
45. Hisada M, Kamiya S, Fujita K, et al. Potent antitumor activity of interleukin-27. Cancer Res 2004; 64(3):1152–1156.
46. Hillinger S, Yang SC, Zhu L, et al. EBV-induced molecule 1 ligand chemokine (ELC/CCL19) promotes IFN-γ-dependent antitumor responses in a lung cancer model. J Immunol 2003;171(12):6457–6465.
47. Stern BV, Boehm BO, Tary-Lehmann M. Vaccination with tumor peptide in CpG adjuvant protects via IFN-γ-dependent CD4 cell immunity. J Immunol 2002;168(12):6099–6105.
48. Hafner M, Zawatzky R, Hirtreiter C, et al. Antimetastatic effect of CpG DNA mediated by type I IFN. Cancer Res 2001;61(14):5523–5528.
49. Riemensberger J, Bohle A, Brandau S. IFN-γ and IL-12 but not IL-10 are required for local tumour surveillance in a syngeneic model of orthotopic bladder cancer. Clin Exp Immunol 2002;127(1):20–26.
50. Chiodoni C, Stoppacciaro A, Sangaletti S, et al. Different requirements for α-galactosylceramide and recombinant IL-12 antitumor activity in the treatment of C-26 colon carcinoma hepatic metastases. Eur J Immunol 2001;31(10):3101–3110.
51. Smyth MJ, Crowe NY, Pellicci DG, et al. Sequential production of interferon-γ by NK1.1(+) T cells and natural killer cells is essential for the antimetastatic effect of α-galactosylceramide. Blood 2002;99(4):1259–1266.
52. Li J, Hu P, Khawli LA, Epstein AL. Complete regression of experimental solid tumors by combination LEC/chTNT-3 immunotherapy and CD25(+) T-cell depletion. Cancer Res 2003;63(23): 8384–8392.
53. Trinchieri G. Interleukin-12: A proinflammatory cytokine with immunoregulatory functions that bridge innate resistance and antigen-specific adaptive immunity. Annu Rev Immunol 1995;13:251–276.
54. Gately MK, Renzetti LM, Magram J, et al. The interleukin-12/interleukin-12-receptor system: Role in normal and pathologic immune responses. Annu Rev Immunol 1998;16:495–521.
55. Bacon CM, Petricoin EF, 3rd, Ortaldo JR, et al. Interleukin 12 induces tyrosine phosphorylation and activation of STAT4 in human lymphocytes. Proc Natl Acad Sci USA 1995;92(16):7307–7311.
56. Brunda MJ, Luistro L, Warrier RR, et al. Antitumor and antimetastatic activity of interleukin 12 against murine tumors. J Exp Med 1993;178(4):1223–1230.
57. Smyth MJ, Taniguchi M, Street SE. The anti-tumor activity of IL-12: Mechanisms of innate immunity that are model and dose dependent. J Immunol 2000;165(5):2665–2670.
58. Cavallo F, Signorelli P, Giovarelli M, et al. Antitumor efficacy of adenocarcinoma cells engineered to produce interleukin 12 (IL-12) or other cytokines compared with exogenous IL-12. J Natl Cancer Inst 1997;89(14):1049–1058.
59. Martinotti A, Stoppacciaro A, Vagliani M, et al. CD4 T cells inhibit in vivo the CD8-mediated immune response against murine colon carcinoma cells transduced with interleukin-12 genes. Eur J Immunol 1995;25(1):137–146.
60. Voest EE, Kenyon BM, O'Reilly MS, Truitt G, D'Amato RJ, Folkman J. Inhibition of angiogenesis in vivo by interleukin 12. J Natl Cancer Inst 1995;87(8):581–586.
61. Gee MS, Koch CJ, Evans SM, et al. Hypoxia-mediated apoptosis from angiogenesis inhibition underlies tumor control by recombinant interleukin 12. Cancer Res 1999;59(19):4882–4889.

62. Duda DG, Sunamura M, Lozonschi L, et al. Direct in vitro evidence and in vivo analysis of the antiangiogenesis effects of interleukin 12. Cancer Res 2000;60(4):1111–1116.

63. Strasly M, Cavallo F, Geuna M, et al. IL-12 inhibition of endothelial cell functions and angiogenesis depends on lymphocyte-endothelial cell cross-talk. J Immunol 2001;166(6):3890–3899.

64. Musiani P, Modesti A, Giovarelli M, et al. Cytokines, tumour-cell death and immunogenicity: A question of choice. Immunol Today 1997;18(1):32–36.

65. Di Carlo E, Rovero S, Boggio K, et al. Inhibition of mammary carcinogenesis by systemic interleukin 12 or p185neu DNA vaccination in Her-2/neu transgenic BALB/c mice. Clin Cancer Res 2001;7(3 Suppl):830s–837s.

66. Noguchi Y, Richards EC, Chen YT, Old LJ. Influence of interleukin 12 on p53 peptide vaccination against established Meth A sarcoma. Proc Natl Acad Sci USA 1995;92(6):2219–2223.

67. Kawano T, Cui J, Koezuka Y, et al. CD1d-restricted and TCR-mediated activation of vα14 NKT cells by glycosylceramides. Science 1997;278(5343):1626–1629.

68. Iinuma T, Homma S, Noda T, Kufe D, Ohno T, Toda G. Prevention of gastrointestinal tumors based on adenomatous polyposis coli gene mutation by dendritic cell vaccine. J Clin Invest 2004;113(9): 1307–1317.

69. Shi X, Cao S, Mitsuhashi M, Xiang Z, Ma X. Genome-wide analysis of molecular changes in IL-12-induced control of mammary carcinoma via IFN-γ-independent mechanisms. J Immunol 2004; 172(7):4111–4122.

70. Smyth MJ, Thia KY, Street SE, et al. Differential tumor surveillance by natural killer (NK) and NKT cells. J Exp Med 2000;191(4):661–668.

71. Noguchi Y, Jungbluth A, Richards EC, Old LJ. Effect of interleukin 12 on tumor induction by 3-methylcholanthrene. Proc Natl Acad Sci USA 1996;93(21):11,798–11,801.

72. Hayakawa Y, Rovero S, Forni G, Smyth MJ. Alpha-galactosylceramide (KRN7000) suppression of chemical- and oncogene-dependent carcinogenesis. Proc Natl Acad Sci USA 2003;100(16): 9464–9469.

73. Boggio K, Nicoletti G, Di Carlo E, et al. Interleukin 12-mediated prevention of spontaneous mammary adenocarcinomas in two lines of Her-2/neu transgenic mice. J Exp Med 1998;188(3):589–596.

74. Roy EJ, Gawlick U, Orr BA, Rund LA, Webb AG, Kranz DM. IL-12 treatment of endogenously arising murine brain tumors. J Immunol 2000;165(12):7293–7299.

75. Altare F, Durandy A, Lammas D, et al. Impairment of mycobacterial immunity in human interleukin-12 receptor deficiency. Science 1998;280(5368):1432–1435.

76. Lo CH, Lee SC, Wu PY, et al. Antitumor and antimetastatic activity of IL-23. J Immunol 2003; 171(2):600–607.

77. Wiley SR, Schooley K, Smolak PJ, et al. Identification and characterization of a new member of the TNF family that induces apoptosis. Immunity 1995;3(6):673–682.

78. Ashkenazi A. Targeting death and decoy receptors of the tumour-necrosis factor superfamily. Nat Rev Cancer 2002;2(6):420–430.

79. Takeda K, Hayakawa Y, Smyth MJ, et al. Involvement of tumor necrosis factor-related apoptosis-inducing ligand in surveillance of tumor metastasis by liver natural killer cells. Nat Med 2001;7(1): 94–100.

80. Smyth MJ, Cretney E, Takeda K, et al. Tumor necrosis factor-related apoptosis-inducing ligand (TRAIL) contributes to interferon γ-dependent natural killer cell protection from tumor metastasis. J Exp Med 2001;193(6):661–670.

81. Zamai L, Ahmad M, Bennett IM, Azzoni L, Alnemri ES, Perussia B. Natural killer (NK) cell-mediated cytotoxicity: Differential use of TRAIL and Fas ligand by immature and mature primary human NK cells. J Exp Med 1998;188(12):2375–2380.

82. Fanger NA, Maliszewski CR, Schooley K, Griffith TS. Human dendritic cells mediate cellular apoptosis via tumor necrosis factor-related apoptosis-inducing ligand (TRAIL). J Exp Med 1999; 190(8): 1155–1164.

83. Griffith TS, Wiley SR, Kubin MZ, Sedger LM, Maliszewski CR, Fanger NA. Monocyte-mediated tumoricidal activity via the tumor necrosis factor-related cytokine, TRAIL. J Exp Med 1999;189(8): 1343–1354.

84. Kayagaki N, Yamaguchi N, Nakayama M, et al. Expression and function of TNF-related apoptosis-inducing ligand on murine activated NK cells. J Immunol 1999;163(4):1906–1913.

85. Kayagaki N, Yamaguchi N, Nakayama M, Eto H, Okumura K, Yagita H. Type I interferons (IFNs) regulate tumor necrosis factor-related apoptosis-inducing ligand (TRAIL) expression on human T cells: A novel mechanism for the antitumor effects of type I IFNs. J Exp Med 1999;189(9): 1451–1460.

86. Takeda K, Cretney E, Hayakawa Y, et al. TRAIL identifies immature natural killer cells in newborn mice and adult mouse liver. Blood 2005;105:2082–2089.

87. Takeda K, Smyth MJ, Cretney E, et al. Involvement of tumor necrosis factor-related apoptosis-inducing ligand in NK cell-mediated and IFN-γ-dependent suppression of subcutaneous tumor growth. Cell Immunol 2001;214(2):194–200.

88. Cretney E, Takeda K, Yagita H, Glaccum M, Peschon JJ, Smyth MJ. Increased susceptibility to tumor initiation and metastasis in TNF-related apoptosis-inducing ligand-deficient mice. J Immunol 2002;168(3):1356–1361.

89. Takeda K, Smyth MJ, Cretney E, et al. Critical role for tumor necrosis factor-related apoptosis-inducing ligand in immune surveillance against tumor development. J Exp Med 2002;195(2): 161–169.

90. Seki N, Hayakawa Y, Brooks AD, et al. Tumor necrosis factor-related apoptosis-inducing ligand-mediated apoptosis is an important endogenous mechanism for resistance to liver metastases in murine renal cancer. Cancer Res 2003;63(1):207–213.

91. Smyth MJ, Thia KY, Street SE, MacGregor D, Godfrey DI, Trapani JA. Perforin-mediated cytotoxicity is critical for surveillance of spontaneous lymphoma. J Exp Med 2000;192(5):755–760.

92. Schmaltz C, Alpdogan O, Kappel BJ, et al. T cells require TRAIL for optimal graft-versus-tumor activity. Nat Med 2002;8(12):1433–1437.

93. Smyth MJ, Takeda K, Hayakawa Y, Peschon JJ, van den Brink MR, Yagita H. Nature's TRAIL—on a path to cancer immunotherapy. Immunity 2003;18(1):1–6.

94. Hersey P, Zhang XD. How melanoma cells evade trail-induced apoptosis. Nat Rev Cancer 2001;1(2): 142–150.

95. Ludwig AT, Moore JM, Luo Y, et al. Tumor necrosis factor-related apoptosis-inducing ligand: A novel mechanism for Bacillus Calmette-Guerin-induced antitumor activity. Cancer Res 2004;64(10): 3386–3390.

96. Ashkenazi A, Dixit VM. Death receptors: Signaling and modulation. Science 1998;281(5381): 1305–1308.

97. Nagane M, Huang HJ, Cavenee WK. The potential of TRAIL for cancer chemotherapy. Apoptosis 2001;6(3):191–197.

98. El-Deiry WS. Insights into cancer therapeutic design based on p53 and TRAIL receptor signaling. Cell Death Differ 2001;8(11):1066–1075.

99. LeBlanc H, Lawrence D, Varfolomeev E, et al. Tumor-cell resistance to death receptor—induced apoptosis through mutational inactivation of the proapoptotic Bcl-2 homolog Bax. Nat Med 2002; 8(3):274–281.

100. Wang Y, Engels IH, Knee DA, Nasoff M, Deveraux QL, Quon KC. Synthetic lethal targeting of MYC by activation of the DR5 death receptor pathway. Cancer Cell 2004;5(5):501–512.

101. Davidson WF, Giese T, Fredrickson TN. Spontaneous development of plasmacytoid tumors in mice with defective Fas-Fas ligand interactions. J Exp Med 1998;187(11):1825–1838.

102. Straus SE, Jaffe ES, Puck JM, et al. The development of lymphomas in families with autoimmune lymphoproliferative syndrome with germline Fas mutations and defective lymphocyte apoptosis. Blood 2001;98(1):194–200.

103. Landowski TH, Qu N, Buyuksal I, Painter JS, Dalton WS. Mutations in the Fas antigen in patients with multiple myeloma. Blood 1997;90(11):4266–4270.

104. Zornig M, Grzeschiczek A, Kowalski MB, Hartmann KU, Moroy T. Loss of Fas/Apo-1 receptor accelerates lymphomagenesis in E mu L-MYC transgenic mice but not in animals infected with MoMuLV. Oncogene 1995;10(12):2397–2401.

105. Peng SL, Robert ME, Hayday AC, Craft J. A tumor-suppressor function for Fas (CD95) revealed in T cell-deficient mice. J Exp Med 1996;184(3):1149–1154.

106. Owen-Schaub LB, van Golen KL, Hill LL, Price JE. Fas and Fas ligand interactions suppress melanoma lung metastasis. J Exp Med 1998;188(9):1717–1723.

107. Hashimoto W, Osaki T, Okamura H, et al. Differential antitumor effects of administration of recombinant IL-18 or recombinant IL-12 are mediated primarily by Fas-Fas ligand- and perforin-induced tumor apoptosis, respectively. J Immunol 1999;163(2):583–589.

108. Nagata S, Golstein P. The Fas death factor. Science 1995;267(5203):1449–1456.

109. Nagata S. Fas-mediated apoptosis. Adv Exp Med Biol 1996;406:119–124.

110. Screpanti V, Wallin RP, Ljunggren HG, Grandien A. A central role for death receptor-mediated apoptosis in the rejection of tumors by NK cells. J Immunol 2001;167(4):2068–2073.

111. Caldwell SA, Ryan MH, McDuffie E, Abrams SI. The Fas/Fas ligand pathway is important for optimal tumor regression in a mouse model of CTL adoptive immunotherapy of experimental CMS4 lung metastases. J Immunol 2003;171(5):2402–2412.

112. MacEwan DJ. TNF receptor subtype signalling: Differences and cellular consequences. Cell Signal 2002;14(6):477–492.

113. Locksley RM, Killeen N, Lenardo MJ. The TNF and TNF receptor superfamilies: Integrating mammalian biology. Cell 2001;104(4):487–501.

114. Carswell EA, Old LJ, Kassel RL, Green S, Fiore N, Williamson B. An endotoxin-induced serum factor that causes necrosis of tumors. Proc Natl Acad Sci USA 1975;72(9):3666–3670.

115. Baxevanis CN, Voutsas IF, Tsitsilonis OE, Tsiatas ML, Gritzapis AD, Papamichail M. Compromised anti-tumor responses in tumor necrosis factor-α knockout mice. Eur J Immunol 2000;30(7): 1957–1966.

116. Smyth MJ, Kelly JM, Baxter AG, Korner H, Sedgwick JD. An essential role for tumor necrosis factor in natural killer cell-mediated tumor rejection in the peritoneum. J Exp Med 1998;188(9): 1611–1619.

117. Moore RJ, Owens DM, Stamp G, et al. Mice deficient in tumor necrosis factor-α are resistant to skin carcinogenesis. Nat Med 1999;5(7):828–831.

118. Suganuma M, Okabe S, Marino MW, Sakai A, Sueoka E, Fujiki H. Essential role of tumor necrosis factor α (TNF-α) in tumor promotion as revealed by TNF-α-deficient mice. Cancer Res 1999;59(18): 4516–4518.

119. Korner H, Cretney E, Wilhelm P, et al. Tumor necrosis factor sustains the generalized lymphoproliferative disorder (gld) phenotype. J Exp Med 2000;191(1):89–96.

120. Battegay EJ, Raines EW, Colbert T, Ross R. TNF-α stimulation of fibroblast proliferation. Dependence on platelet-derived growth factor (PDGF) secretion and alteration of PDGF receptor expression. J Immunol 1995;154(11):6040–6047.

121. Leber TM, Balkwill FR. Regulation of monocyte MMP-9 production by TNF-α and a tumour-derived soluble factor (MMPSF). Br J Cancer 1998;78(6):724–732.

122. Rosen EM, Goldberg ID, Liu D, et al. Tumor necrosis factor stimulates epithelial tumor cell motility. Cancer Res 1991;51(19):5315–5321.

123. Roberts RA, Kimber I. Cytokines in non-genotoxic hepatocarcinogenesis. Carcinogenesis 1999; 20(8):1397–1401.

124. Knight B, Yeoh GC, Husk KL, et al. Impaired preneoplastic changes and liver tumor formation in tumor necrosis factor receptor type 1 knockout mice. J Exp Med 2000;192(12):1809–1818.

125. Kitakata H, Nemoto-Sasaki Y, Takahashi Y, Kondo T, Mai M, Mukaida N. Essential roles of tumor necrosis factor receptor p55 in liver metastasis of intrasplenic administration of colon 26 cells. Cancer Res 2002;62(22):6682–6687.

126. Szlosarek PW, Balkwill FR. Tumour necrosis factor α: A potential target for the therapy of solid tumours. Lancet Oncol 2003;4(9):565–573.

127. Yu P, Lee Y, Liu W, et al. Priming of naive T cells inside tumors leads to eradication of established tumors. Nat Immunol 2004;5(2):141–149.

128. Croft M. Co-stimulatory members of the TNFR family: Keys to effective T-cell immunity? Nat Rev Immunol 2003;3(8):609–620.

129. Dranoff G, Jaffee E, Lazenby A, et al. Vaccination with irradiated tumor cells engineered to secrete murine granulocyte-macrophage colony-stimulating factor stimulates potent, specific, and long-lasting anti-tumor immunity. Proc Natl Acad Sci USA 1993;90(8):3539–3543.

130. Huang AY, Golumbek P, Ahmadzadeh M, Jaffee E, Pardoll D, Levitsky H. Role of bone marrow-derived cells in presenting MHC class I-restricted tumor antigens. Science 1994;264(5161):961–965.

131. Fernandez NC, Lozier A, Flament C, et al. Dendritic cells directly trigger NK cell functions: Cross-talk relevant in innate anti-tumor immune responses in vivo. Nat Med 1999;5(4):405–411.

132. Somers KD, Brown RR, Holterman DA, et al. Orthotopic treatment model of prostate cancer and metastasis in the immunocompetent mouse: Efficacy of flt3 ligand immunotherapy. Int J Cancer 2003;107(5):773–780.

133. Maliszewski C. Dendritic cells in models of tumor immunity. Role of Flt3 ligand. Pathol Biol (Paris) 2001;49(6):481–483.

134. Hung K, Hayashi R, Lafond-Walker A, Lowenstein C, Pardoll D, Levitsky H. The central role of CD4(+) T cells in the antitumor immune response. J Exp Med 1998;188(12):2357–2368.

135. Soiffer R, Lynch T, Mihm M, et al. Vaccination with irradiated autologous melanoma cells engineered to secrete human granulocyte-macrophage colony-stimulating factor generates potent antitumor immunity in patients with metastatic melanoma. Proc Natl Acad Sci USA 1998;95(22): 13,141–13,146.
136. Mach N, Gillessen S, Wilson SB, Sheehan C, Mihm M, Dranoff G. Differences in dendritic cells stimulated in vivo by tumors engineered to secrete granulocyte-macrophage colony-stimulating factor or Flt3-ligand. Cancer Res 2000;60(12):3239–3246.
137. Salgia R, Lynch T, Skarin A, et al. Vaccination with irradiated autologous tumor cells engineered to secrete granulocyte-macrophage colony-stimulating factor augments antitumor immunity in some patients with metastatic non-small-cell lung carcinoma. J Clin Oncol 2003;21(4):624–630.
138. Jaffee EM, Hruban RH, Biedrzycki B, et al. Novel allogeneic granulocyte-macrophage colony-stimulating factor-secreting tumor vaccine for pancreatic cancer: A phase I trial of safety and immune activation. J Clin Oncol 2001;19(1):145–156.
139. Chang AE, Rosenberg SA. Overview of interleukin-2 as an immunotherapeutic agent. Semin Surg Oncol 1989;5(6):385–390.
140. Rosenberg SA. Progress in human tumour immunology and immunotherapy. Nature 2001;411(6835): 380–384.
141. Rosenberg SA, Mule JJ, Spiess PJ, Reichert CM, Schwarz SL. Regression of established pulmonary metastases and subcutaneous tumor mediated by the systemic administration of high-dose recombinant interleukin 2. J Exp Med 1985;161(5):1169–1188.
142. Thompson JA, Peace DJ, Klarnet JP, Kern DE, Greenberg PD, Cheever MA. Eradication of disseminated murine leukemia by treatment with high-dose interleukin 2. J Immunol 1986;137(11): 3675–3680.
143. Mule JJ, Yang JC, Afreniere RL, Shu SY, Rosenberg SA. Identification of cellular mechanisms operational in vivo during the regression of established pulmonary metastases by the systemic administration of high-dose recombinant interleukin 2. J Immunol 1987;139(1):285–294.
144. Papa MZ, Mule JJ, Rosenberg SA. Antitumor efficacy of lymphokine-activated killer cells and recombinant interleukin 2 in vivo: Successful immunotherapy of established pulmonary metastases from weakly immunogenic and nonimmunogenic murine tumors of three district histological types. Cancer Res 1986;46(10):4973–4978.
145. Spiess PJ, Yang JC, Rosenberg SA. In vivo antitumor activity of tumor-infiltrating lymphocytes expanded in recombinant interleukin-2. J Natl Cancer Inst 1987;79(5):1067–1075.
146. Parrish-Novak J, Foster DC, Holly RD, Clegg CH. Interleukin-21 and the IL-21 receptor: Novel effectors of NK and T cell responses. J Leukoc Biol 2002;72(5):856–863.
147. Kasaian MT, Whitters MJ, Carter LL, et al. IL-21 limits NK cell responses and promotes antigen-specific T cell activation: A mediator of the transition from innate to adaptive immunity. Immunity 2002; 16(4):559–569.
148. Parrish-Novak J, Dillon SR, Nelson A, et al. Interleukin 21 and its receptor are involved in NK cell expansion and regulation of lymphocyte function. Nature 2000;408(6808):57–63.
149. Brady J, Hayakawa Y, Smyth MJ, Nutt SL. IL-21 induces the functional maturation of murine NK cells. J Immunol 2004;172(4):2048–2058.
150. Wang G, Tschoi M, Spolski R, et al. In vivo antitumor activity of interleukin 21 mediated by natural killer cells. Cancer Res 2003;63(24):9016–9022.
151. Ma HL, Whitters MJ, Konz RF, et al. IL-21 activates both innate and adaptive immunity to generate potent antitumor responses that require perforin but are independent of IFN-γ. J Immunol 2003;171(2):608–615.
152. Moroz A, Eppolito C, Li Q, Tao J, Clegg CH, Shrikant PA. IL-21 enhances and sustains CD8+ T cell responses to achieve durable tumor immunity: Comparative evaluation of IL-2, IL-15, and IL-21. J Immunol 2004;173(2):900–909.
153. Rosenberg SA. Interleukin-2 and the development of immunotherapy for the treatment of patients with cancer. Cancer J Sci Am 2000;6 Suppl 1:S2–7.
154. Rosenberg SA, Lotze MT, Yang JC, et al. Prospective randomized trial of high-dose interleukin-2 alone or in conjunction with lymphokine-activated killer cells for the treatment of patients with advanced cancer. J Natl Cancer Inst 1993;85(8):622–632.
155. Fisher RI, Rosenberg SA, Fyfe G. Long-term survival update for high-dose recombinant interleukin-2 in patients with renal cell carcinoma. Cancer J Sci Am 2000;6 Suppl 1:S55–57.

156. Atkins MB, Lotze MT, Dutcher JP, et al. High-dose recombinant interleukin 2 therapy for patients with metastatic melanoma: Analysis of 270 patients treated between 1985 and 1993. J Clin Oncol 1999;17(7):2105–2116.

157. Rosenberg SA, Yang JC, Schwartzentruber DJ, et al. Immunologic and therapeutic evaluation of a synthetic peptide vaccine for the treatment of patients with metastatic melanoma. Nat Med 1998;4(3): 321–327.

158. Rosenberg SA, Yang JC, Schwartzentruber DJ, et al. Prospective randomized trial of the treatment of patients with metastatic melanoma using chemotherapy with cisplatin, dacarbazine, and tamoxifen alone or in combination with interleukin-2 and interferon alfa-2b. J Clin Oncol 1999;17(3): 968–975.

159. Dudley ME, Wunderlich JR, Robbins PF, et al. Cancer regression and autoimmunity in patients after clonal repopulation with antitumor lymphocytes. Science 2002;298(5594):850–854.

160. Khatri VP, Fehniger TA, Baiocchi RA, et al. Ultra low dose interleukin-2 therapy promotes a type 1 cytokine profile in vivo in patients with AIDS and AIDS-associated malignancies. J Clin Invest 1998;101(6):1373–1378.

161. Baiocchi RA, Ward JS, Carrodeguas L, et al. GM-CSF and IL-2 induce specific cellular immunity and provide protection against Epstein-Barr virus lymphoproliferative disorder. J Clin Invest 2001;108(6):887–894.

162. Baiocchi RA, Caligiuri MA. Low-dose interleukin 2 prevents the development of Epstein-Barr virus (EBV)-associated lymphoproliferative disease in scid/scid mice reconstituted i.p. with EBV-seropositive human peripheral blood lymphocytes. Proc Natl Acad Sci USA 1994;91(12): 5577–5581.

163. Biron CA. Role of early cytokines, including α and β interferons (IFN-α/β), in innate and adaptive immune responses to viral infections. Semin Immunol 1998;10(5):383–390.

164. Ferbas JJ, Toso JF, Logar AJ, Navratil JS, Rinaldo CR, Jr. CD4+ blood dendritic cells are potent producers of IFN-α in response to in vitro HIV-1 infection. J Immunol 1994;152(9):4649–4662.

165. Siegal FP, Kadowaki N, Shodell M, et al. The nature of the principal type 1 interferon-producing cells in human blood. Science 1999;284(5421):1835–1837.

166. Santini SM, Lapenta C, Logozzi M, et al. Type I interferon as a powerful adjuvant for monocyte-derived dendritic cell development and activity in vitro and in Hu-PBL-SCID mice. J Exp Med 2000;191(10):1777–1788.

167. Le Bon A, Schiavoni G, D'Agostino G, Gresser I, Belardelli F, Tough DF. Type i interferons potently enhance humoral immunity and can promote isotype switching by stimulating dendritic cells in vivo. Immunity 2001;14(4):461–470.

168. Egle A, Villunger A, Kos M, et al. Modulation of Apo-1/Fas (CD95)-induced programmed cell death in myeloma cells by interferon-α 2. Eur J Immunol 1996;26(12):3119–3126.

169. Ishikawa R, Biron CA. IFN induction and associated changes in splenic leukocyte distribution. J Immunol 1993;150(9):3713–3727.

170. Ahmed R. Tickling memory T cells. Science 1996;272(5270):1904.

171. Coughlin CM, Salhany KE, Gee MS, et al. Tumor cell responses to IFNγ affect tumorigenicity and response to IL-12 therapy and antiangiogenesis. Immunity 1998;9(1):25–34.

172. Fallarino F, Gajewski TF. Cutting edge: Differentiation of antitumor CTL in vivo requires host expression of Stat1. J Immunol 1999;163(8):4109–4113.

173. Qin Z, Schwartzkopff J, Pradera F, et al. A critical requirement of interferon gamma-mediated angiostasis for tumor rejection by CD8+ T cells. Cancer Res 2003;63(14):4095–4100.

III

CYTOKINES AND TUMOR STROMA/METASTASIS

13 Cytokines in the Tumor Stroma

Michael C. Ostrowski

1. CYTOKINES AND THE MOLECULAR DIALOGUE BETWEEN STROMA AND TUMOR

In addition to their well-documented roles in leukemia and lymphoma, cytokines and chemokines can directly affect the progression of solid tumors, including carcinomas *(1–3)*. Carcinomas are the most frequent human tumors that arise from the epithelial cells that line the inner surfaces of organs. The conversion of normal epithelial cell to metastatic tumor cell is accepted as a multi-stage process that requires progressive genetic alterations within the epithelial tumor cell and has been the focus of intense investigation over the past three decades *(4,5)*. At the same time, the many other cell types in the tumor microenvironment are increasingly appreciated as components of a complex biologic network akin to an organ system that are critical for tumor progression, and thus may provide new targets for cancer therapy *(3–5)*.

Although it has been appreciated that a molecular dialogue between tumor cells and other cells in the microenvironment is necessary for tumor development, the tumor cells were thought to primarily initiate and orchestrate the conversations with other cell types *(6,7)*. Thus, the microenvironment could be considered a reactive participant in tumor progression, responding to signals initiated by an altered genetic program in the epithelial cell. This view is at odds with what has been learned from studying epithelial cells during embryonic development, where it is clear that mesenchymal cells, for example, fibroblasts and adipocytes, and immune cells, including macrophages and eosinophils, play an active and instructive role in programming epithelial cell structure and function *(8–10)*. The bi-directional molecular dialogue between stromal cells and epithelial cell

From: *Cancer Drug Discovery and Development,*
Cytokines in the Genesis and Treatment of Cancer
Edited by: M. A. Caligiuri and M. T. Lotze © Humana Press Inc., Totowa, NJ

types is critical for normal organ development and function *(8–10)*, and it is highly probable that such interactions are equally important during tumor progression.

A growing body of evidence demonstrates that cytokines and chemokines are key components in the molecular dialogue between tumor cells and other cells types that shape the tumor microenvironment and promote tumor progression and metastasis *(3,11)*. Understanding the role of cytokines and chemokines within the tumor microenvironment is an emerging area of research that clearly has important clinical implications, both for diagnosis and treatment of human carcinoma. Tumor microenvironment cells, and cytokines that modulate their function, may provide an "Achilles heel" to attack cancer cell growth and metastasis, especially in combination with therapies aimed directly at the epithelial tumor cell. Additionally, as documented in other chapters in this book, the use of cytokine immunotherapy for solid tumors is an active area of investigation. Immunotherapy of carcinoma will need to take into account the interactions among microenvironment cells, in particular tumor associated macrophages (TAMs), and tumor cells in order to be successful.

In this chapter, recent evidence demonstrating that cytokines and chemokines can affect discrete stages of carcinoma progression and metastasis by affecting cells in the tumor microenvironment will be highlighted. The focus will be on two types of microenvironment cells, TAMs and stromal fibroblasts, for which the evidence is most compelling. Another obvious stromal cell type to add to this list is the endothelial cell, but the role of cytokines, particularly TNF-α, on the function of endothelial cells in the tumor stroma are discussed at length in Chapter 5.

2. TUMOR-ASSOCIATED MACROPHAGES AND CARCINOMA PROGRESSION

In wound healing and pathogenic inflammatory responses production of cytokines and chemokines signal both recruitment and subsequent activation of immune cells, including macrophages, to the sites of tissue damage *(3,11)*. Macrophages play a critical role in wound healing and inflammatory responses by stimulating cellular immune responses and destroying pathogens, whereas also promoting angiogenesis and tissue repair *(3,11)*. Sites of tumorigenesis can be viewed as a wound or inflammatory site, and many of the same cytokines and chemokines involved in wound healing and pathogen induced inflammation are produced at tumor sites, often directly by the tumor cells *(1–3)*, but also by other cell types present in the tumor microenvironment.

For example, gene expression profiling of several different cell types isolated from primary human breast cancer samples revealed that tumor myoepithelial cells and myofibroblasts differentially express two chemokines, CCL12 (MCP-5) and CCL14 relative to control cells *(12)*. These tumor-induced cytokines can act in an autocrine fashion to stimulate epithelial tumor cell growth *(12)*. However, they can also lead to the recruitment and activation of TAMs, which are major constituents of the carcinoma microenvironment and have been postulated to affect clinical outcome *(3,11,13)*. Somewhat paradoxically, in three different clinical studies of breast cancer, high numbers of TAMs in tumor sections was correlated with poor clinical outcome *(14–16)*. In general, high numbers of TAMs within tumors is associated with poor clinical outcome in several different types of carcinoma *(13)*.

Understanding why TAMs actually promote, instead of inhibit, tumorigenesis has clinical applications. The following sections present experimental data that have begun to dissect the roles of cytokines and TAMs in carcinoma progression.

2.1. Colony Stimulating Factor-1 (CSF-1), TAMs, and Tumor Metastasis in Breast Cancer

CSF-1 (also known as macrophage colony stimulating factor, M-CSF) is a cytokine that regulates growth, differentiation and survival of monocytes and macrophages *(17)*. CSF-1 is also a chemotactic factor for monocytes and macrophages *(17)*. Expression of CSF-1 has been detected in more than 70% of human breast cancers and is correlated with poor clinical prognosis *(18)*. Although there is some evidence that CSF-1 can act in an autocrine/paracrine fashion to directly affect the growth of breast tumor cells *(19)*, a more critical role likely involves the recruitment and differentiation of the monocytes that become TAMs.

Work from Jeffrey Pollard's group has demonstrated a critical action of CSF-1 and TAMs in breast tumor metastasis *(20)*. This work used the *osteopetrotic (op)* mutant mouse model that was caused by a spontaneous mutation in the CSF-1 gene. As a consequence of this mutation, homozygous *op/op* mice lack CSF-1 and contain only low levels of most types of tissue macrophages *(21)*. When the *op* mutation was combined with the MMTV-Polyoma virus middle T (PyMT) transgene, a transgene that induces breast tumors and lung metastasis in 100% of affected mice, TAMS were decreased but tumor onset and tumor growth were not affected. Strikingly, lung metastasis of mammary tumor cells was decreased by 70% in the PyMT;*op/op* mice. Lung metastasis could be restored, in fact increased, by adding a CSF-1 transgene to the mammary epithelial cells *(20)*.

How do TAMs exert this striking affect on breast cancer metastasis in this model? First, CSF-1 is known to regulate expression of extracellular proteases like uPA and MMP9 in macrophages *(11,20)*, and these types of enzymes can contribute to remodeling of the extracellular matrix and to tumor cell invasiveness. Second, activated TAMs can produce pro-angiogenic factors, including TNF-α and vascular endothelial growth factor, and by this mechanism promote tumor angiogenesis *(11,13)*. Macrophages are especially believed to be a major source of pro-angiogenic factors within the hypoxic environment of carcinoma *(13)*.

Recent experimental evidence provides a third more provocative role for macrophages in tumor metastasis *(22)*. These studies used an elegant in vivo approach, combining a chemotaxis-based in vivo invasion assay and multiphoton-based intravital imaging, to show that the interaction between macrophages and tumor cells facilitates the migration of carcinoma cells within the primary tumor. Macrophages produce epidermal growth factors that are chemoattractive for tumor cells, and tumor cells produce CSF-1, setting up a paracrine loop that is required for tumor cell migration.

Therefore, macrophages appear to affect the tumor microenvironment to promote basement membrane remodeling, angiogenesis and tumor cell migration.

2.2. The Pro-inflammatory NF-κB pathway, TAMs and Colon Tumor Initiation and Progression

As argued above, many cytokines and chemokines are activated within the tumor microenvironment and these can play multiple roles in both tumor cells and other cell types within the microenvironment. A pathway that many of these cytokines converge on within all target cells is the NF-κB pathway *(23)*. NF-κB is a transcription factor composed of two nonidentical subunits that regulates downstream target genes required for inflammatory responses *(23)*. In resting cells, NF-κB is retained in the cytoplasm through association with specific inhibitors, the IκB proteins *(23)*. Activation of cells by pro-inflammatory signals activates the IKK kinase complex that subsequently phosphorylates and inactivates IκB proteins, thus leading to the nuclear translocation of NF-κB. Defining the action of NF-κB signaling in different cell types within the tumor microenvironment can provide a general view of the mechanisms by which cytokines regulate tumor progression.

Genetic analyses of the NF-κB pathway by Michael Karin's group provide experimental evidence for the importance of NF-κB signaling in a mouse model for colitis-associated cancer *(24)*. In humans, colitis-associated cancer arises in patients with inflammatory bowel disease and comprises about 5% of all colorectal cancers *(25)*. Anti-inflammatory therapy with nonsteroidal anti-inflammatory drugs reduces the risk of colitis-associated cancer by about 80% *(26)*. In addition, activated NF-κB was detected in macrophages and epithelial cells from biopsy specimens or in cultured cells of patients *(27)*. These data suggest that inflammation dependent on the NF-κB pathway may contribute to either initiation or progression of colitis-associated cancer.

To specifically test the role of the NF-κB pathway within these two cell types, mouse loxP/Cre genetic technology was used to conditionally delete IKKβ kinase within either the tumor epithelial cells or the TAMs in the murine colitis associated cancer model *(24)*. Deletion of this kinase would render cells unresponsive to inflammatory stimuli. The result of these experiments demonstrated that removing the NF-κB pathway in either epithelial cells or TAMs significantly decreased tumor initiation and progression, but by different mechanisms. Removing the NF-κB pathway within the tumor cells resulted in a small, but significant, reduction in tumor number and size and correlated with increased apoptosis of tumor epithelial cells. In contrast, removing NF-κB in macrophages resulted in a larger decrease in tumor number and size by a mechanism that involved decreased tumor cell proliferation. The decrease in tumor cell proliferation correlated with down-regulated expression of pro-inflammatory cytokines and chemokines in TAMs, including TNF-α, IL-1β and MIP-2, leading to the possibility that such factors may directly increase proliferation of tumor cells *(24)*. An alternative explanation might be that these cytokines indirectly affect tumor growth by stimulating expression of growth factors within other cell types present in the tumor microenvironment. A third possibility might be that activated TAMs produce reactive oxygen species (ROS) that act as a mutagen in epithelial cells, thus leading directly to the mutation of genes, oncogenes and tumor suppressors, that control cell growth within the tumor cells *(11,13)*.

2.3. Prospects for Anti-TAM Therapies

The studies described above demonstrate a role for TAMs in both the initiation and early progression phases of carcinoma as well as in the later stages that involve tumor angiogenesis and metastasis. Combined with available clinical data indicating a general relationship between TAMs and poor clinical prognosis *(11,13)*, TAMs would appear to provide an attractive clinical target for treatment of carcinoma.

However, an important question that needs to answered before considering specific anti-TAM therapies is why TAMs promote tumor growth and metastasis, instead of eliminating tumors. One explanation for the persistent inflammatory response seen in cancer is that tumor cells disrupt the fine balance of cytokines that are necessary for correct regulation of the inflammatory response (3). In this view, normal inflammation is by definition self-limiting. At a molecular level, the action of pro-inflammatory cytokines is ultimately balanced by the action of anti-inflammatory cytokines. Inflammation thus has clear beginning, middle and end phases, and specific cytokine signatures mark each of these chapters. In cancer, the pro-inflammatory phase persists because this balance is disrupted. In this view, targeting common aspects of inflammation, for example by using available anti-inflammatory agents like nonsteroidal anti-inflammatory drugs and anti-COX2 inhibitors, might provide a strategy to inhibit the influence of TAMs in most types of carcinoma (3). Another strategy would be to target the molecules known to be generally important for the action of macrophages in inflammation, for example, TNF-α or proteases like MMP9 (3).

A second possibility that might explain this persistent response during tumorigenesis is that this response reflects a developmental program that is distinct from wound healing and pathogen-induced inflammation (11). For example, experiments in the *op/op* mouse model demonstrate a critical action of macrophages in mammary gland development, but not a general role in all organ systems (10). Specifically, during mammary gland development macrophages appear to be necessary for epithelial cell proliferation and invasion into adjacent stroma that lead to formation of terminal end buds as well as the subsequent branching of the ducts that results from end bud formation (10). This normal developmental process shares more than passing similarities to the interaction of TAMs and mammary tumor epithelial cells. In this view, breast tissue macrophages, either during normal development or tumorigenesis, may be "educated" by their local environment and programmed to carry out a certain set of tasks. This also implies that during normal development there must be mechanisms to eliminate these macrophages after they have completed their task, a process that is not active in neoplasia.

Understanding the molecular differences among tissue macrophages isolated from different sites might be critical in understanding the behavior of these cells, both during normal development and during tumor progression. For example, directly targeting CSF-1 or signaling pathways activated by this cytokine that lead to activation of key target genes may be an effective strategy for breast cancer, but not for colon cancer (28). In this regard, one specific target might be the paracrine loop between mammary tumor cells and TAMs that appears to be critical for tumor cell invasiveness and metastasis (22). This may be a tractable target because it involves interactions of soluble ligands and cell surface receptors.

3. TUMOR STROMAL FIBROBLAST
AND CARCINOMA INITIATION AND PROGRESSION

Mesenchymal cells, in particular stromal fibroblasts, are another cell type within the tumor microenvironment that can affect tumor cell progression. As argued above, there is clear evidence from studies of organ development that fibroblast-epithelial interactions are critical for normal development (8,9). Experiments from Gerald Cuhna's lab were seminal in establishing an active role for tumor fibroblasts in the progression of prostate tumors (29). These experiments used an organ culture system in which prostate mesenchymal and epithelial interactions could be studied in vivo. Results from this approach clearly demonstrated that tumor stromal fibroblasts, but not normal prostatic fibroblasts, could increase tumorigenicity of immortal prostatic epithelial cells genetically "primed" for tumorigenesis by oncogene expression *(29)*. These experiments indicated that the tumor stromal fibroblast was stably altered when compared to the normal fibroblast, and that the change(s) was necessary for epithelial cell tumorigenicity. In this section, evidence supporting the role of TGF-β1 signaling pathways in tumor stromal fibroblasts is presented.

3.1. Genetic Evidence for TGF-β Receptor 1 Action From Stromal Fibroblasts in Tumor Initiation

TGF-β and components in the major signaling pathway through which this cytokine exerts its' effects are recognized tumor suppressors in many different types of human carcinoma, including in prostate and gastric cancer *(30)*. Evidence to date indicates that, as would be expected for a tumor suppressor, mutations in these genes occur in epithelial cells *(30)*.

In contrast to this accepted view, work from Hal Moses and collaborators, performed in mouse genetic models, demonstrated that disruption of TGF-β signaling in stromal fibroblasts could be an initiating event for prostate and gastric carcinoma *(31;* and Chapter 5). In these experiments, "floxed" alleles for the TGF-β receptor type II (TGFRII) were combined with a Cre transgene specific for stromal fibroblasts in several different organs, including prostate and stomach. This was accomplished by using the promoter for Fibroblast Specific Protein-1 (Fsp-1). The gene for Fsp-1 was originally cloned in a differential screen to identify fibroblast specific genes and its' promoter has been extensively characterized in transgenic experiments *(32)*. The conditional deletion of TGF-β signaling in fibroblasts resulted in preneoplastic lesions in the epithelium of prostate and invasive squamous cell carcinoma of the forestomach, both associated with an increased number of stromal cells. That deletion of TGFRII was specific to the stromal fibroblasts was confirmed by in situ measurement of TGFRII expression, as well as by examining the status of the gene in fibroblasts or epithelium in the affected tissues obtained from laser capture microdissection.

Studying biomarkers of cancer progression in affected epithelial cells in this model revealed that c-myc expression was upregulated and that the cdk inhibitors p21 and p27 were downregulated in forestomach in FSP-Cre/TGFRII floxed mice relative to controls. Further, the tyrosine kinase receptor c-met was hyper-phosphorylated in the same epithelial cells, and the ligand for this receptor, Hepatocyte Growth Factor/Scatter Factor (HGF) was upregulated in the stromal fibroblast compartment. The activation of this paracrine loop between stromal fibroblasts and epithelial cells provides a possible mechanism to explain these results.

These results provide additional evidence for an active role of stromal fibroblasts in carcinoma initiation and progression, and identify TGF-β as part of the molecular dialogue among these different cell types. An interesting question that remains is why deletion of the TGFRII in stromal fibroblasts in other organs, for example kidney, lung or mammary gland, did not result in fibroblast proliferation or neoplastic progression. It will also be interesting to see results of experiments in which the stromal TGFRII conditional knockout is combined with initiating events, for example expression of onco-transgenes, within the epithelial cells. Intriguingly, these studies also provide experimental support for the idea that genetic alterations in cell types other than epithelial cells could be the initiating event for neoplastic progression, a topic that will be considered in more detail in Section 4 below.

3.3. TGF-β Action From Stromal Fibroblasts in Tumor Progression

In addition to its' action as tumor suppressor, TGF-β can also act as a dominant gene to promote tumor cell growth and metastasis *(30)*. A likely explanation for this anomalous behavior is that TGF-β signaling plays different roles during different stages of cancer progression, as a tumor suppressor during initiation and preneoplastic phases, but as a promoter of tumor growth during later stages *(30;* and Chapter 6). In this latter context, TGF-β expression in stromal fibroblasts may be important for tumor progression, as demonstrated by recent work from Robert Weinberg's group.

This work used a novel xenotransplant model that produces "humanized" mouse mammary glands that contain both human stromal fibroblasts and mammary epithelial cells *(33)*. In this model, human mammary epithelial cells (obtained from normal individuals following elective reduction mammoplasty) were placed into mammary glands of immune compromised NOD/SCID mice, from which endogenous epithelial cells have been removed. Human mammary cells alone did not undergo normal differentiation. However, if normal human mammary fibroblasts were first engrafted into these cleared mouse mammary glands, the subsequent introduction of human mammary epithelial cells led to development of human breast ducts within the chimeric fat pad. These human epithelial structures were capable of responding to hormonal cues with milk production. In the second part of the experiments, mammary stromal fibroblasts were first modified to express either TGF-β or HGF. The altered stroma led to the growth of structures resembling benign neoplasia, and in the case of a sample from one patient, a malignant lesion. These experiments demonstrate that stromal alterations can directly promote tumor progression and provide a model to directly study the interactions of human stromal fibroblasts and epithelial cells.

In another type of xenotransplant model developed by David Rowley's lab, similar results were obtained for prostate cancer cells *(34)*. In this model, the prostate cancer cell line LNAcNP does not grow when injected subcutaneously into immune compromised mice, but grows efficiently when injected along with a stromal fibroblast cell line *(35)*. In addition to promoting tumor growth, the stromal fibroblasts increased angiogenesis at the site of tumor injection. Inclusion of TGF-β blocking agents, either a neutralizing antibody or TGF-β latency-associated peptide, resulted in markedly reduced tumor growth and angiogenesis *(34)*.

Taken together, these results support an active role for TGF-β produced by stromal fibroblasts in tumor progression, and suggest increased angiogenesis may be a result of production of this cytokine by fibroblasts.

4. FUTURE DIRECTIONS FOR TUMOR-STROMAL CELL RESEARCH

For the past two decades the focus has been on the epithelial tumor cell, and defining the genetic and molecular mechanisms that contribute to tumor cell initiation, progression and metastasis. However, it is becoming more widely accepted that understanding the contribution of other cell types in the tumor microenvironment to all stages of tumorigenesis will be critical to taking the next steps to improved cancer diagnosis and treatment.

Although the bi-directional conversations between tumor stromal cells and epithelial tumor cells, and the essential role of cytokines in this discourse, have been clearly established, our understanding of the molecular mechanisms underlying this communication remain rudimentary. Some of the same approaches that have been successful in studying tumor cells will undoubtedly be useful for increasing our understanding of tumor stromal cell biology, but the potential complexity of tumor-stromal interactions indicate that new strategies and techniques will have to be developed to study the interactions of multiple cell types in the tumor microenvironment. The next sections discuss three areas of development that will be essential for increasing our understanding of tumor stromal cell interactions.

4.1. Isolation and Characterization of Distinct Cell Types From the Tumor Stroma

An increased focus on isolation and characterization of distinct cell types from within both tumors and normal organs is one crucial area for development in this field. Isolation of as many cell types as possible should be emphasized, as there are relatively few cell types, mainly fibroblasts and endothelial cells, that have been studied in any detail thus far.

Mouse models will be especially useful in this regard, because transgenic expression of GFP in different cell types allows the rapid purification of highly enriched cell populations using existing high speed fluorescent cell sorting (FACS) technology *(36,37)*. However, enrichment of human cell populations must also be a priority *(12)*. This will require a more systemic effort to identify a large number of cell surface markers, as has already been accomplished for hematopoietic cells. As in the hematopoietic system, a greater range of cell surface markers will allow more precise distinction of the various cell types in the microenvironment. Technical advancements in cell sorting techniques are also likely to be required for studies with human cells, as the amount of material available for fractionation will in most cases be very small. Continued improvement in FACS and automation of other techniques, for example magnetic bead technologies, would facilitate purification of human cell types.

Once sufficient quantities of highly enriched cell populations are available systematic molecular phenotyping should be a priority. Both high throughput microarray and proteomic approaches will provide molecular signatures that will allow basic questions to be addressed. For example, are breast cancer TAMs more related to TAMs isolated from other tumor sites, or are they more related to resident mammary gland macrophages? What genes do breast stromal fibroblasts and colon stromal fibroblasts both express, and what genes are expressed uniquely only in breast stromal fibroblasts? This type of molecular cataloging will lead to specific hypotheses that can then be addressed experimentally.

Isolated cell types can also be used for cell biologic assays, and can also be used to set up xenotransplantation or in vitro assays designed to study interactions of different cell types in controlled settings.

4.2. Model Systems for Studying Tumor Stromal Interactions

Development of improved mouse models to study the genetic interactions between tumor and stromal cells is a second area that will require increased attention. In initial phases, this will involve development of specific regulatory regions to precisely deliver

Cre not just to tumor epithelial cells, but also to other cell types in the microenvironment. For example, the FSP-Cre system discussed above *(31)* is a first step in this direction, but a system that targets specifically only prostate stromal fibroblasts would be a
much more useful tool. Improvements in this area will depend on progress in isolating
and characterizing stromal cells from different organs, as discussed above, to identify
stromal genes that are expressed in an organ or tissue specific fashion, or even a tumor
specific fashion. For example, the regulatory sequences of a gene that was activated in
TAMs from multiple tumor sites could be very useful in mouse models for both breast
and colon cancer.

The next stage of model development would provide the ability to remove two different genes in two different cell types. This could be accomplished for example, by
expression of both Cre recombinase and Frt recombinase *(38)* under the control of regulatory sequences specific for different cell compartments within the same mouse.
Models that more accurately mimic human tumor-microenvironment genetic interactions would be possible with such model systems.

Improved transplantation models, including "humanized" xenotransplantation models *(33)*, will provide a complementary approach to the mouse genetic models. Moreover,
continued efforts to develop in vitro models that more accurately reflect in vivo architecture will provide avenues for studying both genetic and cellular interactions, for
example improved 3-D culture systems for studying mammary gland development and
tumorigenesis *(39)*. Improvement and innovation will be linked to the ability to obtain
pure populations of stromal cells.

4.3. Human Genetic Studies to Identify Genes
That Act From Stromal Cell Compartments

One important unanswered question is what are the genes that act from the tumor
stroma during the progression of human carcinoma? An assumption is that these will be
the same genes that are altered within the tumor cells themselves, but this could well be
faulty reasoning. Isolation and characterization of human tumor stromal cells as
described above might give clues as to genes that should be studied, however the information would provide only indirect evidence.

Human genetic studies would provide one approach to directly identify genes that act
from tumor stromal cells. For example, studies from Charis Eng's lab have demonstrated
that mutations and LOH can be detected in p53 and PTEN tumor suppressors in human
mammary tumor stromal fibroblasts isolated by laser capture microdissection *(40)*.
Genome wide surveys to detect and compare LOH in human mammary tumor epithelial cells and stromal fibroblasts have revealed distinct patterns and frequencies of LOH
in the two cell compartments, as well as three LOH events that are more frequent in the
stromal compartment *(41)*. Extending this technique could reveal genes that are mutated
preferentially in stromal cells, and that can subsequently be modeled in mouse systems.

The hypothesis that genetic alterations in stromal cells can contribute directly to epithelial cell malignant transformation and progression remains controversial but has been independently confirmed in breast cancer *(42,43)*, and has also been detected in bladder and
colon cancer *(43–45)*. Additionally, experimental results demonstrating that that deletion of
the TGFIIR gene in stromal fibroblasts can lead to neoplastic disease in prostate and
fore stomach in mice can be interpreted to provide experimental evidence for the role of

stromal mutations in cancer progression *(31)*. These results are potentially paradigm shifting. Although it is generally accepted that progressive genetic alterations within the tumor cell are responsible for tumor initiation and progression, the possibility that such mutations can occur in different cell types in the tumor microenvironment would call for a radical shift in current thinking about tumor progression and the role of stromal components in this process. Clearly, increased and intensive investigations in this area are warranted.

In conclusion, whereas the importance of the stroma in tumor progression has been realized for several decades, we are only recently entering a stage where the exact mechanisms that underlie tumor-stromal interactions can be examined. This area of research holds great promise for increasing our basic understanding of cancer, and perhaps even shifting existing models for the molecular basis of cancer. These findings also hold great promise for improving clinical diagnosis and treatment of carcinoma.

REFERENCES

1. Balkwill F, Mantovani A. Inflammation and cancer: back to Virchow? Lancet 2001; 357:539–545.
2. Balkwill F. Cancer and the chemokine network. Nat Rev Cancer 2004; 4:540–550.
3. Coussens LM, Werb Z. Inflammation and cancer. Nature 2002; 420:860–867.
4. Hanahan D, Weinberg RA. The hallmarks of cancer. Cell 2000; 100:57–70.
5. Cunha GR, Matrisian LM. It's not my fault, blame it on my microenvironment. Differentiation 2002; 70:469–472.
6. Ronnov-Jessen L, Petersen OW, Bissell MJ. Cellular changes involved in conversion of normal to malignant breast: importance of the stromal reaction. Physiol Rev 1996; 76:69–125.
7. Rowley DR. What might a stromal response mean to prostate cancer progression? Cancer Metastasis Rev 1998; 17:411–419.
8. Cunha GR, Alarid ET, Turner T, Donjacour AA, Boutin EL, Foster BA. Normal and abnormal development of the male urogenital tract. Role of androgens, mesenchymal-epithelial interactions, and growth factors. J Androl 1992; 13:465–475.
9. Robinson GW, Karpf AB, Kratochwil K. Regulation of mammary gland development by tissue interaction. J Mammary Gland Biol Neoplasia 1999; 4:9–19.
10. Gouon-Evans V, Rothenberg ME, Pollard JW. Postnatal mammary gland development requires macrophages and eosinophils. Development 2000; 127:2269–2282.
11. Pollard JW. Tumour-educated macrophages promote tumour progression and metastasis. Nat Rev Cancer 2004; 4:71–78.
12. Allinen M, Beroukhim R, Cai L, et al. Molecular characterization of the tumor microenvironment in breast cancer. Cancer Cell 2004; 6:17–32.
13. Bingle L, Brown NJ, Lewis CE. The role of tumour-associated macrophages in tumour progression: implications for new anticancer therapies. J Pathol 2002; 196:254–265.
14. Leek RD, Lewis CE, Whitehouse R, Greenall M, Clarke J, Harris AL. Association of macrophage infiltration with angiogenesis and prognosis in invasive breast carcinoma. Cancer Res 1996; 56: 4625–4629.
15. Lee AH, Happerfield LC, Bobrow LG, Millis RR. Angiogenesis and inflammation in invasive carcinoma of the breast. J Clin Pathol 1997; 50:669–673.
16. Goede V, Brogelli L, Ziche M, Augustin HG. Induction of inflammatory angiogenesis by monocyte chemoattractant protein-1. Int J Cancer 1999; 82:765–770.
17. Pixley FJ, Stanley ER. CSF-1 regulation of the wandering macrophage: complexity in action. Trends Cell Biol 2004; 14:628–638.
18. Scholl SM, Pallud C, Beuvon F, et al. Anti-colony-stimulating factor-1 antibody staining in primary breast adenocarcinomas correlates with marked inflammatory cell infiltrates and prognosis. J Natl Cancer Inst 1994; 86:120–126.
19. Kacinski BM. CSF-1 and its receptor in breast carcinomas and neoplasms of the female reproductive tract. Mol Reprod Dev 1997; 46:71–74.

20. Lin EY, Nguyen AV, Russell RG, Pollard JW. Colony-stimulating factor 1 promotes progression of mammary tumors to malignancy. J Exp Med 2001; 193:727–740.

21. Cecchini MG, Dominguez MG, Mocci S, et al. Role of colony stimulating factor-1 in the establishment and regulation of tissue macrophages during postnatal development of the mouse. Development 1994; 120:1357–1372.

22. Wyckoff J, Wang W, Lin EY, et al. A paracrine loop between tumor cells and macrophages is required for tumor cell migration in mammary tumors. Cancer Res 2004; 64:7022–7029.

23. Ghosh S, Karin M. Missing pieces in the NF-kappaB puzzle. Cell 2002; 109 Suppl:S81–96.

24. Greten FR, Eckmann L, Greten TF, et al. IKKbeta links inflammation and tumorigenesis in a mouse model of colitis-associated cancer. Cell 2004; 118:285–296.

25. Chung DC. The genetic basis of colorectal cancer: insights into critical pathways of tumorigenesis. Gastroenterology 2000; 119:854–865.

26. Eaden J. Review article: The data supporting a role for aminosalicylates in the chemoprevention of colorectal cancer in patients with inflammatory bowel disease. Aliment Pharmacol Ther 2003; 18 Suppl 2:15–21.

27. Rogler G, Brand K, Vogl D, et al. Nuclear factor kappaB is activated in macrophages and epithelial cells of inflamed intestinal mucosa. Gastroenterology 1998; 115:357–369.

28. Aharinejad S, Paulus P, Sioud M, et al. Colony-stimulating factor-1 blockade by antisense oligonucleotides and small interfering RNAs suppresses growth of human mammary tumor xenografts in mice. Cancer Res 2004; 64:5378–5384.

29. Olumi AF, Grossfeld GD, Hayward SW, Carroll PR, Tlsty TD, Cunha GR. Carcinoma-associated fibroblasts direct tumor progression of initiated human prostatic epithelium. Cancer Res 1999; 59:5002–5011.

30. Wakefield LM, Roberts AB. TGF-beta signaling: positive and negative effects on tumorigenesis. Curr Opin Genet Dev 2002; 12:22–29.

31. Bhowmick NA, Chytil A, Plieth D, et al. TGF-beta signaling in fibroblasts modulates the oncogenic potential of adjacent epithelia. Science 2004; 303:848–851.

32. Okada H, Danoff TM, Fischer A, Lopez-Guisa JM, Strutz F, Neilson EG. Identification of a novel cis-acting element for fibroblast-specific transcription of the FSP1 gene. Am J Physiol 1998; 275:F306–314.

33. Kuperwasser C, Chavarria T, Wu M, et al. Reconstruction of functionally normal and malignant human breast tissues in mice. Proc Natl Acad Sci U S A 2004; 101:4966–4971.

34. Tuxhorn JA, McAlhany SJ, Yang F, Dang TD, Rowley DR. Inhibition of transforming growth factor-beta activity decreases angiogenesis in a human prostate cancer-reactive stroma xenograft model. Cancer Res 2002; 62:6021–6025.

35. Tuxhorn JA, McAlhany SJ, Dang TD, Ayala GE, Rowley DR. Stromal cells promote angiogenesis and growth of human prostate tumors in a differential reactive stroma (DRS) xenograft model. Cancer Res 2002; 62:3298–3307.

36. Motoike T, Loughna S, Perens E, et al. Universal GFP reporter for the study of vascular development. Genesis 2000; 28:75–81.

37. Sasmono RT, Oceandy D, Pollard JW, et al. A macrophage colony-stimulating factor receptor-green fluorescent protein transgene is expressed throughout the mononuclear phagocyte system of the mouse. Blood 2003; 101:1155–1163.

38. Branda CS, Dymecki SM. Talking about a revolution: The impact of site-specific recombinases on genetic analyses in mice. Dev Cell 2004; 6:7–28.

39. Gudjonsson T, Ronnov-Jessen L, Villadsen R, Bissell MJ, Petersen OW. To create the correct microenvironment: three-dimensional heterotypic collagen assays for human breast epithelial morphogenesis and neoplasia. Methods 2003; 30:247–255.

40. Kurose K, Gilley K, Matsumoto S, Watson PH, Zhou XP, Eng C. Frequent somatic mutations in PTEN and TP53 are mutually exclusive in the stroma of breast carcinomas. Nat Genet 2002; 32:355–357.

41. Fukino K, Shen L, Matsumoto S, Morrison CD, Mutter GL, Eng C. Combined total genome loss of heterozygosity scan of breast cancer stroma and epithelium reveals multiplicity of stromal targets. Cancer Res 2004; 64:7231–7236.

42. Moinfar F, Man YG, Arnould L, Bratthauer GL, Ratschek M, Tavassoli FA. Concurrent and independent genetic alterations in the stromal and epithelial cells of mammary carcinoma: implications for tumorigenesis. Cancer Res 2000; 60:2562–2566.

43. Wernert N, Locherbach C, Wellmann A, Behrens P, Hugel A. Presence of genetic alterations in microdissected stroma of human colon and breast cancers. Anticancer Res 2001; 21:2259–2264.
44. Paterson RF, Ulbright TM, MacLennan GT, et al. Molecular genetic alterations in the laser-capture-microdissected stroma adjacent to bladder carcinoma. Cancer 2003; 98:1830–1836.
45. Matsumoto N, Yoshida T, Yamashita K, Numata Y, Okayasu I. Possible alternative carcinogenesis pathway featuring microsatellite instability in colorectal cancer stroma. Br J Cancer 2003; 89:707–712.

14 Cytokines and Tumor Angiogenesis

Sharmila Roy-Chowdhury and Charles K. Brown

CONTENTS

1. INTRODUCTION

1.1. Historical Perspectives

The term *angiogenesis* was first coined by John Hunter, a British surgeon, to describe blood vessel formation in reindeer antlers in 1787. The first histologic description of angiogenesis was presented by Arthur Tremain Hertig in 1935, detailing the formation of placental blood vessels. In 1939, based on observations of tumors transplanted to transparent chambers in in vivo animal models, A. G. Ide and colleagues proposed the existence of a tumor-derived factor capable of stimulating blood vessel formation *(1)*. In 1945, G. H. Algire and his co-workers at the National Cancer Institute (NCI) recognized that the blood supply of tumors was derived from the host and was essential for tumor growth *(2)*. The findings of Algire et al. offered the first evidence supporting the association between tumor vasculature and tumor growth. In 1948, I. C. Michaelson postulated that a diffusible angiogenic factor produced by the retina conferred the neovascularization phenotype observed during proliferative diabetic retinopathy and named this soluble factor as "Factor X" *(3)*. Twenty years later, Greenblatt and Shubik *(4)* and Ehrmann and Knoth *(5)* demonstrated independently that tumor cells could stimulate vasoproliferation through transfilter diffusion experiments and confirmed the notion of a diffusible angiogenic factor elaborated by tumor cells. In 1971, Judah Folkman further refined the view on the relationship between tumor and its vasculature by hypothesizing that the growth of cancer from a few cell layers thick into a gross tumor requires angiogenic stimuli which are mediated by substances produced by the tumor. He proposed that anti-angiogenic therapy, therefore, might be an effective approach to treating human cancers *(6–8)*. This view on

From: *Cancer Drug Discovery and Development,*
Cytokines in the Genesis and Treatment of Cancer
Edited by: M. A. Caligiuri and M. T. Lotze © Humana Press Inc., Totowa, NJ

tumor angiogenesis was provocative and contrary to the prevailing thoughts of the time. Despite not being accepted by the scientific community, Dr. Folkman endeavored along this line of research and initiated the effort that lead to the isolation of the first angiogenic cytokine, basic fibroblast growth factor (bFGF) *(9)*. Findings from his work have come to form the foundation in the molecular understanding of tumor angiogenesis and Dr. Folkman is often regarded as the "father of angiogenesis".

The first angiogenesis inhibitor was discovered in the cartilage by Henry Brem and Judah Folkman in 1975 *(10)*. As presented above, the first angiogenic cytokine discovered was bFGF and was purified by Yuen Shing and Michael Klagsbrun at Harvard Medical School in 1984 *(9)*. Vascular endothelial growth factor (VEGF), one of the most important angiogenic cytokines, was discovered independently by Napoleone Ferrara and Jean Plouet in 1989 *(11,12)*. This newly discovered VEGF cytokine turned out to be identical to a previously characterized molecule called vascular permeability factor (VPF), which was discovered by Donald Senger and Harold Dvorak in 1983 *(13)*. Because of these initial discoveries, over 30 natural angiogenesis inhibitors and over 20 angiogenic growth factors have been characterized.

1.2. Tumor Angiogenesis

Angiogenesis is a fundamental process essential for the normal physiologic functions of reproduction, embryogenesis and wound healing. It is defined as the growth of new blood vessels from pre-existing vasculature and is a highly regulated process under ordinary conditions. However, many pathologic conditions such as arthritis, diabetic retinopathy, and cancer are associated with persistent and uncontrolled angiogenesis, suggesting increased levels of angiogenic and decreased levels of angiostatic factors mediating the progression of these pathologies *(14)*.

Angiogenesis is essential for tumor growth beyond 2–3 mm^3 size, as it allows for an increased supply of nutrients and oxygen to the tumor, as well as, the outflow of waste products from the tumor. Tumors lacking adequate blood supply undergo apoptosis *(15)* or necrosis *(16)*. Conversely, tumors that have undergone neovascularization enter a phase of rapid growth and acquire the potential to metastasize as the new vasculature provides a mean for tumor cells to gain access into the blood stream and to travel to distant sites, such as liver, lungs, or bones *(17)*. As such, extensive neovascularization has been correlated to be a poor prognostic variable in several forms of human malignancies *(18–31)*.

The induction of angiogenesis is an important step in carcinogenesis *(32)*. The angiogenic cascade can be divided into a prevascular phase—the so called "angiogenic switch" *(14,33)* and a vascular phase *(34)*. The activation of this switch appears to be necessary for the rapid growth that is seen in tumors. Once activated, the normal balance between the proangiogenic and the antiangiogenic signals becomes disrupted. Cytokine stimulation of endothelial cells is integral to the activation of the "angiogenic switch." The stimulated endothelial cells then migrate to the extracellular matrix where they proliferate and form vascular buds. In the second phase of angiogenesis, the vascular or formation phase, the vascular buds from the migrating endothelial cells give rise to capillaries, thereby extending the circulatory system into the tumor microenvironment.

The structural features of the tumor vasculature are determined by the expression and interaction of angiogenic factors produced by the tumor. Stimulated by angiogenic cytokines, endothelial cells proliferate rapidly and produce large broad vessels that circulate blood at slow flow rates. The tumor vessel walls formed during tumor angiogenesis are unable to recruit pericytes and adventitial smooth muscle cells.

Table 1
Major Angiogenic and Angiostatic Factors[a,b]

	Pro-angiogenic factors	Anti-angiogenic factors
Directly-acting factors	VEGF Family	Angiostatin
	FGF Family	Matrix Protein Fragments
	aFGF	Endostatin
	bFGF	Tumsatin
	ELR(+) CXC Chemokines	Canstatin
	IL-8	Arresten
	GRO	ELR(–) CXC Chemokines
	MCP-1	PF-4
	TGF Family	IP-10
	TGF-α	MIG
	TGF-β	
	PDGF-BB	
Indirectly-acting factors	TNF-α	IFN Family
	Angiogenin	IFN-α
	Angiopoietins	IFN-β
	Angiopoietin-1	IFN-γ
	Angiopoietin-2	Thrombospondins
		TSP-1
		TSP-2

[a]The table lists some of the major angiogenic and angiostatic cytokines. These factors are grouped according to their angiogenic functions (stimulatory vs inhibitory) and their actions on endothelial cells (direct- vs indirect-acting).

[b]VEGF, vascular endothelial growth factor; FGF, fibroblast growth factor; ELR, Glu-Leu-Arg motif; IL, interleukin; GRO, growth regulated oncogene; MCP-1, monocyte chemo-attractant protein-1; TGF, transforming growth factor; PDGF, platelet derived growth factor; TNF-α, tumor necrosis factor-α; PF-4, platelet factor-4; IP-10, interferon-inducible protein-10; MIG, monokine-induced by interferon-γ; IFN, interferon; TSP, thrombospondins.

Additionally, the basement membrane is discontinuous and punctuated by large gaps among the endothelial cells *(35)*. The combined result of the slow flow and the abnormal leaky vasculature is to promote metastasis by allowing tumor cell access into the circulatory system and assisting the distant dissemination of cancer.

Tumor angiogenesis is regulated by a balance between positive and negative factors of neovascularization, as tumor cells mediate production of not only angiogenic factors but also angiostatic molecules that act specifically on endothelial cells. Stimulation of tumor angiogenesis has been demonstrated to increase tumor growth and metastasis *(36–40)*, whereas angiogenesis inhibition has been shown to prevent tumor growth and in some instances, cause tumor regression in experimental tumor models *(41–47)*. Most of the factors that mediate angiogenesis are *cytokines,* which are soluble proteins secreted by one cell and influence another cell or cells in an autocrine, paracrine or endocrine fashion. Numerous cytokines that mediate angiogenesis have been identified with the most relevant molecules belonging to the VEGF, FGF, and CXC chemokine families. Cytokines are classified as *direct-acting* or *indirect-acting* mediators of angiogenesis based on the effect exerted on endothelial cells; some of the more common cytokines relevant to the angiogenesis biology are shown in Table 1.

2. VASCULAR ENDOTHELIAL GROWTH FACTOR

VEGF is one of the most potent stimulators of angiogenesis and its identification was the result of independent and unrelated lines of research. This cytokine was first isolated from the ascites secreted by hepatocellular carcinoma in guinea pigs and was named vascular permeability factor (VPF) as it increased the permeability of peritumoral vessels *(13)*. Later, a factor isolated from the pituitary-derived folliculostellate cells was found to have mitogenic properties for endothelial cells and was named vascular endothelial growth factor (VEGF) *(11)*. The amino acid sequences of VPF and VEGF were subsequently found to be identical and VEGF was adopted as the common name for this important angiogenic cytokine.

2.1. VEGF Properties

VEGF is a heparin-binding homodimeric glycoprotein with the monomers bound by two disulfide bonds and a molecular weight of 34–46 kDa *(11)*. It is directly involved in tumor angiogenesis and activates this process through stimulation of endothelial cell proliferation, migration and differentiation. VEGF acts specifically on endothelial cells *(48)* and many of its properties appear to make it the primary molecule responsible for angiogenesis under many physiologic and pathologic conditions. VEGF has the capacity to induce nitric oxide production that lead to vasodilatation and increased blood flow, early processes that are necessary before the initiation of angiogenesis *(49,50)*. It is a mitogen and a chemotactic factor for endothelial cells *(48)*. It induces the production of proteases such as urokinase-type plasminogen activator *(51)* and interstitial collagenase by endothelial cells *(52)* and thus supports the remodeling of the perivascular matrix *(51)*. VEGF increases the permeability of normal blood vessels to plasma proteins by acting on small capillaries and venules, without causing a significant inflammatory response, endothelial cell injury, or mast cell degranulation *(53)*.

VEGF is also a survival factor for endothelial cells and can prevent apoptosis in these cells. Normally, cells under starvation conditions in vitro will undergo apoptosis. However, VEGF can reverse this phenotype by inducing the expression of anti-apoptotic proteins Bcl-2 *(54)*, XIAP *(55)*, and survivin *(56)* in endothelial cells. VEGF has been shown to maintain the viability of the endothelium by its ability to induce these same anti-apoptotic factors in proliferating endothelial cells *(57,58)*.

2.2. VEGF Family of Cytokines

Human VEGF, sometimes referred to as **VEGF-A**, is encoded by a gene located on chromosome 6p21.3 and contains eight exons and seven introns *(59–61)*. Since cloning of the VEGF gene in the early 1980s, eight isoforms of the VEGF protein have been characterized (Table 2) *(60–63)*. These VEGF isomers differ in the number of amino acids and are the results of differential splicing. The most common isomers contain 121, 165, 189, and 206 amino acids, and are named $VEGF_{121}$, $VEGF_{165}$, $VEGF_{189}$, and $VEGF_{206}$, respectively. $VEGF_{189}$ and $VEGF_{206}$ are highly basic proteins that bind heparin with high affinity and are found predominantly bound to the endothelial cell surface and extracellular matrix *(64)*. These sequestered isomers are released into solubility by heparinase, which cleaves heparin to release the cytokines, or by plasmin, which cleaves $VEGF_{189}$ and $VEGF_{206}$ to release the first 110 amino-terminus residues, $VEGF_{110}$ *(65)*. $VEGF_{121}$ is an acidic protein that lacks the basic amino acids encoded by exons 6 and 7. The lack of basic residues allows $VEGF_{121}$ to exist as a freely soluble protein rather than

Table 2
VEGF Family of Cytokines[a,b]

VEGF Isoforms	$VEGF_{110}$
	$VEGF_{121}{}^c$
	$VEGF_{145}$
	$VEGF_{162}$
	$VEGF_{165}{}^c$
	$VEGF_{165b}$
	$VEGF_{183}$
	$VEGF_{189}{}^c$
	$VEGF_{206}{}^c$
VEGF Homologues	PlGF-1
	PlGF-2
	VEGF-B
	VEGF-C
	VEGF-D
	VEGF-E

[a]The table lists the various VEGF isoforms generated from differential splicing of VEGF transcripts, as well as, cytokines belonging to the VEGF family evidenced by gene and amino acid sequence homologies.

[b]VEGF, vascular endothelial growth factor; PlGF, placental growth factor.

[c]Common VEGF isomers.

heparin-bound. $VEGF_{165}$, the predominant form secreted by the majority of normal and tumor cells, lacks residues encoded by exon 6 and have properties intermediate to the acidic ($VEGF_{121}$) and basic ($VEGF_{189}$ and $VEGF_{206}$) isomers. Therefore, a significant portion of $VEGF_{165}$ is also found bound to the endothelial cell surface and extracellular matrix (66). The loss of the heparin-binding domains has been shown to decrease the mitogenic activity of VEGF molecules and these findings suggest that the properties of $VEGF_{165}$ should confer the optimal bioavailability and biologic activity of all VEGF isomers (67). This notion is supported by the observations that VEGF[-/-] homozygous tumor cells can only be fully rescued from its tumorigenic phenotype by $VEGF_{165}$ (68) and transgenic mice expressing exclusively $VEGF_{121}$ will all die within 2 wk after birth (69).

Based on their primary structures and biologic functions, several genes homologous to VEGF have been identified and their protein products (placental growth factor-1 (PlGF-1), PlGF-2, VEGF-B, VEGF-C, VEGF-D, and VEGF-E) have been added to the VEGF family of cytokines (70–75). Although the mitogenic effects of these homologues are lower than potency of the VEGF isomers, these homologous proteins, nevertheless, play important roles in the regulation of angiogenesis and their functions will be discussed in the next section along with the VEGF receptors.

2.3. VEGF Receptors

The biologic effects of the VEGF cytokine family are mediated through four cell surface receptors: Flt-1(VEGFR-1), Flk-1/KDR (VEGFR-2), Flt-4(VEGFR-3), and neuropilin-1 (NP-1). VEGFR-1, VEGFR-2, and VEGFR-3 are classical tyrosine kinase receptors (76–78), while NP-1 belongs to the collapsing/semaphorin proteins, a family

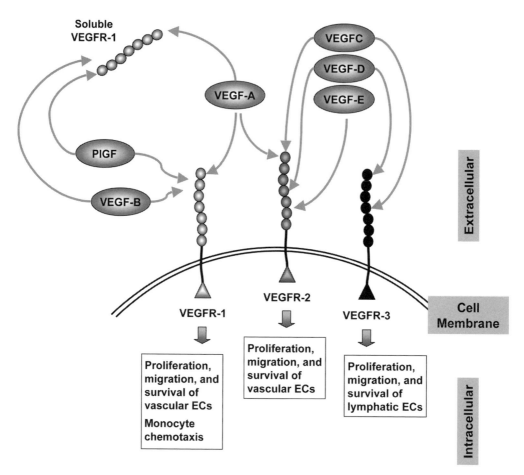

Fig. 1. Function and binding specificity of VEGF receptors to their ligands. Structural similarity and ligands for the three VEGF receptors are depicted. VEGFR1 binds ligands VEGF/VEGF-A, VEGF-B and PlGF. VEGFR2, the major proangiogenic receptor for VEGF binds VEGF/VEGF-A, VEGF-C, VEGF-D, and VEGF-E. VEGFR3, the major receptor regulating lymphatic endothelial cells, binds VEGF-C and VEGF-D. VEGF, vascular endothelial growth factor; VEGFR, VEGF receptor; PlGF, placental growth factor; ECs, endothelial cells.

of molecules that influence the growth and guidance of neuronal processes *(79)*. VEGF-1 and VEGFR-2 are receptors for VEGF, while VEGFR-3, a related receptor tyrosine kinase, does not bind VEGF and is a receptor for VEGF-C and VEGF-D *(80)*. Based on the interactions of the VEGF cytokines with the individual VEGF receptors, differential biologic responses on endothelial cells and angiogenesis are produced.

VEGFR-1 and VEGFR-2 are two highly related receptors found on the surface of activated endothelial cells *(80)*, as well as, certain bone marrow-derived mononuclear phagocytes *(81)*. These receptors have seven immunoglobulin (Ig)-like extracellular domains, a single transmembrane region, and a consensus intracellular tyrosine kinase sequence (Fig. 1) *(82–84)*. VEGFR-1 will bind VEGF, as well as, PlGF and VEGF-B *(85-86)*, and this binding site has been mapped to the second Ig-like domain on VEGFR-1 *(87–89)*. Alternative splicing generates a soluble VEGFR-1, which has been demonstrated to be an inhibitor of VEGF activity *(90)*. VEGFR-1 expression is up-regulated by low oxygen tension via the hypoxia-inducible factor-1 (HIF-1) mechanism *(91)*. VEGFR-1 plays a dual role in angiogenesis by acting as a positive and negative regulator under different conditions. Normally, VEGFR-1 catalyzes a weak tyrosine kinase autophosphorylation in response to VEGF *(92–93)*, and has been proposed to be a decoy receptor for VEGF by sequestering this cytokine from VEGFR-2, the major mediator of VEGF's mitogenic activity *(85)*. Under pathologic conditions of VEGFR-1 ligand overexpression, as in tumor angiogenesis, VEGFR-1 acts as a positive regulator and stimulates proliferation of endothelial cells *(94–95)*. A third ligand for VEGFR-1 is VEGF-B, and binding of this cytokine to VEGFR-1 promotes migration of endothelial cells *(96)*. In hematopoietic cells, the binding of VEGFR-1 stimulates monocyte chemotaxis *(97)*.

Although Flk-1/VEGFR-2 binds VEGF with lower affinity than VEGFR-1, this receptor is the major mediator of the mitogenic, chemotactic and prosurvival signals of VEGF *(98–100)*. Four ligands have been identified that bind VEGFR-2: VEGF, VEGF-C, VEGF-D, and VEGF-E (Fig. 1). Binding of VEGFR-2 with its ligands activates the Raf-Mek-Erk signaling pathway through protein kinase C and result in endothelial cell proliferation *(101,102)*.

Two additional receptors have also been described to mediate the functions of the VEGF family of cytokines. Flt-4/VEGFR-3 is found on the surface of various cells, particularly on the endothelium of lymphatic capillaries *(77)*. VEGFR-3 does not bind VEGF, but rather the ligands for VEGFR-3 are VEGF-C and VEGF-D. Activation of VEGFR-3 by its ligands stimulates lymphangiogenesis of the lymphatic capillaries *(72,103)*. The neuropilin (NP-1) receptor is present on the surface of neuronal cells *(79)*. It is an isoforms-specific receptor that binds $VEGF_{165}$ but not $VEGF_{121}$. Overexpression of NP-1 receptor results in enhanced binding of $VEGF_{165}$ to VEGFR-2, leading to increased proliferation and chemotaxis.

2.4. Regulation of VEGF Expression

VEGF expression is regulated by many factors including hypoxia, inflammatory cytokines, hormones and oncogenes. Hypoxia is one of the most potent inducer of VEGF expression by tumor cells and often occurs in tumors during their growth phase *(104–106)*. Hypoxia stimulates the expression of HIF-1, a key mediator of cellular hypoxic responses *(107)*. The upstream promoter of the VEGF gene contains a 28 base-pair enhancer element that binds HIF-1 *(108,109)*. HIF-1 induction of VEGF gene expression is modulated by the von Hippel-Lindau (VHL) tumor suppressor *(110)* and in VHL-deficient cell lines, HIF-1 is constitutively activated *(111)*. VHL mediates many cellular functions, one of which is that it is part of the ubiquitin ligase complex that targets proteins for proteosomal degradation. Under normal oxygen tensions, HIF-1 is hydroxylated by oxygen and this hydroxylated form is recognized by the VHL tumor suppressor and targeted for degradation *(112,113)*. Under hypoxic conditions, HIF-1 is not inactivated and stimulates VEGF gene transcription.

VEGF gene expression is stimulated by cytokines and growth factors which include interleukin-1(IL-1) *(114)*, interleukin-6 (IL-6) *(115)*, tumor necrosis factor-α (TNF-α), transforming growth factor-α (TGF-α) and TGF-β *(116)*, epidermal growth factor (EGF) *(117)*, and platelet-derived growth factor (PDGF) *(117,118)*. Hormones are also important mediators of VEGF gene expression, especially in tumor cells. Thyroid stimulating hormone (TSH) has been shown to induce VEGF expression in several thyroid carcinoma

Table 3
FGF Super Family[a]

FGF subfamily	FGF molecule
I	FGF-1
	FGF-2
II	FGF-3
	FGF-5
III	FGF-11
	FGF-12
	FGF-13
	FGF-14
IV	FGF-4
	FGF-6
V	FGF-9
	FGF-16
	FGF-20
VI	FGF-7
	FGF-10
VII	FGF-8
	FGF-17
	FGF-18

FGF, fibroblast growth factor.

[a]There are 22 FGF molecules with sequence homology ranging from 17% to 72% that belong to the FGF super gene family. Based on these sequence homologies, the FGF factors can be grouped to one of seven subfamilies.

cell lines. Additionally, sex steroid such as androgens and estrogens have been implicated as stimuli in VEGF production by prostate *(119)* and endometrial carcinomas *(120)*, respectively. Lastly, modulation of VEGF gene transcriptional has been linked with specific transforming events mediated by oncogenes. Mutations or amplifications of raf *(121)*, ras *(121)*, fos *(122)*, and src *(123)* oncogenes haven been demonstrated to result in VEGF gene upregulation.

3. FIBROBLAST GROWTH FACTORS

FGF was among the first cytokines that was demonstrated to have a role in stimulation of angiogenesis. It was first isolated as two polypeptides from extracts of the bovine brain and pituitary body: acidic FGF (16 kDa) or FGF-1and basic FGF (18 kDa) or FGF-2. These two polypeptides have 55% similarity in their amino acid sequence, but differ in their acidic and basic properties, in which FGF-1 has a pH of 5 and FGF-2 has a pH of 9.6 *(124)*. To date, 22 human FGF proteins ranging in molecular weight of 7 kDa to 38 kDa have been characterized and constitute the FGF superfamily *(125,126)*. Members of this superfamily are generated from gene duplication and differential splicing, and based on amino acid sequence homology (17–72%) are further grouped into seven subfamilies (Table 3) *(127)*. Despite their respective heterogeneity, all FGF molecules contain a conserved 120 amino acid core region that contains six identical, interspersed amino acids *(127–130)*. FGFs are extracellular cytokines that act through four tyrosine kinase FGF receptors. These receptors exhibit varying specificities for all FGFs, which accounts for similar effects generated by different FGF molecules on common cell types *(131,132).*

3.1. FGF Function and Mechanism of Action

The functions of FGFs are not limited to the stimulation of cell growth. These cytokines have been demonstrated to be involved in the regulation of the proliferation, differentiation and migration of various cells of mesodermal and neuroetodermal origins, including endothelial cells, fibroblasts and other cell types *(133).*

The role of FGF-2 in angiogenesis was first shown in cultures of endothelial and smooth muscle cells. Its role in tumor angiogenesis was identified when it was isolated as the main angiogenic factor from chondrosarcoma *(134).* FGF-2 is a major mitogenic factor for endothelial cells. Additionally, FGF-2 increases endothelial cell migration by reversibly decreasing cell adhesion and increasing cell membrane mobility through reorganization of intracellular contractile apparatus *(135–137).* Lastly, FGF-2 has also been demonstrated to stimulate extracellular matrix proteolysis and, therefore, plays an important role in extracellular matrix remodeling *(138).*

At least seven species of FGF-2 have been identified, and differences in function are in part owing to differential intracellular compartmentalization of these isomers. Endothelial cell proliferation is stimulated by high molecular weight (HMW) isoforms of FGF (22, 22.5, 24 and 34 kDa), which are found in the nucleus and increase cell proliferation through stimulation of ribosomal gene transcription *(139).* The HMW isomers are generated by four upstream alternate CUG (leucine) start codons that provide amino terminal extension to the 18 kDa FGF-2 core molecule *(140,141).* Imbedded within the extended amino termini are localization sequences that direct the nuclear trafficking of the HMW species *(142).*

3.2. FGF Receptors

The normal biologic effects of FGF molecules are mediated through four structurally similar FGF receptors 1–4 (FGFR 1–4), which are widely distributed on the surface of various cell types. Although the roles of these receptors in tumor angiogenesis is not yet clear, an association between angiogenesis and increased expression of FGFR1 has been found.

The binding of FGF with its receptor(s) is aided by the presence of heparin. Heparan sulfate binds several FGF molecules and stabilizes FGFs from denaturation and proteolysis. Additionally, FGF diffusion and release into the interstitial space is limited by the heparin interaction *(143).* The resulting cytokine-heparin mixture is presented to the FGFRs *(144).* FGF cytokine binding to their receptors causes receptor dimerization and activation of the tyrosine kinase. These kinases phosphorylate each other and initiate downstream signaling.

There are three components to this downstream signaling (Fig. 2). The first and main component is activation of the *ras* G-protein and mitogen-activated protein kinase (MAPK) cascade to stimulate gene expression *(145).* A second signal involves the phosphorylation of STAT-1 (signal transducer and activator of transcription-1) and its subsequent translocation into the nucleus for transcriptional activation *(146).* Lastly, the activated FGFR stimulates phospholipase C to split PIP_2 (phosphatidylinositol-4,5-bisphosphate) into IP_3 (inositol 1,4,5-trisphosphate) and diacylglycerol. IP_3 causes release of Ca^{++} from intracellular stores and effecting signal transduction *(145).*

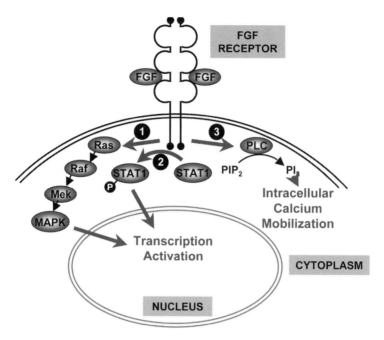

Fig. 2. Mechanisms of FGF receptor signal transduction. Signal transduction from the FGF receptor can be mediates through one of three pathways 1) activation of the ras G-protein and MAP kinase cascade to stimulate gene expression; 2) transcription factor STAT1 phosphorylation and translocation into the nucleus; or 3) activation of phospholipase C, which metabolizes PIP_2 to generate IP_3 and mobilization of intracellular calcium ions. FGF, fibroblast growth factor; MAPK, mitogen-activated protein kinase; STAT, signal transducer and activator of transcription; PLC, phospholipase C; PIP_2, phosphatidylinositol-4,5-bisphosphate; IP_3, inositol 1,4,5-trisphosphate.

4. CXC CHEMOKINES

Chemokines belong to a unique family of small protein molecules that are classified according to the spacing of conserved cysteine (C) residues into CC, CXC, CX_3C, and C chemokines *(147)*. CXC chemokines are heparin binding proteins that are less than 10 kDa in their monomeric forms and can regulate angiogenesis in a disparate manner based on their structures. These cytokines have four highly conserved cysteine amino acid residues, with the first two residues separated by one nonconserved amino acid residue *(148,149)*. Since the mid-1980's, at least 12 different CXC chemokines have been identified and genes for nine of the CXC chemokine family are clustered on human chromosome 4.

Although the CXC motif distinguishes these chemokines from other families, their angiogenic potential is determined by a second structural domain. The amino-terminus of the majority of the CXC chemokines contains three amino acid residues (glutamate-leucine-arginine: the ELR motif), which precede the first cysteine amino acid residue of the primary structure of these chemokines. Those family members, which contain the ELR motif, have enhanced neutrophil binding capabilities and are angiogenic *(150)*. In contrast, those members which do not contain the ELR motif are angiostatic (Table 4).

4.1. ELR(+) CXC Chemokines

The role of the ELR motif in mediating angiogenesis was studied by Strieter et al. in 1998 *(150)*. Endothelial cell migration was increased in the presence ELR(+)CXC

Table 4
CXC[a] Chemokines With Angiogenesis Activity

ELR(+) CXC chemokines[b]	ELR(−) CXC chemokines
Interleukin-8 (IL-8)	Platelet Factor-4 (PF-4)
Growth-Related Oncogene-α (GRO-α)	Growth-Related Oncogene-β (GRO-β)[c]
Growth-Related Oncogene-γ (GRO-γ)	Interferon-γ-Inducible Protein-10 (IP-10)
Epithelial Neutrophil Activating	Monokine Induced by Interferon-γ (MIG)
Protein-78 (ENA-78)	
Granulocyte Chemotactic Protein-2 (GCP-2)	
Platelet Basic Protein (PBP)	
Connective Tissue Activating Protein-III	
(CTAP-III)	
β-Thromboglobulin (β-TG)	
Neutrophil Activating Protein-2 (NAP-2)	

[a]CXC chemokines constitute one of the largest groups of chemokines with demonstrated angiogenic activity. In general, CXC chemokines that contain a glutamate-leucine-arginine motif (ELR) within its amino acid sequence stimulate angiogenesis, while those chemokines lacking the ELR motif are angiostatic. There are exceptions to this rule.
[b]ELR, glutamate-leucine-arginine.
[c]Angiogenic CXC chemokine that does not contain the ELR motif.

chemokines (interleukin-8 [IL-8] and epithelial neutrophil activating protein-78 [ENA-78]) in a dose dependent manner. Other ELR(+)CXC chemokines, granulocyte chemotactic protein-2 (GCP-2), growth related oncogene (GRO)-α, β, and γ, platelet basic protein (PBP), connective tissue activating protein-III (CTAP-III), and neutrophil activating protein-2 (NAP-2), when tested showed a similar ability to induce endothelial cell migration. In contrast, ELR(−) chemokines (platelet factor 4 [PF4] and interferon-γ-inducible protein-10 [IP-10]) did not induce endothelial cell chemotaxis. Moore et al. further proved that ELR(−) chemokines were inhibitors of angiogenesis by performing endothelial cell chemotaxis in response to ELR(+)CXC chemokines (IL-8 or ENA-78) or bFGF with varying concentrations of ELR(−) chemokines (PF4, IP-10 or monokine induced by interferon-γ (MIG)) *(151)*. The endothelial cell migration in response to the ELR(+) CXC chemokines was significantly inhibited by the ELR(−) CXC chemokines (PF4, IP-10 or MIG). Interestingly, neither IP-10 nor MIG inhibited IL-8 induced neutrophil chemotaxis *(150)*. These studies were also done in vivo using the cornea micro-pocket assay of neovascularization and similar results were demonstrated with the ELR(+) and ELR(−) factors.

4.1.1. INTERLEUKIN 8

IL-8 was shown to be an angiogenic factor in 1992 *(152–154)*. Kitadai et al. found high levels of IL-8 in six of eight gastric carcinoma cell lines and 32 of 39 gastric carcinoma specimens as compared to normal mucosal controls. The levels of IL-8 correlated strongly with the specimen vascularity *(155)*. IL-8 was shown to be the major inducer of neovascularization of squamous cell carcinomas by Lingen et al. *(156)*.

Moore et al. demonstrated that IL-8 is a positive regulator of tumor formation in severe combined immunodeficiency (SCID) mice injected with the prostate cancer cell line PC-3 *(157)*. Patients with prostate cancer have been found to have high serum levels of IL-8 and these levels correlated with the stage of the disease. Additionally, in prostate cancer, serum IL-8 levels have been determined to be an independent prognostic variable from the serum levels of free and total prostate-specific antigen (PSA) *(158)*. The combined use of free and total PSA ratio and IL-8 levels has been found to be more accurate in distinguishing between prostate cancer and benign prostatic hypertrophy.

IL-8 has been found also to play a significant role in other cancers by mediating angiogenesis and tumorigenesis. IL-8 was found to be expressed at high levels in ovarian cancer cells and expression was correlated with tumorigenicity *(159)*. In nonsmall-cell lung cancer, serum IL-8 is significantly elevated in tumor-bearing mice and this level correlated with the vessel density of these tumors *(160)*. When tumor-bearing animals were treated with neutralizing antibodies to IL-8, a 40% reduction in tumor growth and spontaneous metastases to the lungs was observed *(161)*. This reduction in tumor growth and metastases correlated directly with reduced angiogenesis of the lesions.

4.1.2. GROWTH-RELATED ONCOGENE CHEMOKINES

There are three members of the GRO chemokines that mediate processes of angiogenesis: GRO-α, β, and γ. GRO-α, or melanoma growth stimulatory activity (MGSA), was first discovered as a product of oncogene-transfected cell lines and as a growth factor for melanoma cell lines. Luan et al. showed that GRO-α is expressed in 70% of human melanoma lesions examined. GRO-β is an exception to the "ELR rule" in that it is an angiogenic CXC chemokine but lacks the ELR motif. GRO-α, β, and γ genes have been transfected into mouse Melan-A melanocytes and resulted in 100% tumor formation when these clones were injected into Nude or SCID mice *(162,163)*. The tumors were very vascular, similar to the B16 melanoma tumor controls. When these tumors are depleted of GRO chemokines, a significant decrease in tumor angiogenesis was observed *(162,163)*.

4.2. ELR(–)CXC Chemokines

4.2.1. PLATELET FACTOR 4

PF-4 targets to the tumor endothelium of active angiogenesis following systemic injection of fluoroscein isothiocyanate-labeled PF-4 *(164,165)*. It was originally described for its ability to bind heparin and inactivate heparin's anticoagulation function. Its high affinity for heparin and other glycosaminoglycans appears to be important in its inhibitory activity of heparin-binding cytokines, such as bFGF and VEGF. PF-4 has been demonstrated to inhibit endothelial cell migration, proliferation and angiogenesis in response to bFGF and $VEGF_{165}$ by forming heterodimers with these cytokines and preventing them from binding to their cognate receptors *(166–168)*. $VEGF_{121}$ is not a heparin binding protein *(64,166,169)* and PF-4 does not inhibit its ability to bind to VEGF receptors on endothelial cells. It does, however, inhibit $VEGF_{121}$-induced endothelial cell proliferation through other unrecognized mechanisms.

A definitive PF-4 receptor has yet to be identified. However, the existence of such a receptor is supported by evidence of binding of this ligand to endothelial cells and direct inhibition of endothelial cell cycle by preventing S-phase entry *(170)*.

4.2.2. ELR(–)CXC CHEMOKINES REGULATED BY INTERFERONS

MIG (monokine induced by interferon-γ), IP-10 (interferon-γ-inducible protein-10) and ITAC (interferon inducible T-cell-α chemo-attractant) are three CXC chemokines of which their expressions are influenced by interferons (IFNs). MIG and ITAC are primarily induced by IFN-γ, whereas IP-10 expression is stimulated by all three IFNs (α, β, and γ) *(149,171–177)*.

IP-10 was shown to be an endogenous inhibitor of tumor formation in mouse tumor models. Squamous cell lung carcinomas, which grow poorly when xeno-transplanted into SCID mice, were found to have high levels of IP-10 *(178)*. Tumor formation was increased if a neutralizing antibody to IP-10 was given during the growth of the tumor *(178)*. Additionally, IP-10 and MIG were found to be higher in Burkitt lymphomas that demonstrated spontaneous regression and this correlated directly with impaired angiogenesis *(179)*. ITAC, similar to IP-10 and MIG, inhibits neovascularization in the rat corneal micro-pocket assay of angiogenesis in response to either ELR(+)CXC chemokines or VEGF. Overall, these findings suggest that all interferon-inducible ELR(–)CXC chemokines are potent inhibitors of angiogenesis.

4.2.3. CXC Chemokine Receptors

Although high affinity binding sites for most CXC chemokines have been demonstrated in primary endothelial cells and vasculatures of normal and neoplastic tissues, the identification of receptors for these ligands has been unsuccessful for many years, mainly owing to lack of reagents that led to conflicting results from several laboratories *(180,181)*. The recent introduction of specific monoclonal antibodies and sensible RNA probe-based assays, have allowed for the detection of previously unidentified receptors. Despite these recent advances, the specific receptors that convey the angiogenic signals mediated by individual CXC chemokines remain to be determined. In general, candidate CXC chemokine receptors (CXCRs) responsible for angiogenic stimulation include CXCR1, CXCR2 and CXCR4, while inhibitory signaling is likely mediated by CXCR3 and CXCR5 (Table 5).

Currently, five CXCRs have been identified. IL-8 and GCP-2 bind specifically to CXCR1, whereas all the other ELR(+)CXC chemokines bind to CXCR2 *(182–183)*. IP-10 and MIG (ELR(–)) bind to CXCR3 and SDF-1 binds to CXCR4 *(184–185)*. B-cell-attracting chemokine-1 (BCA-1), a newly described CXC chemokine expressed on lymphoid tissues that is chemotactic for B-lymphocytes, has been demonstrated to bind CXCR5 *(186)*. A definite receptor has yet to be identified for PF-4.

5. INDIRECT MODULATORS OF ANGIOGENESIS

Several factors regulate tumor angiogenesis *indirectly* by either stimulating or inhibiting the pro-angiogenic or angiostatic factors. Common *indirect promoters of angiogenesis* include tumor necrosis factor-α (TNF-α) and transforming growth factor β. TNF-α promotes angiogenesis by different mechanisms. First, it stimulates urokinase secretion by endothelial cells and promotes endothelial cell migration. Second, TNF-α stimulates the expression of intercellular adhesion molecules (ICAM-1) on the surface of endothelial cells and promotes the formation of blood vessels. Third, TNF-α induces the secretion of angiogenic growth factor bFGF and thus promotes angiogenesis indirectly *(187–188)*.

TGF-β is a cytokine that inhibits normal angiogenesis through inhibition of endothelial cell proliferation and migration *(189)*. However, despite this apparent negative role in normal angiogenesis, TGF-β is a powerful stimulator of tumor angiogenesis. It is secreted by tumor cells and attracts monocytes, macrophages, and lymphocytes to the neoplastic tissue. When present, these inflammatory cells secrete angiogenic cytokines and may serve as a mechanism for stimulating tumor angiogenesis *(190)*.

Notable *indirect inhibitors of angiogenesis* are interferons (IFN α, β, and γ) and interleukins (IL-1, 4, 10, 12, and 18). Inhibition of angiogenesis by the interferons is

Table 5
Function of CXC Chemokines and Their Receptors[a,b,c]

Chemokine	Receptor	Angiogenic function
GCP-2	CXCR1	+
IL-8	CXCR1, CXCR2	+
GRO-α	CXCR2	+
GRO-β	CXCR2	+
GRO-γ	CXCR2	+
ENA-78	CXCR2	+
MIG	CXCR3	−
IP-10	CXCR3	−
ITAC	CXCR3	−
SDF-1	CXCR4	+
BCA-1	CXCR5	−
PF-4	Unknown	−

[a]CXC chemokines mediate contrasting processes of angiogenesis based on binding to specific receptors. Currently, five CXC chemokine receptors have been described. In general, CXCR1, 2, and 4 transduce signals that lead to stimulation of angiogenesis, while CXCR3 and 5 likely mediate inhibitory signals.

[b]Angiogenic function stimulatory (+), inhibitory (−).

[c]GCP-2, granulocyte chemotactic protein-2; GRO, growth-related oncogene; IL-8, interleukin-8. ENA-78, epithelial neutrophil activating protein-78, MIG, monokine induced by interferon-γ; IP-10, interferon-γ-inducible protein-10; ITAC, interferon inducible T-cell alpha chemo-attractant; SDF-1, stromal-derived factor-1; BCA-1, B-cell-attracting chemokine-1; PF-4, platelet factor-4; CXCR, CXC chemokine receptor.

accomplished through multiple mechanisms. First, interferons induce the production of angiostatic factors: IFN-γ induces the production of MIG, while IP-10 is induced by IFN-β, and γ. Second, interferons inhibit angiogenesis by augmenting the production of proangiogenic factors: IFN-α and β inhibit FGF-2 expression, while IFN-γ attenuates the expression of angiogenic factors IL-8, GRO-α, and ENA-78 *(191,192)*. Similarly, interleukins inhibits the function of proangiogenic factors in order to mediate their angiostatic effects. VEGF- and FGF-stimulated angiogenesis is inhibited by IL-4, while VEGF expression is inhibited by IL-10 *(193–195)*.

6. CONCLUSION

Angiogenesis is an indispensable process that plays an extremely important role in the normal progression of embryogenesis, wound healing, and the female reproductive cycle. It is equally important in pathologic states of inflammation and cancer, and the central role of angiogenesis driving metastatic tumor progression has been recognized through studies of the past few decades. Since Judah Folkman's first articulation of the therapeutic implication of tumor angiogenesis, we have seen a striking increase in our knowledge of molecular mediators involved in the angiogenic process. An understanding of these elements has revealed a complex system encompassing a multitude of cytokines with overlapping functions and is the basis of ongoing development of various anticancer agents. The evolution of angiogenesis into a modality of therapy was achieved when the US Food and Drug Administration approved Avastin, a VEGF inhibitory antibody, for the first-line treatment of metastatic colorectal cancer. Prospects of other angiogenic and angiostatic agents currently in clinical trials yield optimisms of potential applications in numerous diseases including tissue repair and regeneration, as well as, anti-cancer therapeutics. However, current understanding of angiogenesis remains incomplete and realization of this goal will demand center stage of research efforts in the coming decades.

REFERENCES

1. Ide AG, Baker NH, Warren SL. Vascularization of the Brown Pearce rabbit epithelioma transplant as seen in transparent ear chamber. Am J Roentgenol 1939;42:891–899.
2. Algire GH, Chalkley HW, Legallais FY, Park HD. Vascular reactions of normal and malignant tissues in vivo. I. Vascular reactions of mice to wounds and to normal and neoplatic transplants. J Natl Cancer Inst 1945;6:73–85.
3. Michaelson IC. The mode of development of the vascular system of the retina with some observations on its significance for certain retinal disorders. Trans Ophthalmol Soc UK 1948;68: 137–180.
4. Greenblatt M, Shubik P. Tumor angiogenesis: Transfilter diffusion studies in the hamster by the transparent chamber technique. J Natl Cancer Inst 1968;41:111–124.
5. Ehrmann RL, Knoth M. Choriocarcinoma. Transfilter stimulation of vasoproliferation in the hamster cheek pouch. Studied by light and electron miscroscopy. J Natl Cancer Inst 1968;41:1329–1341.
6. Folkman J. Tumor angiogenesis: Therapeutic implications. N Engl J Med 1971;2851182–1186.
7. Folkman, J. What is the evidence that tumors are angiogenesis dependent? J Natl Cancer Inst 1990; 824–6.
8. Folkman, J. Anti-angiogenesis new concept for therapy of solid tumors. Ann Surg 1972;175409–416.
9. Shing Y, Folkman J, Sullivan R, Butterfield C, Murray J, Klagsbrun M. Heparin affinity purification of a tumor-derived endothelial cell growth factor. Science 1984;2231296–1299.
10. Brem H, Folkman J. Inhibition of tumor angiogenesis mediated by cartilage. J Exp Med 1975;141427–439.
11. Ferrara N, Henzel WJ. Pituitary follicular cells secrete a novel heparin-binding growth factor specific for vascular endothelial cells. Biochem Biophys Res Commun 1989;161851–858.
12. Plouet J, Moukadiri H. Specific binding of vasculotropin to bovine brain capillary endothelial cells. Biochimie 1990;7251–55.
13. Senger DR, Galli SJ, Dvorak AM, et al. Tumor cells secrete a vascular permeability factor that promotes accumulation of ascites fluid. Science 1983;219983–985.
14. Hanahan D, Folkman J. Patterns and emerging mechanisms of the angiogenic switch during tumorigenesis. Cell 1996;86353–364.
15. Holmgren L, O'Reilly MS, and Folkman J. Dormancy of micrometastases balanced proliferation and apoptosis in the presence of angiogenesis suppression. Nat Med 1995;1149–153.
16. Brem S, Brem H, Folkman J, et al. Prolonged tumor dormancy by prevention of neovascularization in the vitreous. Cancer Res 1976;362807–2812.
17. Folkman J, Shing Y. Angiogenesis. J Biol Chem 1992;26710931–10934.
18. Weidner N, Semple JP, Welch WR, Folkman J. Tumor angiogenesis and metastasis—correlation in invasive breast carcinoma. N Engl J Med 1991;3241–8.
19. Barnhill RL, Levy MA. Regressing thin cutaneous malignant melanomas (< or = 1.0 mm) are associated with angiogenesis. Am J Pathol 1993;14399–104.
20. Li VW, Folkerth RD, Wantanabe H, et al. Microvessel count and cerebrospinal fluid basic fibroblast growth factor in children with brain tumor. Lancet 1994;34482–86.
21. Hall MC, Tronocoso P, Pollack A, et al. Significance of tumor angiogenesis in clinically localized prostate carcinoma treated with external beam radiotherapy. Urology 1994;44869–875.
22. Zatterstrom UK, Brun E, Willen R, et al. Tumor angiogenesis and prognosis in squamous cell carcinoma of the head and neck. Head Neck 1995;17312–318.
23. Frank RE, Saclarides TJ, Leurgans S, et al. Tumor angiogenesis as a predictor of recurrence and survival in patient with node-negative colon cancer. Ann Surg 1995;222695–699.
24. Kirschner CV, Alanis-Amezcua JM, Martin VG, et al. Angiogenesis factor in endometrial carcinoma a new prognostic indicator? Am J Obstet Gynecol 1996;1741879–1882.
25. Angeletti CA, Lucchi M, Fontanini G, et al. Prognostic significance of tumoral angiogenesis in completely resected late stage lung carcinoma (stage IIA-N2). Impact of adjuvant therapies in a subset of patients at high risk of recurrence. Cancer 1996;78409–415.

26. Inoue K, Ozeki Y, Suganuma T, et al. Vascular endothelial growth factor expression in primary esophageal squamous cell carcinoma. Association with angiogenesis and tumor progression. Cancer 1997;79206–213.

27. Tanigawa N, Matsumura M, Amaya H, et al. Tumor vascularity correlates with the prognosis of patients with esophageal squamous cell carcinoma. Cancer 1997;79220-225.

28. Abulafia O, Triest WE, Sherer DM. Angiogenesis in primary and metastatic epithelial ovarian carcinoma. Am J Obstet Gynecol 1997;17754–1-547.

29. Nativ O, Sabo E, Reiss A, et al. Clinical significance of tumor angiogenesis in patients with localized renal cell carcinoma. Urology 1998;51693–696.

30. Danko M, Ilic I, Cepulic M, et al. Tumor angiogenesis and outcome in osteosarcoma. Pediatr Hematol Oncol 2004;21611–619.

31. Sun XY, Wu ZD, Liao XF, Yuan JY. Tumor angiogenesis and its clinical significance in pediatric malignant liver tumor. World J Gastroenterol 2005;11741–743.

32. Folkman J, Watson K, Ingber D, et al. Induction of angiogenesis during the transition from hyperplasia to neoplasia. Nature 1989;33958–61.

33. Pepper MS, Montesano R, Mandriota SJ, et al. Angiogenesis a paradigm for balanced extracellular proteolysis during cell migration and morphogenesis. Enzyme Protein 1996;49138–162.

34. Kurz H. Physiology of angiogenesis. J Neurooncol 2000;5017–35.

35. Less JR, Skalak TC, Sevick EM, et al. Microvascular architecture in a mammary carcinoma branching patterns and vessel dimensions. Cancer Res 1991;51265–273.

36. Czubayko F, Smith RV, Chung HC, Wellstein A. Tumor growth and angiogenesis induced by a secreted binding protein for fibroblast growth factors. J Biol Chem 1994;26928243–28248.

37. Kondo Y, Arii S, Mori A, et al. Enhancement of angiogenesis, tumor growth, and metastasis by transfection of vascular endothelial growth factor into LoVo human colon cancer cell line. Clin Cancer Res 2000;6622–630.

38. Hu YL, Tee MK, Goetzl EJ, et al. Lysophosphatidic acid induction of vascular endothelial growth factos expression in human ovarian cancer cells. J Natl Cancer Inst 2001;93762–768.

39. Guo P, Fang Q, Tao HQ, et al. Overexpression of vascular endothelial growth factor by MCF-7 breast cancer cells promotes estrogen-independent tumor growth in vivo. Cancer Res 2003;634684–4691.

40. Furuhashi M, Sjoblom T, Abramsson A, et al. Platelet-derived growth factor production by B16 melanoma cells leads to increased pericyte abundance in tumors and an associated increase in tumor growth rate. Cancer Res 2004;642725–2733.

41. Zugmaier G, Lippman ME, Wellstein A. Inhibition by pentosan polysulfate (PPS) of heparin-binding growth factors released from tumor cells and blockage by PPS of tumor growth in animals. J Natl Cancer Inst 1992;841716–1724.

42. Strawn LM, McMahon G, App H, et al. Flk-1 as a target for tumor growth inhibition. Cancer Res 1996;563540–3545.

43. Dhanabal M, Ramchandran R, Volk R, et al. Endostatin yeast production, mutants, and antitumor effects in renal cell carcinoma. Cancer Res 1999;59189–197.

44. Masferrer JL, Leahy KM, Koki AT, et al. Antiangiogenic and antitumor activities of cyclooxygenase-2 inhibitors. Cancer Res 2000;601306–1311.

45. Guba M, von Breitenbuch P, Steinbauer M, et al. Rapamycin inhibits primary and metastatic tumor growth by antiangiogenesis involvement of vascular endothelial growth factor. Nat Med 2002;8128–135.

46. Levin EG, Sikora L, Ding L, et al. Suppression of tumor growth and angiogenesis in vivo by a truncated form of 24-kd fibroblast growth factor (FGF)-2. Am J Pathol 2004;1641183–1190.

47. Sun J, Blaskovich MA, Jain RK, et al. Blocking angiogenesis and tumorigenesis with GFA-116, a synthetic molecule that inhibits binding of vascular endothelial growth factor to its receptor. Cancer Res 2004;643586–3592.

48. Leung DW, Cachianes G, Kuang WJ, et al. Vascular endothelial growth factor is a secreted angiogenic mitogen. Science 1989;2461306–1309.

49. Ku DD, Zaleski JK, Liu S, Brock TA. Vascular endothelial growth factor induces EDRF-dependent relaxation in coronary arteries. Am J Physiol 1993;265H586–H592.

50. Kohn S, Nagy JA, Dvorak HF, Dvorak AM. Pathways of macromolecular tracer transport across venules and small veins. Structural basis for the hyperpermeability of tumor blood vessels. Lab Invest 1992;67596–607.

51. Pepper MS, Ferrara N, Orci L, Montesano R. Vascular endothelial growth factor (VEGF) induces plasminogen activators and plasminogen activator inhibitor-1 in microvascular endothelial cells. Biochem Biophys Res Commun 1991;181902-906.

52. Unemori EN, Ferrara N, Bauer EA, Amento EP. Vascular endothelial growth factor induces interstitial collagenase expression in human endothelial cells. J Cell Physiol 1992;153557–562.
53. Senger DR, Van de Water L, Brown LF, Nagy JA, et al. Vascular permeability factor (VPF, VEGF) in tumor biology. Cancer Metastasis Rev 1993;12303–324.
54. Gerber HP, Dixit V, Ferrara N. Vascular endothelial growth factor induces expression of the antiapoptotic proteins Bcl-2 and A1 in vascular endothelial cells. J Biol Chem 1998;27313,313–13,316.
55. Tran J, Rak J, Sheehan C, et al. Marked induction of the IAP family antiapoptotic proteins survivin and XIAP by VEGF in vascular endothelial cells. Biochem Biophys Res Commun 1999;264781–788.
56. Tran J, Master Z, Yu JL, et al. A role for survivin in chemresistance of endothelial cells mediated by VEGF. Proc NatlAcad Sci USA 2002;994349–4354.
57. Alon T, Hemo I, Itin A, Pe'er J, et al. Vascular endothelial growth factor acts as a survival factor for newly formed retinal vessels and has implications for retinopathy of prematurity. Nat Med 1995; 11024–1028.
58. Benjamin LE, Keshet E. Conditional switching of vascular endothelial growth factor (VEGF) expression in tumors induction of endothelial cell shedding and regression of hemangioblastoma-like vessels by VEGF withdrawal. Proc Natl Acad Sci USA 1997;948761–8766.
59. Vincenti V, Cassano C, Rocchi M, Persico G. Assignment of the vascular endothelial growth factor gene to human chromosome 6p21.3. Circulation 1996;931493–1495.
60. Houck KA, Ferrara N, Winer J, et al. The vascular endothelial growth factor family identification of a fourth molecular species and characterization of alternative splicing of RNA. Mol Endocrinol 1991;51806–1814.
61. Tischer E, Mitchell R, Hartman T, et al. The human gene for vascular endothelial growth factor. Multiple protein forms are encoded through alternative exon splicing. J Biol Chem 1991; 26611,947–11,954.
62. Poltorak Z, Cohen T, Sivan R, et al. VEGF145, a secreted vascular endothelial growth factor isoform that binds to extracellular matrix. J Biol Chem 1997;2727151–7158.
63. Bates DO, Cui TG, Doughty JM, et al. VEGF(165)b, an inhibitory splice variant of vascular endothelial growth factor, is down-regulated in renal cell carcinoma. Cancer Res 2002;624123–4131.
64. Houck KA, Leung DW, Rowland AM, et al. Dual regulation of vascular endothelial growth factor bioavailability by genetic and proteolytic mechanisms. J Biol Chem 1992;26726,031–26,037.
65. Ferrara N. Vascular endothelial growth factor basic science and clinical progress. Endocr Rev 2004;25581–611.
66. Park JE, Keller GA, Ferrara N. The vascular endothelial growth factor (VEGF) isoforms differential deposition into the subepithelial extracellular matrix and bioactivity of extracellular matrix-bound VEGF. Mol Biol Cell 1993;41317–1326.
67. Keyt BA, Berleau LT, Nguyen HV, et al. The carboxyl-terminal domain (111-165) of vascular endothelial growth factor is critical for its mitogenic potency. J Biol Chem 1996;2717788–7795.
68. Grunstein J, Masbad JJ, Hickley R, et al. Isoforms of vascular endothelial growth factor act in a coordinated fashion to recruit and expand tumor vasculature. Mol Cell Biol 2000;207282–7291.
69. Carmeliet P, Ng Y-S, Nuyens D, et al. Impaired myocardial angiogenesis and ischemic cardiomyopathy in mice lacking the vascular endothelial growth factor isoforms VEGF164 and VEGF188. Nat Med 1999;5495–502.
70. Olofsson B, Pajusola K, Kaipainen A, von Euler G, et al. Vascular endothelial growth factor B, a novel growth factor for endothelial cells. Proc Natl Acad Sci USA 1996;932576–2581.
71. Grimmond S, Lagercrantz J, Drinkwater C, Silins G, et al. Cloning and characterization of a novel human gene related to vascular endothelial growth factor. Genome Res 1996;6124–131.
72. Joukov V, Pajusola K, Kaipainen A, et al. A novel vascular endothelial growth factor, VEGF-C, is a ligand for the Flt4 (VEGFR-3) and KDR (VEGFR-2) receptor tyrosine kinases. EMBO J 1996; 15290–298.
73. Maglione D, Guerriero V, Viglietto G, et al. Isolation of a human placenta cDNA coding for a protein related to the vascular permeability factor. Proc Natl Acad Sci USA 1991;889267–9271.
74. Yamada Y, Nezu J, Shimane M, Hirata Y. Molecular cloning of a novel vascular endothelial growth factor, VEGF-D. Genomics 1997;42483–488.
75. Meyer M, Clauss M, Lepple-Wienhues A, et al. A novel vascular endothelial growth factor encoded by Orf virus, VEGF-E, mediates angiogenesis via signaling through VEGFR-2 (KDR) but not VEGFR-1 (Flt-1) receptor tyrosine kinases. EMBO J 1999;18363–374.
76. Terman BI, Dougher-Vermazen M, Carrion ME, et al. Identification of the KDR tyrosine kinase as a receptor for vascular endothelial cell growth factor. Biochem Biophys Res Commun 1992; 1871579–1586.

77. Pajusola K, Aprelikova O, Korhonen J, et al. FLT4 receptor tyrosine kinase contains seven immunoglobulin-like loops and is expressed in multiple human tissues and cell lines. Cancer Res 1992;525738–5743.

78. de Vries C, Escobedo JA, Ueno H, et al. The fms-like tyrosine kinase, a receptor for vascular endothelial growth factor. Science 1992;255989–991.

79. Kolodkin AL, Levengood DV, Rowe EG, et al. Neuropilin is a semaphorin III receptor. Cell 1997;90753–762.

80. Veikkola T, Karkkainen M, Claesson-Welsh L, Alitalo K. Regulation of angiogenesis via vascular endothelial growth factor receptors. Cancer Res 2000;60203–212.

81. Shen H, Clauss M, Ryan J, et al. Characterization of vascular permeability factor/vascular endothelial growth factor receptors on mononuclear phagocytes. Blood 1993;812767–2773.

82. Shibuya M, Yamaguchi S, Yamane A, et al. Nucleotide sequence and expression of a novel human receptor-type tyrosine kinase (flt) closely related to the fms family. Oncogene 1990;8519–527.

83. Matthews W, Jordan CT, Gavin M, et al. A receptor tyrosine kinase cDNA isolated from a population of enriched primitive hematopoietic cells and exhibiting close genetic linkage to c-kit. Proc Natl Acad Sci USA 1991;889026–9030.

84. Terman BI, Carrion ME, Kovacs E, et al. Identification of a new endothelial cell growth factor receptor tyrosine kinase. Oncogene 1991;61677–1683.

85. Park JE, Chen HH, Winer J, et al. Placenta growth factor. Potentiation of vascular endothelial growth factor bioactivity, in vitro and in vivo, and high affinity binding to Flt-1 but not Flk-1/KDR. J Biol Chem 1994;26925,646–25,654.

86. Olofsson B, Korpelainen E, Pepper MS, et al. Vascular endothelial growth factor B (VEGF-B) binds to VEGF receptor-1 and regulates plasminogen activator activity in endothelial cells. Proc Natl Acad Sci USA 1998;9511,709–11714.

87. Davis-Smyth T, Chen H, Park J, et al. The second immunoglobulin-like domain of the VEGF tyrosine kinase receptor Flt-1 determines ligand binding and may initiate a signal transduction cascade. EMBO J 1996;154919–4927.

88. Barleon B, Totzke F, Herzog C, et al. Mapping of the sites for ligand binding and receptor dimerization at the extracellular domain of the vascular endothelial growth factor receptor FLT-1. J Biol Chem 1997;27210382–10388.

89. Davis-Smyth T, Presta LG, Ferrara N. Mapping the charged residues in the second immunoglobulin-like domain of the vascular endothelial growth factor/placenta growth factor receptor Flt-1 required for binding and structural stability. J Biol Chem 1998;273L3216–3222.

90. Kendall RL, Thomas KA. Inhibition of vascular endothelial cell growth factor activity by an endogenously encoded soluble receptor. Proc Natl Acad Sci USA 1993;9010705–10.709.

91. Gerber HP, Condorelli F, Park J, Ferrara N. Differential transcriptional regulation of the two VEGF receptor genes. Flt-1, but notFlk-1/KDR, is up-regulated by hypoxia. J Biol Chem 1997;27223,659–23,667.

92. de Vries C, Escobedo JA, Ueno H, et al. The fms-like tyrosine kinase, a receptor for vascular endothelial growth factor. Science 1992;255989–991.

93. Waltenbverger J, Claesson Welsh L, Siegbahn A, et al. Different signal transduction properties of KDR and FLt-1, two receptors for vascular endothelial growth factor. J Biol Chem 1994;26926,988–26,995.

94. Hiratsuka S, Maru Y, Okada A, et al. Involvement of Flt-1 tyrosine kinase (vascular endothelial growth factor receptor-1) in pathological angiogenesis. Cancer Res 2001;611207–1213.

95. McMahon G. VEGF receptor signaling in tumor angiogenesis. Oncologist 2000;5 (Suppl 1) 3–10.

96. Huang K, Andersson C, Roomans GM, et al. Signaling properties of VEGF receptor-1 and -2 homo- and heterodimers. Int J Biochem Cell Biol 2001;33315–324.

97. Barleon B, Sozzani S, Zhou D, et al. Migration of human monocytes in response to vascular endothelial growth factor (VEGF) is mediated via the VEGF receptor flt-1. Blood 1996;873336–3343.

98. Terman BI, Dougher Vermazen M, Carrion ME, et al. Identification of the KDR tyrosine kinase as a receptor for vascular endothelial growth factor. Biochem Biophys Res Commun 1992;1871579–1586.

99. Quinn TP, Peters KG, De Vries C, et al. Fetal liver kinase 1 is a receptor for vascular endothelial growth factor and is selectively expressed in vascular endothelium. Proc Natl Acad Sci USA 1993;907533–7537.

100. Millauer B, Wizigmann Voos S, Schnurch H, et al. High affinity VEGF binding and developmental expression suggest Flk-1 as a mjor regulator of vasculogenesis and angiogenesis. Cell 1993; 72835–846.

101. Takahashi T, Ueno H, Shibuya M. VEGF activates protein kinase C-dependent, but ras-independent Raf-MEK-MAP kinase pathway for DNA synthesis in primary endothelial cells. Oncogene 1999;182221–2230.

102. Wu LW, Mayo LD, Dunbar JD, et al. Utilization of distinct signaling pathways by receptors for vascular endothelial cell growth factor and other mitogens in the induction of endothelial cell proliferation. J Biol Chem 2000;2755096–5103.

103. Kaipainen A, Korhonen J, Mustonen T, et al. Expression of the fms-like tyrosine kinase 4 gene becomes restricted to lymphatic endothelium during development. Proc Natl Acad Sci USA 1995; 923566–3570.

104. Minchenko A, Salceda S, Bauer T, Caro J. Hypoxia regulatory elements of the human vascular endothelial growth factor gene. Cell Mol Biol Res 1994;4035–39.

105. Minchenko A, Bauer T, Salceda S, Caro J. Hypoxic stimulation of vascular endothelial growth factor expression in vitro and in vivo. Lab Invest 1994;71374–379.

106. Shweiki D, Itin A, Soffer D, Keshet E. Vascular endothelial growth factor induced by hypoxia may mediate hypoxia-initiated angiogenesis. Nature 1992;359843–845.

107. Semenza G. Signal transduction to hypoxia-inducible factor 1. Biochem Pharmacol 2002;64993–998.

108. Levy AP, Levy NS, Wegner S, Goldberg MA. Transcriptional regulation of the rat vascular endothelial growth factor gene by hypoxia. J Biol Chem 1995;27013,333–13,340.

109. Liu Y, Cox SR, Morita T, Kourembanas S. Hypoxia regulates vascular endothelial growth factor gene expression in endothelial cells. Identification of a 5' enhancer. Circ Res 1995;77638–643.

110. Mole DR, Maxwell PH, Pugh CW, Ratcliffe PJ. Regulation of HIF by the von Hippel-Lindau tumour suppressor implication for cellular oxygen sensing. IUBMB 2001;5243–47.

111. Maxwell PH, Wiesener MS, Chang GW, et al. The tumour suppressor protein VHL targets hypoxia-inducible factors for oxygen-dependent proteolysis. Nature 1999;399271–275.

112. Jaakkola P, Mole DR, Tian YM, et al. Targeting of HIF-α to the von Hippel-Lindau ubiquitylation complex by O_2-regulated prolyl hydroxylation. Science 2000;1292468–472.

113. Ivan M, Kondo K, Yang H, et al. HIF-α targeted for VHL-mediated destruction by proline hydroxylation implications for O_2 sensing. Science 2001;292464–468.

114. Li J, Perrella MA, Tsai JC, et al. Induction of vascular endothelial growth factor gene expression by interleukin-1 beta in rat aortic smooth muscle cells. J Biol Chem 1995;270308–312.

115. Cohen T, Nahari D, Cerem LW, et al. Interleukin 6 induces the expression of vascular endothelial growth factor. J Biol Chem 1996;271736–741.

116. Pertovaara L, Kaipainen A, Mustonen T, et al. Vascular endothelial growth factor is induced in response to transforming growth factor-beta in fibroblastic and epithelial cells. J Biol Chem 1994;2696271–6274.

117. Goldman CK, Kim J, Wong WL, et al. Epidermal growth factor stimulates vascular endothelial growth factor production by human malignant glioma cells a model of glioblastoma multiforme pathophysiology. Mol Biol Cell 1993;4121–133.

118. Stavri GT, Hong Y, Zachary IC, et al. Hypoxia and platelet-derived growth factor-BB synergistically upregulate the expression of vascular endothelial growth factor in vascular smooth muscle cells. FEBS Lett 1995;358311–315.

119. Stewart RJ, Panigrahy D, Flynn E, Folkman J. Vascular endothelial growth factor expression and tumor angiogenesis are regulated by androgens in hormone responsive human prostate carcinoma evidence for androgen dependent destabilization of vascular endothelial growth factor transcripts. J Urol 2001;165688–693.

120. Mueller MD, Vigne JL, Pritts EA, et al. Progestins activate vascular endothelial growth factor gene transcription in endometrial adenocarcinoma cells. Fertil Steril 2003;79386–392.

121. Grugel S, Finkenzeller G, Weindel K, et al. Both v-Ha-Ras and v-Raf stimulate expression of the vascular endothelial growth factor in NIH 3T3 cells. J Biol Chem 1995;27025,915–25,919.

122. Saez E, Rutberg SE, Mueller E, et al. c-fos is required for malignant progression of skin tumors. Cell 1995;82721–732.

123. Mukhopadhyay D, Tsiokas L, Sukhatme VP. Wild-type p53 and v-Src exert opposing influences on human vascular endothelial growth factor gene expression. Cancer Res 1995;556161–6165.

124. Gospodarowicz D, Moran JS. Mitogenic effect of fibroblast growth factor on early passage cultures of human and murine fibroblasts. J Cell Biol 1975;66451–457.

125. Powers CJ, McLeskey SW, Wellstein A. Fibroblast growth factors, their receptors and signaling. Endocr Relat Cancer 2000;7165–197.

126. Dow JK, deVere White RW. Fibroblast growth factor 2 its structure and property, paracrine function, tumor angiogenesis, and prostate-related mitogenic and oncogenic functions. Urology 2000; 55800–806.

127. Nishimura T, Nakatake Y, Konishi M, Itoh N. Identification of a novel FGF, FGF-21, preferentially expressed in the liver. Biochim Biophys Acta 2000;1492203–206.

128. Fernig DG, Gallagher JT. Fibroblast growth factors and their receptors an information network controlling tissue growth, morphogenesis and repair. Prog Growth Factor Res 1994;5353–377.

129. Dickson C, Deed R, Dixon M, Peters G. The structure and function of the int-2 oncogene. Prog Growth Factor Res 1989;1123–132.

130. Kirikoshi H, Sagara N, Saitoh T, et al. Molecular cloning and characterization of human FGF-20 on chromosome 8p21.3-p22. Biochem Biophys Res Commun 2000;274337–343.

131. Ornitz DM, Xu J, Colvin JS, et al. Receptor specificity of the fibroblast growth factor family. J Biol Chem 1996;27115,292–15,297.

132. Partanen J, Vainikka S, Korhonen J, et al. Diverse receptors for fibroblast growth factors. Prog Growth Factor Res 1992;469–83.

133. Basilico C, Moscatelli D. The FGF family of growth factors and oncogenes. Adv Cancer Res 1992; 59115–165.

134. Baird A, Mormede P, Bohlen P. Immunoreactive fibroblast growth factor (FGF) in a transplantable chondrosarcoma inhibition of tumor growth by antibodies to FGF. J Cell Biochem 1986;3079–85.

135. Pepper MS, Montesano R, Orci L, Vassalli JD. Plasminogen activator inhibitor-1 is induced in migrating endothelial cells. J Cell Physio 1992;153129–139.

136. Presta M, Maier JA, Rusnati M, Ragnotti G. Basic fibroblast growth factor production, mitogenic response, and post-receptor signal transduction in cultured normal and transformed fetal bovine aortic endothelial cells. J Cell Physiol 1989;141517–526.

137. Schweigerer L, Neufeld G, Friedman J, et al. Capillary endothelial cells express basic fibroblast growth factor, a mitogen that promotes their own growth. Nature 1987;325257–259.

138. Pepper MS, Belin D, Montesano R, et al. Transforming growth factor-beta 1 modulates basic fibroblast growth factor-induced proteolytic and angiogenic properties of endothelial cells in vitro. J Cell Biol 1990;111743–755.

139. Arese M, Chen Y, Florkiewicz RZ, et al. Nuclear activities of basic fibroblast growth factor potentiation of low-serum growth mediated by natural or chimeric nuclear localization signals. Mol Biol Cell 1999;101429–1444.

140. Arnaud E, Touriol C, Boutonnet C, et al. A new 34-kilodalton isoform of human fibroblast growth factor 2 is cap dependently synthesized by using a non-AUG start codon and behaves as a survival factor. Mol Cell Biol 1999;19505–514.

141. Florkiewicz RZ, Shibata F, Barankiewicz T, et al. Basic fibroblast growth factor gene expression. Ann N Y Acad Sci 1991;638109–126.

142. Quarto N, Finger FP, Rifkin DB. The NH2-terminal extension of high molecular weight bFGF is a nuclear targeting signal. J Cell Physiol 1991;147311–318.

143. Ornitz DM. FGFs, heparan sulfate and FGFRs complex interactions essential for development. BioEssays 2000;22108–112.

144. Spivak-Kroizman T, Lemmon MA, Dikic I, et al. Heparin-induced oligomerization of FGF molecules is responsible for FGF receptor dimerization, activation, and cell proliferation. Cell 1994;791015–1024.

145. Chambard JC, Paris S, L'Allemain G, Pouyssegur J. Two growth factor signalling pathways in fibroblasts distinguished by pertussis toxin. Nature 1987;326800–803.

146. Johnson MR, Valentine C, Basilico C, Mansukhani A. FGF signaling activates STAT1 and p21 and inhibits the estrogen response and proliferation of MCF-7 cells. Oncogene 1998;162647–2656.

147. Rossi D, Zlotnik A. The biology of chemokines and their receptors. Annu Rev Immunol 2000; 18217–242.

148. Strieter RM, Lukacs NW, Standiford TJ, Kunkel SL. Cytokines. 2. Cytokines and lung inflammation mechanisms of neutrophil recruitment to the lung. Thorax 1993;48765–769.

149. Farber JM. Mig and IP-10 CXC chemokines that target lymphocytes. J Leukoc Biol 1997;61246–257.

150. Strieter RM, Polverini PJ, Kunkel SL, et al. The functional role of the ELR motif in CXC chemokine-mediated angiogenesis. J Biol Chem. 1995;27027,348–27,357.

151. Moore BB, Arenberg DA, Addison CL, et al. Tumor angiogenesis is regulated by CXC chemokines. J Lab Clin Med 1998;13297–103.

152. Strieter RM, Kunkel SL, Elner VM, et al. Interleukin-8. A corneal factor that induces neovascularization. Am J Pathol 1992;1411279–1284.

153. Koch AE, Polverini PJ, Kunkel SL, et al. Interleukin-8 as a macrophage-derived mediator of angiogenesis. Science 1992;2581798–1801.

154. Hu DE, Hori Y, Fan TP. Interleukin-8 stimulates angiogenesis in rats. Inflammation 1993; 17135–143.

155. Kitadai Y, Haruma K, Sumii K, et al. Expression of interleukin-8 correlates with vascularity in human gastric carcinomas. Am J Pathol 1998;15293–100.

156. Lingen MW, Polverini PJ, Bouck NP. Retinoic acid induces cells cultured from oral squamous cell carcinomas to become anti-angiogenic. Am J Pathol 1996;149247–258.

157. Moore BB, Arenberg DA, Stoy K, et al. Distinct CXC chemokines mediate tumorigenicity of prostate cancer cells. Am J Pathol 1999;1541503–1512.

158. Veltri RW, Miller MC, Zhao G, et al. Interleukin-8 serum levels in patients with benign prostatic hyperplasia and prostate cancer. Urology 1999;53139–147.

159. Yoneda J, Kuniyasu H, Crispens MA, et al. Expression of angiogenesis-related genes and progression of human ovarian carcinomas in nude mice. J Natl Cancer Inst 1998;90447–454.

160. Smith DR, Polverini PJ, Kunkel SL, et al. Inhibition of interleukin 8 attenuates angiogenesis in bronchogenic carcinoma. J Exp Med 1994;1791409–1415.

161. Arenberg DA, Kunkel SL, Polverini PJ, et al. Inhibition of interleukin-8 reduces tumorigenesis of human non-small cell lung cancer in SCID mice. J Clin Invest 1996;972792–2802.

162. Luan J, Shattuck-Brandt R, Haghnegahdar H, et al. Mechanism and biological significance of constitutive expression of MGSA/GRO chemokines in malignant melanoma tumor progression. J Leukoc Biol 1997;62588–597.

163. Owen JD, Strieter R, Burdick M, et al. Enhanced tumor-forming capacity for immortalized melanocytes expressing melanoma growth stimulatory activity/growth-regulated cytokine beta and gamma proteins. Int J Cancer 1997;7394–103.

164. Hansell P, Maione TE, Borgstrom P. Selective binding of platelet factor 4 to regions of active angiogenesis in vivo. Am J Physiol 1995;269H829–836.

165. Borgstrom P, Discipio R, Maione TE. Recombinant platelet factor 4, an angiogenic marker for human breast carcinoma. Anticancer Res 1998;184035–4041.

166. Gengrinovitch S, Greenberg SM, Cohen T, et al. Platelet factor-4 inhibits the mitogenic activity of VEGF121 and VEGF165 using several concurrent mechanisms. J Biol Chem 1995;27015,059–15,065.

167. Jouan V, Canron X, Alemany M, et al. Inhibition of in vitro angiogenesis by platelet factor-4-derived peptides and mechanism of action. Blood 1999;94984–993.

168. Perollet C, Han ZC, Savona C, et al. Platelet factor 4 modulates fibroblast growth factor 2 (FGF-2) activity and inhibits FGF-2 dimerization. Blood 1998;913289–3299.

169. Houck KA, Ferrara N, Winer J, et al. The vascular endothelial growth factor family identification of a fourth molecular species and characterization of alternative splicing of RNA. Mol Endocrinol 1991;51806–1814.

170. Gupta SK, Singh JP. Inhibition of endothelial cell proliferation by platelet factor-4 involves a unique action on S phase progression. J Cell Biol 1994;1271121–1127.

171. Luster AD. Chemokines—chemotactic cytokines that mediate inflammation. N Engl J Med 1998;338436–445.

172. Farber JM. HuMig a new human member of the chemokine family of cytokines. Biochem Biophys Res Commun 1993;192223–230.

173. Farber JM. A macrophage mRNA selectively induced by gamma-interferon encodes a member of the platelet factor 4 family of cytokines. Proc Natl Acad Sci USA 1990;875238–5242.

174. Farber JM. A collection of mRNA species that are inducible in the RAW 264.7 mouse macrophage cell line by gamma interferon and other agents. Mol Cell Biol 1992;121535–1545.

175. Luster AD, Unkeless JC, Ravetch JV. Gamma-interferon transcriptionally regulates an early-response gene containing homology to platelet proteins. Nature 1985;315672–676.

176. Luster AD, Ravetch JV. Biochemical characterization of a gamma interferon-inducible cytokine (IP-10). J Exp Med 1987;1661084–1097.

177. Cole KE, Strick CA, Paradis TJ, et al. Interferon-inducible T cell alpha chemoattractant (I-TAC) a novel non-ELR CXC chemokine with potent activity on activated T cells through selective high affinity binding to CXCR3. J Exp Med 1998;1872009–2021.

178. Arenberg DA, Kunkel SL, Polverini PJ, et al. Interferon-gamma-inducible protein 10 (IP-10) is an angiostatic factor that inhibits human non-small cell lung cancer (NSCLC) tumorigenesis and spontaneous metastases. J Exp Med 1996;184981–992.

179. Sgadari C, Angiolillo AL, Cherney BW, et al. Interferon-inducible protein-10 identified as a mediator of tumor necrosis in vivo. Proc Natl Acad Sci USA 1996;9313791–13796.

180. Schonbeck U, Brandt E, Petersen F, et al. IL-8 specifically binds to endothelial but not to smooth muscle cells. J Immunol 1995;1542375–2383.

181. Petzelbauer P, Watson CA, Pfau SE, Pober JS. IL-8 and angiogenesis evidence that human endothelial cells lack receptors and do not respond to IL-8 in vitro. Cytokine 1995;7267–272.

182. Leong SR, Lowman HB, Liu J, et al. IL-8 single-chain homodimers and heterodimers interactions with chemokine receptors CXCR1, CXCR2, and DARC. Protein Sci 1997;6609–617.

183. Wuyts A, Van Osselaer N, Haelens A, et al. Characterization of synthetic human granulocyte chemotactic protein 2 usage of chemokine receptors CXCR1 and CXCR2 and in vivo inflammatory properties. Biochemistry 1997;362716–2723.

184. Farber JM. Mig and IP-10 CXC chemokines that target lymphocytes. J Leukoc Biol 1997;61243–257.

185. Ueda H, Siani MA, Gong W, et al. Chemically synthesized SDF-1alpha analogue, N33A, is a potent chemotactic agent for CXCR4/Fusin/LESTR-expressing human leukocytes. J Biol Chem 1997;27224,966–24,970.

186. Legler DF, Loetscher M, Roos RS, et al. B cell-attracting chemokine 1, a human CXC chemokine expressed in lymphoid tissues, selectively attracts B lymphocytes via BLR1/CXCR5. J Exp Med 1998;187655–660.

187. Yoshida K, Gage FH. Cooperative regulation of nerve growth factor synthesis and secretion in fibroblasts and astrocytes by fibroblast growth factor and other cytokines. Brain Res 1992;56914–25.

188. Zhang QX, Duenas M, Rosengart T. Effect of tumor necrosis factor-alpha on a cell line transformed by a secreted form of human fibroblast growth factor-1 gene and on its parental cell line. Cancer Lett 1995;8949–54.

189. Muller G, Behrens J, Nussbaumer U, et al. Inhibitory action of transforming growth factor beta on endothelial cells. Proc Natl Acad Sci USA 1987;845600–5604.

190. Kim IY, Kim MM, Kim SJ. Transforming growth factor-beta biology and clinical relevance. J Biochem Mol Biol 2005;381–8.

191. Gusella GL, Musso T, Bosco MC, et al. IL-2 up-regulates but IFN-gamma suppresses IL-8 expression in human monocytes. J Immunol 1993;1512725–2732.

192. Schnyder-Candrian S, Strieter RM, Kunkel SL, Walz A. Interferon-alpha and interferon-gamma down-regulate the production of interleukin-8 and ENA-78 in human monocytes. J Leukoc Biol 1995;57929–935.

193. Lee IY, Kim J, Ko EM, et al. Interleukin-4 inhibits the vascular endothelial growth factor- and basic fibroblast growth factor-induced angiogenesis in vitro. Mol Cells 2002;14115–121.

194. Kohno T, Mizukami H, Suzuki M, et al. Interleukin-10-mediated inhibition of angiogenesis and tumor growth in mice bearing VEGF-producing ovarian cancer. Cancer Res 2003;635091–5094.

195. Huang S, Xie K, Bucana CD, et al. Interleukin 10 suppresses tumor growth and metastasis of human melanoma cells potential inhibition of angiogenesis. Clin Cancer Res 1996;21969–1979.

15 | Chemokine and Receptor Expression in Tumor Progression

Paola Allavena, Federica Marchesi, and Alberto Mantovani

CONTENTS

INTRODUCTION
TUMORS PRODUCE CHEMOKINES
ROLE OF TUMOR-DERIVED CHEMOKINES IN ATTRACTING LEUKOCYTES
ROLE OF CHEMOKINES IN TUMOR SPREAD AND PROGRESSION
TUMOR CELLS EXPRESS CHEMOKINE RECEPTORS
CONCLUSIONS
REFERENCES

1. INTRODUCTION

Chemotactic cytokines (chemokines) are a family of small proteins (8–10 kDa) inducing directed cell migration (chemotaxis) along a chemical gradient *(1–5)*. Chemokines tightly regulate the positioning of leukocytes in secondary lymphoid organs (e.g., in lymph nodes and thymus), and are key determinants of the recruitment of leukocytes at sites of inflammation and tumor tissues. Besides hematopoietic cells, chemokines affect several other cell types, such as epithelial and endothelial cells, fibroblasts and tumor cells. Chemokines play an important role in immune and inflammatory reactions; in addition most of these molecules affect other important cell functions such as angiogenesis, collagen production, activation of enzymes and regulation of cell growth and apoptosis. Forty-seven chemokines have been identified so far in man. Based on a cystein motif, different subfamilies: CXC, CC, C and CX3C have been classified (Table 1). The chemokine scaffold consists of an N-terminal loop connected via Cys bonds to the more structured core of the molecule (three b sheets) with a C terminal a helix *(1–4)*.

Chemokines interact with seven transmembrane domains, G-protein coupled receptors. Ten CC (CCR1-10), six CXC (CXCR1-6), one CX3C (CX3CR1) and one XCR (CXR1) receptors have been identified *(3–6)*. Receptor expression is a crucial determinant of the spectrum of action of chemokines. Regulation of receptor transcription, as well as receptor signalling, is tightly regulated during cell differentiation and activation.

From: *Cancer Drug Discovery and Development,*
Cytokines in the Genesis and Treatment of Cancer
Edited by: M. A. Caligiuri and M. T. Lotze © Humana Press Inc., Totowa, NJ

Table 1
Chemokine and Receptor Classification[a]

Chemokine Ligands	Other Names	Chemokine Receptors
CXC Subfamily		
CXCL1	GROα/MGSA-α	CXCR2>CXCR1
CXCL2	GROβ/MGSA-β	CXCR2
CXCL3	GROγ/MGSA-γ	CXCR2
CXCL4	PF4	Unknown
CXCL5	ENA-78	CXCR2
CXCL6	GCP-2	CXCR1, CXCR2
CXCL7	NAP-2	CXCR2
CXCL8	IL-8	CXCR1, CXCR2
CXCL9	Mig	CXCR3
CXCL10	IP-10	CXCR3
CXCL11	I-TAC	CXCR3
CXCL12	SDF1 α/β	CXCR4
CXCL13	BCA-1	CXCR5
CXCL14	BRAK/bolekine	Unknown
(CXCL15)	Unknown	Unknown
CXCL16		CXCR6
C Subfamily		
XCL1	Lymphotactin/SCM-1α/ATAC	XCR1
XCL2	SCM-1β	XCR1
CX3C Subfamily		
CX3CL1	Fractalkine	CX3CR1
CC Subfamily		
CCL1	I-309	CCR8
CCL2	MCP-1/MCAF/ TDCF	CCR2
CCL3	MIP-1α/LD78α	CCR1, CCR5
CCL3L1	LD78β	CCR1, CCR5
CCL4	MIP-1β	CCR5
CCL5	RANTES	CCR1, CCR3, CCR5
(CCL6)	Unknown	Unknown
CCL7	MCP-3	CCR1, CCR2, CCR3
CCL8	MCP-2	CCR3, CCR5
(CCL9/10)	Unknown	CCR1
CCL11	Eotaxin	CCR3
(CCL12)	Unknown	CCR2
CCL13	MCP-4	CCR2, CCR3
CCL14	HCC-1	CCR1, CCR5
CCL15	HCC-2/Lkn-1/MIP-1δ	CCR1, CCR3
CCL16	HCC-4/LEC/LCC-1	CCR1, CCR2
CCL17	TARC	CCR4
CCL18	DC-CK1/PARC/AMC-1	Unknown
CCL19	MIP-3β/ELC/exodus-3	CCR7
CCL20	MIP-3α/LARC/exodus-1	CCR6
CCL21	6Ckine/SLC/exodus-2	CCR7
CCL22	MDC/STCP-1	CCR4
CCL23	MPIF-1/CKβ8/CKβ8-1	CCR1
CCL24	Eotaxin-2/MPIF-2	CCR3
CCL25	TECK	CCR9
CCL26	Ecotaxin-3	CCR3
CCL27	CTACK/ILC	CCR10
CCL28	MEC	CCR3/CCR10

[a]In parenthesis: only mouse ligand identified.

Because the discovery of chemokines, the field was strongly connected to cancer biology. This connection is illustrated by the identification of monocyte chemotactic protein-1, now called CCL2, in culture supernatants of tumor cell lines *(7)*. Indeed tumor cells have represented an invaluable tool for the identification and characterization of chemokines. In the tumor microenvironment chemokines are produced both by stromal cells (fibroblasts, endothelial cells, and infiltrating leukocytes) and by the tumor itself. The field of chemokines in tumor biology has dramatically developed in the last decade and has expanded from the regulation of leukocyte attraction within the tumor mass to the promotion of tumor cell survival, proliferation, and mobilization *(8)*. In this chapter we will review the current knowledge on the field of chemokines and their relationship with cancer biology.

2. TUMORS PRODUCE CHEMOKINES

In the early 1980s it had been noted that tumor supernatants contained chemo-attractants active on monocytes *(9)*. The first tumor-derived chemotactic factor identified turned out to be human CCL2. CCL2 is probably the CC chemokine most frequently found in tumors. Human tumors shown to express CCL2 in vivo include sarcomas, gliomas, lung tumors, carcinomas of the breast, cervix and ovary, melanoma, and pancreas *(8)*. Several lines of evidence, including correlation between production and infiltration in murine and human tumors, passive immunization, and gene modification, indicate that CCL2 plays a pivotal role in the recruitment of monocytes in neoplastic tisues, as discussed below *(8,10,11)*.

A variety of other chemokines have been detected in neoplastic tissues as products of tumor cells or stromal elements. These include CCL5, CXCL12, CXCL8, CXCL1, CXCL13, CCL17 and CCL22. CCL5 is produced by breast carcinoma and melanoma *(12,13)*. In breast cancer CCL5 expression by tumor cells correlates with a more advanced stage of disease, suggesting that CCL5 may be involved in breast cancer progression *(13,14)*. Melanoma is probably the most studied cancer type in which CXC chemokines and in particular CXCL1 and related molecules (CXCL2, CXCL3, CXCL8 or IL-8) have been demonstrated to play a role in tumor progression *(15)*. They do so by direct stimulation of neoplastic growth, promotion of inflammation, and induction of angiogenesis. CXCL1 was initially identified and purified from supernatants of melanoma cell lines and characterized as an autocrine growth factor *(16,17)*. Blocking of CXCL1, or its receptor CXCR2, with specific antibodies inhibited the growth of melanoma cells in vitro *(18)*. Conversely, the over-expression of CXCL1 *(19)*, CXCL2, or CXCL3 *(20)*; in various melanoma cell lines increased their ability to form colonies in soft agar and their tumorigenicity in nude mice. A few other studies have proposed a similar role for CXCL8 related chemokines in head and neck *(21)*, pancreas *(22)*, and nonsmall-cell lung cancer (NSCLC) *(23)*.

Autocrine and paracrine expression of CCL20 has been reported in pancreatic cancer *(24)*. CXCL13 is a B-cell chemokine and is highly expressed in *Helicobacter pylori*-induced lymphoma *(25)*. A role for CXCL13 in the localization of tumor cells has been suggested.

Chemokine production can be constitutive or inducible by environmental stimuli. Although constitutive chemokines control the homeostatic trafficking of leukocytes under steady state conditions, inducible chemokines are produced under conditions of inflammation and immune reactions. Tumors are generally characterized by the constitutive expression of chemokines belonging to the inducible realm. The molecular mechanism accounting for constitutive expression have been defined only for CXCL1 and involved NFκB activation. Melanoma cells display high expression of NF-κB-inducing kinase (NIK) (26) and this phenotype is responsible for constitutive activation of IκB kinase activity and MAPK signaling cascades, as well as for constitutive activation of NF-κB (27,28). This may represent a general mechanism undelying constitutive expression of inflammatory chemokines in tumors.

3. ROLE OF TUMOR-DERIVED CHEMOKINES IN ATTRACTING LEUKOCYTES

Tumors are composed of tumor cells and stromal cells, which sometimes are very developed and can even outnumber cancer cells. Besides fibroblasts and endothelial cells, leukocytes (especially macrophages and T-lymphocytes) are the most represented cell types.

3.1. Monocyte-Macrophages

Tumor-associated macrophages (TAM) derive from monocytic precursors circulating in the blood (29). Several studies have indicated that CCL2 is primarily responsible for the recruitment of monocytes at the tumor site. Indeed, CCL2 levels correlated with the abundance of TAM in several types of adenocarcinoma, including ovarian, breast, and pancreas (30–35). Interestingly, CCL2 production has been detected also in TAM, indicating the existence of an amplification loop for their recruitment (34). Other CC chemokines related to CCL2, such as CCL7 and CCL8 are also produced by tumors and shown to recruit monocytes (36).

TAM have an ambiguous role in their relationship with tumor cells, as described in the macrophage balance hypothesis (10,28,37). Although they can potentially display tumor cytotocity, they are believed to have primarily protumor functions (see Chapter 14) (10,38).

TAM produce several factors that can promote angiogenesis, such as basic fibroblast growth factor (bFGF), vascular endothelial growth factor (VEGF), and several proteases (Fig.1). They also possess procoagulant activity through fibrin deposition, which indirectly enhances blood vessel formation. Indeed it was observed that the density of blood microvessels correlates with the extent of macrophage infiltration in breast cancer (39,40). TAM are also a source of IL-10 and PGE_2, two potent immuno-modulating molecules contributing to immunosuppression (10,41,42). On the basis of this functional profile TAM have been considered to be M2 type macrophages, like macrophages activated by Th2-cytokines and IL-10 (10). A recent review of the prognostic significance of TAM levels in human tumors concluded that in 10 of 15 studies macrophage infiltration was associated with worse prognosis (43).

In accordance with the potential dual role of TAM, the gene transfer of CCL2 into tumors had contrasting effects. At least three reports indicated reduced tumorigenicity (44–46). The results of another study pointed to an opposite effect: the number of spontaneous lung metastases was augmented in animals injected with CCL2-transfectants compared to those injected with parental cells (47,48). The impact of CCL2 on tumor growth in a nontumorigenic melanoma system revealed a biphasic effect. Low-level CCL2 secretion, with "physiologic" accumulation of TAM promoted

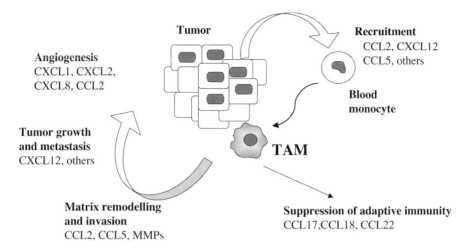

Fig. 1. Relevance of the chemokine network in the tumor micro-environment and in the pro-tumoral function of tumor-associated macrophages (TAM). Tumor-derived chemokines actively recruit circulating blood monocytes at the tumor site. Chemokines participate in several pro-tumoral functions of TAM, including promotion of angiogenesis, tissue remodeling and invasion, activation of matrix-metalloproteases (MMPs) and direct tumor growth. Selected chemokines attract T-helper 2 (Th2)-polarized lymphocytes and T-regulatory cells, which are ineffective in ictumor immunity and suppress ictumor responses.

tumor formation, whereas high CCL2 secretion resulted in massive macrophage infiltration into the tumor mass and in its destruction *(48)*. Similarly, a high inoculum of CCL-2-transfected melanoma cells showed retarded tumor growth, whereas a small inoculum was more tumorigenic *(38)*. These results are consistent with the "macrophage balance" hypothesis *(10,29)*.

As mentioned above, in addition to being a target for chemokines, TAM are a source of a selected set of these mediators (CCL2, CCL17, CCL18, and CCL22) (Fig.1). CCL18 was recently identified as the most abundant chemokine in human ovarian ascites fluid *(49)*. When the source of CCL18 was investigated, it was tracked to TAM, with no production by ovarian carcinoma cells. CCL18 is a CC chemokine produced constitutively by immature DC and inducible in macrophages by IL-4, IL-13 and IL-10. Because IL-4 and IL-13 are not expressed in substantial amounts in ovarian cancer, it is likely that IL-10, produced by tumor cells and macrophages themselves, accounts for CCL18 production by TAM. CCL18 is an attractant for naive T-cells by interacting with an unidentified receptor *(3,5)*. Attraction of naive T-cells in a peripheral microenvironment dominated by M2 macrophages and immature DC is likely to induce T-cell anergy.

3.2. Neutrophils

CXCL8 and related chemokines act primarily on neutrophils. In spite of constitutive production of these ligands by tumor cells, neutrophils are not a major and obvious constituent of the leukocyte infiltrate. However, these cells, though present in minute numbers, may play a key role in triggering and sustaining the inflammatory cascade, for instance by releasing angiogenic molecules *(50)*. Interestingly, IL-4 and IL-13 render monocytes exquisitely sensitive to CXCL8 and CXCL1 *(51)*. Therefore, in the tumor microenvironment, where IL-4/IL-13-producing, polarized type II T-cells can be present,

CXCL8 and related chemokines may contribute to guide the positioning and to regulate the function of macrophages.

3.3. Lymphocytes

Most of our knowledge on the role of chemokines in the recruitment of T- and NK-cells is derived fron studies using chemokine-transfected tumor cells. Trasduction of CCL5 in tumor cells resulted in loss of tumorigenicity owing to activation of ictumor immunity *(52)*. Similar activity was shown by CCL3. These ligands of CCR5 are expressed, for instance, in nasopharingeal and ovarian carcinoma and have been proposed to regulate T-cell infiltration *(30,52)*. Despite these evidences, in vivo expression of CCL5 is associated with advanced disease in breast and cervical cancer *(13,53)*.

Expression of CXCL9 has been associated with heavy infiltration of T-lymphocytes in human melanoma *(54)* and in mouse tumor models *(55–57)*. CXCL10 was reported to be an important factor for IL-12-mediated ictumor response through the recruitment and activation of CD8 lymphocytes *(58)* and NK cells *(59)*. The chemokine CCL21 recruits dendritic cells and lymphocytes (naive T, NK cells, and a subset of memory T-cells), and displays icneoplastic effects when transduced in tumor cells *(60–62)* or injected locally *(63)*. Similar results were reported for CCL19, which shares with CCL21 the same receptor CCR7 *(64)*.

Chemokines are part of amplification and regulation systems of polarized T-cell responses. Some chemokines may enhance innate and specific host immunity against tumors but on the other hand other chemokines may contribute to escape from the immune system, by recruiting Th2 effectors and regulatory T-cells *(65,66)*. Work in gene-modified mice has shown that CCL2 can orient specific immunity in a Th2 direction. Although the exact mechanism for this action has not been defined, it may include stimulation of IL-10 production in macrophages *(67)*.

Reed-Sternberg cells in Hodgkin's lymphoma have been shown to express CCL22 and CCL17 *(68,69)*. These chemokines recognize CCR4 which is preferentially expressed on Th2 lymphocytes and on T-regulatory cells (Treg) *(2,70)*. Interestingly, in the same tumor, stromal cells produce CCL11, which attracts eosinophils and Th2 cells. Therefore, in this human tumor, neoplastic elements and stroma use complementary tools to recruit immunocompetent cells associated with polarized type II responses, unable to mediate ictumor immunity.

In the same vein of driving polarized Th2 cells into tumors, the oncogenic virus human herpesvirus 8 (HHV8), involved in the pathogenesis of Kaposi sarcoma and hematologic malignancies, encodes three CC chemokines (vMIPI, II and III) which interact with CCR3, CCR4, and CCR8 expressed on Th2 cells and T-regulatory cells *(70)*. Consistently with these in vitro observations, Kaposi sarcoma is infiltrated by CD8+ and, to a lesser extent, CD4+ cells with a predominant Th2 phenotype. Therefore, HHV8 virus-encoded chemokines represent a strategy to subvert antiviral/antitumor immunity by favouring the recruitment of inefficient cells and cells with suppressive activity.

In addition to viral chemokines, HHV8 encodes for a chemokine receptor homologue, ORF74, also known as KSHV vGPCR, showing similiarity with CXCR2 *(71,72)*. This receptor triggers a constitutive signal which is further increased by CXCL8 and CXCL1, providing a good example of a direct role of chemokines and receptors in neoplastic transformation. Indeed, over-expression of KSHV vGPCR alone resulted in the development of lesions resembling Kaposi sarcoma *(71)*.

3.4. Dendritic Cells

It has been clearly shown that chemokines tightly control the tissue trafficking of myeloid dendritic cells (DC) in their migration to secondary lymphoid organs *(73–77)*. Chemokines are also involved in the recruitment of DC at the tumor site *(78,79)*. Although usually rare cells, DC have been detected in several tumor types, including lung, prostate, nasopharynx, kidney, thyroid, breast, ovary, and melanoma *(80–89)*. Although TAM are, usually, dispersed evenly within the tumor mass. Tumor-associated DC (TADC) localize in specific areas. In papillary carcinoma of the thyroid, DC were found at the invasion edge of the tumor *(120)*. In breast carcinoma, DC with a mature phenotype (DC-LAMP+) were localized in peri-tumoral areas, whereas immature DC were inside the tumor *(80)*. A few chemokines are more restricted for DC. CCL20 interacts with CCR6, a receptor expressed by Langerhans cells but not by monocyte-derived DC. Infiltration of Langerhans-like DC, positive for the marker Langerin, was noted in breast cancer expressing CCL20 *(80)*.

The presence of plamacytoid DC (P-DC), a distinct DC subset of lymphoid origin, is a recent finding. P-DC have been shown to accumulate in breast metastatic lymph nodes *(90)* and in ovarian cancer in correlation with the expression of CXCL12 to which they respond *(89)*. Primary melanoma is infiltrated with both myeloid and P-DC *(91,92)*.

The significance of active recruitment of antigen-presenting cells in the tumor, especially whether it is a sign of active immune response, is not clear. DC are well equipped to pick up tumor antigens and cross-present them to T-lymphocytes, as documented by several studies *(77,83,94)*. However DC can also potently induce tolerance *(95,96)* and, as mentioned above, the tumor microenvironment contains immuno-suppressive factors that have been shown to hamper dendritic cell differentiation and activation (Fig. 2).

In several tumor models where chemokine-induced tumor regression was established, the presence of DC was documented, but their exact role has not been investigated. The chemokines involved in these studies included CCL7, CCL16, CCL21 CCL20, CCL19, and CXCL12 *(60–64,97–99)*. Therefore the role of intratumoral DC in the establishment of ictumor immunity, or in the induction of tolerance, remains to be elucidated.

4. ROLE OF CHEMOKINES IN TUMOR SPREAD AND PROGRESSION

It has long been known that tumor-derived proteases can cleave the extracellular matrix molecules and lead to the dissolution of the basement membrane, thus facilitating the process of tumor cell invasion. A variety of proteolytic enzymes, in particular the tissue type plasminogen activator (t-PA), the urokinase-type plasminogen activators (u-PA) and the large family of matrix-metalloproteinases (MMPs) have been implicated in this degradation *(100–102)*. The activity of these enzymes has been associated with more aggressive neoplastic behaviour. For example, t-PA and u-PA and their respective receptors, annexin II and u-PAR, were demonstrated to contribute to the invasive behavior of pancreatic cancer *(103)*. MMP-2 expression is increased in several tumors and strongly correlates with nodal status and tumor stage *(104)*. Chemokines are potent inducers of enzymes and receptors which degrade the extracellular matrix and favor tumor invasion. In a gene expression analysis, the chemokine CCL5 specifically induced gene expression of various MMPs, especially MMP9, along with the uPA receptor *(105)*.

Blood   **Tumor micro-environment**

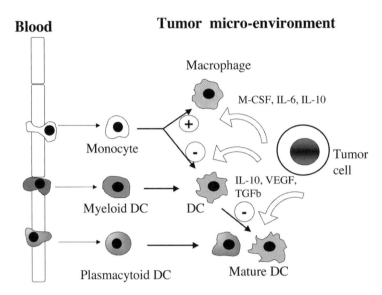

Fig. 2. Immune-suppressive effects of the tumor micro-environment. Tumor cells produce several cytokines which affect the outcome of a potential ictumor response. Cytokines like IL-10, vascular endothelial growth factor (VEGF) and transforming growth factor (TGFb) inhibit the differentiation of monocytes into dendritic cells (DC), as well as the maturation of DC precursors into immunocompetent mature DC. Cytokines like IL-10, IL-6, and monocyte colony stimulating factor (M-CSF), favor the differentiation of monocytes into M2 type macrophages, which, at the tumor site, may have pro-tumoral functions. (*See* Chapters 5, 8, 9, and 13 for further details).

Macrophages can produce proteases and strong evidence demonstrates that chemokines activate TAM to release MMPs in the tumor micro-environment (Fig.1). In particular, MMP9 derived from hematopoietic cells of host origin, has been shown to contribute to skin carcinogenesis *(100)*. In addition, MMP9 has complex effects beyond matrix degradation, including promotion of angiogenesis and release of growth factors *(106)*.

Angiogenesis is a key event in tumor growth and progression. Chemokines have a major impact on the regulation of neovascularization in tumor tissues (Table 2). The NH2-terminus of several CXC chemokines contains a highly conserved amino acid motif (Glu-Leu-Arg: ELR motif), which immediately preceeds the first cystein *(107–109)*. ELR+ chemokines have potent angiogenic activity. The angiogenic members include CXCL1 through CXCL8, with the exception of CXCL4. These chemokines act through a common receptor, CXCR2. Although some ELR+ chemokines bind both CXCR1 and CXCR2, it is widely accepted that only CXCR2 mediates the angiogenic activity and, accordingly, endothelial cells express only CXCR2 *(110)*. Another important ligand-receptor pair is CXCL12 and CXCR4. Even if CXCL12 is a non-ELR chemokine, its activity has been inplicated in neo-angiogenesis *(111,112)*. The importance of ELR+ chemokines in supporting angiogenesis during the neoplastic progression has been established in a variety of tumor cell types, including prostate and ovarian carcinoma and NSCLC *(113–116)*.

Both in mouse tumor models and in surgical specimens obtained from tumor patients, expression of CXCL5 and CXCL8 was associated with increased neovascularization and inversely correlated with survival. Conversely, depletion of CXCL5 resulted in attenuation of tumor growth and angiogenesis. The finding of the unique use of

Table 2
Regulation of Angiogenesis by Chemokines[a]

Promoting angiogenesis		
ELR*+ chemokines	CXCL1	
	CXCL2	
	CXCL3	
	CXCL5	
	CXCL6	
	CXCL7	
	CXCL8	
ELR- Chemokine	CXCL12	
Inhibiting angiogenesis		
ELR- chemokine	CXCL4	
	CXCL9	Interferon-inducible
	CXCL10	Interferon-inducible
	CXCL11	Interferon-inducible

[a]ELR: highly conserved amino acid motif defining a subgroup of CXC chemokines.

CXCR2 receptor, despite the redundancy of ELR+ chemokines, provides a good opportunity to target this receptor for therapeutic interventions.

On the other hand, another series of CXC chemokines lacking the ELR motif (non-ELR) are characterized by the ability to block or inhibit angiogenesis. The angiostatic members are CXCL4, CXCL9, CXCL10, and CXCL11. The three latter chemokines are interferon-inducible, and their biologic functions are directly relevant to the function of Th1 stimulating cytokines, like IL-12, IL-18, and IL-23, that induce the production of IFN-γ (109). CXCL9, CXCL10, and CXCL11 bind the CXCR3 receptor (1,108). Recent observation has demonstrated that CXCR3 exists in two different isoforms: CXCR3A and CXCR3B, which differ in their NH$_2$ terminus (117). CXCR3B, which is more expressed than CXCR3A in endothelial cells, appears to mediate the angiostatic activity of IFN-inducible chemokines. In addition, CXCL4 was shown to bind to CXCR3B (117).

Non-ELR CXC chemokines have been shown to inhibit angiogenesis in several tumor models. Over-expression of CXCL9 and CXL10 in tumor cells leads to spontaneous tumor regression in lymphoma cells (118,119), NSCLC (120) and melanoma (121).

Therefore, the balance of ELR+ vs non-ELR chemokines produced in the tumor microenvironment may determine the degree of angiogenesis surrounding and inside the tumor tissue and the consequent tumor progression.

Macrophages play a central role in tissue remodeling and repair during ontogeny and adult life. They exert a dual influence on blood vessel formation and function: on the one hand macrophages produce molecules that are pro-angiogenic, on the other hand they can express anti-angiogenic molecules and damage the integrity of blood vessels. In general, in the tumor micro-environment, the pro-angiogenic functions of TAM prevail (Fig. 1). TAM produce a host of growth factors that affect tumor cell proliferation, angiogenesis, and the deposition and dissolution of connective tissues. In several studies, TAM accumulation in human cancer has been associated with high neovascularization and with the production of angiogenic factors such as VEGF and platelet-derived endothelial cell growth factor, fibroblast and epidermal growth factor (EGF, FGF), and chemokines (10,40,43).

Uneven vascularization and hypoxia are characteristics of neoplastic tissues. TAM accumulate preferentially in the poorly vascularized regions of tumors with low oxygen tension. Under hypoxic conditions TAM are stimulated to express hypoxia-inducible genes, such as VEGF, bFGF and CXL8. Therefore, macrophages recruited *in situ* represent an indirect pathway of amplification of angiogenesis, in concert with angiogenic molecules directly produced by tumor cells.

5. TUMOR CELLS EXPRESS CHEMOKINE RECEPTORS

Chemokines act through specific 7-transmembrane receptors coupled to G proteins *(1)*. Whereas the expression of chemokines in human and experimental tumors had been the object of intense investigation, the expression of chemokine receptors has been pursued to a much lesser extent, until very recently.

Earlier studies already pointed out that tumor cells express functional chemokine receptors. Some tumor cell lines migrated in response to CXCL8 and related chemokines, and antibodies against CXCR2 were able to inhibit the growth of melanoma cells in vitro *(18)*. Other inflammatory chemokines have been tested and induced motility of malignant cells of hematopoietic and epithelial origin *(122,123)*. The most potent chemoattractants for human breast adenocarcinoma cell lines were CCL3, CCL4, CCL5, and CCL2.

Breast carcinoma cells also express CXCR4, the receptor for CXCL12, and this receptor has recently been implicated in the process of metastatization *(124)*. Since then, many other tumors of different histologies have been evaluated and shown to express chemotactic receptors (Table 3).

Although cancer cells may express different receptor repertoire, the most common receptor is, by far, CXCR4. Several different tumor types of hematologic, epithelial, and mesenchimal origin express this receptor. For instance CXCR4 was found in acute lymphoblastic and myeloblastic leukemia, in non-Hodgkin lymphoma, in tumors derived from the ovaries, lung, kidney, pancreas, and prostate, as well as in melanoma, neuroblastoma, and rhabdomyosarcoma *(8)*.

In addition to CXCR4, other receptors have been detected. In human pancreatic cancer, expression of CCR6 and its ligand CCL20, was reported *(24)*. Melanoma cells express CCR7, (receptor for CCL19 and CCL21) *(124)*. as well as CCR10 (receptor for CCL27) *(124)*. Gastric tumors express CCR7 and this receptor was associated with lymph node metastasis and poorer prognosis in two different studies *(125,126)*. In one retrospective analysis of patients with NSCLC, expression of CCR7 correlated with increased lymph node metastatic involvement *(127)*. These results found further support in experimental tumor models: transduction of tumor cells with CCR7 conferred improved ability to metastasize to regional lymph nodes *(128)*, whereas CXCR4-transfected celle preferentially migrated to the lung *(129)*. NSCLC also express CXCR4 *(130–132)*. In immunodeficient mice inoculated with CXCR4-positive human NSCLC, the administration of specific neutralizing anti-CXCL12 antibodies abrogated organ metastases *(133)*. Overall these results support the concept that chemokines and their receptors may be involved in the control of cancer dissemination.

Several lines of evidence show that the chemokine CXCL12 may also be involved in promoting tumor cell survival and growth. In several types of cancer, including glioma, melanoma, NSCLC, renal, and thyroid, CXCL12 can stimulate the proliferation and/or survival of CXCR4-expressing tumor cells *(8)*.

Table 3
Chemokine Receptors Expressed by Human Tumor Cells

Tumor type	Chemokine receptor expressed	
	Most frequent	*Other Receptors*
Breast	CXCR4	CCR7
Ovary	CXCR4	CCR9
Prostate	CXCR4	CCR9
Melanoma	CXCR4	CXCR3, CCR7, CCR10
NSCLC	CXCR4	CCR7

Production of CXCL12, both at mRNA and at protein level, has been detected in several tumors, including CXCR4-positive tumors, thus suggesting that autocrine or paracrine loops of growth may be feasible.

6. CONCLUSIONS

A complex network of chemokines and receptors exists in the tumor microenvironment. Chemokines are crucial determinant of the leukocyte infiltrate of tumors. Strong evidence suggest that tumor-associated macrophages may promote tumor progression via the release of angiogenic factors, proteolytic enzymes, and immune-suppressive molecules, which would enhance tumor growth, dissemination and evasion from immune control. In addition, ELR+ chemokines have direct angiogenic activity. Tumor cells themselves express chemokine receptors, in particular CXCR4, which possibly supports tumor cell survival and invasion.

If chemokine and receptor expression is an advantage for tumor cells, it is possible that these molecules will become target of therapeutic interventions. Chemokine and receptor antgonists are being developed and actively investigated. In several murine cancer models and in preliminary clinical studies, these molecules have shown activity both as inhibitors of leukocyte recruitment, as well as inhibitors of angiogenesis and metastatic spreading *(8,134–136)*.

The chemokine network definitely affects tumor development, but its ultimate significance is still poorly understood. Further studies in primary and metastatic tumors are needed, and will possibly lead to new approaches to treatment.

REFERENCES

1. Rossi D, Zlotnik A. The biology of chemokines and their receptors. Annu Rev Immunol 2000; 18:217–242.
2. Mantovani A. The chemokine system: redundancy for robust outputs. Immunol Today 1999; 20: 254–157.
3. Murphy PM, Baggiolini M, Charo IF, et al. International union of pharmacology. XXII. Nomenclature for chemokine receptors. Pharmacol Rev 2000; 52:145–176.
4. Rollins BJ. Chemokines. Blood 1997; 90:909–928.
5. Mackay CR. Chemokines: immunology's high impact factors. Nat Immunol 2001; 2:95–101.
6. Zlotnik A, Yoshie O. Chemokines: a new classification system and their role in immunity. Immunity 2000; 12:121–127.
7. Bottazzi B, Polentarutti N, Acero R, et al. Regulation of the macrophage content of neoplasms by chemoattractants. Science 1983; 220:210–212.
8. Balkwill F. Cancer and the chemokine network. Nat Rev Cancer 2004; 4:540–550.

9. Meltzer MS, Stevenson MM, Leonard EJ. Characterization of macrophage chemotaxins in tumor cell cultures and comparison with lymphocyte-derived chemotactic factors. Cancer Res 1977; 37:721–715.

10. Mantovani A, Sozzani S, Locati M, Allavena P, Sica A. Macrophage polarization: tumor-associated macrophages as a paradigm for polarized M2 mononuclear phagocytes. Trends Immunol 2002; 23:549–555.

11. Mantovani A. Chemokines in neoplastic progression. Semin Cancer Biol 2004; 14.

12. Mrowietz U, Schwenk U, Maune S, et al. The chemokine RANTES is secreted by human melanoma cells and is associated with enhanced tumour formation in nude mice. Br J Cancer 1999; 79: 1025–1031.

13. Luboshits G, Shina S, Kaplan O, et al. Elevated expression of the CC chemokine regulated on activation, normal T cell expressed and secreted (RANTES) in advanced breast carcinoma. Cancer Res 1999; 59:4681–4687.

14. Azenshtein E, Luboshits G, Shina S, et al. The CC chemokine RANTES in breast carcinoma progression: regulation of expression and potential mechanisms of promalignant activity. Cancer Res 2002; 62:1093–1102.

15. Haghnegahdar H, Du J, Wang D, et al. The tumorigenic and angiogenic effects of MGSA/GRO proteins in melanoma. J Leukoc Biol 2000; 67:53–62.

16. Richmond A, Thomas HG. Purification of melanoma growth stimulatory activity. J Cell Physiol 1986; 129:375–384.

17. Bordoni R, Fine R, Murray D, Richmond A. Characterization of the role of melanoma growth stimulatory activity (MGSA) in the growth of normal melanocytes, nevocytes, and malignant melanocytes. J Cell Biochem 1990; 44:207–219.

18. Norgauer J, Metzner B, Schraufstatter I. Expression and growth-promoting function of the IL-8 receptor beta in human melanoma cells. J Immunol 1996; 156:1132–1137.

19. Balentien E, Mufson BE, Shattuck RL, Derynck R, Richmond A. Effects of MGSA/GRO alpha on melanocyte transformation. Oncogene 1991; 6:1115–1124.

20. Owen JD, Strieter R, Burdick M, et al. Enhanced tumor-forming capacity for immortalized melanocytes expressing melanoma growth stimulatory activity/growth-regulated cytokine beta and gamma proteins. Int J Cancer 1997; 73:94–103.

21. Richards BL, Eisma RJ, Spiro JD, Lindquist RL, Kreutzer DL. Coexpression of interleukin-8 receptors in head and neck squamous cell carcinoma. Am J Surg 1997; 174:507–512.

22. Takamori H, Oades ZG, Hoch OC, Burger M, Schraufstatter IU. Autocrine growth effect of IL-8 and GROalpha on a human pancreatic cancer cell line, Capan-1. Pancreas 2000; 21:52–56.

23. Olbina G, Cieslak D, Ruzdijic S, et al. Reversible inhibition of IL-8 receptor B mRNA expression and proliferation in non-small cell lung cancer by antisense oligonucleotides. Anticancer Res 1996; 16: 3525–3530.

24. Kleeff J, Kusama T, Rossi DL, et al. Detection and localization of Mip-3alpha/LARC/Exodus, a macrophage proinflammatory chemokine, and its CCR6 receptor in human pancreatic cancer. Int J Cancer 1999; 81:650–657.

25. Mazzucchelli L, Blaser A, Kappeler A, et al. BCA-1 is highly expressed in Helicobacter pylori-induced mucosa-associated lymphoid tissue and gastric lymphoma. J Clin Invest 1999; 104:R49–54.

26. Yang J, Richmond A. Constitutive IkappaB kinase activity correlates with nuclear factor-kappaB activation in human melanoma cells. Cancer Res 2001; 61:4901–4909.

27. Dhawan P, Richmond A. A novel NF-kappa B-inducing kinase-MAPK signaling pathway up-regulates NF-kappa B activity in melanoma cells. J Biol Chem 2002; 277:7920–7928.

28. Richmond A. Nf-kappa B, chemokine gene transcription and tumour growth. Nat Rev Immunol 2002; 2:664–674.

29. Mantovani A, Bottazzi B, Colotta F, Sozzani S, Ruco L. The origin and function of tumor-associated macrophages. Immunol Today 1992; 13:265–270.

30. Negus RP, Stamp GW, Hadley J, Balkwill FR. Quantitative assessment of the leukocyte infiltrate in ovarian cancer and its relationship to the expression of C-C chemokines. Am J Pathol 1997; 150:1723–1734.

31. Negus RP, Stamp GW, Relf MG, et al. The detection and localization of monocyte chemoattractant protein-1 (MCP-1) in human ovarian cancer. J Clin Invest 1995; 95:2391–2396.

32. Monti P, Leone BE, Marchesi F, et al. The CC chemokine MCP-1/CCL2 in pancreatic cancer progression: regulation of expression and potential mechanisms of antimalignant activity. Cancer Res 2003; 63:7451–7461.

33. Valkovic T, Lucin K, Krstulja M, Dobi-Babic R, Jonjic N. Expression of monocyte chemotactic protein-1 in human invasive ductal breast cancer. Pathol Res Pract 1998; 194:335–340.

34. Ueno T, Toi M, Saji H, et al. Significance of macrophage chemoattractant protein-1 in macrophage recruitment, angiogenesis, and survival in human breast cancer. Clin Cancer Res 2000; 6:3282–3289.

35. Silzle T, Kreutz M, Dobler MA, Brockhoff G, Knuechel R, Kunz-Schughart LA. Tumor-associated fibroblasts recruit blood monocytes into tumor tissue. Eur J Immunol 2003; 33:1311–1320.

36. Van Damme J, Proost P, Lenaerts JP, Opdenakker G. Structural and functional identification of two human, tumor-derived monocyte chemotactic proteins (MCP-2 and MCP-3) belonging to the chemokine family. J Exp Med 1992; 176:59–65.

37. Balkwill F, Mantovani A. Inflammation and cancer: back to Virchow? Lancet 2001; 357:539–545.

38. Bottazzi B, Walter S, Govoni D, Colotta F, Mantovani A. Monocyte chemotactic cytokine gene transfer modulates macrophage infiltration, growth, and susceptibility to IL-2 therapy of a murine melanoma. J Immunol 1992; 148:1280–1285.

39. Jonjic N, Valkovic T, Lucin K, et al. Comparison of microvessel density with tumor associated macrophages in invasive breast carcinoma. Anticancer Res 1998; 18:3767–3770.

40. Leek RD, Lewis CE, Whitehouse R, Greenall M, Clarke J, Harris AL. Association of macrophage infiltration with angiogenesis and prognosis in invasive breast carcinoma. Cancer Res 1996; 56: 4625–4629.

41. Elgert KD, Alleva DG, Mullins DW. Tumor-induced immune dysfunction: the macrophage connection. J Leukoc Biol 1998; 64:275–290.

42. Pollard JW. Tumour-educated macrophages promote tumour progression and metastasis. Nat Rev Cancer 2004; 4:71–78.

43. Bingle L, Brown NJ, Lewis CE. The role of tumour-associated macrophages in tumour progression: implications for new anticancer therapies. J Pathol 2002; 196:254–265.

44. Hoshino Y, Hatake K, Kasahara T, et al. Monocyte chemoattractant protein-1 stimulates tumor necrosis and recruitment of macrophages into tumors in tumor-bearing nude mice: increased granulocyte and macrophage progenitors in murine bone marrow. Exp Hematol 1995; 23:1035–1039.

45. Huang S, Singh RK, Xie K, et al. Expression of the JE/MCP-1 gene suppresses metastatic potential in murine colon carcinoma cells. Cancer Immunol Immunother 1994; 39:231–238.

46. Rollins BJ, Sunday ME. Suppression of tumor formation in vivo by expression of the JE gene in malignant cells. Mol Cell Biol 1991; 11:3125–3131.

47. Nakashima E, Mukaida N, Kubota Y, et al. Human MCAF gene transfer enhances the metastatic capacity of a mouse cachectic adenocarcinoma cell line in vivo. Pharm Res 1995; 12:1598–1604.

48. Nesbit M, Schaider H, Miller TH, Herlyn M. Low-level monocyte chemoattractant protein-1 stimulation of monocytes leads to tumor formation in nontumorigenic melanoma cells. J Immunol 2001; 166:6483–6490.

49. Schutyser E, Struyf S, Proost P, et al. Identification of biologically active chemokine isoforms from ascitic fluid and elevated levels of CCL18/pulmonary and activation-regulated chemokine in ovarian carcinoma. J Biol Chem 2002; 277:24584–24593.

50. Strieter RM, Belperio JA, Phillips RJ, Keane MP. Chemokines: angiogenesis and metastases in lung cancer. Novartis Found Symp 2004; 256:173–184; discussion 184–188, 259–269.

51. Bonecchi R, Facchetti F, Dusi S, et al. Induction of functional IL-8 receptors by IL-4 and IL-13 in human monocytes. J Immunol 2000; 164:3862–3869.

52. Mule JJ, Custer M, Averbook B, et al. RANTES secretion by gene-modified tumor cells results in loss of tumorigenicity in vivo: role of immune cell subpopulations. Hum Gene Ther 1996; 7:1545–1553.

53. Niwa Y, Akamatsu H, Niwa H, Sumi H, Ozaki Y, Abe A. Correlation of tissue and plasma RANTES levels with disease course in patients with breast or cervical cancer. Clin Cancer Res 2001; 7:285–289.

54. Kunz M, Toksoy A, Goebeler M, Engelhardt E, Brocker E, Gillitzer R. Strong expression of the lymphoattractant C-X-C chemokine Mig is associated with heavy infiltration of T cells in human malignant melanoma. J Pathol 1999; 189:552–558.

55. Luster AD, Leder P. IP-10, a -C-X-C- chemokine, elicits a potent thymus-dependent antitumor response in vivo. J Exp Med 1993; 178:1057–1065.

56. Dobrzanski MJ, Reome JB, Dutton RW. Immunopotentiating role of IFN-γ in early and late stages of type 1 CD8 effector cell-mediated tumor rejection. Clin Immunol 2001; 98:70–84.

57. Sun H, Kundu N, Dorsey R, Jackson MJ, Fulton AM. Expression of the Chemokines IP-10 and Mig in IL-10 Transduced Tumors. J Immunother 2001; 24:138–143.

58. Pertl U, Luster AD, Varki NM, et al. IFN-γ-inducible protein-10 is essential for the generation of a protective tumor-specific CD8 T cell response induced by single-chain IL-12 gene therapy. J Immunol 2001; 166:6944–6951.

59. Yao L, Sgadari C, Furuke K, Bloom ET, Teruya-Feldstein J, Tosato G. Contribution of natural killer cells to inhibition of angiogenesis by interleukin-12. Blood 1999; 93:1612–1621.

60. Vicari AP, Ait-Yahia S, Chemin K, Mueller A, Zlotnik A, Caux C. Antitumor effects of the mouse chemokine 6Ckine/SLC through angiostatic and immunological mechanisms. J Immunol 2000; 165:1992–2000.

61. Nomura T, Hasegawa H, Kohno M, Sasaki M, Fujita S. Enhancement of anti-tumor immunity by tumor cells transfected with the secondary lymphoid tissue chemokine EBI-1-ligand chemokine and stromal cell-derived factor-1alpha chemokine genes. Int J Cancer 2001; 91:597–606.

62. Sharma S, Stolina M, Luo J, et al. Secondary lymphoid tissue chemokine mediates T cell-dependent antitumor responses in vivo. J Immunol 2000; 164:4558–4563.

63. Kirk CJ, Hartigan-O'Connor D, Nickoloff BJ, et al. T cell-dependent antitumor immunity mediated by secondary lymphoid tissue chemokine: augmentation of dendritic cell-based immunotherapy. Cancer Res 2001; 61:2062–2070.

64. Braun SE, Chen K, Foster RG, et al. The CC chemokine CK beta-11/MIP-3 beta/ELC/Exodus 3 mediates tumor rejection of murine breast cancer cells through NK cells. J Immunol 2000; 164:4025–4031.

65. Watanabe K, Jose PJ, Rankin SM. Eotaxin-2 generation is differentially regulated by lipopolysaccharide and IL-4 in monocytes and macrophages. J Immunol 2002; 168:1911–1918.

66. Bonecchi R, Bianchi G, Bordignon PP, et al. Differential expression of chemokine receptors and chemotactic responsiveness of type 1 T helper cells (Th1s) and Th2s. J Exp Med 1998; 187:129–134.

67. Gu L, Tseng S, Horner RM, Tam C, Loda M, Rollins BJ. Control of TH2 polarization by the chemokine monocyte chemoattractant protein-1. Nature 2000; 404:407–411.

68. Cossman J, Annunziata CM, Barash S, et al. Reed-Sternberg cell genome expression supports a B-cell lineage. Blood 1999; 94:411–416.

69. van den Berg A, Visser L, Poppema S. High expression of the CC chemokine TARC in Reed-Sternberg cells. A possible explanation for the characteristic T-cell infiltratein Hodgkin's lymphoma. Am J Pathol 1999; 154:1685–1691.

70. Iellem A, Mariani M, Lang R, et al. Unique chemotactic response profile and specific expression of chemokine receptors CCR4 and CCR8 by CD4(+)CD25(+) regulatory T cells. J Exp Med 2001; 194:847–853.

71. Yang TY, Chen SC, Leach MW, et al. Transgenic expression of the chemokine receptor encoded by human herpesvirus 8 induces an angioproliferative disease resembling Kaposi's sarcoma. J Exp Med 2000; 191:445–454.

72. Alcami A. Viral mimicry of cytokines, chemokines and their receptors. Nat Rev Immunol 2003; 3:36–50.

73. Sozzani S, Allavena P, D'Amico G, et al. Differential regulation of chemokine receptors during dendritic cell maturation: a model for their trafficking properties. J Immunol 1998; 161:1083–86.

74. Steinman RM, Hawiger D, MC. N. Tolerogenic dendritic cells. Annu Rev Immunol. 2003; 21:685–711.

75. Shortman K, Liu YJ. Mouse and human dendritic cell subtypes. Nature Rev Immunol 2002; 2: 151–161.

76. Lanzavecchia A, Sallusto F. Regulation of T cell immunity by dendritic cells. Cell 2001;106: 263–266.

77. Banchereau J, Paczesny S, Blanco P, et al. Dendritic cells: controllers of the immune system and a new promise for immunotherapy. Ann N Y Acad Sci 2003; 987:180–187.

78. Allavena P, Sica A, Vecchi A, Locati M, Sozzani S, Mantovani A. The chemokine receptor switch paradigm and dendritic cell migration: its significance in tumor tissues. Immunol Rev 2000; 177:141-9.

79. Vicari AP, Caux C. Chemokines in cancer. Cytokine Growth Factor Rev 2002; 13:143–154.

80. Bell D, Chomarat P, Broyles D, et al. In breast carcinoma tissue, immature dendritic cells reside within the tumor, whereas mature dendritic cells are located in peritumoral areas. J Exp Med 1999; 190:1417–1426.

81. Giannini A, Bianchi S, Messerini L, et al. Prognostic significance of accessory cells and lymphocytes in nasopharyngeal carcinoma. Pathol Res Pract 1991; 187:496–502.

82. Zeid NA, Muller HK. S100 positive dendritic cells in human lung tumors associated with cell differentiation and enhanced survival. Pathology 1993; 25:338–343.

83. Enk AH, Jonuleit H, Saloga J, Knop J. Dendritic cells as mediators of tumor-induced tolerance in metastatic melanoma. Int J Cancer 1997; 73:309–316.

84. Troy A, Davidson P, Atkinson C, Hart D. Phenotypic characterisation of the dendritic cell infiltrate in prostate cancer. J Urol 1998; 160:214–219.

85. Scarpino S, Stoppacciaro A, Ballerini F, et al. Papillary carcinoma of the thyroid: hepatocyte growth factor (HGF) stimulates tumor cells to release chemokines active in recruiting dendritic cells. Am J Pathol 2000; 156:831–837.

86. Schwaab T, Schned AR, Heaney JA, et al. In vivo description of dendritic cells in human renal cell carcinoma. J Urol 1999; 162:567–573.

87. Tsujitani S, Kakeji Y, Watanabe A, Kohnoe S, Maehara Y, Sugimachi K. Infiltration of dendritic cells in relation to tumor invasion and lymph node metastasis in human gastric cancer. Cancer 1990; 66:2012–2016.

88. Lespagnard L, Gancberg D, Rouas G, et al. Tumor-infiltrating dendritic cells in adenocarcinomas of the breast: a study of 143 neoplasms with a correlation to usual prognostic factors and to clinical outcome. Int J Cancer 1999; 84:309–314.

89. Zou W, Machelon V, Coulomb-L'Hermin A, et al. Stromal-derived factor-1 in human tumors recruits and alters the function of plasmacytoid precursor dendritic cells. Nat Med 2001; 7:1339–1346.

90. Reya T, Morrison SJ, Clarke MF, Weissman IL. Stem cells, cancer, and cancer stem cells. Nature 2001; 414:105–111.

91. Vermi W, Bonecchi R, Facchetti F, et al. Recruitment of immature plasmacytoid dendritic cells (plasmacytoid monocytes) and myeloid dendritic cells in primary cutaneous melanomas. J Pathol 2003; 200:255–268.

92. Salio M, Cella M, Vermi W, et al. Plasmacytoid dendritic cells prime IFN-γ-secreting melanoma-specific CD8 lymphocytes and are found in primary melanoma lesions. Eur J Immunol 2003; 33:1052–1062.

93. Ardavin C, Amigorena S, Reis e Sousa C. Dendritic cells: immunobiology and cancer immunotherapy. Immunity 2004; 20:17–23.

94. Schuler G, Schuler-Thurner B, Steinman RM. The use of dendritic cells in cancer immunotherapy. Curr Opin Immunol 2003; 15:138–147.

95. Steinman RM, Hawiger D, Nussenzweig MC. Tolerogenic dendritic cells. Annu Rev Immunol 2003; 21:685–711.

96. Vicari AP, Caux C, Trinchieri G. Tumour escape from immune surveillance through dendritic cell inactivation. Semin Cancer Biol 2002; 12:33–42.

97. Fioretti F, Fradelizi D, Stoppacciaro A, et al. Reduced tumorigenicity and augmented leukocyte infiltration after monocyte chemotactic protein-3 (MCP-3) gene transfer: perivascular accumulation of dendritic cells in peritumoral tissue and neutrophil recruitment within the tumor. J Immunol 1998; 161:342–346.

98. Fushimi T, Kojima A, Moore MA, Crystal RG. Macrophage inflammatory protein 3alpha transgene attracts dendritic cells to established murine tumors and suppresses tumor growth. J Clin Invest 2000; 105:1383–1393.

99. Giovarelli M, Cappello P, Forni G, et al. Tumor rejection and immune memory elicited by locally released LEC chemokine are associated with an impressive recruitment of APCs, lymphocytes, and granulocytes. J Immunol 2000; 164:3200–3206.

100. Egeblad M, Werb Z. New functions for the matrix metalloproteinases in cancer progression. Nat Rev Cancer 2002; 2:161–174.

101. Nagase H, Woessner JF, Jr. Matrix metalloproteinases. J Biol Chem 1999; 274:21,491–21,494.

102. Van den Steen PE, Dubois B, Nelissen I, Rudd PM, Dwek RA, Opdenakker G. Biochemistry and molecular biology of gelatinase B or matrix metalloproteinase-9 (MMP-9). Crit Rev Biochem Mol Biol 2002; 37:375–536.

103. Nagakawa Y, Aoki T, Kasuya K, Tsuchida A, Koyanagi Y. Histologic features of venous invasion, expression of vascular endothelial growth factor and matrix metalloproteinase-2 and matrix metalloproteinase-9, and the relation with liver metastasis in pancreatic cancer. Pancreas 2002; 24:169–178.

104. Krecicki T, Zalesska-Krecicka M, Jelen M, Szkudlarek T, Horobiowska M. Expression of type IV collagen and matrix metalloproteinase-2 (type IV collagenase) in relation to nodal status in laryngeal cancer. Clin Otolaryngol 2001; 26:469–472.

105. Locati M, Deuschle U, Massardi ML, et al. Analysis of the gene expression profile activated by the CC chemokine ligand 5/RANTES and by lipopolysaccharide in human monocytes. J Immunol 2002; 168:3557–3562.

106. Heissig B, Hattori K, Friedrich M, Rafii S, Werb Z. Angiogenesis: vascular remodeling of the extra-cellular matrix involves metalloproteinases. Curr Opin Hematol 2003; 10:136–141.

107. Strieter RM, Polverini PJ, Kunkel SL, et al. The functional role of the ELR motif in CXC chemokine-mediated angiogenesis. J Biol Chem 1995; 270:27348–27357.

108. Luster AD. Chemokines—chemotactic cytokines that mediate inflammation. N Engl J Med 1998; 338:436–445.

109. Strieter RM, Belperio JA, Phillips RJ, Keane MP. CXC chemokines in angiogenesis of cancer. Semin Cancer Biol 2004; 14:195–200.

110. Heidemann J, Ogawa H, Dwinell MB, et al. Angiogenic effects of interleukin 8 (CXCL8) in human intestinal microvascular endothelial cells are mediated by CXCR2. J Biol Chem 2003; 278: 8508–8515.

111. Bachelder RE, Wendt MA, Mercurio AM. Vascular endothelial growth factor promotes breast carci-noma invasion in an autocrine manner by regulating the chemokine receptor CXCR4. Cancer Res 2002; 62:7203–7206.

112. Salcedo R, Wasserman K, Young HA, et al. Vascular endothelial growth factor and basic fibroblast growth factor induce expression of CXCR4 on human endothelial cells: In vivo neovascularization induced by stromal-derived factor-1alpha. Am J Pathol 1999; 154:1125–1135.

113. Yoneda J, Kuniyasu H, Crispens MA, Price JE, Bucana CD, Fidler IJ. Expression of angiogenesis-related genes and progression of human ovarian carcinomas in nude mice. J Natl Cancer Inst 1998; 90:447–454.

114. Gawrychowski K, Skopinska-Rozewska E, Barcz E, et al. Angiogenic activity and interleukin-8 con-tent of human ovarian cancer ascites. Eur J Gynaecol Oncol 1998; 19:262–264.

115. Arenberg DA, Keane MP, DiGiovine B, et al. Epithelial-neutrophil activating peptide (ENA-78) is an important angiogenic factor in non-small cell lung cancer. J Clin Invest 1998; 102:465–472.

116. Veltri RW, Miller MC, Zhao G, et al. Interleukin-8 serum levels in patients with benign prostatic hyperplasia and prostate cancer. Urology 1999; 53:139–147.

117. Lasagni L, Francalanci M, Annunziato F, et al. An alternatively spliced variant of CXCR3 mediates the inhibition of endothelial cell growth induced by IP-10, Mig, and I-TAC, and acts as functional receptor for platelet factor 4. J Exp Med 2003; 197:1537–1549.

118. Sgadari C, Angiolillo AL, Cherney BW, et al. Interferon-inducible protein-10 identified as a media-tor of tumor necrosis in vivo. Proc Natl Acad Sci U S A 1996; 93:13,791–13,796.

119. Sgadari C, Farber JM, Angiolillo AL, et al. Mig, the monokine induced by interferon-γ, promotes tumor necrosis in vivo. Blood 1997; 89:2635–2643.

120. Addison CL, Arenberg DA, Morris SB, et al. The CXC chemokine, monokine induced by interferon-gamma, inhibits non-small cell lung carcinoma tumor growth and metastasis. Hum Gene Ther 2000; 11:247–261.

121. Feldman AL, Friedl J, Lans TE, et al. Retroviral gene transfer of interferon-inducible protein 10 inhibits growth of human melanoma xenografts. Int J Cancer 2002; 99:149–153.

122. Menten P, Saccani A, Dillen C, et al. Role of the autocrine chemokines MIP-1alpha and MIP-1beta in the metastatic behavior of murine T cell lymphoma. J Leukoc Biol 2002; 72:780–789.

123. Youngs SJ, Ali SA, Taub DD, Rees RC. Chemokines induce migrational responses in human breast carcinoma cell lines. Int J Cancer 1997; 71:257–266.

124. Muller A, Homey B, Soto H, et al. Involvement of chemokine receptors in breast cancer metastasis. Nature 2001; 410:50–56.

125. Mashino K, Sadanaga N, Yamaguchi H, et al. Expression of chemokine receptor CCR7 is associated with lymph node metastasis of gastric carcinoma. Cancer Res 2002; 62:2937–2941.

126. Yan C, Zhu ZG, Yu YY, et al. Expression of vascular endothelial growth factor C and chemokine receptor CCR7 in gastric carcinoma and their values in predicting lymph node metastasis. World J Gastroenterol 2004; 10:783–790.

127. Takanami I. Overexpression of CCR7 mRNA in nonsmall cell lung cancer: correlation with lymph node metastasis. Int J Cancer 2003; 105:186–189.

128. Wiley HE, Gonzalez EB, Maki W, Wu MT, Hwang ST. Expression of CC chemokine receptor-7 and regional lymph node metastasis of B16 murine melanoma. J Natl Cancer Inst 2001; 93:1638–1643.

129. Murakami T, Maki W, Cardones AR, et al. Expression of CXC chemokine receptor-4 enhances the pulmonary metastatic potential of murine B16 melanoma cells. Cancer Res 2002; 62:7328–7334.

130. Kijima T, Maulik G, Ma PC, et al. Regulation of cellular proliferation, cytoskeletal function, and sig-nal transduction through CXCR4 and c-Kit in small cell lung cancer cells. Cancer Res 2002; 62: 6304–6311.

131. Oonakahara K, Matsuyama W, Higashimoto I, Kawabata M, Arimura K, Osame M. Stromal-derived factor-1alpha/CXCL12-CXCR 4 axis is involved in the dissemination of NSCLC cells into pleural space. Am J Respir Cell Mol Biol 2004; 30:671–677.
132. Spano JP, Andre F, Morat L, et al. Chemokine receptor CXCR4 and early-stage non-small cell lung cancer: pattern of expression and correlation with outcome. Ann Oncol 2004; 15:613–617.
133. Phillips RJ, Burdick MD, Lutz M, Belperio JA, Keane MP, Strieter RM. The stromal derived factor-1/CXCL12-CXC chemokine receptor 4 biological axis in non-small cell lung cancer metastases. Am J Respir Crit Care Med 2003; 167:1676–1686.
134. Proudfoot AE, Buser R, Borlat F, et al. Amino-terminally modified RANTES analogues demonstrate differential effects on RANTES receptors. J Biol Chem 1999; 274:32,478–32,485.
135. Robinson SC, Scott KA, Wilson JL, Thompson RG, Proudfoot AE, Balkwill FR. A chemokine receptor antagonist inhibits experimental breast tumor growth. Cancer Res 2003; 63:8360–8365.
136. Zeelenberg IS, Ruuls-Van Stalle L, Roos E. Retention of CXCR4 in the endoplasmic reticulum blocks dissemination of a T cell hybridoma. J Clin Invest 2001; 108:269–277.

16 The Biology of Cancer Cachexia and the Role of TNF-α

Denis C. Guttridge

CONTENTS

1. INTRODUCTION

Cachexia, or wasting, is the most common syndrome resulting from human malignancies, estimated to contribute to nearly a quarter of all cancer deaths. Although cachexia has been clinically diagnosed for more than a century, it is only relatively recently that investigators have begun unraveling the molecular mechanisms underlying the wasting state that predominates in adipose and skeletal muscle tissues. Tumor necrosis factor-α, or TNF-α is considered a leading mediator or cancer cachexia. This cytokine is produced by tumor, immune, and stromal cells to provide a growth and survival advantage within the tumor microenvironment. It also functions in an autocrine and paracrine fashion in adipose and skeletal muscles to regulate tissue breakdown. TNF-induced fat catabolism is largely regulated through the feeding response and through the control of gene expression to differentiate and maintain the homeostasis of adipose tissue. Regulation of skeletal muscle catabolism in cachexia is regulated by the ubiquitin–proteasome system, whose activity may also be controlled by TNF. Elucidation of the TNF signaling pathway has provided further insight into the regulation of cancer cachexia. One effector of this pathway in particular, NF-κB, appears to be essential for TNF-mediated fat and skeletal muscle decay. Understanding the mechanisms by which NF-κB functions in cancer cachexia may reveal still other novel therapeutic targets of wasting that may be used in combination with currently existing anti-TNF therapy.

From: *Cancer Drug Discovery and Development,*
Cytokines in the Genesis and Treatment of Cancer
Edited by: M. A. Caligiuri and M. T. Lotze © Humana Press Inc., Totowa, NJ

2. FEATURES OF CANCER CACHEXIA

Cachexia derives from the Greek words, *kekos* that stands for "bad" and *hexis*, standing for "condition." This syndrome is most pronounced in end stage diseases that tend to associate with chronic inflammation, such as in cancer, AIDS, chronic heart failure, sepsis, tuberculosis, and severe burns *(1–3)*. Cachexia is a complex metabolic disorder, which is most often characterized as a wasting process resulting in severe weight loss. In actuality however, cachexia is more than simply weight loss. This disease state also encompasses features of anorexia, anemia, lipolysis, acute phase response, and insulin resistance. Unlike simple starvation, which causes the depletion of fat while preserving protein content mainly from skeletal muscle, in cachexia neither tissue is spared *(4)*. This may be one reason to explain why in cachectic patients, nutritional supplements alone are sufficient to restore transient weight gain through the accumulation of fat, but is mostly ineffective in restoring lean body mass *(5)*. The chronic consumption or wasting of muscle protein, combined with an absence of compensatory production of new protein, culminates in conditions of asthenia, immobility, and eventual death *(2)*. Cachexia is one of the most prevalent adverse effects of cancer. It has been estimated that over 50% of cancer patients suffer from cachexia, and 20% of mortalities are thought to result from cachexia complications rather than the direct tumor burden *(3,6)*. Weight loss as small as 5% of the usual body weight can significantly worsen prognosis. The wasting condition can also drastically lower tumor responsiveness to chemo and radiotherapy. Patients diagnosed as cachectic must therefore receive lower doses of treatment, and even under such conditions often develop dose-limited toxicity *(7)*.

The degree of cachexia and resulting decrease in lean mass appears to correlate tightly to tumor types that generally divide themselves into three classes *(8,9)*. The first class, represented by such cancers as lymphoma, sarcoma, and breast tumors, exhibit the smallest fraction of weight loss. In only a minority of patients suffering from these tumor types does weight loss exceed 10% of the original body weight before the onset of disease. The second class of tumors represented by colon, prostate, small cell and nonsmall-cell lung cancer promote greater than 10% weight loss in approx 15% of patients. However, tumor progression can eventually lead to enhanced loss of lean mass, and lung cancer patients have been reported to lose as much as 30% of their pre-illness stable weight. The third class, exhibiting the highest incidence of cachexia, is represented by upper gastrointestinal cancers such as pancreas and gastric. It has been estimated in these tumors over 30% of patients have greater than 10% reduction of body weight. One study has even reported that at time of diagnosis, 85% of patients with pancreatic carcinoma exhibited some degree of weight loss, and multiple cases were reported where patients lost 25% of their original body weight near time of death *(10)*. Perhaps not surprising, it is also this third class of tumor types that exhibit the lowest median survival rates. Why certain classes of tumors are more prone to developing cachexia is not clear, but this likely derives from the specificity as well as the concentration of cachectic factors produced from both tumor and host cells.

Cancer cachexia is foremost a metabolic condition that ensues as a direct consequence of the growth and survival of tumor cells. Tumor development is fueled at the expense of the host, thus creating an energy imbalance that underlies the wasting state *(11)* (Fig. 1). Glucose is the major source of fuel, which tumor cells obtain from the breakdown of adipose and skeletal muscle. Fat wasting or lipolysis generates free fatty

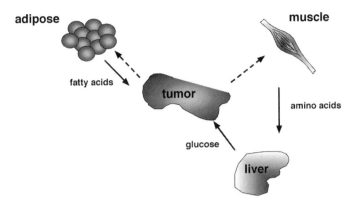

Fig. 1. Factors secreted from tumor cells induce the breakdown of adipose and skeletal muscle tissues releasing fatty acids and amino acids, respectively. These substances are used directly by the tumor or can be converted to glucose via the liver only to be reused by tumor cells.

acids and glycerol, which are directly used by the cancer cells, or otherwise converted to glucose to be subsequently reabsorbed by the tumor *(12,13)*. Because of insufficient oxygen, the Kreb cycle and oxidative phosphorylation are not favored processes in tumor cells. Rather, glucose is converted to lactate, which is then transported to the liver. There, the carbon skeleton is metabolized to resynthesize glucose, only to be imported back to the tumor (the Cori cycle). The free fatty acids that are also imported in tumor cells can be converted to prostaglandins or products of the lipoxygenase pathways that may serve as cofactors in the regulation of gene expression. Fatty acids can also function as stimulants for tumor growth by possibly providing anti-apoptotic activity to dividing cells.

Given that skeletal muscle is the most abundant tissue in the human body, it is understandable why that such a tissue would be used as a major fuel source for the benefit of a growing tumor. A minor fraction of this energy is provided by glucose, whereas the majority derives from amino acids resulting from the breakdown of myofibrillar proteins and from free pools that are not used owing to an inhibition in protein synthesis *(14)*. Of the amino acids transported from skeletal muscle, approx 50% are represented by glutamine and alanine *(15)*. Tumor cells use glutamine as a source of nitrogen for the synthesis of purine and pyrimidine bases, whereas it is thought that alanine is used as a vehicle of nitrogen transport. Other amino acids are recycled via the liver and converted to glucose, which essentially insures the continuing supply of energy to the tumor at the expense of the host.

3. MECHANISMS OF MUSCLE WASTING

Several mechanisms have been proposed to account for cancer induced muscle wasting. Wasting may first result from a reduced rate of protein synthesis, either from dietary restriction, or from the lack of available amino acid precursors that have been competed for from tumor cells *(3,16)*. The inhibition of protein synthesis may also result from a reduction of total RNA content. In one study, tumor induced muscle wasting in mice correlated with a 30% reduction in protein synthesis that was associated with a 20% decline in total RNA content *(17)*. However, whether RNA downregulation occurs by a transcriptional or post-transcriptional mechanism has yet to be fully defined.

Muscle catabolism may also result from the activation of several proteolytic pathways *(14,16)*. One is the lysosomal system, whereby endocytosed plasma proteins or membrane receptors undergo degradation by acid-activated cathepsin proteases B, H, and D. These enzymes may also be responsible for the degradation of cytosolic proteins that become taken up by autophagic vacuoles that are subsequently fused to lysosomes *(18)*. Although cathepsins have been shown to contribute to muscle breakdown, it remains argumentative whether these enzyme are truly involved in the breakdown of myofibrillar proteins, and little evidence exist to support their role in muscle wasting associated with cancer cachexia *(19)*. The second of these pathways functions in the cytosol and is referred to as the calcium-dependent calpain proteolytic system *(20)*. Calpains are calcium activated cysteine proteases which exist as m-calpain, μ-calpain, and the muscle specific form p94. The activity of these proteases is regulated by the inhibitor calpastatin *(21)*. Although a link between this pathway and muscle wasting has not formally been established, the regulation of p94 has been described in an experimental animal cancer cachexia model, and at least in sepsis-induced wasting, calpain activity was associated with the release of myofibrillar filaments from the sarcomere *(22)*.

The third, and by far the best studied of these proteolytic systems, is the cytosolic, ATP-dependent ubiquitin proteasome pathway *(3)*. This system is thought to play a prominent role not only in cancer cachexia, but has also been implicated in muscle wasting associated in sepsis, weightlessness, starvation, and denervation atrophy *(16)*. In this pathway, proteins are marked for degradation through the covalent binding of ubiquitin, a small heat-stable polypeptide. Conjugation of ubiquitin is regulated by ubiquitin E1-activating, E-2 carrier, and E-3 ligase enzymes, which regulate the polyubiquination of proteins marked for degradation *(23)*. Targeted degradation is regulated by the proteasome, a multimeric complex consisting of the central 20S catalytic core and the 19S terminal regulatory domains. Proteins entering the proteasome are cleaved by a cyclical "bite–chew" mechanism of proteolysis. These cleavage "bites" are regulated by the chymotrypsin-like activity of the 20S core, which is proceeded by the "chew" of a caspase like activity *(24)*. The major targets of degradation in muscle are thought to be the myofibrillar proteins. The four core myofibrillar proteins including, myosin heavy chain, actin, tropomyosin, and troponin, constitute the sarcomere or the basic contractile unit of skeletal muscle *(25)*. Multiple adjoining sarcomeres form myofibrils which multimerizes to fill a skeletal muscle fiber. Myosin heavy chain alone consists of 40% of myofibrillar proteins. Elegant in vitro studies were performed to demonstrate that each of core myofibrillar proteins served as substrates for ATP dependent proteasome degradation *(26)*. However, it was also shown that pre-assembled myofibrils were resistant to this degradative activity, suggesting that disassembly of the sarcomere is the rate-limiting step of ATP-dependent proteolysis. More recent work showed that release of the myofibril and their subsequent disassociation is a calcium–calpain-dependent process *(22)*. Isolated muscles from tumor-bearing animals have been shown to undergo proteolysis in an ATP-dependent fashion, which could be blocked by proteasome inhibitors *(27)*. Similar levels of proteolysis were not blocked by lysosomal or calcium inhibitors *(16)*. Furthermore, muscles from tumor-bearing animals showed an increased mRNA expression for ubiquitin and several subunits of the proteosome, whereas the overall RNA content in cachectic muscles decreased by approx 30% *(28)*. Taken together, these studies indicate that tumor regulated muscle wasting is largely dependent on the activity of the ubiquitin-proteosome pathway, but most likely also involves calcium dependent proteolysis and mechanisms regulating the inhibition of protein synthesis either at the transcriptional or post-transcriptional level.

4. CYTOKINES AS MEDIATORS OF CANCER CACHEXIA

Much of the past two decades of cancer cachexia research have been devoted to identifying the mediators of wasting, with the hope that this would lead us to novel and effective therapies for end-stage disease patients. To date however, this search continues and whether one or more cachectic factors are sufficient to initiate and sustain the wasting condition in human malignancies remains a point of controversy. Nevertheless, active research in this field has yielded the identification of several key mediators of cachexia that fall into two groups. The first are synthesized and secreted specifically from tumor cells, such as lipid mobilizing factor, that targets adipose tissue and degrades fatty acids, and proteolysis inducing factor (PIF) that induces protein degradation in skeletal muscle via the ubiquitin proteasome pathway (2,3). The second are pro-inflammatory cytokines, including TNFα, IL-1β, IL-6, and IFNγ, which are secreted from the tumor or more classically synthesized from immune cells in response to the tumor (1). In contrast to tumor-specific cachectic factors, the pro-inflammatory cytokines appear to contribute to cancer cachexia at multiple nodes. For the purpose of this chapter, focus will be placed on the regulation of cancer cachexia by pro-inflammatory cytokine TNF-α (previously designated cachectin, but here on referred to only as TNF).

5. TNF PRODUCTION IN CANCER

Macrophages are the predominant producers of TNF, but this cytokine is also expressed from a range of biologically diverse cell types including monocytes, fibroblasts, keratinocytes, adipocytes, skeletal myoblasts, and other cells that individually or in combination have been thought to influence the development of an oncogenic state (29–32). Secretion of TNF from the epithelial, stromal, or immune cell compartments may also function in autocrine and paracrine fashions. In the miroenvironment of tumor cell progression, TNF is thought to contribute to the growth and survival of these cells (32). This may occur through the activation of growth stimulatory signaling pathways such as MAP kinase (33), or can involve the PI3K/Akt survival pathway (34) shown to function through the NF-κB transcription factor to regulate anti-apoptotic gene expression (30,35). In addition, TNF can stimulate the secretion of chemokines that function in the recruitment of infiltrating immune cells (36), as well as the expression of metalloproteinases that function in the remodeling of the surrounding cellular matrix (37). At appropriate concentrations, TNF may also promote the expression of angiogenic factors that facilitate the transport of nutrients to the tumor milieu (38). The chronic expression of TNF from tumor and surrounding cell types allow systemic levels of TNF to rise and promote its pro-cachectic effects on distant tissues. The wasting of these tissues provide the needed nutrients to favor tumor progression. The mechanisms by which TNF induces wasting on adipose and skeletal muscle are described in Sections 5.1. and 5.2.

5.1. TNF Regulation of Adipocyte Metabolism

Adipose tissue represents one of the largest energy storage sites in the body. Similar to muscle, adipose homeostasis is thus largely dependent on the sustained balance between energy intake and energy expenditure (31). Intake is regulated by the import of free fatty acids from the circulation to adipose cells, and their subsequent conversion to triglycerides; a process referred to as lipogenesis. Expenditure, or lipolysis, breaks down triglycerides to glycerol and free fatty acids, which are secreted into the circulation to be used as energy sources for other tissues or reabsorbed into fat cells. In cachexia, the rate of energy expenditure vastly exceeds the rate of energy intake thus creating the wasting state *(1)*.

TNF has been shown to regulate adipose homeostasis at multiple nodes, which most likely explains why this cytokine is considered to be a leading mediator of hyperlipidemia and fat wasting in cancer cachexia (Fig. 2). Both in vitro and in vivo studies show that TNF inhibits fatty-acid uptake by suppressing the synthesis of lipoprotein lipase, which facilitate the import process *(39–41)*. TNF has also been found to decrease the expression of FATP and FAT proteins that also function in the transport of free fatty acids into adipose cells *(42)*. Another node of TNF action is its ability to prevent lipogenesis. Studies show that TNF down regulates the expression of key enzymes such as acetyl-CoA carboxylase *(43)* and fatty acid synthase *(44)* that function in the synthesis of triglycerides. Yet a third node of TNF action is its ability to stimulate lipolysis or breakdown of adipose tissue. Though in vitro and in vivo studies clearly support the role of TNF in degenerative process *(45,46)*, the molecular mechanisms underlying this regulation remains undefined. To date, there is little evidence to support that lipolysis is mediated through the induced expression of lipolytic genes responsive to TNF. In contrast, studies performed in fat cell cultures or in predifferentiated adipocyte cell lines show that TNF-mediated degeneration of fat correlates with the pronounced reduction of transcription factors such as PPARγ and C/EBPα *(47,50)*, whose functions are known to be essential for the maintenance of fat *(51,52)*. Such results infer that TNF-induced lipolysis results from the inhibition of mature adipose genes as a direct consequence of the reduction of their upstream regulators, PPARγ and C/EBPα. Indeed, treatment of cells with activators of PPARγ, such as thiazolinediones and 15dPGJ2, was demonstrated to block TNF-induced lipolysis *(53,54)*. How these drugs function in this capacity is not yet established, but it is likely to relate to the inhibition of TNF action rather than a direct increase in PPARγ activity, given that the addition of such compounds were shown to block the IκB kinase complex *(55)* recognized as an essential component of the TNF signaling pathway *(see* TNF Signaling Section 5.3.).

Although not as well studied, TNF-mediated lipolysis may also be related to the inability of pre-adipocytes to undergo differentiation in response to an injury signal. Studies, mainly using 3T3-L1 pre-adipocyte cultures, have shown that TNF is an extremely potent inhibitor of adipocyte differentiation *(31,45)*. Adipogenesis is regulated by a group of temporally expressed transcription factors that function in orchestrating the growth arrest, survival, and expression of fat specific genes required for differentiation *(52,56)*. To date, TNF has been shown to have its greatest effects on the downregulation of PPARγ and C/EBPα that not only sustain fat as mentioned above, but also known to be essential in the fat differentiation *(57,58)*. The induction of these transcription factors occurs relatively late in the differentiation program under the control of earlier expressed transcription factors, C/EBPβ, C/EBPδ, and SREBP1c/ADD1 *(59,60)*. Interestingly, regulation of these early expressed transcription factors has not been observed to be significantly affected by TNF treatment. This suggests that PPARγ and C/EBPα are direct targets of TNF action. However, because C/EBPα has been shown to regulate PPARγ expression *(61)*, it is possible that the downregulation of PPARγ by TNF is mediated through the inhibition of C/EBPα. Currently, the mechanism by which TNF suppresses

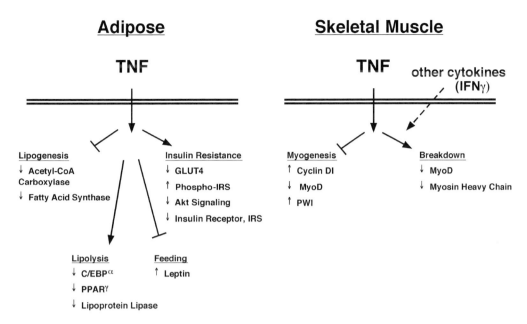

Fig. 2. TNF uses various mechanisms to induce adipose and skeletal muscle wasting. In adipose tissue, TNF modulates adipogenesis and feeding response while inducing lipolysis and insulin resistance. In skeletal muscle, TNF inhibits muscle differentiation or myogenesis, and alone or in the presence of other cytokines such as IFN-γ induces the breakdown of mature muscle by inhibiting the expression of muscle specific gene products.

C/EBPα transcription is not well defined, and it would be interesting to study how the levels of this transcription factor is potentially affected in mice lacking TNF expression.

Another node by which TNF is involved in cancer cachexia is how it effects feeding. Anorexia, or the loss of appetite, is a classic feature of cachexia, but as mentioned above is not a process in cachexia that is easily reversible by nutritional supplementation *(3)*. TNF is thought to directly impinge on feeding by controlling the expression of leptin. This hormone is expressed by fat cells and functions to reduce feeding response by acting through its receptor expressed in neurons of the hypothalamus *(62)*. Leptin knockout mice display an obese phenotype supporting the function of this hormone in feeding response. Leptin is also thought to function by suppressing the synthesis of a major anabolic effector in the hypothalamus, namely neuropeptide Y *(63)*. Several groups have observed that TNF can increase the production of leptin from fat cells *(64,65)*, which has led to the hypothesis that elevated levels of TNF in the circulation can promote an anorexic state by increasing leptin and concomitantly reducing levels of neuropeptide Y *(62)*.

Yet another node of TNF action relevant to adipocyte homeostasis and cancer cachexia is the involvement of this cytokine in the regulation of insulin resistance *(66)*. Here again studies support that TNF is capable of regulating this cellular process by multiple mechanisms that either individually or in combination result in the modulation of the insulin receptor and its signaling pathway. One of these mechanisms involves the reduction of GLUT4 expression, a protein that functions in glucose transport. A study performed using predifferentiated apidocyte cultures has shown that TNF-induced loss of GLUT4 expression occurs at the transcriptional level *(67)*, but the factors responsible for this transcriptional repression have not yet been identified. TNF may also act directly on the insulin receptor-signaling pathway. This can occur through the phosphorylation of the receptor substrate protein, IRS-1 (68). Post-translational modification of this protein inhibits the interaction of the insulin receptor with its binding partner, phosphotidylinositol (PI) 3-kinase, which entails leads to the loss of Akt/PDK activity (69). To date, the kinases involved in regulating the phosphorylation of IRS proteins are unknown, but some studies support the role of PKC and its various isoforms, such as PKCε, which were demonstrated to enhance TNF-mediated inhibition of insulin receptor signaling (70). There is also data suggesting that TNF can modulate insulin receptor signaling by causing the downregulated expression of the receptor itself or the IRS associated proteins (71).

5.2. TNF Regulation of Muscle Wasting

Although the role of TNF in muscle wasting is less established than that compared to adipocyte metabolism, there is nevertheless a substantial body of evidence to suggest that TNF is an important contributing factor of muscle wasting in cancer (Fig. 2). Early studies showed that chronic administration of recombinant TNF caused a reduction in muscle mass, which corresponded to a decrease in myofibrillar gene expression (72). Similar results were obtained in animals administered TNF producing tumor cells (73). The decline in muscle mass was shown to be specific to TNF because body weight could be sustained in mice lacking the TNF receptor (74).

Mechanistically, TNF is thought to induce muscle wasting by activating the ubiquitin/proteasome pathway. This activation is mediated at the RNA level of various genes of the ubtiquitin ligase and proteasome system. Administration of TNF in animals has been shown to induce the expression of ubiquitin, as well as genes coding for various subunits of the 19S proteasome complex (75). Similar results with respect to ubiquitin expression were obtained in cancer cachexia models (76,77) whose activity was shown to be associated with TNF (78). Validation that TNF regulates ubiquitin gene expression in vivo was demonstrated with using anti-TNF treatment (79) and by using mice deleted for the TNF receptor (74). Recently, a more direct role for TNF regulation of the ubiquitin/proteasome pathway was demonstrated. In both cultured myotubes and mouse muscles, investigators showed that TNF treatment caused the induction of the E2 ubiquitin ligase, UbcH2/E2(20k) (80). TNF regulation of UbcH2 was shown to occur at the RNA level. Furthermore, these same investigators showed that TNF was capable of inducing the polyubiquitination of whole muscle protein. Which muscle proteins are targeted for degradation by the ubiquitin/proteasome pathway in a TNF dependent manner has not been established. Owing to their abundance and functional relevance in muscle architecture, it has been largely presumed that such targets are the myofibrillar proteins, myosin heavy chain, actin, troponin and tropomyosin. Data showing that chronic administration of TNF in animals decreased myosin heavy chain expression (72), supporting the notion that TNF-dependent polyubiquitination of myosin heavy chain is possible, additional in vivo evidence is clearly required to validate these results.

An additional mechanism by which TNF may regulate muscle wasting is by modulating the ability of myogenic precursor cells to undergo differentiation. Approximately 5% of adult skeletal musculature is composed of quiescent satellite cells. In response to injury, these cells are activated and enter cell cycle to undergo several rounds of DNA division. It is believed that a set number of daughter cells re-enter a quiescent state while others are programmed to differentiate and replace myotubes lost during injury (81).

Using cultured myoblasts, several groups of investigators have demonstrated that TNF functions as a potent inhibitor of myogenesis, and various mechanisms have been proposed to account for such an activity *(82–84)*. One mechanism by which TNF blocks differentiation is by functioning as a mitogen. Myoblasts treated with TNF possessed a higher rate of proliferation compared to control cells, and were therefore unable to properly exit from cell cycle in response to differentiation conditions. TNF induced suppression of cell cycle withdrawal correlated with sustained levels of cyclin D1 *(85)*. TNF has also been shown to inhibit differentiation by suppressing the synthesis of the myogenic transcription factor, MyoD *(82)*. Proliferating myoblasts express MyoD in an inactive form. The switch to differentiation causes the activation of MyoD which leads to the induction of numerous genes important in the regulation of cell cycle arrest, fusion, and contractile function *(86,87)*. Estimates from recent microarray data suggest that MyoD directly regulates 1% of genes involved in skeletal myogenesis *(88)*. TNF was shown to downregulate MyoD at the RNA level, and this regulation was further demonstrated to be dependent on the NF-κB transcriptional factor *(82)* (*see* section on NF-κB below). Furthermore, TNF-mediated inhibition of differentiation was shown to be specific to MyoD because overexpression of this bHLH transcription factor rescued the TNF phenotype. Yet a third manner in which TNF prevents differentiation is through the activation of the PW1 protein *(89)*, which was shown to positively regulate the pro-apoptotic activity of predifferentiated myoblasts. Possibly in this mechanism, inhibition of differentiation occurs by a TNF-induced stress response controlled by the PW1 protein. Interestingly, the ability of TNF to suppress differentiation was abrogated in cells that lacked the pro-apoptotic gene, Bax. Furthermore, PW1 inhibition of differentiation in response to TNF was independent of NF-κB activation or the loss of MyoD. Collectively, these data demonstrate that TNF is capable of negatively regulating myogenesis by diverse mechanisms. However, whether this regulation of myogenesis is relevant in response to injury has recently come under question. Using a standard muscle injury model, investigators showed that rates of muscle regeneration were unaltered in TNF knockout mice *(90)*. If TNF indeed functioned as a negative regulator of differentiation, one would have predicted that the rate of regeneration would have increased in mice lacking this cytokine. Such data argue against a role for TNF in differentiation in response to injury. However, it is possible that inhibition of myogenic differentiation by TNF may manifest itself only in injury conditions associated with chronic inflammation, and not in a physiologic condition as currently tested. Under such an inflammatory condition, one may envision that persistent TNF production in the local environment of muscle cells would compromise the differentiation of newly formed myoblasts. It is also possible that TNF regulation of myogenesis occurs in embryogenesis or in early postnatal maturation of skeletal muscle. Similar regulation has been observed with the protein myostatin, which is known to induce severe muscle wasting, and whose expression has also been detected in early developing muscle cells *(91)*.

5.3. The TNF Signaling Pathway

To better understand the mechanisms by which TNF functions in adipose and skeletal muscle, it is important to understand the intracellular effectors that mediate the actions of this cytokine. Insight into the identification and biology of these effectors may lead to the development of drug targets for cancer cachexia. TNF is synthesized as a 24-kDa transmembrane protein, it is proteolyzed by the TACE protein to yield a soluble form of 17 kDa

(29). Intriguingly, both membrane and soluble forms are capable of regulating biologic response. TNF belongs to a family of cytokines whose immediate members include lymphotoxin, Fas ligand, receptor-activator of NF-κB ligand (RANKL), TNF-related apoptosis-inducing ligand (TRAIL), and CD40 *(92)*. Each of these cytokines function as homotrimers that recognize selective receptors to elicit diverse biologic responses (Fig. 3). TNF trimerization consists of 157 amino acids recognized by two distinct cell surface receptors, TNF-R1 and TNF-R2 *(93)*. These receptors differ in their cell type expression and association with intracellular signaling factors. In most cells, TNF action is mediated through its interaction with the TNF-R1. Binding of TNF to its receptor causes receptor trimerization that recruit adapter proteins to initiate the signaling pathway *(30,93)*. The TNF receptor-associated death domain (TRADD) protein is the first to be associated with TNF-RI, which functions to recruit additional adapter proteins, Fas-associated death domain (FADD), TNF receptor-associated factor-2 (TRAF2), and receptor-interacting protein (RIP). These proteins themselves recruit other factors that specify distinct branches in the TNF signaling pathway. For instance, FADD recruitment of caspase-8 to the TNF-R1 leads to the activation of the caspase cascade resulting in cellular apoptosis. TRAF-2 binding to TRADD recruits anti-apoptotic factors, c-IAP1 and c-IAP2 that function to modulate caspase activity, but also serve to activate the NF-κB transcription factor. Recently, the c-IAP2 protein was shown to function as an E3 ligase that is capable of polyubiquitination of the gamma or NEMO subunit of the IκB kinase complex (IKK), that itself directly activates NF-κB *(94)*. TRAF-2 also associates with mitogen-activated protein kinases (MAPK) triggering a cascade of MAPK activities resulting in the activation of p38 and JNK, the latter of which causes the phosphorylation of c-Jun in the AP-1 transcription complex *(30)*. Whereas NF-κB activation is only mildly affected in TRAF-2 deficient fibroblasts, JNK activation is completely abolished in these cells in response to TNF *(95)*. This suggests that other TNF-R1 adapter proteins are necessary for the activation of NF-κB. Indeed, one of these factors was identified to be the RIP protein, whose expression in cells was shown to be essential for TNF-mediated NF-κB activation *(96)*. Interestingly, although RIP contains a serine/threonine kinase domain, this activity is dispensable for NF-κB activation.

6. THE ROLE OF NF-κB IN CANCER CACHEXIA

Although TNF activation of JNK and p38 are likely to contribute in some aspect to cancer cachexia, most of TNF activity relevant to wasting appears to signal through NF-κB. The NF-κB transcription factor belongs to the Rel family of proteins that in mammalian cells consist of RelA (p65), c-Rel, RelB, p50 (derived from p105 precursor), and p52 (from the p100 precursor) *(35,97,98)*. Each of these proteins contain the Rel homology domain which specifies DNA binding, protein–protein interaction, and a nuclear localization sequence. In contrast to p50 and p52 subunits, RelA (p65), c-Rel, and RelB proteins contain transactivation domains in their carboxy-terminus. NF-κB activity is maintained as protein dimers, and although in vitro each of the subunits is capable of forming homo or heterodimers, in most cells NF-κB consists of a p50/p65 complex. NF-κB predominantly resides in the cytoplasmic compartment of cells, maintained as an inactive complex bound to its inhibitor protein IκB. These proteins function as inhibitors by masking the nuclear localization sequence within the Rel domain of NF-κB family members. Nuclear translocation, and thus activation of NF-κB, occurs through the degradation of IκB

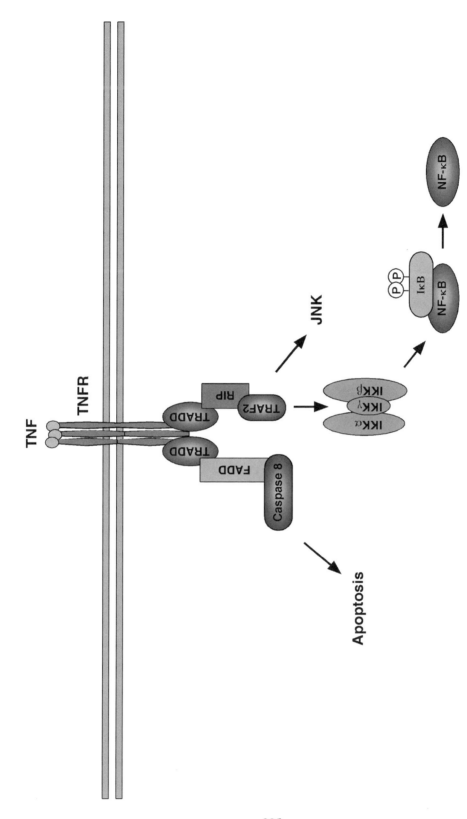

Fig. 3. TNF binding to its receptor induces the recruitment of TRADD (TNF receptor associated death domain), which leads to FADD (Fas associated death domain) binding and subsequent caspase 8 activation. Alternatively, RIP binding to TRADD recruits TRAF2, which activates JNK or NF-κB.

proteins, which as eluded to above is regulated by the IκB kinase (IKK) complex *(99)*. The activation of NF-κB occurs via IKK phosphorylation of IκB inhibitor proteins on two serine residues, causing polyubiquitination on neighboring lysine residues. These ordered post-translational modifications lead to IκB proteolysis by the 26S proteasome. Once in the nucleus NF-κB binds to its canonical DNA binding site and interacts with transcriptional co-activators to regulate gene expression *(100)*.

Recently, microarray analysis was performed using TNF treated predifferentiated adipocytes *(101)*. Most significant was that of the 142 genes found induced by TNF and of the 78 genes repressed by this cytokine, nearly every one was observed to depend on the activity of NF-κB. This data is consistent with a previously microarray study performed with TNF treated wild type or p65 null fibroblasts *(102)*. These works established for the first time the relevance of NF-κB activity in TNF signaling, and for adipose metabolism and its implication in cachexia, it provided strong evidence that this transcription factor was most likely to mediate many of the effects previously reported by TNF in vitro and in vivo.

Although similar microarray analyses have not been performed in TNF treated skeletal muscle, several groups have nevertheless demonstrated that TNFα inhibition of myogenesis is indeed mediated through the activity of NF-κB. The most plausible mechanism currently proposed is that this regulation occurs through the repressed synthesis of MyoD *(82)*. NF-κB inhibition of MyoD was shown to occur via the p65 subunit. Specifically, activation of p65 caused the destabilization of the MyoD mature mRNA. In addition, it was shown that this regulation required the transactivation function of the p65 subunit, and that p65 could not directly downregulate the MyoD transcript. Based on these results, the authors predicted that activation of p65 by TNF caused the induction of an unknown gene with possible RNase activity to cause the destabilization of MyoD transcripts. Loss of MyoD was shown to be sufficient for TNF mediated inhibition of differentiation. TNF has also been shown to modulate myogenesis by stabilizing cyclin D1 expression under differentiation conditions *(85)*. Cyclin D1 is itself a known negative regulator of skeletal muscle differentiation *(103)*. Because cyclin D1 was shown to be a transcriptional target of NF-κB *(85,104)*, it is likely that the activation of NF-κB by TNF is responsible for maintaining cyclin D1 expression in C2C12 myoblasts.

NF-κB may also contribute as a negative regulator of myogenesis through the synthesis of its own activator, TNF. The TNF gene contains NF-κB binding sites in its promoter and has been shown in several cell types to be regulated by NF-κB *(105–107)*. It is therefore possible that a positive feedback loop exists between TNF and NF-κB that may be relevant in the regulation of a cachectic state. Studies using cultured myotubes have clearly demonstrated that TNF-induced muscle damage requires the activity of NF-κB *(82,108)*. It was further demonstrated that activation of NF-κB in response to TNF is mediated through the production of reactive oxygen species *(109)*. Interestingly, investigators have demonstrated that chronic administration of TNF in nude mice led to muscle wasting that was reversible with antioxidant treatments *(73)*. Although NF-κB activity was not explored in this model, others have reported that inhibition of NF-κB activity in tumor cells could reduce the incidence of muscle cachexia *(110)*. In vivo, NF-κB activity has been shown to be elevated in skeletal muscles subjected to various forms of injury including ischemia/reperfusion *(111)*, disuse *(112)*, and mechanical stress of normal as well as dystrophin deficient muscles *(113)*. There is also evidence that absence of NF-κB activity in muscle fibers, owing to a defect in calpain 3 signaling, may contribute to pathophysiologic state of limb girdle muscular dystrophy *(114)*. Collectively, these data are highly consistent with the notion that NF-κB functions in cancer-induced muscle wasting.

7. CYTOKINES IN CANCER CACHEXIA

Whether TNF alone is sufficient to induce the cachetic phenotype in cancer remains in question. Certainly with relevance to adipose tissue, both in vitro and in vivo studies support the role of TNF in fat wasting. In regards to muscle wasting however, the consequence of chronic TNF signaling is less clear *(115)*. Although administration of TNF in animals leads to a reduction in muscle mass *(72,116)*, other investigators were unable to demonstrate any depletion in muscle protein when cultured muscle explants were treated with the cytokine *(117)*. TNF treatment of cultured myotubes was also seen to have little effect on the regulation of myosin heavy chain, a myofibrillar protein considered a standard marker of muscle wasting *(82,118)*. In contrast, other investigators using similar myotube cultures have reposted reductions of myosin levels by TNF *(108)*. Why such an apparent discrepancy exist is not yet clear, but it suggests that other pro-cachetic factors may function in addition to, or in combination with, TNF to regulate muscle wasting. Like TNF, chronic injection of IL-1 in animals was also shown to cause a redistribution of body proteins *(72)*. IL-6 has also been strongly implicated in regulating the cachetic phenotype in cancer *(119)*. This cytokine is known to regulate the expression of hepatic acute phase proteins, which themselves are considered cachetic factors of skeletal muscle. A clear role for IL-6 in cachexia was demonstrated using a tumor model of cachexia in IL-6 knockout mice. In this study, investigators reported a marked attenuation in wasting in these animals as compared to tumor bearing mice deleted in TNF, IL-1, or IFN-γ genes *(120)*. However, because inhibition of wasting was measured in body weight rather than in lean mass, it is difficult to interpret the essentialness of IL-6 for muscle wasting in this tumor model. In addition to these factors, tumors expressing IFN-γ *(121)* or LIF *(122)* also indicate a role of these cytokines in wasting. However, whether these cytokines alone are sufficient to induce both fat and skeletal muscle breakdown remains enigmatic. Evidence of cytokine synergism was demonstrated on cultured myotubes and intact muscles treated with TNF and IFN-γ *(82,118)*. The addition of these factors at physiologic concentrations caused the pronounced reduction of myosin heavy chain as well as MyoD (Fig. 2), but not other myofibrillar proteins, α-actin, troponin, or tropomyosin *(123)*. In contrast, combinatorial treatments of TNF with either IL-1 or IL-6 had relatively little effect on myosin levels, which suggested that muscle breakdown is highly dependent on which combinations of cytokines are present in the muscle microenvironment. Importantly, the regulation of myosin by TNF plus IFN-γ required NF-κB activity. Thus, NF-κB appears to play several roles in muscle decay. On one hand its activation by TNF in myoblasts is sufficient to suppress MyoD expression to inhibit the maturation of these cells. On the other hand, its activation by TNF and IFN-γ promotes myofibrillar protein loss. Recently, it was discovered that TNF treatment in myotubes was sufficient to sustain NF-κB activity *(118)*. This implies that NF-κB is required but not sufficient to mediate the cachetic effects of TNF and IFN-γ. This cooperative factor of NF-κB has yet to be elucidated, but it is likely to involve STAT proteins which are known to be tightly regulated by IFN-γ.

8. SUMMARY

Since the discovery of TNF or cachectin in the early 1980's, much has been learned regarding how this pleotropically acting cytokine participates in whole body wasting. Studies in culture as well as in animals have revealed the anti-adipogenic and antimyogenic activities of TNF. It is believed that TNF alone has the ability to control fat metabolism by effecting feeding, modulating adipogenesis, and promoting insulin resistance and lipolysis. For muscle, in vitro evidence suggest that TNF is sufficient to block muscle differentiation, but it is less clear whether other factors, possibly cytokines, are required in addition to TNF to stimulate muscle decay. Given these activities and its association in cancer, there is good reason to classify TNF as a leading mediator of cachexia and a genuine therapeutic target. Anti-TNF therapy has proved success in such chronic inflammatory disease states as Crohn disease and rheumatoid arthritis *(123)*. The efficacy of two drugs in particular, infliximab and etanercept, have been validated in clinical trial studies for these types of diseases. Infliximab is an IgG chimeric mouse-human chimeric antibody against TNF, whereas etanercept is a fusion protein between the human TNF receptor and a human IgG. The elucidation of the TNF receptor signaling pathway, and the specific effectors that are thought to regulate the cachectic phenotype provide novel targets for cancer cachexia treatment. Compounds such as inhibitors to the IKK proteins are currently available *(124,125)*, and their potential benefit in cachexia treatment, along with anti-TNF therapies, should be addressable in the near future.

REFERENCES

1. Argiles JM, Lopez-Soriano FJ. The role of cytokines in cancer cachexia. Med. Res. Rev. 1999; 19:223–248.
2. Tisdale MJ. Biology of cachexia. J. Nat. Cancer Instit. 1997; 89:1763–1773.
3. Tisdale MJ. Cachexia in cancer patients. Nature Rev. Cancer 2002; 2:862–871.
4. Body JJ. The Syndrome of Anorexia-Cachexia. Curr. Opin. Oncol. 1999; 11:255–260.
5. Evans WK, Makuch R, Clamon GH, et al. Limited impact of total parenteral nutrition on nutritional status during treatment for small cell lung cancer. Cancer R. 1985; 45:3347–3353.
6. van Eys J. Nutrition and cancer: physiological interrelationships. Annu. Rev. Nutr. 1985; 5:435–461.
7. Andreyev HJ, Norman AR, Oates J, Cunningham D. Why do patients with weight loss have a worse outcome when undergoing chemotherapy for gastrointestinal malignancies? Eur. J. Cancer 1998; 34:503–509.
8. Dewys WD, Begg C, Lavin PT, et al. Prognostic effect of weight loss prior to chemotherapy in cancer patients. Eastern Cooperative Oncology Group. Am. J. Med. 1980; 69:491–497.
9. DeWys W. Management of cancer cachexia. Semin. Oncol. 1985; 12:452–460.
10. Wigmore SJ, Plester CE, Richardson RA, Fearon KC. Changes in nutritional status associated with unresectable pancreatic cancer. Br. J. Cancer 1997; 75:106–109.
11. Giordano A, Calvani M, Petillo O, Carteni M, Melone MR, Peluso G. Skeletal muscle metabolism in physiology and in cancer disease. J. Cell. Biochem. 2003; 90:170–186.
12. Beutler B, Greenwald D, Hulmes JD, et al. Identity of tumour necrosis factor and the macrophage-secreted factor cachectin. Nature 1985; 316:552–554.
13. Beutler B. Cachexia: a fundamental mechanism. Nut. Rev. 1988; 46:369–373.
14. Hasselgren PO, Fischer JE. Muscle cachexia: current concepts of intracellular mechanisms and molecular regulation. Ann. Sur. 2001; 233:9–17.
15. Felig P. Amino acid metabolism in man. Ann. Rev. Biochem. 1975; 44:933–955.
16. Lecker SH, Solomon V, Mitch WE, Goldberg AL. Muscle protein breakdown and the critical role of the ubiquitin-proteasome pathway in normal and disease states. J. Nut. 1999; 129:227S–237S.
17. Emery PW, Lovell L, Rennie MJ. Protein synthesis measured in vivo in muscle and liver of cachectic tumor-bearing mice. Cancer Res. 1984; 44:2779–2784.

18. Dice JF. Peptide sequences that target cytosolic proteins for lysosomal proteolysis. Tren. Biochem. Sci. 1990; 15:305–309.
19. Jagoe RT, Redfern CP, Roberts RG, Gibson GJ, Goodship TH. Skeletal muscle mRNA levels for cathepsin B, but not components of the ubiquitin-proteasome pathway, are increased in patients with lung cancer referred for thoracotomy. Clin. Sci. 2002; 102:353–361.
20. Huang J, Forsberg NE. Role of calpain in skeletal-muscle protein degradation. Proc. Nat. Acad. Sci. USA 1998; 95:12,100–12,105.
21. Murachi T, Tanaka K, Hatanaka M, Murakami T. Intracellular Ca2+-dependent protease (calpain) and its high-molecular-weight endogenous inhibitor (calpastatin). Advances Enz. Reg. 1980; 19:407–424.
22. Williams AB, Decourten-Myers GM, Fischer JE, Luo G, Sun X, Hasselgren PO. Sepsis stimulates release of myofilaments in skeletal muscle by a calcium-dependent mechanism. FASEB J. 1999; 13:1435–1443.
23. Ciechanover HA. The ubiquitin system. Ann. Rev. Biochem. 1998; 67:425–479.
24. Kisselev AF, Akopian TN, Castillo V, Goldberg AL. Proteasome active sites allosterically regulate each other, suggesting a cyclical bite-chew mechanism for protein breakdown. Mol. Cell 1999; 4:395–402.
25. Clark KA, McElhinny AS, Beckerle MC, Gregorio CC. Striated muscle cytoarchitecture: an intricate web of form and function. Ann. Rev. Cell Dev. Biol. 2002; 18:637–706.
26. Solomon V, Goldberg AL. Importance of the ATP-ubiquitin-proteasome pathway in the degradation of soluble and myofibrillar proteins in rabbit muscle extracts. J. Biol. Chem. 1996; 271: 26,690–26,697.
27. Tawa NE, Jr., Odessey R, Goldberg AL. Inhibitors of the proteasome reduce the accelerated proteolysis in atrophying rat skeletal muscles. J. Clin. Invest. 1997; 100:197–203.
28. Baracos VE, DeVivo C, Hoyle DH, Goldberg AL. Activation of the ATP-ubiquitin-proteasome pathway in skeletal muscle of cachectic rats bearing a hepatoma. Am. J. Physiol. 1995; 268:E996–1006.
29. Tracey KJ, Cerami A. Tumor necrosis factor: a pleiotropic cytokine and therapeutic target. Ann. Rev. of Med. 1994; 45:491–503.
30. Baud V, Karin M. Signal transduction by tumor necrosis factor and its relatives. Tren. Cell Biol. 2001; 11:372–377.
31. Sethi JK, Hotamisligil GS. The role of TNF alpha in adipocyte metabolism. Sem. Cell Dev. Biol. 1999; 10:19–29.
32. Wilson J, Balkwill F. The role of cytokines in the epithelial cancer microenvironment. Sem. Cancer Biol. 2002; 12:113–120.
33. Kan H, Xie Z, Finkel MS. TNF-α enhances cardiac myocyte NO production through MAP kinase-mediated NF-κB activation. Am. J. Phy. 1999; 277:H1641–1646.
34. Sandra F, Matsuki NA, Takeuchi H, et al. TNF inhibited the apoptosis by activation of Akt serine/threonine kinase in the human head and neck squamous cell carcinoma. Cell. Sig. 2002; 14:771–778.
35. Baldwin AS. Control of oncogenesis and cancer therapy resistance by the transcription factor NF-κB. J Clin Invest. 2001; 107:241–246.
36. Negus RP, Turner L, Burke F, Balkwill FR. Hypoxia down-regulates MCP-1 expression: implications for macrophage distribution in tumors. J. Leuko. Biol. 1998; 63:758–765.
37. Leber TM, Balkwill FR. Regulation of monocyte MMP-9 production by TNF-α and a tumour-derived soluble factor (MMPSF). Br. J. Cancer 1998; 78:724–732.
38. Fajardo LF, Kwan HH, Kowalski J, Prionas SD, Allison AC. Dual role of tumor necrosis factor-α in angiogenesis. Am. J. Path. 1992; 140:539–544.
39. Hauner H, Petruschke T, Russ M, Rohrig K, Eckel J. Effects of tumour necrosis factor alpha (TNF alpha) on glucose transport and lipid metabolism of newly-differentiated human fat cells in cell culture. Diabetologia 1995; 38:764–771.
40. Cornelius P, Enerback S, Bjursell G, Olivecrona T, Pekala PH. Regulation of lipoprotein lipase mRNA content in 3T3-L1 cells by tumour necrosis factor. Biochem. J. 1988; 249:765–769.
41. Semb H, Peterson J, Tavernier J, Olivecrona T. Multiple effects of tumor necrosis factor on lipoprotein lipase in vivo. J. Biol. Chem. 1987; 262:8390–8394.
42. Memon RA, Feingold KR, Moser AH, Fuller J, Grunfeld C. Regulation of fatty acid transport protein and fatty acid translocase mRNA levels by endotoxin and cytokines. Am. J. Physiol. 1998; 274:E210–217.
43. Pape ME, Kim KH. Effect of tumor necrosis factor on acetyl-coenzyme A carboxylase gene expression and preadipocyte differentiation. Mol. Endo. 1988; 2:395–403.

44. Doerrler W, Feingold KR, Grunfeld C. Cytokines induce catabolic effects in cultured adipocytes by multiple mechanisms. Cytokine 1994; 6:478–484.

45. Torti FM, Dieckmann B, Beutler B, Cerami A, Ringold GM. A macrophage factor inhibits adipocyte gene expression: an in vitro model of cachexia. Science 1985; 229:867–869.

46. Oliff A, Defeo-Jones D, Boyer M, et al. Tumors secreting human TNF/cachectin induce cachexia in mice. Cell 1987; 50:555–563.

47. Meng L, Zhou J, Sasano H, Suzuki T, Zeitoun KM, Bulun SE. Tumor necrosis factor alpha and inter-leukin 11 secreted by malignant breast epithelial cells inhibit adipocyte differentiation by selectively down-regulating CCAAT/enhancer binding protein alpha and peroxisome proliferator-activated receptor gamma: mechanism of desmoplastic reaction. Cancer R. 2001; 61:2250–2255.

48. Xing H, Northrop JP, Grove JR, Kilpatrick KE, Su JL, Ringold GM. TNF alpha-mediated inhibition and reversal of adipocyte differentiation is accompanied by suppressed expression of PPARgamma without effects on Pref-1 expression. Endocrinol. 1997; 138:2776–2783.

49. Zhang B, Berger J, Hu E, et al. Negative regulation of peroxisome proliferator-activated receptor-gamma gene expression contributes to the antiadipogenic effects of tumor necrosis factor-α. Mol. Endocrinol. 1996; 10:1457–1466.

50. Ron D, Brasier AR, McGehee RE, Jr., Habener JF. Tumor necrosis factor-induced reversal of adipocytic phenotype of 3T3-L1 cells is preceded by a loss of nuclear CCAAT/enhancer binding pro-tein (C/EBP). J. Clin. Invest. 1992; 89:223–233.

51. Rosen ED, Sarraf P, Troy AE, et al. PPAR gamma is required for the differentiation of adipose tissue in vivo and in vitro. Mol. Cell 1999; 4:611–617.

52. Rosen ED, Walkey CJ, Puigserver P, Spiegelman BM. Transcriptional regulation of adipogenesis. Genes Dev. 2000; 14:1293–1307.

53. Feingold KR, Doerrler W, Dinarello CA, Fiers W, Grunfeld C. Stimulation of lipolysis in cultured fat cells by tumor necrosis factor, interleukin-1, and the interferons is blocked by inhibition of prostaglandin synthesis. Endocrinol. 1992; 130:10–16.

54. Souza SC, Yamamoto MT, Franciosa MD, Lien P, Greenberg AS. BRL 49653 blocks the lipolytic actions of tumor necrosis factor-α: A potential new insulin-sensitizing mechanism for thiazolidine-diones. Diabetes 1998; 47:691–695.

55. Straus DS, Pascual G, Li M, et al. 15-deoxy-delta 12,14-prostaglandin J2 inhibits multiple steps in the NF-κ B signaling pathway. Pro. Nat. Acad. Sci., USA 2000; 97:4844–4849.

56. Hwang CS, Loftus TM, Mandrup S, Lane MD. Adipocyte differentiation and leptin expression. Ann. Rev. Cell Dev. Biol. 1997; 13:231–259.

57. Lowell BB. PPARgamma: an essential regulator of adipogenesis and modulator of fat cell function. Cell 1999; 99:239–242.

58. Wang ND, Finegold MJ, Bradley A, et al. Impaired energy homeostasis in C/EBP alpha knockout mice. Science 1995; 269:1108–1112.

59. Yeh WC, Cao Z, Classon M, McKnight SL. Cascade regulation of terminal adipocyte differentiation by three members of the C/EBP family of leucine zipper proteins. Genes Dev. 1995; 9:168–181.

60. Kim JB, Spiegelman BM. ADD1/SREBP1 promotes adipocyte differentiation and gene expression linked to fatty acid metabolism. Genes Dev. 1996; 10:1096–1107.

61. Wu Z, Rosen ED, Brun R, et al. Cross-regulation of C/EBP alpha and PPAR gamma controls the tran-scriptional pathway of adipogenesis and insulin sensitivity. Mol. Cell 1999; 3:151–158.

62. Loftus TM. An adipocyte-central nervous system regulatory loop in the control of adipose homeosta-sis. Sem. Cell Dev. Biol. 1999; 10:11–18.

63. Schwartz MW, Baskin DG, Bukowski TR, et al. Specificity of leptin action on elevated blood glucose levels and hypothalamic neuropeptide Y gene expression in ob/ob mice. Diabetes 1996; 45:531–535.

64. Grunfeld C, Zhao C, Fuller J, et al. Endotoxin and cytokines induce expression of leptin, the ob gene product, in hamsters. J. Clin. Invest. 1996; 97:2152–2157.

65. Kirchgessner TG, Uysal KT, Wiesbrock SM, Marino MW, Hotamisligil GS. Tumor necrosis factor-α contributes to obesity-related hyperleptinemia by regulating leptin release from adipocytes. J. Clin. Invest. 1997; 100:2777–2782.

66. McCall JL, Tuckey JA, Parry BR. Serum tumour necrosis factor alpha and insulin resistance in gas-trointestinal cancer. Br. J. Sur. 1992; 79:1361–1363.

67. Stephens JM, Pekala PH. Transcriptional repression of the C/EBP-α and GLUT4 genes in 3T3-L1 adipocytes by tumor necrosis factor-α. Regulations is coordinate and independent of protein synthe-sis. J. Biol. Chem. 1992; 267:13580–13584.

68. Hotamisligil GS, Peraldi P, Budavari A, Ellis R, White MF, Spiegelman BM. IRS-1-mediated inhibition of insulin receptor tyrosine kinase activity in TNF-α- and obesity-induced insulin resistance. Science 1996; 271:665–668.

69. Hotamisligil GS, Murray DL, Choy LN, Spiegelman BM. Tumor necrosis factor alpha inhibits signaling from the insulin receptor. Proc. Nat. Acad. Sci., USA 1994; 91:4854–4858.

70. Kellerer M, Mushack J, Mischak H, Haring HU. Protein kinase C (PKC) epsilon enhances the inhibitory effect of TNF alpha on insulin signaling in HEK293 cells. FEBS Lett. 1997; 418:119–122.

71. Stephens JM, Lee J, Pilch PF. Tumor necrosis factor-α-induced insulin resistance in 3T3-L1 adipocytes is accompanied by a loss of insulin receptor substrate-1 and GLUT4 expression without a loss of insulin receptor-mediated signal transduction. J. Biol. Chem. 1997; 272:971–976.

72. Fong Y, Moldawer LL, Marano M, et al. Cachectin/TNF or IL-1 alpha induces cachexia with redistribution of body proteins. Amer. J. Physiol. 1989; 256:R659–665.

73. Buck M, Chojkier M. Muscle wasting and dedifferentiation induced by oxidative stress in a murine model of cachexia is prevented by inhibitors of nitric oxide synthesis and antioxidants. EMBO J. 1996; 15:1753–1765.

74. Llovera M, Garcia-Martinez C, Lopez-Soriano J, et al. Role of TNF receptor 1 in protein turnover during cancer cachexia using gene knockout mice. Mol. Cell. Endo. 1998; 142:183–189.

75. Llovera M, Garcia-Martinez C, Agell N, Lopez-Soriano FJ, Argiles JM. TNF can directly induce the expression of ubiquitin-dependent proteolytic system in rat soleus muscles. Biochem. Biophy. Res. Comm. 1997; 230:238–241.

76. Llovera M, Garcia-Martinez C, Agell N, Marzabal M, Lopez-Soriano FJ, Argiles JM. Ubiquitin gene expression is increased in skeletal muscle of tumour-bearing rats. FEBS Lett. 1994; 338:311–318.

77. Llovera M, Garcia-Martinez C, Agell N, Lopez-Soriano FJ, Argiles JM. Muscle wasting associated with cancer cachexia is linked to an important activation of the ATP-dependent ubiquitin-mediated proteolysis. Int. J. Cancer 1995; 61:138–141.

78. Garcia-Martinez C, Llovera M, Agell N, Lopez-Soriano FJ, Argiles JM. Ubiquitin gene expression in skeletal muscle is increased by tumour necrosis factor-α. Biochem. Biophys. Res. Commun. 1994; 201:682–686.

79. Costelli P, Carbo N, Tessitore L, et al. Tumor necrosis factor-α mediates changes in tissue protein turnover in a rat cancer cachexia model. J. Clin. Invest. 1993; 92:2783–2789.

80. Li YP, Lecker SH, Chen Y, Waddell ID, Goldberg AL, Reid MB. TNF-α increases ubiquitin-conjugating activity in skeletal muscle by up-regulating UbcH2/E220k. FASEB J. 2003; 17:1048–1057.

81. Seale P, Rudnicki MA. A new look at the origin, function, and "stem-cell" status of muscle satellite cells. Dev. Biol. 2000; 218:115–124.

82. Guttridge DC, Mayo MW, Madrid LV, Wang CY, Baldwin AS, Jr. NF-κB-induced loss of MyoD messenger RNA: possible role in muscle decay and cachexia.[see comment]. Science 2000; 289:2363–2366.

83. Langen RC, Schols AM, Kelders MC, Wouters EF, Janssen-Heininger YM. Inflammatory cytokines inhibit myogenic differentiation through activation of nuclear factor-κB. FASEB J. 2001; 15:1169–1180.

84. Layne MD, Farmer SR. Tumor necrosis factor-α and basic fibroblast growth factor differentially inhibit the insulin-like growth factor-I induced expression of myogenin in C2C12 myoblasts. Exper. Cell R. 1999; 249:177–187.

85. Guttridge DC, Albanese C, Reuther JY, Pestell RG, Baldwin AS, Jr. NF-κB controls cell growth and differentiation through transcriptional regulation of cyclin D1. Mol. Cell. Biol. 1999; 19:5785–5799.

86. Lassar AB, Skapek SX, Novitch B. Regulatory mechanisms that coordinate skeletal muscle differentiation and cell cycle withdrawal. Curr. Opin. Cell Biol. 1994; 6:788–794.

87. Black BL, Olson EN. Transcriptional control of muscle development by myocyte enhancer factor-2 (MEF2) proteins. Annu. Rev. Cell Dev. Biol. 1998; 14:167–196.

88. Bergstrom DA, Penn BH, Strand A, Perry RL, Rudnicki MA, Tapscott SJ. Promoter-specific regulation of MyoD binding and signal transduction cooperate to pattern gene expression. Mol. Cell 2002; 9:587–600.

89. Coletti D, Yang E, Marazzi G, Sassoon D. TNFalpha inhibits skeletal myogenesis through a PW1-dependent pathway by recruitment of caspase pathways. EMBO J. 2002; 21:631–642.

90. Collins RA, Grounds MD. The role of tumor necrosis factor-α (TNF-α) in skeletal muscle regeneration. Studies in TNF-α(-/-) and TNF-α(-/-)/LT-α(-/-) mice. J. Histochem. Cytochem. 2001; 49:989–1001.

91. McPherron AC, Lawler AM, Lee SJ. Regulation of skeletal muscle mass in mice by a new TGF-beta superfamily member. Nature 1997; 387:83–90.

92. Aggarwal BB. Signalling pathways of the TNF superfamily: a double-edged sword. Nature Rev. Immunol. 2003; 3:745–756.

93. Chen G, Goeddel DV. TNF-R1 signaling: a beautiful pathway. Science 2002; 296:1634–1635.

94. Tang ED, Wang CY, Xiong Y, Guan KL. A role for NF-κB essential modifier/IκB kinase-gamma (NEMO/IKKgamma) ubiquitination in the activation of the IκB kinase complex by tumor necrosis factor-α. J. Biol. Chem. 2003; 278:37,297–37,305.

95. Lee SY, Reichlin A, Santana A, Sokol KA, Nussenzweig MC, Choi Y. TRAF2 is essential for JNK but not NF-κB activation and regulates lymphocyte proliferation and survival. Immun. 1997; 7:703–713.

96. Kelliher MA, Grimm S, Ishida Y, Kuo F, Stanger BZ, Leder P. The death domain kinase RIP mediates the TNF-induced NF-κB signal. Immunity 1998; 8:297–303.

97. Verma IM, Stevenson JK, Schwartz EM, Van Antwerp D, Miyamoto S. Rel/NF-kB/IkB family: intimate tales of association and dissociation. Genes Dev. 1995; 9:2723–2735.

98. Baldwin AS, Jr. The NF-κ B and I κ B proteins: new discoveries and insights. Ann. Rev. Imm. 1996; 14:649–683.

99. Karin M, Ben-Neriah Y. Phosphorylation meets ubiquitination: the control of NF-[κ]B activity. Ann. Rev. Immun. 2000; 18:621–663.

100. Zhong H, May MJ, Jimi E, Ghosh S. The phosphorylation status of nuclear NF-κ B determines its association with CBP/p300 or HDAC-1. Mol. Cell 2002; 9:625–636.

101. Ruan H, Hacohen N, Golub TR, Van Parijs L, Lodish HF. Tumor necrosis factor-α suppresses adipocyte-specific genes and activates expression of preadipocyte genes in 3T3-L1 adipocytes: nuclear factor-κB activation by TNF-α is obligatory. Diabetes 2002; 51:1319–1336.

102. Hoffmann A, Horwitz BH, Baltimore D. Genetic analysis of the NFkB/IkB regulatory network: multiple roles and specificity in transcriptional control, NFkB Regulation and Function: From Basic Research to Drug Development, Tahoe City, California, 2002. Keystone Symposia.

103. Skapek SX, Rhee J, Spicer DB, Lassar AB. Inhibition of myogenic differentiation in proliferating myoblasts by cyclin D1-dependent kinase. Science 1995; 267:1022–1024.

104. Hinz M, Krappmann D, Eichten A, Heder A, Scheidereit C, Strauss M. NF-kB Function in Growth Control: Regulation of Cyclin D1 Expression and G0/G1-to-S-Phase Transition. Mol. Cell. Biol. 1999; 19:2690–2698.

105. Yao J, Mackman N, Edgington TS, Fan ST. Lipopolysaccharide induction of the tumor necrosis factor-α promoter in human monocytic cells. Regulation by Egr-1, c-Jun, and NF-κB transcription factors. J. Biol. Chem. 1997; 272:17,795–17,801.

106. Swantek JL, Christerson L, Cobb MH. Lipopolysaccharide-induced tumor necrosis factor-α promoter activity is inhibitor of nuclear factor-κB kinase-dependent. J. Biol. Chem. 1999; 274:11,667–11,671.

107. Steer JH, Kroeger KM, Abraham LJ, Joyce DA. Glucocorticoids suppress tumor necrosis factor-α expression by human monocytic THP-1 cells by suppressing transactivation through adjacent NF-κ B and c-Jun-activating transcription factor-2 binding sites in the promoter. J. Biol. Chem. 2000; 275:18,432–18,440.

108. Li YP, Reid MB. NF-κB mediates the protein loss induced by TNF-α in differentiated skeletal muscle myotubes. Amer. J. Physiol. 2000; 279:R1165–1170.

109. Li YP, Schwartz RJ, Waddell ID, Holloway BR, Reid MB. Skeletal muscle myocytes undergo protein loss and reactive oxygen-mediated NF-κB activation in response to tumor necrosis factor alpha. FASEB J. 1998; 12:871–880.

110. Kawamura I, Morishita R, Tomita N, et al. Intratumoral injection of oligonucleotides to the NF κ B binding site inhibits cachexia in a mouse tumor model. Gene Ther. 1999; 6:91–97.

111. Lille ST, Lefler SR, Mowlavi A, et al. Inhibition of the initial wave of NF-κB activity in rat muscle reduces ischemia/reperfusion injury. Muscle Nerve 2001; 24:534–541.

112. Hunter RB, Stevenson E, Koncarevic A, Mitchell-Felton H, Essig DA, Kandarian SC. Activation of an alternative NF-κB pathway in skeletal muscle during disuse atrophy. FASEB J. 2002; 16:529–538.

113. Kumar A, Lnu S, Malya R, et al. Mechanical stretch activates nuclear factor-κB, activator protein-1, and mitogen-activated protein kinases in lung parenchyma: implications in asthma. FASEB J. 2003; 17:1800–1811.

114. Baghdiguian S, Richard I, Martin M, et al. Pathophysiology of limb girdle muscular dystrophy type 2A: hypothesis and new insights into the IκBalpha/NF-κB survival pathway in skeletal muscle. J. Mol. Med. 2001; 79:254–261.

115. Spiegelman BM, Hotamisligil GS. Through thick and thin: wasting, obesity, and TNF alpha. Cell 1993; 73:625–627.

116. Goodman MN. Tumor necrosis factor induces skeletal muscle protein breakdown in rats. Amer. J. Physiol. 1991; 260:E727–730.
117. Moldawer LL, Svaninger G, Gelin J, Lundholm KG. Interleukin 1 and tumor necrosis factor do not regulate protein balance in skeletal muscle. Am. J. Physiol. 1987; 253:C766–773.
118. Ladner KJ, Caligiuri MA, Guttridge DC. Tumor necrosis factor-regulated biphasic activation of NF-κ B is required for cytokine-induced loss of skeletal muscle gene products. J. Biol. Chem. 2003; 278: 2294–2303.
119. Barton BE. IL-6-like cytokines and cancer cachexia: consequences of chronic inflammation. Immunol. Res. 2001; 23:41–58.
120. Cahlin C, Korner A, Axelsson H, Wang W, Lundholm K, Svanberg E. Experimental cancer cachexia: the role of host-derived cytokines interleukin (IL)-6, IL-12, interferon-gamma, and tumor necrosis factor alpha evaluated in gene knockout, tumor-bearing mice on C57 Bl background and eicosanoid-dependent cachexia. Cancer Res. 2000; 60:5488–5493.
121. Matthys P, Dijkmans R, Proost P, et al. Severe cachexia in mice inoculated with interferon-gamma-producing tumor cells. Int. J. Cancer 1991; 49:77–82.
122. Mori M, Yamaguchi K, Honda S, et al. Cancer cachexia syndrome developed in nude mice bearing melanoma cells producing leukemia-inhibitory factor. Cancer R. 1991; 51:6656–6659.
123. Acharyya S, Ladner KJ, Nelsen LL, et al. Cancer cachexia is regulated by selective targeting of skeletal muscle gene products. J Clin Invest 2004; 114:370–378.
124. Suryaprasad AG, Prindiville T. The biology of TNF blockade. Autoimm. Rev. 2003; 2:346–357.
125. Burke JR, Pattoli MA, Gregor KR, et al. BMS-345541 is a highly selective inhibitor of I κ B kinase that binds at an allosteric site of the enzyme and blocks NF-κ B-dependent transcription in mice. J. Biol. Chem. 2003; 278:1450–1456.
126. Castro AC, Dang LC, Soucy F, et al. Novel IKK inhibitors: beta-carbolines. Bioorg. Med. Chem. Lett. 2003; 13:2419–2422.

IV CYTOKINES IN THE TREATMENT OF CANCER

17 Interleukin-2 and Cancer Therapy

Kim Margolin and Joseph Clark

1. INTRODUCTION AND HISTORY: THE PROMISE OF IL-2 AS A T-CELL GROWTH FACTOR

IL-2 was originally isolated as a soluble factor with the property of enhancing T-lymphocyte proliferation in studies of the human immunodeficiency virus (1). The earliest studies of its activity in the cellular therapy of cancer used partially-purified IL-2 from the Jurkat human T-cell line. Subsequent studies used recombinant IL-2 produced in *E. coli*, an unlimited source of this valuable cytokine that has been used more than any other immunologic agent for laboratory and clinical investigations of immunotherapy for malignant and nonmalignant disease. Proof of concept for the potent activity of IL-2-activated killer cells (termed lymphokine-activated killer, or LAK cells) against established malignancy in animal models was provided in the extensive series of reports from Rosenberg and the Surgery Branch of the National Cancer Institute beginning in the mid-1980s (2–4). The earliest human studies used Jurkat-derived IL-2 and *ex vivo*-activated autologous LAK cells derived from leukapheresis of patients with advanced cancer. These patients initially received intravenous IL-2 before mononuclear cell collections and then received additional IL-2 following the re-infusion of autologous lymphocytes that had undergone further exposure to IL-2 *ex vivo* for several days. The encouraging level of activity against renal cancer and melanoma, including a 5–7% rate

From: *Cancer Drug Discovery and Development,*
Cytokines in the Genesis and Treatment of Cancer
Edited by: M. A. Caligiuri and M. T. Lotze © Humana Press Inc., Totowa, NJ

of durable complete remission, was particularly gratifying in light of the marked resistance of these two malignancies to chemotherapy and other biologic agents such as interferon. Subsequent clinical trials demonstrated that *ex vivo* exposure of patient cells to IL-2 was not necessary, as the in vivo exposure appeared to be associated with a comparable likelihood of antitumor response *(5)*. At the same time, the success of this approach at centers outside of the National Cancer Institute was confirmed with a series of studies by the Cytokine Working Group and other institutions *(6–9)*.

2. TOXICITIES OF IL-2 AND ATTEMPTS TO MITIGATE THEM WITH SELECTIVE AGENTS

The animal models of IL-2 in the treatment of cancer suggested a close relationship between the amount of IL-2 exposure, the number of LAK cells re-infused, and the overall clinical benefit of this approach. Phase I clinical studies confirmed these DLTs and demonstrated the potential of IL-2 to cause severe, dose-related multi-organ toxicities with nearly all toxicities resolving completely within hours to days following the last exposure to IL-2. The common mechanism appeared to be a "capillary leak syndrome" that allowed for the movement of plasma and activated lymphocytes into the interstitial spaces of nearly all organs examined. A common pattern of initial profound vasodilatation, resulting in hypotension, followed by fluid retention and evidence of "third-space" accumulation of the excess volume resulting from support of the intravascular volume using intravenous crystalloid was experienced by all patients. Individual toxicities that limited the cumulative exposure to IL-2 included hypotension with hypoperfusion of end-organs exacerbated by the use of vasopressors to support the arterial blood pressure, acidosis and renal insufficiency, pulmonary insufficiency, cardiac arrhythmias or myocarditis, dermatitis and occasional mucositis, and central nervous system dysfunction. After randomized and nonrandomized trials in patients with various malignancies suggested the equivalence of high-dose IL-2 alone and IL-2 plus LAK cells, the subsequent elimination of the *ex vivo* LAK cell component, increasing experience with high-dose IL-2, and a trend to decreasing total IL-2 administration, resulted in an improved overall safety profile, particularly with regard to pulmonary, acid-base and hemodynamic toxicities *(10)*.

Although the vast majority of high-dose IL-2 toxicities are completely reversible, occasional patients in the early investigations developed evidence of myocardial damage manifested by myocardial dysfuntion, EKG changes, chemical evidence of myocarditis, and in the rare fatal cases, pathologic evidence of a lymphocytic myocardial infiltrate believed to be responsible for the damage *(10–16)*. The incidence of this type of toxicity is now rare, presumably owing to continued use of rigorous screening to exclude patients at risk for cardiovascular complications, as well as the general trend to reduced IL-2 exposure in recent series. The other irreversible toxicity, although nonlife-threatening, is the common development of thyroid dysfunction, usually hypothyroidism, in patients who survive for prolonged intervals following IL-2 therapy. The etiology of thyroid dysfunction is presumed to be an autoimmune thyroiditis resulting from IL-2-mediated dysregulation of a thyroid-reactive T-cell clone or some form of cross-reactivity between thyroid and tumor antigens stimulated by IL-2 *(17–22)*. All of the other toxicities of IL-2, whereas challenging to patients undergoing therapy and the physicians who manage them, are reversible within a few hours to several days and represent varying degrees of sensitivity to capillary leakage or direct infiltration by IL-2-activated lymphocytes or the secondary effects of other cytokines induced by lymphocytes in response to IL-2. These include dermatitis, usually a diffuse, maculo-papular erythema resembling a drug eruption and sometimes intensely pruritic; GI toxicities ranging from nausea, emesis, diarrhea and occasional stomatitis to mild to moderate hepatobiliary dysfunction (variable enzyme and bilirubin elevation, synthetic dysfunction as well as hepatomegaly, sometimes tender); flu-like symptoms including the "first-dose" occurrence of chills and fever followed variably by fatigue, malaise, and occasional arthralgias and myalgias. Most patients experience some degree of alteration of mental status, ranging from mild confusion to the rare development of visual hallucinations, severe depression and delirium or combative behavior. Asymptomatic but occasionally dose-limiting hematologic alterations include lymphopenia, eosinophilia, anemia and thrombocytopenia sometimes requiring transfusion support, and a "rebound" lymphocytosis following discontinuation of IL-2 (reviewed in refs. *23,24*). Paradoxical increases in the susceptibility to bacterial infection during and after IL-2 therapy result from a cytokine-induced neutrophil chemotactic dysfunction and the susceptibility of tissues lacking their usual barriers to infection such as the skin and gastrointestinal tract *(25,26)*.

3. CURRENT STATUS OF HIGH-DOSE IL-2 IN RENAL CANCER

The original experience using high-dose IL-2 in patients with cancer was reviewed by Dr. Steven Rosenberg, who had pioneered this approach with colleagues at the National Cancer Institute, Surgery Branch *(4)*. This pooled series of 652 patients contained 155 patients who received high-dose IL-2 alone, 214 with LAK cells, 66 with tumor-infiltrating lymphocytes cultured from patient tumors and reinfused with high-dose IL-2, and 128 with α-interferon. A smaller number of patients received IL-2 with chemotherapy or other cytokines. Two hundred seven patients in this series had renal cancer, and the response rate, which varied from 22 to 35%, appeared to favor the inclusion of LAK cells. However, subsequent randomized trials and sequential comparative trials in which patients were rigorously screened using the same eligibility criteria did not suggest a benefit for this component *(5,27)*. The use of other cell types such as TIL (tumor-infiltrating lymphocytes *[28]*) and the use of other cytokines such as α-interferon *(29–34)* added to the complexities and toxicities of the regimens without apparent benefit, so the regimen approved in 1992 by the FDA and used as the "gold standard" for achieving durable complete responses and long-term survivals in renal cancer is high-dose IL-2 alone. Subsequent series and pooled databases have demonstrated the reproducible level of activity and provided a basis for the design of regimens with reduced toxicity or improved therapeutic efficacy *(35,36)*.

A series of such studies was carried out by the Cytokine Working Group (previously known as the Extramural NCI-LAK Working Group, based on an initial contract to 6 cancer centers to reproduce the clinical results of Rosenberg and colleagues at the Surgery Branch *(4,37)*. In summary, the Cytokine Working Group confirmed the activity, including durable complete remissions in a small fraction of patients, of high-dose IL-2 in advanced renal cancer. This group also demonstrated the lack of benefit associated with alternative schedules such as continuous intravenous infusion (less activity *[38]*) and the use of chemotherapy-containing combinations (more unfavorable therapeutic index *[39]*). Using novel methods to assess the impact of potential modulators of

IL-2 toxicity, this group also showed that inhibitors of tumor necrosis factor, inter-leukin-1, lipid-mediators of inflammatory signal transduction, and cytokine-inducible nitric oxide synthase did not provide significant toxicity reduction *(40–45)*.

The results of this group's most recent study, a large Phase III randomized trial of inpatient high-dose IL-2 versus a popular, fairly well-tolerated outpatient combination of lower-dose IL-2 and α-interferon, have been analyzed and are the basis for several correlative analyses of pathology, immunologic and metabolic parameters in predicting the benefit of high-dose IL-2 *(46–48)*. Overall, responses were more than twice as frequent in the group receiving high-dose inpatient IL-2 (23 vs 9%), but the primary endpoints of overall and progression-free survival were not significantly impacted by the treatment arm. At the time of trial design, prestratifications were limited to performance status, sites of disease and presence of the primary renal cancer. At the conclusion of the study, the groups were analyzed by separating the patients in each treatment arm into additional categories based on more recently-identified factors. The unanticipated finding was that patients with the most unfavorable characteristics (primary tumor in place, hepatic and/or osseous metastases) benefited significantly from treatment with high-dose, inpatient IL-2, whereas those with the more favorable characteristics did equally well with either regimen. The outcomes from this study have also been analyzed with respect to new information regarding pathologic prognostic and predictive features for patients with advanced renal cancer undergoing IL-2-based therapy, and the results are currently undergoing validation testing in Phase III trials of IL-2-based therapy with other biologic agents.

The need for high-dose IL-2, with its associated toxicities, expense, and the need for experienced physicians in specialized centers, has also been investigated in a novel Phase III trial design by Yang and colleagues at the NCI Surgery Branch. In the first part of this randomized trial, patients were assigned to receive high-dose IL-2 on the standard regimen or 0.1 of the standard dose, using the same schedule and route of administration. After initial analysis of the data suggested the lack of a significant benefit of high-dose IL-2 over the low-dose regimen *(49)*, a third treatment arm was added, consisting of outpatient subcutaneous IL-2 using a regimen that had been reported in European multicenter studies to be effective and tolerable when self-administered. The final results of this trial, reported in 2003, confirmed that the response rate to high-dose IL-2 at the Surgery Branch was now predictably in the same range reported outside of the National Cancer Institute. Patients randomized to receive low-dose intravenous IL-2 or the outpatient subcutaneous regimen had a lower response rate, but their survival that did not differ significantly from that of the patients assigned to high-dose therapy *(50)*. Although the overall activity of high-dose IL-2 remains disappointing, the results of this trial also confirmed that durable complete remissions were achieved more frequently with high-dose therapy.

In addition to the need for better identification of patients who will benefit from IL-2 for advanced renal cancer, there is a desperate need for effective adjuvant therapy for patients with resected disease who are at a high risk of recurrence. The Cytokine Working Group recently reported the results of a small Phase III trial to assess the benefit of a single course (two 5-day cycles) of high-dose IL-2 for patients with renal cancer at risk of recurrence following nephrectomy. In view of the toxicities of high-dose IL-2, the trial was designed to detect a large benefit that would justify further manipulations of the regimen in larger, more definitive trials. Further, the endpoint of progression-free rather than overall survival was chosen because of the high likelihood that patients would receive IL-2-based therapy at the time of relapse, thus potentially negating the survival impact of adjuvant IL-2. The results of this study, which accrued 44 primary nephrectomy patients and another 25 who were randomized following surgical excision of a single or limited number of metastases, did not demonstrate a benefit in progression-free interval for patients assigned to IL-2 *(51)*. It is likely that with the emergence of new therapies for renal cancer, IL-2 will become a component of combination regimens containing agents with complementary mechanisms of antitumor activity and minimally overlapping toxicities.

4. CURRENT STATUS OF HIGH-DOSE IL-2 IN MELANOMA

Like renal cancer, melanoma is a tumor with minimal responsiveness to chemotherapies or other cytokines that has been the focus of extensive study using IL-2-based approaches. Initial studies in melanoma were designed exactly like those used for renal cancer, which are summarized above. In the 1989 Rosenberg/NCI Surgery Branch review, 270 of the 652 pooled patients had advanced melanoma. The results of their treatment with high-dose IL-2 and LAK cells (66 patients), IL-2 alone (60 patients), or one of the other combinations (with α-interferon, tumor necrosis factor, antibody, cyclophosphamide or tumor-infiltrating lymphocytes) mirrored those of the patients with advanced renal cancer receiving IL-2 alone, again suggesting that there is a maximum achievable response rate in the range of 20% (about 1/3 of which are durable complete responses) for IL-2 alone that is not enhanced by the addition of other agents *(4)*.

Investigators working in the field of IL-2-based immunotherapy of malignancy have taken advantage of important differences in the biology of renal cancer and melanoma. The two most important features of melanoma that lend themselves to the development of innovations in IL-2-based therapy include 1) the availability of chemotherapeutic agents with activity against melanoma that possess only partially overlapping toxicities with those of IL-2, and 2) the availability of well-characterized tumor antigens in melanoma that have been studied in combination with IL-2 and other immunostimulatory agents in both the advanced disease and the adjuvant setting. Although many chemotherapy combinations with IL-2 with or without other cytokines (often called "biochemotherapy") appeared promising when first reported, recent data from randomized studies have nearly all shown disappointing results suggesting the lack of benefit for using complex multi-agent regimens containing one or more chemotherapies and IL-2 with or without α-interferon *(52)*. Although these results were not surprising, in view of the more empiric than rational design of the regimens used, there has continued to be a dedicated group of investigators who have applied cutting-edge principles from the explosive growth in cancer immunology to design regimens more likely to succeed in human advanced cancer. Examples of such immunotherapeutic strategies designed to "break tolerance" include the combination of high-dose IL-2 with melanoma-specific peptides *(53,54)* or the administration of high-dose, nonmyeloablative chemotherapy followed by the reinfusion of highly-selected T-cell "clones" with reactivity against known melanoma peptide antigens *(55)*. The chemotherapy in this case was designed to reduce the number of regulatory T-cells that are believed to quench the activity of the cytolytic CD8 cells with peptide-specific, HLA-restricted antitumor activity. Confirmatory trials of this approach are ongoing, and further studies of the mechanisms of resistance and escape from immune control will be an important correlate of these investigations.

5. IL-2-BASED THERAPY OF HEMATOLOGIC MALIGNANCIES

During the time that IL-2-based therapies for solid tumors were under intense investigation, the potential of IL-2 for the treatment of hematologic malignancies was also explored. In the case of leukemias and lymphomas, additional opportunities included the study of effector T-cells and NK cells in the marrow and stem cell compartment as well as the differentiation of hematopoietic precursor cells into dendritic cells, yielding a population of cells that could present its own antigens and be a target for immunotherapeutic eradication. Based on this extensive body of preclinical data, clinical trials were carried out at several centers to assess the feasibility of IL-2 with or without *ex vivo* IL-2-activated cells in the primary and adjunctive treatment of leukemia and lymphoma *(56–69)*; there was at that time also a renewed interest in the potential role of IL-2-activated hematopoietic cells as a component of regimens using high-dose chemotherapy with stem cell support for solid tumors *(61,62)*. The latter approach has largely been abandoned owing to the lack of sufficient evidence for efficacy of the cytoreductive "conditioning" regimen against solid tumors, although other approaches to cellular immunotherapy for these diseases remain under active investigation. However, the results of ongoing or recently-completed randomized controlled trials are eagerly awaited: the first was a Children's Oncology Group trial assessing IL-2 consolidation for acute myelogenous leukemia in remission *(63)*; the second is a recently-completed Southwest Oncology Group trial assessing IL-2 following autologous stem cell transplant for intermediate-grade B-cell non-Hodgkin lymphoma in second remission (J.A. Thompson/SWOG 9438, manuscript in preparation). IL-2 has also been evaluated for its ability to enhance antibody-dependent cellular cytotoxicity, specifically in combination with rituximab, a chimeric monoclonal antibody widely used in the treatment of indolent and aggressive B-cell lymphomas; a randomized trial of rituximab with or without IL-2 is expected to begin accrual in 2004 (D. Hurst, personal communication), and its potential for combination with other antibodies to produce additive or synergistic benefit will likely follow.

6. IL-2 IN OTHER MALIGNANCIES

The value of IL-2 or IL-2-containing combinations in other tumor types has been little-studied, because 1) most other tumors are more responsive to cytotoxic therapies than melanoma and renal cancer, 2) most of these cytotoxic therapies have predictable toxicities that are better tolerated by a higher fraction of patients than IL-2 in patients with these malignancies, and 3) there has been inadequate study of the potential important interactions between IL-2 and other agents like cytotoxic drugs, other cytokines, or other biologic molecules with potentially complementary mechanisms. It may well turn out that the most important activity of IL-2 is as an adjuvant to other types of immunotherapy. These may be antigen-specific (as with the rituximab combination as well as in combination with tumor-derived peptides that elicit an antigen-specific T-cell response). Alternatively, they may occur via stimulation of the "innate" branch of the immune system (i.e., natural killer cell-mediated cytotoxicity, which is governed by very different intercellular interactions than T-cell responses) and may be based on

IL-2 alone or in synergistic combinations with agents that possess different mechanisms, such as inhibitors of angiogenesis or cell signaling pathways.

7. ALTERNATIVE IL-2 MOLECULES

Many investigators and biotechnology corporations have endeavored to design a "better" IL-2, particularly because the disappointing results of several modulator trials were published (32–37). Efforts have included single amino acid substitutions resulting in preferential binding to the IL-2 receptor of T-cells over that of NK cells (64) or chemical modification of IL-2 to produce a molecule with markedly prolonged half-life that enhances overall exposure while minimizing the episodes of high peak concentrations that might be associate more with toxicity than benefit (65,66). IL-2 has also been covalently linked to an antibody molecule that targets or traffics the IL-2 to the site where effector cells can be concentrated for both sensitization to tumor antigen as well as for optimal cytotoxic activity following activation by IL-2 (67).

8. IL-2 AND OTHER BIOLOGIC AGENTS

Except for the extensive experience with interferon combinations, primarily alpha but also gamma, the use of IL-2 in combination with other cytokines has been limited. With the interferons, the successful development of a combination based on agents with only partially-overlapping toxicities has not been realized. Furthermore, the antitumor activity of such combinations has not been superior to that of either agent alone, and the only IL-2-containing combination that has achieved even moderate acceptance in the community setting is in the outpatient, subcutaneously-administered regimen detailed above. The role of other combinations, such as with IL-6, IL-10, IL-12, IL-15, IL-18, IL-21, and probably many others, remains to be further elucidated by carefully-designed protocols with a solid preclinical and clinical rationale, a proven record of safety and tolerability, and appropriate correlative laboratory studies.

9. CONCLUSIONS

In the nearly 2 decades since the discovery of IL-2, the expansion of its role in various approaches to the biologic therapy of malignant disease has taken several promising directions. Although the original application of IL-2 in supraphysiologic doses continues to provide remissions, sometimes durable, in a small fraction of patients with advanced renal cancer and melanoma, its mechanisms of action remain speculative, ranging from antigen-driven T-cell-based effects to nonspecific activation of NK cells against tumor. IL-2 continues to be an essential element of more precisely defined strategies such as vaccines that involve dendritic cells and other methods of optimized antigen presentation to induce cytolytic T-cell responses in an antigen-specific, HLA-restricted fashion. Promising combinations of IL-2 with other cytokines, chemotherapeutic agents, angiogenesis inhibitors and small molecules with defined molecular targets are likely to find a niche in the near future. More innovative approaches such as bispecific IL-2-containing molecules that retarget effector lymphocytes and derivative molecules that provide enhanced activity and/or reduced toxicity are also in development. Experience with the design of translational studies of IL-2 over the past 20 years has provided the framework for the study of other immunotherapies, which will continue to evolve as the field expands into the 21st century.

REFERENCES

1. Smith, KA Interleukin-2: inception, impact, and implications. Science: 27; 240(4856): 1169–76 (1988).
2. Rosenberg SA, Lotze MT, Muul, LM, et al. Observations on the systemic administration of autologous lymphokine-activated killer cells and recombinant interleukin-2 to patients with metastatic cancer. N Engl J Med (Special Report): 313:23; 1485 (1985).
3. Rosenberg SA, Lotze MT, Muul LM, et al. A progress report on the treatment of 157 patients with advanced cancer using lymphokine-activated killer cells and interleukin-2 or high-dose interleukin-2 alone. N Engl J Med. 9;316(15):889–97 (1987).
4. Rosenberg SA, Lotze MT, Yang JC, et al. Experience with the use of high-dose interleukin-2 in the treatment of 652 cancer patients. Ann Surg. 210(4):474–84; discussion 484-5 (1989).
5. Law, TM, Motzer, RJ, Mazumdar, M, et al. Phase III randomized trial of interleukin-2 with or without lymphokine-activated killer cells in the treatment of patients with advanced renal cell carcinoma. Cancer 76:5;827 (1995).
6. Dutcher JP, Creekmore S, Weiss GR, Margolin K, et al. A phase II study of interleukin-2 and lymphokine-activated killer cells in patients with metastatic malignant melanoma. J Clin Oncol. 7(4):477–85 (1989).
7. Weiss GR, Margolin KA, Aronson FR, et al. A randomized phase II trial of continuous infusion interleukin-2 or bolus injection interleukin-2 plus lymphokine-activated killer cells for advanced renal cell carcinoma. J Clin Oncol. 10(2):–81 (1992).
8. Hawkins MJ, Atkins MB, Dutcher JP, et al. A phase II clinical trial of interleukin-2 and lymphokine-activated killer cells in advanced colorectal carcinoma. J Immunother. 15 (1):74–8. (1994).
9. Sparano JA, Fisher RI, Weiss GR, Margolin K, et al. Phase II trials of high-dose interleukin-2 and lymphokine-activated killer cells in advanced breast carcinoma and carcinoma of the lung, ovary, and pancreas and other tumors. J Immunother Emphasis Tumor Immunol. 16(3):216–23 (1994).
10. Kammula US, White DE, Rosenberg SA, et al. Trends in the safety of high dose bolus interleukin-2 administration in patients with metastatic cancer. Cancer. Aug 15;83(4): 797–805 (1998).
11. Du Bois JS, Udelson JE, Atkins MB, et al. Severe reversible global and regional ventricular dysfunction associated with high-dose interleukin-2 immunotherapy. J Immunother Emphasis Tumor Immunol. 18(2):119–23 (1995).
12. White RL Jr, Schwartzentruber DJ, Guleria A, et al. Cardiopulmonary toxicity of treatment with high dose interleukin-2 in 199 consecutive patients with metastatic melanoma or renal cell carcinoma. Cancer. 15;74(12):3212–22 (1994).
13. Zhang J, Yu ZX, Hilbert SL, et al. Cardiotoxicity of human recombinant interleukin-2 in rats. A morphological study. Circulation. 87(4):1340–53 (1993).
14. Marshall ME, Cibull ML, Pearson T, et al. Human recombinant interleukin-2 provokes infiltration of lymphocytes into myocardium and liver in rabbits. J Biol Response Mod. 9(3):279–87 (1990).
15. Samlowski WE, Ward, JH, Craven CM, et al. Severe myocarditis following high-dose interleukin-2 administration. Arch Pathol Lab Med. 113(8):838–41 (1989).
16. Kragel AH, Travis WD, Feinberg L, et al. Pathologic findings associated with interleukin-2-based immunotherapy for cancer: A postmortem study of 19 patients.Hum Pathol. 21(5):493–502 (1990).
17. Krouse RS, Royal RE, Heywood G, et al. Thyroid dysfunction in 281 patients with metastatic melanoma or renal carcinoma treated with interleukin-2 alone. J Immunother Emphasis Tumor Immunol. 18(4):272–8 (1995).
18. Vialettes B, Guillerand MA, Viens P, et al. Incidence rate and risk factors for thyroid dysfunction during recombinant interleukin-2 therapy in advanced malignancies. Acta Endocrinol (Copenh). 129(1):31–8 (1993).
19. Kruit WH, Bolhuis RL, Goey SH, Interleukin-2-induced thyroid dysfunction is correlated with treatment duration but not with tumor response. J Clin Oncol. 11(5):921–4 (1993).
20. Schwartzentruber DJ, White DE, Zweig MH, et al. Thyroid dysfunction associated with immunotherapy for patients with cancer. Cancer. 1;68(11):2384–90 (1991).
21. Pichert G, Jost LM, Zobeli L, Thyroiditis after treatment with interleukin-2 and interferon alpha-2a. Br J Cancer. 62(1):100–4 (1990).
22. Atkins MB, Mier JW, Parkinson DR, et al. Hypothyroidism after treatment with interleukin-2 and lymphokine-activated killer cells. N Engl J Med. 318(24):1557–63 (1988).

23. Margolin, K. The Clinical Toxicities of High-Dose Interleukin-2. *In: Therapeutic Applications of Interleukin-2.* M.B. Atkins and J.W. Mier, eds., Marcel Dekker, Inc., New York, NY, Ch. 17: pp 331–362, 1993.

24. Siegel JP, Puri RK. Interleukin-2 toxicity. J Clin Oncol. 9(4):694–704 (1991).

25. Klempner, MS, Noring, R, Mier, JW, et al. An acquired chemotactic defect in neutrophils from patients receiving interleukin-2 immunotherapy. N Engl J Med. 5;322(14):959–65 (1990).

26. Pockaj BA, Topalian SL, Steinberg SM, et al. Infectious complications associated with interleukin-2 administration: a retrospective review of 935 treatment courses. J Clin Oncol. 11(1):136–47 (1993).

27. Fyfe G, Fisher RI, Rosenberg SA, et al. Results of treatment of 255 patients with metastatic renal cell carcinoma who received high-dose recombinant interleukin-2 therapy. J Clin Oncol. 3:688–96 (1995).

28. Yannelli JR, Hyatt C, McConnell S, et al. Growth of tumor-infiltrating lymphocytes from human solid cancers: summary of a 5-year experience. Int J Cancer. 65(4):413–21 (1996).

29. Ilson DH, Motzer RJ, Kradin RL, et al. A phase II trial of interleukin-2 and interferon alfa-2a in patients with advanced renal cell carcinoma. J Clin Oncol (11):1822 (1992).

30. Atkins MB, Sparano J, Fisher RI, et al. Randomized phase II trial of high-dose interleukin-2 either alone or in combination with interferon alfa-2b in advanced renal cell carcinoma. J Clin Oncol. 1993 11(4):661–70, (1993).

31. Vogelzang NJ, Lipton A, Figlin RA, et al. Subcutaneous interleukin-2 plus interferon alfa-2a in metastatic renal cancer: an outpatient multicenter trial. J Clin Oncol (9): 1809–16, (1993).

32. Marincola FM, White DE, Wise AP, Rosenberg SA, et al. Combination therapy with interferon alfa-2a and interleukin-2 for the treatment of metastatic cancer. J Clin Oncol (5):1110–22, (1995).

33. Negrier S, Escudier B, Lasset C, et al. Recombinant human interleukin-2, recombinant human interferon alfa-2a, or both in metastatic renal-cell carcinoma. Groupe Francais d' Immunotherapie, N Engl J Med 338(18):1272–1278 (1998).

34. Dutcher JP, Atkins M, Fisher R, et al. Interleukin-2-based therapy for metastatic renal cell cancer: The Cytokine Working Group Experience, 1989-1997. Cancer J Sci Am. 3 Suppl 1:S73–S78 (1997).

35. Atkins MB, Lotze MT, Dutcher JP, et al. Margolin Seminars in Oncology 2002 IL-2 in RCC High-dose recombinant interleukin 2 therapy for patients with metastatic melanoma: analysis of 270 patients treated between 1985 and 1993. J Clin Oncol. 17(7):2105–16 (1999).

36. Atkins MB, Dutcher J, Weiss G, et al. Kidney cancer: the Cytokine Working Group experience (1986-2001): part I. IL-2-based clinical trials. Med Oncol.18(3):197–207. (2001).

37. Fisher RI, Coltman CA, Doroshow JH, et al. Metastatic renal cancer treated with interleukin-2 and lymphokine-activated killer cells. Ann Intern Med 108: 518–523, (1988).

38. Weiss GR, Margolin KA, Aronson FR, et al. A randomized phase II trial of continuous infusion interleukin-2 or bolus injection interleukin-2 plus lymphokine-activated killer cells for advanced renal cell carcinoma. J Clin Oncol. 10(2):275–81 (1992).

39. Dutcher JP, Logan T, Gordon M, et al. Phase II trial of interleukin 2, interferon alpha, and 5-fluorouracil in metastatic renal cell cancer: a cytokine working group study. Clin Cancer Res. 6(9): 3442–50 (2000).

40. Sosman, JA, Weiss GR, Margolin KA, et al. Phase IB clinical trial of anti-CD3 followed by high-dose bolus interleukin-2 in patients with metastatic melanoma and advanced renal cell carcinoma: clinical and immunologic effects. J Clin Oncol, 11:8;1496–1505 (1993).

41. Margolin KM, Atkins M, Sparano J, et al. Prospective randomized trial of lisofylline for the prevention of toxicities of high-dose interleukin 2 therapy in advanced renal cancer and malignant melanoma. Clinical Cancer Research, 3:565–572 (1997).

42. Trehu EG, Mier JW, Dubois JS, et al. Phase I trial of interleukin 2 in combination with the soluble tumor necrosis factor receptor p75 IgG chimera. Clin Cancer Res. 2:1341–1351, (1996).

43. Du Bois JS, Trehu EG, Mier JW, et al. Randomized placebo-controlled clinical trial of high-dose interleukin-2 in combination with a soluble p75 tumor necrosis factor receptor immunoglobulin g chimera in patients with advanced melanoma and renal cell carcinoma. J Clin Oncol, 15:3;1052–1062 (1997).

44. McDermott DF, Trehu EG, Mier JW, et al. A two-part phase I trial of high-dose interleukin 2 in combination with soluble (Chinese hamster ovary) interleukin 1 receptor. Clin Cancer Res, 5:1203–1213, (1998).

45. Atkins MB, Redman B, Mier J, et al. A phase I study of CNI-1493, an inhibitor of cytokine release, in combination with high-dose interleukin-2 in patients with renal cancer and melanoma. Clin Cancer Res, 7:486–492, (2001).

46. McDermott DF, Parker RA, Youmans AL, The effect of recent nephrectomy on treatment with high-dose interleukin-2 (HD IL-2) or subcutaneous (SC) IL-2/interferon alfa-2b (IFN) in patients with metastatic renal cell carcinoma (RCC). ASCO, 22:1547;385, (2003).
47. Zea AH, Atkins MB, McDermont D, et al. Role of CD35 expression and arginase activity in predicting response and survival in metastatic renal cell carcinoma (mRCC) patients receiving IL-2. ASCO, 22;2535 (2004).
48. Upton MP, Parker RA, Youmans A, et al. Histologic predictors of renal cell carcinoma (RCC) response to interleukin-2-based therapy. J Immunother 28:488–495 (2005).
49. Yang JC, Topalian SL, Parkinson D, et al. Randomized comparison of high-dose and low-dose intravenous interleukin-2 for the therapy of metastatic renal cell carcinoma: an interim report. J Clin Oncol. 12(8):1572–6 (1994).
50. Yang JC, Sherry RM, Steinberg SM, et al. Randomized study of high-dose and low-dose interleukin-2 in patients with metastatic renal cancer. J Clin Oncol. 15;21(16):3127–32 (2003).
51. Clark JI, Atkins MB, Urba WJ, et al. Adjuvant high-dose bolus interleukin-2 for patients with high-risk renal cell carcinoma: A cytokine working group randomized trial. J Clin Oncol. 2003 Aug 15;21(16):3133–40. Epub (2003).
52. Margolin K Biochemotherapy of melanoma: rational therapeutics in the search for weapons of melanoma destruction. Cancer 101(3):435–438 (2004).
53. Rosenberg SA, et al. Immunologic and therapeutic evaluation of a synthetic peptide vaccine for the treatment of patients with metastatic melanoma. Nat Med 4:321–327 (1998).
54. Gollob J. Flaherty L, Smith J, et al. A Cytokine Working Group (CWG) phase II trial of a modified gp100 melanoma petide (gp100 (209M)) and high dose interleukin-2 (HD IL-2) administered q3 weeks in patients with stage IV melanoma: Limited anti-tumor activity. Proc Am Soc Clin Oncol 20:A1423 (2001).
55. Dudley ME, Wunderlich JR, Robbins PF, et al. Cancer regression and autoimmunity in patients after clonal repopulation with antitumor lymphocytes. Science. 25;298(5594): 850–4. Epub (2002).
56. Stein AS, O'Donnell MR, Slovak ML, et al. Interleukin-2 After Autologous Stem-Cell Transplantation for Adult Patients with Acute Myeloid Leukemia in First Complete Remission. J Clin Oncol 21:4;615–623 (2003).
57. Blaise D, Attal M, Reiffers J, et al. Randomized study of recombinant interleukin-2 after autologous bone marrow transplantation for acute leukemia in first complete remission. European Cytokine Network, 11:1;91–8 (2000).
58. Margolin, K.A., Negrin, R.S., Wong, K.K., et al. Cellular immunotherapy and autologous transplantation for hematologic malignancy. Immunol Rev, 157:231 (1997).
59. Margolin KM, Forman SJ. Immunotherapy with interleukin-2 after hematopoietic cell transplantation for hematologic malignancy. Cancer J Sci Am, 6[suppl. 1]:S33–S38, (2000).
60. Van Besien K, Mehra R, Wadehra N, et al. Phase II study of autologous transplantation with interleukin-2-incubated peripheral blood stem cells and posttransplantation interleukin-2 in relapsed or refractory non-Hodgkin lymphoma. Biol Bone Marrow Transpl 10:386–394 (2004)
61. Sosman JA, Stiff P, Moss SM, et al. Pilot trial of interleukin-2 with granulocyte colony-stimulating factor for the mobilization of progenitor cells in advanced breast cancer patients undergoing high-dose chemotherapy: expansion of immune effectors within the stem-cell graft and post-stem-cell infusion. J Clin Oncol. 1;19(3):634–44 (2001).
62. Meehan KR, Verma UN, Cahill R, et al. Interleukin-2-activated hematopoietic stem cell transplantation for breast cancer: investigation of dose level with clinical correlates. Bone Marrow Transplant. 20(8): 643–51 (1997).
63. Sievers EL, Lange BJ, Sondel PM, et al. Children's Cancer Group trials of Interleukin-2 therapy to prevent relapse of acute myelogenous leukemia. Cancer J Sci Am 1:S39–44 (2000)
64. Hartmann G. Technology evaluation: BAY-50-4798, Bayer. Curr Opin Mol Ther. 2:221–7.
65. Meyers FJ, Paradise C, Scudder SA, et al. A phase I study including pharmacokinetics of polyethylene glycol conjugated interleukin-2. Clin Pharmacol Ther 49(3):307–313 (1999).
66. Yao Z, Dai W, Perry J, et al. Effect of albumin fusion on the biodistribution of interleukin-2. Cancer Immunol Immunother. 53(5):404–10 (2003).
67. Lode HN, Reisfeld RA. Targeted cytokines for cancer immunotherapy. Immunol Res. 21(2-3):279–88.

18   Interleukin-12 and Cancer Therapy

Timothy E. Bael and Jared A. Gollob

1. INTRODUCTION

Although the ability of IL-2 to induce sustained tumor regression in patients with renal cell cancer and melanoma established a clinical role for cytokine therapy in fighting cancer, the severe toxicity seen in early trials limited its application to a select group of patients *(1)*. In 1989 cytotoxic lymphocyte maturation factor, later termed IL-12, was discovered *(2)*. IL-12 plays a central role in interferon gamma (IFN-γ) production and the development of a Th1 type immune response, thereby playing a role in both innate and adaptive immunity. In mouse models, IL-12 can inhibit tumor growth and metastasis. Early clinical trials of rhIL-12 in melanoma and renal cell cancer were complicated by severe toxicity and attenuation of the immune response over time. Revised dosing schedules, alternate routes of administration, and the use of combination cytokine therapy have led to improved tolerability and more sustained immune activation, but have resulted in only modest clinical activity. Current clinical trials continue to explore new ways to augment the antitumor activity of IL-12 in lymphoma and other potentially responsive malignancies.

2. BIOLOGY OF IL-12

2.1. A Heterodimeric Cytokine

The IL-12 family of cytokines, which includes IL-12, IL-23 and IL-27, have a unique heterodimeric structure that is central to their regulation and function. IL-12 is composed of 35 kDa and 40 kDa subunits termed p35 and p40, respectively. The p35 subunit is 197 amino acids long with α-helix domains and is homologous to granulocyte-colony stimulating factor (G-CSF) and IL-6 *(3,4)*. The p40 subunit is 306 amino acids long and is

From: *Cancer Drug Discovery and Development,*
Cytokines in the Genesis and Treatment of Cancer
Edited by: M. A. Caligiuri and M. T. Lotze © Humana Press Inc., Totowa, NJ

homologous to the extracellular portion of the alpha chain of the IL-6 receptor *(5,3)*. p40 and p35 covalently bind together and circulate as biologically active IL-12p70. p35 mRNA has been found in peripheral blood mononuclear cells, normal murine tissues, and tumor cell lines. Conversely, the transcription of p40 is more restricted, seen only in cells that produce biologically active IL-12p70. The regulation of IL-12p70 production is thought to occur primarily through regulation of the p40 promoter *(6)*.

2.2. The IL-12 Receptor

In 1994, Chua et al. identified a transmembrane receptor with low affinity binding to IL-12 *(7)*. IL-12Rβ1 is a 662 amino acid glycoprotein with a 591 amino acid extracellular domain and a 91 amino acid intracellular tail. A member of the hemopoietin receptor superfamily, IL-12Rβ1 is homologous to gp130 and the G-CSF receptor *(7)*, and it interacts with the p40 subunit of IL-12p70 *(8)*. Although antibody blocking experiments demonstrated that IL-12Rβ1 is required for IL-12 signaling, the lack of high affinity binding or a clear signal transduction domain led to the search for a second IL-12 receptor *(9)*. IL-12Rβ2 was identified in 1996 by Presky et al. (10). IL-12Rβ2 is an 862 amino acid protein with a 595 amino acid extracellular domain and a 216 amino acid cytoplasmic domain containing three tyrosine residues *(10)*. The extracellular domain of IL-12Rβ2, like IL-12Rβ1, is homologous to the β-hemopoietin receptors, but IL-12Rβ2 binds to both the p35 and p40 subunits of IL-12p70 *(8)*. IL-12Rβ2 expression alone, as with IL-12Rβ1, leads to low affinity IL-12 binding, but high affinity binding is seen with IL-12Rβ1 and β2 coexpression *(10)*. Although IL-12Rβ1 is expressed on resting lymphocytes, regulation of IL-12 responsiveness occurs largely through the expression of IL-12Rβ2, present on resting NK cells and on a small subset of circulating T-cells. The regulation of IL-12Rβ2 expression is also central to the IFN-γ producing Th1 phenotype *(11–13)*.

2.3. IL-12 Signal Transduction:
Janus Family Kinases, p38 MAPK, and STATs

As shown in Fig. 1, IL-12 signal transduction occurs through both p38 MAP kinase and the JAK/STAT pathway *(9,14)*. Although the IL-12 receptor itself has no protein kinase domain, it is closely associated at the cell membrane with JAK2 and TYK2 *(9,14)*. TYK2 interacts directly with the IL-12Rβ1 subunit and JAK2 with both IL-12Rβ1 and β2 subunits *(9)*. Activated by IL-12p70 binding to the IL-12 receptor, JAK2 and TYK2 phosphorylate each other and phosphorylate the tyrosine residues on IL-12Rβ2. IL-12Rβ2 phosphorylation provides docking sites for the SH2 domain of signal transducer and activator of transcription (STAT) proteins, which are then phosphorylated by JAK2 and TYK2 on C-terminal tyrosine residues *(15,16)*. Tyrosine phosphorylation allows for dimer formation, nuclear translocation and DNA binding *(16,17)*. STAT proteins are also phosphorylated on serine residues by p38 MAPK, which augments the response to IL-12 by further stimulating transcriptional activation *(18,19)*.

STAT4 has been most clearly demonstrated as central to the T and NK cell response to IL-12. STAT4 knockout mice have dampened IFN-γ production and NK cell-mediated cytotoxicity after exposure to IL-12, and mice lacking STAT4 also lose the ability to develop Th1 type helper T-cells *(20,21)*. However, STAT1, STAT3 and STAT5 also play a role in T-cell IL-12 responsiveness. This has been demonstrated in a subset of cirulating T-cells (CD8+ CD18[bright] T-cells) that can be activated by combined stimulation with

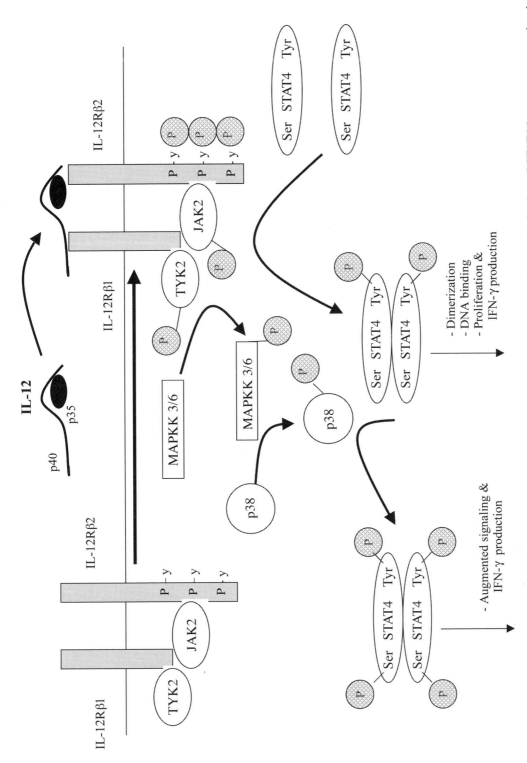

Fig. 1. Model showing how IL-12R-mediated signal transduction involves the phosphoryation and activation of STAT4 by receptor -associated Janus kinases and by p38 MAP kinase.

319

IL-12 and IL-2 without ligation of the TCR/CD3 complex *(22)*. In this T-cell population, costimulation with IL-2 and IL-12 induces MKK 3 and 6 and p38 MAPK activation and leads to STAT1 and STAT3 serine phosphorylation. Inhibition of p38 MAP kinase blocks serine phosphorylation of STAT1 and STAT3 and blocks T-cell activation to IL-12 and IL-2 *(19)*. A functional role for STAT1, 3 and 5 was also demonstrated in a patient with recurrent sinusitis and atypical mycobacterial infections characteristic of IL-12 deficiency syndrome. This patient was shown to have a muted IL-12 response despite normal IL-12Rβ1 and IL-12Rβ2 and intact STAT4 activation. However, T-cells from this patient were unable to activate STAT 1, 3, or 5 in response to IL-12 *(23)*.

2.4. Immune Activation by IL-12

IL-12 is central to the development of a Th1 immune response. Antigen presenting cells (APC) drive development of Th0 CD4+ T-cells towards the Th1 phenotype by combining antigen presentation and activation of the TCR with secretion of IL-12 *(6,24)*. This leads to CD4+ T-cell proliferation, upregulation of IL-12Rβ2, and the production of IFN-γ and IL-2 *(24,25)*. CD4+ Th1 cells then induce antigen specific proliferation of CD8+ cells and the development of cytotoxic T-lymphocytes (CTL, or Tc1 cells). Additionally, IL-12 induces NK cell proliferation and IFN-γ production *(26)*, B-cell IgG production *(27)*, and activation of neutrophils *(28)*. IFN-γ produced in response to IL-12 induces the upregulation of MHC molecules *(29,30)*, and activates macrophages and NK cells *(31–33)*.

2.5. Regulation of the IL-12 Response

The Th1 immune response induced by IL-12 is dependent on T-cell and APC costimulatory signaling and is modulated by multiple cytokines. In addition to the activation of the TCR, several studies have also shown that ligation of either CD2 or CD28, both expressed on T-cells, augments the response to IL-12. CD2 binds to CD58 on APCs. Antibodies blocking the CD2 adhesion domain or CD58 markedly reduce T-cell IL-12 responsiveness *(34)*. CD28 binds to B7 on APCs, and ligation of CD28 with the TCR increased Janus kinase and STAT4 phosphorylation and IFN-γ production by T-cells after exposure to IL-12 *(35)*. Conversely, ligation of APC CD40 via CD40L on T-cells augments APC activation and IL-12 secretion *(36)*.

Multiple cytokines, including IL-2, IL-15, IL-18 and IFN-γ have been shown to augment the response to IL-12. Expression of IL-12Rβ2 is increased by IFN-γ and IL-12, and is downregulated by IL-4 *(22,34)*. As discussed previously, IL-2 augments the IL-12 response by up-regulating serine phosphorylation of STAT1 and STAT3 *(19)*. IL-18 and IL-15, both produced by activated monocytes, are also synergistic with IL-12. IL-15, like IL-12, is secreted early in the immune response. In mouse models, IL-15 augments IL-12 induced IFN-γ production by T-cells, upregulates the IL-12 receptor, and stimulates NK cells *(37,38)*. Human PBMC show a greater increase in proliferation and IFN-γ production after being cultured with IL-12 plus IL-2 or IL-15 than when cultured with IL-12 alone *(22)*. In mouse models, IL-18 acts synergistically with IL-12 as a potent stimulator of IFN-γ production, and upregulates the IL-12 receptor *(39)*. IL-18 and IL-12 synergistically induce both IFN-γ production by murine CD4+ T-cells and regression of mouse SCK tumors (40). Also, IL-12 production by the APC is increased by several costimulatory cytokines, including IFN-γ, IL-15, and IL-12 *(39,41,42)*.

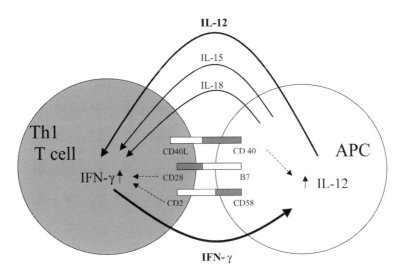

Fig. 2. IL-12 and IFN-γ form a positive feedback loop between T cells and APCs. Model shows how the production of costimulatory cytokines and the engagement of costimulatory molecules are central to Th1 development and the activation of APCs.

Production of IL-18 binding protein and IL-10 dampen the response to IL-12. IFN-γ produced in response to IL-12 induces monocytes to produce IL-18 binding protein, *a* isoform (IL-18BPa) *(43)*. IL-18BPa then binds and neutralizes IL-18, preventing it from synergizing with IL-12 to further induce IFN-γ production. IL-10 is a potent inhibitor of the IL-12 mediated immune response. Secreted by activated macrophages and IL-12 stimulated T-cells, IL-10 downregulates the production of both IL-12 and IFN-γ *(6,44,45)*.

As shown in Fig. 2, the complex regulation of T-cell IL-12 responsiveness and the need for costimulatory signaling underscores the importance of the interaction between APCs and T-cells. APCs combine antigen presentation with the ligation of costimulatory adhesion molecules and the production of costimulatory cytokines to drive the T-cell Th1 response. In turn, T-cell and NK cell derived IFN-γ, as well as IL-12; contribute to dendritic cell and monocyte activation.

2.6. IL-23 and IL-27: Newly Discovered Cytokines

Recently, two additional cytokines have been characterized that are closely related to IL-12: IL-23 and IL-27. Secreted by dendritic cells, IL-23 is a heterodimeric cytokine composed of the p40 subunit of IL-12 bound to a second glycoprotein, p19 *(46)*. p19 has 4 α-helix domains and is structurally similar to p35 and G-CSF *(46)*. Like p35, p19 is not biologically active by itself but only as a heterodimer with p40 *(46)*. IL-23 shares the IL-12Rβ1 receptor with IL-12p70, but signaling occurs via a unique receptor chain, IL-23Rβ3 *(9)*. The actions of IL-12 and IL-23 are overlapping but distinct. Both activate STAT4 and induce Th1 differentiation and IFN-γ production *(46,47)*. As with p40 and p35, transgenic expression of both p19 and p40 in mice can cause an uncontrolled inflammatory process *(47)*. However, in both mouse and human models, IL-23 is a less potent stimulator of IFN-γ than IL-12, and in mice IL-23 is more potent than IL-12 in activating memory T-cells *(46)*.

IL-27 is composed of two glycoproteins, p28 and Epstein-Barr virus-induced gene 3 (EBI3). The p28 protein is 243 amino acids long with 4 α-helix domains. EBI3 was first detected in the supernatant of EBV infected B-cells and is homologous to p40. The IL-27 receptor is a heterodimer composed of WSX-1 and glycoprotein 130 (gp130) that can induce signaling through STAT1 and STAT3 *(48)*. Although IL-27 is secreted primarly by activated monocytes, WSX-1/gp130 mRNA has been found in a wide array of cells including monocytes, T-cells and mast cells, indicating a potentially broad role for IL-27 in the immune response (49, 48). IL-27 may regulate the T-cell response to IL-12, and is synergistic with IL-12 in producing high levels of IFN-γ by T and NK cells *(49,50)*. IL-27 is also a potent stimulus for proliferation of human naïve, but not memory, T-cells *(49)*.

3. IL-12 AS AN ANTITUMOR AGENT

Brunda et al first demonstrated in vivo antitumor activity of IL-12 in mouse models *(51)*. Mice injected simultaneously with B16F10 melanoma cells and IL-12 had a dose dependent inhibition of metastasis formation after 22 d. IL-12 given 7 d after the injection of tumor cells reduced the tumor volume. These experiments together demonstrated effectiveness in preventing both new metastases and growth of existing tumors. Activity for IL-12 has also been demonstrated against reticulum cell sarcoma, Renca renal cell adenocarcinoma, C26 colon cancer, and TSA mammary adenocarcinoma cell lines *(51–53)*.

3.1. Cell Populations Mediating Antitumor Effects of IL-12

CD8+ cytotoxic T-cells play a clear role in the antitumor immune response to IL-12, and CD8+ T-cells have been shown to infiltrate tumors both in mouse models and in humans after treatment with rhIL-12 *(54,52)*. In mouse models, Brunda et al demonstrated that the antitumor effect of IL-12 was lost with CD8+ T-cell depletion. Conversely, NK cell and CD4+ T-cell depletion had little to no effect in that system *(51)*. In mice injected with TSA mammary cell line tumors, CD8+ T-cell depletion mitigated the antitumor action of systemic IL-12 therapy on both sc and lung metastases, whereas depletion of CD4+ T-cells or NK cells did not *(52)*. In humans, a study analyzing PBMC from patients treated with sc rhIL-12 identified a subset of CD8+ cells strongly expressing CD18 (CD18[bright]) that expanded in vivo and upregulated the IL-12 receptor in response to rhIL-12 therapy. CD8+ T-cells with low level expression of CD18 (CD18[dim]) were unaffected by rhIL-12. The CD18[bright] T-cells also differed from CD18[dim] cells in their expression of costimulatory cell adhesion molecules, and were morphologically similar to NK cells. Unlike CD18[dim] cells, CD18[bright] cells were capable of IFN-γ production as well as both non-MHC-restricted and CD3- mediated cytotoxic activity after exposure to IL-12 and IL-2 in vitro *(22)*.

Vα14 NKT cells may also play a role in IL-12 mediated tumor rejection *(55)*. Vα14 NKT cells represent a subpopulation of CD8 negative T-cells with a distinct lineage and are identifiable by a unique and invariant TCRα chain. Cui et al. demonstrated that selective depletion of Vα14 NKT cells without manipulation of CD8+ or NK cells resulted in loss of IL-12 mediated immunity in three mouse tumor models. Furthermore, tumor immunity mediated through Vα14 NKT cells persisted despite inhibition of IFN-γ and depletion of CD8+ cells, indicating that NKT cells alone may be sufficient for tumor rejection by IL-12 *(55)*. However, the singular role of Vα14 NKT cells has not been consistently reproduced in other studies. In a recent study using a similar mouse tumor model, IL-12 had an equivalent antitumor effect in both wild-type and Vα14 NKT-deficient mice, whereas other mouse studies have shown a unique role for NKT cells as well as other lymphocyte populations, such as NK cells, in IL-12 mediated antitumor immunity *(56,57)*.

The role of NK cells in IL-12 induced tumor immunity is unclear. Several studies in mice have indicated that in the context of an otherwise normal immune system, NK cells are not essential for an IL-12 induced antitumor response. Treatment of NK deficient or phenotypically normal beige mice with IL-12 produced an equivalent immune response against B16 melanoma cells, and antibody mediated depletion of NK cells in mice injected with TSA mammary cells had little impact on survival after IL-12 therapy *(51,52)*. However, it has also been shown that in the absence of T and NKT cells, NK cells effectively mediate an antitumor response after IL-12 stimulation. RAG-2 –/– mice (lacking T-cells, B-cells and NKT-cells) were shown to have an antitumor response to IL-12 equivalent to wild type mice, but antitumor immunity was lost with NK cell depletion *(58)*. A clear role for NK cells was also seen after treatment with IL-12 and Cyclophosphamide in mice with large, established tumors *(56)*.

As with NK cells, CD4+ T-cells are not central to the IL-12 response in otherwise immunocompetent mice. Selective depletion in mice of CD4+ cells has little effect on the tumor response to IL-12 therapy *(51)*. However, like NK cells, CD4+ cells have a role in immune modified mouse tumor models. Removal of CD4+ cells from CD8+ depleted mice further attenuates the effectiveness of IL-12 in controlling tumors *(59)*. CD4+ T-cells are required for an antitumor response to IL-12 in IFN-γ knockout mice *(53,59)*.

Finally, neutrophils may also play a role in the antitumor effect of IL-12. IL-12 has been shown to bind to neutrophils and cause Ca^{+2} mediated activation and increased production of reactive oxygen metabolites *(28)*. In chimpanzees, neutrophil activation occurs within 24 hrs of IL-12 therapy *(60)*. Cavallo et al. demonstrated neutrophil infiltrates in subcutaneous TSA mammary tumors in mice treated with IL-12 and showed that neutrophil depletion decreased the effect of IL-12 on survival *(52)*.

3.2. IFN-γ and Other Cytokines in Antitumor Effects of IL-12

IFN-γ is central to the IL-12 response and has been shown to have multiple antineoplastic effects through the activation of immune effector cells, the induction of secondary cytokines and chemokines, and a direct effect on tumor cells in murine tumor models. In vivo neutralization of IFN-γ abolishes the antitumor effect of IL-12 *(53,61)*. IFN-γ mediated antitumor immunity occurs through the activation of macrophages and dendritic cells, the augmentation of NK cell and NKT effector cell function, *(31,33)* as well as facilitation of the Th1 immune response. IFN-γ upregulates expression of IL-12βR2 on T and NK cells, increases IL-12 production by macrophages and dendritic cells *(22,42)*, and increases expression of tumor MHC molecules *(62,63)*.

IFN-γ also induces the production of three chemokines with antiangiogenic properties: IFN-inducible 10-kDa protein (IP-10), monokine induced by IFN (Mig), and IFN-inducible T-cell-chemokine (I-TAC) *(64–66)*. Collectively termed CXC3 chemokines, they bind the CXC3 receptor found on intraepithelial lymphocytes, macrophages, dendritic cells, and endothelial cells *(67)*. The two potential antitumor effects of the CXC3 chemokines include facilitating T-cell migration and inhibiting angiogenesis. Evidence for their ability to induce chemotaxis includes studies showing that tumor cells engineered to secret

IP-10 grow normally in culture but then elicit a T-cell-dependent inflammatory infiltrate in vivo *(68)*. Also, administering IL-12 to mice with Renca tumors causes T-cell infiltration into the tumors that is inhibited by the administration of anti-Mig and anti-IP-10 antibodies *(69)*. CXC3 chemokines are also anti-angiogenic. In mouse models, both IP-10 and Mig induce tumor necrosis associated with vascular damage when injected directly into tumors *(70,71)*. Although IL-12 and IP-10 both inhibit bFGF-induced Matrigel neovascularization, the ability of IL-12 to inhibit neovascularization is neutralized by anti IFN-γ or anti IP-10 antibodies *(72,73)*. In other studies, SCK mammary and K1735 tumors engineered to be unresponsive to IFN-γ were more tumorigenic and less sensitive to IL-12 therapy. This was not attributable to differences in immunologic rejection; instead, it was found that IL-12 could inhibit angiogenesis only in IFN-γ responsive tumors. The authors hypothosized that this may be owing to the loss of IFN-γ induced tumor secretion of antiangiogenic factors such as IP-10.

IFN-γ also has several potential direct antitumor effects through STAT mediated signaling *(75–77)*. IFN-γ enhances STAT1 signaling decreases cell proliferation by increasing expression of Cyclin-Dependent Kinase Inhibitor p21, and induces apoptosis via up-regulation of caspase 1 in A431 and HeLa cells *(76,77)*. In melanoma cells, increased JAK-STAT signaling, mediated via the up-regulation of STAT1 expression by IFN-γ, led to increased sensitivity to the antitumor effects of IFN-α *(75)*.

A model for the antitumor effects of IL-12 administered systemically is shown in Fig. 3. In this model administration of IL-12 augments production of IL-15 and IL-18 by APCs. IL-12 combines with IL-15 and IL-18 to induce IFN-γ production by circulating NK cells and CD8+ CD18[bright] T-cells. IFN-γ then contributes to the development of innate and adaptive antitumor immunity by fostering Th1 T-cell development, activating NK cells and monocytes, inducing the production of chemokines with anti-angiogenic lymphocyte chemotaxic effects, and exerting direct effects on tumor cells that fosters immune recognition and apoptosis.

4. CLINICAL TRIALS OF IL-12

4.1. Intravenous IL-12 in Renal Cell Cancer and Melanoma

There have been numerous clinical trials of iv recombinant human (rh) IL-12 in patients with melanoma and renal cell cancer (Table 1). In the first phase I trial, rhIL-12 was given as a test dose on day 1 followed by a 13 d rest period during which pharmacokinetic studies were performed *(78)*. Intravenous infusions at the same dose level were then administered for the first 5 d of a 21-d course. Patients with stable or responding disease could continue treatment for six courses. Forty patients were enrolled, 32 had renal cell cancer or melanoma, and 25 had received prior systemic therapy, including 14 treated with high dose IL-2. Dose levels ranged from 3 ng/kg/d to 1000 ng/kg/d, and 14 patients were treated at the maximum tolerated dose (MTD) of 500 ng/kg/d. The most common grade-3 toxicities were elevated AST (three patients) and bilirubin (six patients), and neutropenia (five patients). Additionally, one patient had an upper gastrointestinal bleed and one patient died of *Clostridium perfringens* sepsis from an unknown source, likely bowel. The half life of rhIL-12 at 500 ng/kg measured after the test dose was 9.6 h, significantly longer than other cytokines such as IL-2. IFN-γ production was induced in a dose-dependent manner during cycle 1, with dual peaks 24 h after the test dose and then on day 3 of week 1 before levels declined on days 4 and 5

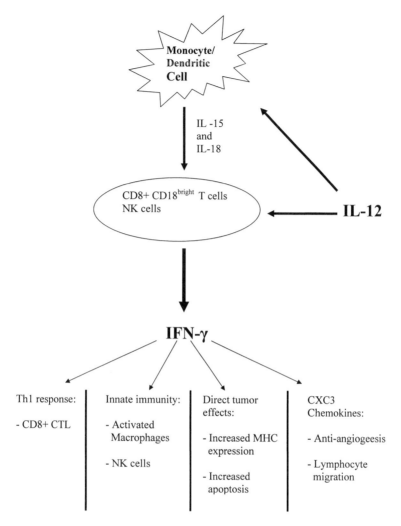

Fig. 3. Mechanisms of IL-12-mediated antitumor activity, showing the central role of IFN-γ.

despite continued rhIL-12 infusions. Unfortunately, the IFN- γ response appeared transient with little IFN-γ produced during subsequent cycles of rhIL-12 regardless of the dose level. Two patients in the trial had objective responses, including one patient with a CR that lasted 4 wk and another with a PR continuing for over 22 mo *(78)*.

In addition to inducing IFN-γ production, rhIL-12 had numerous measurable effects on the immune system. Grade 4 lymphopenia occurred at all dose levels. Lymphocyte counts nadired on day 2 and then during the first 5-d course, returning to normal within 72 h. NK cells declined most dramatically, nadiring at 6% of their baseline levels, whereas CD4+ and CD8+ T-cells declined to 15% and 29% of their baseline levels, respectively *(26)*. There was no rebound lymphocytosis as seen after therapy with high dose IL-2 *(79)*. Unlike the production of IFN-γ, the effect of rhIL-12 on lymphocytes was observed through multiple dosing cycles. Additionally, there was a several fold increase in the expression of NK cell adhesion molecules, including CD56, CD2, CD11a/CD18, and CD 54, and enhanced NK cell cytotoxicity towards K562 cells *(26)*. These effects

Table 1
Select Published Trials of Intravenous IL-12 in Melanoma and Renal Cell Cancer[a]

Author	Year	Phase	Number of patients	Dose	Schedule	Test dose	Grade III/IV toxicity	Objective[1] responses	Comments
Atkins, MB (78)	1997	I	40	Escalation to MTD of 500 ng/kg/ day	days 1–5 of 21-day cycle	Yes	LFT elevations Neutropenia Anemia, Orthostasis Infection	1 PR, 1CR	32 patients with melanoma and renal cell cancer, 8 with other malignancies.
Leonard, JP (81)	1997	II	17	500 ng/kg/day	days 1–5 of 21-day cycle	No	LFT elevations Neutropenia, GI Hemorrhage, Dyspnea Fatigue, Death	Not Assessable	Stopped early for severe Grade IV toxicity and two unexpected deaths.
Gollob, JA (82)	2000	I	28	Escalation to 500 ng/kg/ day	BIW for 6-week cycle	No	LFT elevations Neutropenia, Anemia, Fever, Orthostasis	1 PR	Objective response occurred after 4 cycles.
Gollob, JA (83)	2003	I	28	Escalation to MTD of 500 ng/kg/ day of IL-12 and 3 MU/ m² SQ of IL-2	IL-12 BIW for 6 week cycle, and IL-2 SQ 1 hour before and 20 hours after IL-12 starting with dose number six.	No	LFT elevations Leukopenia, Anemia, Hypotension	1 PR	Achieved sustained IFN-γ and IP-10 response with additionof SQ IL-2.

[a]CR, complete response; PR, partial response

were seen during lymphocyte recovery, but then were absent 2 wk after therapy. Additionally, T-cells were found to have enhanced proliferation after CD3 ligation post therapy with rhIL-12. Unlike the effects on NK cells, the T-cell effects were not seen during the lymphocyte recovery phase but rather on day 14 after the test dose. These results are consistent with mouse models demonstrating a transient macrophage-induced down regulation of T-cell mediated immunity immediately after IL-12 exposure *(80)*.

The acceptable toxicity of rhIL-12 at dose levels with demonstrable biologic effects led to the initiation of a phase II trial of iv rhIL-12. Seventeen patients were given 500 ng/kg/d for days 1 through 5 of a 21-d cycle without the test dose used during the phase-I trial *(81)*. Unfortunately, there was severe unexpected toxicity and the trial was closed early with no patients receiving more than one cycle of therapy. A high proportion of patients experienced grade-3 or -4 fatigue, dyspnea, stomatitis, leukopenia, and hepatic toxicity. Twelve of the 17 patients were hospitalized and two died from rhIL-12 related toxicity, including hemorrhagic colitis and intestinal ulceration. The only significant difference between the phase-I and phase-II trials was the use of a rhIL-12 test dose. Peak IFN-γ levels measured in patients in the phase-II trial were several fold higher than IFN-γ levels among patients receiving 500 ng/kg in the phase-I trial. Subsequent studies performed in mice demonstrated that the use of a test dose prevented the marked elevation of IFN-γ seen during the five daily IL-12 infusions and significantly decreased IL-12 related toxicity *(81)*. Several subsequent phase II trials of rhIL-12 with daily dosing for 5 d at 500 ng/kg/d following a test dose were subsequently performed. Toxicity was tolerable, but there was minimal to no clinical efficacy (unpublished data).

One possible reason for the failure of rhIL-12 administered as a daily injection for 5 d to show more potent antitumor activity was the inability of rhIL-12 to consistently induce IFN-γ production. In an attempt to achieve a more sustained IFN-γ response, a phase-I dose escalation trial of twice weekly iv rhIL-12 without a test dose was initiated *(82)*. Successive cohorts of patients were treated with doses ranging from 30 ng/kg to 700 ng/kg. Twenty-eight patients were enrolled; 23 had received prior immunotherapy. The MTD was 500 ng/kg, with 2 of 14 patients treated at that dose experiencing DLTs, one with orthostatic hypotension and another with agranulocytosis. Five patients were treated at 700 ng/kg, with two experiencing DLTs (grade-3 elevation of hepatic transaminases, and grade-3 Coombs negative hemolytic anemia). There was one objective response, a PR in a patient treated at 500 ng/kg, and two other patients had stable disease for over 6 mo *(82)*.

Serial IFN-γ measurements were taken during cycle 1 in 10 patients treated at or above the MTD with twice weekly iv rhIL-12 *(82)*. Several patterns of IFN-γ production were seen. All patients had peak IFN-γ levels during the first week and then most showed near complete attenuation of IFN-γ production by week 4. One subgroup of patients continued to produce IFN-γ during week 4 of therapy at a level similar to what was seen in week 1 *(82)*. All of the clinical responses as well as the side effects of hemolytic anemia and agranulocytosis were seen in this subgroup of patients with sustained IFN-γ production *(82)*. Lymphocyte cytokine responsiveness was also evaluated in vitro using patient PBMCs collected before therapy and on week 4 of rhIL-12 treatment. PBMC isolated before and after rhIL-12 exposure maintained the proliferative response to either IL-12 alone or IL-12 combined with IL-2 or IL-15. IFN-γ production at week 4 was seen only in response to IL-12 when it was combined with IL-2 or IL-15, and was strongest at week 4 in the patients who had a sustained IFN-γ response in vivo (82). In this study, investigators also measured pharmacokinetics of IL-12 after repeated dosing. Although the peak serum IL-12 levels remained constant, $t_{1/2}$ decreased over time. This is a recurrent finding in rhIL-12 clinical trials. However, the decreased $t_{1/2}$ did not account for the changes in IFN-γ response, as serum rhIL-12 levels did not correlate with the magnitude or pattern of IFN-γ production *(82)*. Other cytokines measured, including IL-10, were consistently induced by IL-12 both during week 1 and 4 of therapy *(82)*.

In a recently published phase-I trial, consistent induction of IFN-γ was achieved by combining iv rhIL-12 with sc IL-2 *(83)*. Twenty-eight patients with metastatic melanoma and renal cell cancer were treated with biweekly infusions of rhIL-12, at dose levels of 300 or 500 ng/kg/day, combined with 0.5 to 6.0 MU/m² of IL-2 given subcutaneously 1 h before and 20 h after the rhIL-12, starting with rhIL-12 dose number six. Eleven patients were treated at the MTD (500 ng/kg of rhIL-12 and 3.0 MU/m² of IL-2). There were no grade-4 toxicities, but several patients experienced grade-3 lab abnormalities including elevated AST/ALT and various cytopenias. After an initial waning of the IFN-γ response by dose 5 of rhIL-12 alone, the addition of IL-2 led to IFN-γ production comparable to that seen after the first dose of rhIL-12. This augmented IFN-γ production was sustained through week 6 of therapy. IP-10 was also measured and was induced in a pattern similar to IFN-γ. There were several measurable responses in this study. One patient with melanoma had a partial response and two melanoma patients had regression of skin metastases. Four patients with renal cell cancer and one patient with ocular melanoma had prolonged periods of stable disease *(83)*. Although this trial achieved the goal of a sustained IFN-γ response, the clinical effectiveness of rhIL-12 remained modest, with few objective responses.

4.2 Subcutaneous IL-12 in Renal Cell Cancer and Melanoma

Bajetta et al. in 1998 published the first trial of sc rhIL-12 *(see* Table 2). Ten patients with melanoma were treated with 500 ng/kg/d on days 1, 8, and 15 of a 28-d cycle *(84)*. The regimen was well tolerated with flu like symptoms in all patients but only one patient with a grade-3 toxicity (neutropenia). Peak IFN-γ production occurred after the first rhIL-12 dose, with subsequent attenuation of response in most patients. The magnitude of the IFN-γ response was much smaller than that seen with iv rhIL-12, with serum IFN-γ levels being one-fifth the level seen after a similar iv dose *(82,84)*. Subcutaneous rhIL-12 did induce lymphocyte activation in a manner similar to what was seen after iv therapy, with NK cells being most affected. Correlative studies also demonstrated increased expression of T-cell adhesion and homing molecules (CD11a, CD18, CD49d and CD44), and several excised cutaneous metastases that were responding to IL-12 were found to have CD8+/CD45RO+ memory T-cell infiltrations. Also, in vitro studies of PBMCs showed an increased tumor-specific cytotoxic T-cell response to autologous tumor cell lines after rhIL-12 therapy *(54)*. Three patients in the trial had minor responses, two with resolution of cutaneous lesions and one with resolution of a hepatic mass *(84)*.

The pharmacokinetics of rhIL-12 after sc dosing differed from that of iv dosing. rhIL-12 peaked 8–12 h after sc injection. The $t_{1/2}$ was similar to that of the iv infusion after dose one (8–10 h), but with repeated dosing serum levels did not rise to a detectable level in most patients *(84)*. This was hypothesized to be the result of a lack of accumulation of rhIL-12 in the serum owing to increased clearance rather than a change in absorption. The investigators looked for but did not find anti rhIL-12 antibodies.

Table 2
Select Published Trials of Subcutaneous IL-12 in Melanoma and Renal Cell Cancer

Author	Year	Phase	Number of patients	Dose	Schedule	Test dose	Grade III/IV toxicity	Objective[a] responses	Comments
Bajetta, E (84)	1998	II	10	500 ng/kg/day	days 1,8,15 of 28 day cycle	No	Neutropenia	None	There were 3 minor responses
Portielje, JEA (85)	1999	I	28	Escalation to MTD of 1000 ng/kg/day	TIW for 2 weeks of 4 week cycle	Yes[b]	Neutropenia	1 PR	
Ohno, R (87)	2000	I	15	Escalation to MTD of 300 ng/kg/day	TIW for 2 weeks of 3-week cycle	No	LFT elevations Leukopenia	1 CR 1 PR	
Motzer, RJ (88)	1998	I	51	Escalation to MTD of 1000–1500 ng/kg on day 15[c]	days 1, 8, 15 of 28-day cycle	No	LFT elevations Leukopenia Pulmonary toxicity	1 CR	
Motzer, RJ (89)	2001	II	30	1500 ng/kg on day 15[d]	days 1, 8, 15 of 28-day cycle	No	LFT elevations Leukopenia Stomatitis Ascites	2 PR	Randomized phase II trial, 16 additional patients treated with IFN-α2a
Hutson, TE (90)	2001	I	11	Escalation to MTD of 500 ng/kg/day of IL-12 and 1.0 MU/m^2 of IFN-α2a	BIW TIW	No	Fatigue Neutropenia	None	Preliminary results

[a]PR , partial response, CR, complete response.
[b]MTD for test dose was 500 ng/kg.
[c]24 patients treated with fixed weekly dosing with MTD of 1000 ng/kg/day; 27 patients with intracycle dose escalation schema with MTD of 100 ng/kg day 1, 500 ng/kg d8, and 1500 ng/kg day 15.
[d]Dose escalation regimen for rhIL–12 taken from Motzer, RJ 1998: of 100 ng/kg day 1, 500 ng/kg day 8, and 1500 ng/kg day 15.

In trials administering sc rhIL-12 three times a week, a higher cumulative dose of rhIL-12 could be given, but the resulting immune response was not consistently improved. Twenty-eight patients were treated in a phase-I study of sc rhIL-12 administered as a test dose on day 1 and then three times a week for the first 2 wk of a 28-d cycle *(85)*. The MTD was 500 ng/kg for the test dose and 1000 ng/kg for the thrice-weekly dosing. There were few grade-3 or -4 toxicities. Peak serum rhIL-12 levels were higher than those seen with weekly sc rhIL-12, but unfortunately this did not translate into a more sustained IFN-γ response. Even at 1250 ng/kg, rhIL-12 failed to induce IFN-γ production beyond the first week of therapy *(86)*. A second phase-I dose escalation study in Japan of thrice weekly sc rhIL-12 eliminated the test dose and treated patients for 2 out of every 3 wk *(87)*. The MTD was 300 ng/kg/d. The results of this study differed significantly from previous trials of sc rhIL-12. The serum half life of rhIL-12 after the first injection was close to 25 h, almost three times higher then had been previously observed, and neither $t_{1/2}$ or peak concentration decreased with repeated dosing. Although the peak IFN-γ levels were seen after the first dose, unlike other studies, there was a continued measurable IFN-γ response even after the sixth dose of the third cycle *(87)*. Fourteen patients were enrolled in the trial and there were two responses, one CR and one PR, each lasting about 4 mo *(87)*.

The largest trials of sc rhIL-12 were performed by Motzer et al. in renal cell cancer *(88,89)*. A phase-I trial enrolling 51 heavily pretreated patients used two separate dosing schemes, one with fixed and one with escalating weekly doses *(88)*. In the fixed arm, 24 patients were treated with the same dose of rhIL-12 on days 1, 8, and 15 of a 28-d cycle. The MTD was 1000 ng/kg/d, with elevated transaminases on day 8 being the most common toxicity *(88)*. In an effort to avoid this transient liver toxicity, 27 patients were treated with escalating doses of rhIL-12 during cycle 1, and then continued on the highest dose for subsequent cycles. The MTD in this regimen was 100 ng/kg on day 1, 500 ng/kg on day 8, and 1500 ng/kg on day 15. The DLTs were grade 3 and grade 4 hepatic transaminase elevations at 1500 ng/kg. Measurements of IFN-γ demonstrated brisk induction on day 15 in patients treated with dose escalation. There was one objective response, a CR in a patient treated with dose escalation to 1500 ng/kg, and 34 of 49 evaluable patients had varying periods of stable disease *(88)*.

A modification of this dosing regimen was carried to a randomized trial of rhIL-12 vs IFN-α2a as first line therapy in patients with metastatic renal cell cancer *(89)*. Forty-six patients were randomized in a 2:1 ratio favoring rhIL-12. Thirty were treated with sc rhIL-12 with dose escalation up to 1250 ng/kg on day 15, and 16 patients were treated with sc IFN-α2a 9 million units three times per week. There was significant induction of IFN-γ after dosing on day 15 of both cycle one and two of rhIL-12. However, despite a sustained IFN-γ, response the overall clinical response rate was low. With only two partial responses seen among the 29 evaluable patient treated in the rhIL-12 arm, the study was closed early *(89)*.

Based on the synergy between IFN-γ and IFN-α in augmenting JAK-STAT signaling and inducing IP-10 and Mig, Hutson et al. conducted a phase I trial of concurrent sc rhIL-12 and sc IFN-α2b in patients with renal cell cancer or melanoma *(90)*. As of 2001, 11 patients were enrolled and treated with escalating doses of up to 500 ng/kg of rhIL-12 twice per week and 1.0 MU/m^2 of IFN-α2b three times a week *(90)*. At the time of their interim report the MTD had not been reached and 9 of the 11 patients had stable disease. No follow up report has yet been published. A phase-II trial in melanoma was initiated by CALGB giving iv rhIL-12 300 ng/kg on day 1 and IFN-α2b 3.0 MU/m^2

on days 2 through 6 of a 14-d cycle (CALGB 500001). Unfortunately, this trial was closed early after the planned interim analysis showed no meaningful responses (William Carson, M.D., personal communication).

4.3. The Use of rhIL-12 in Other Malignancies

4.3.1. LYMPHOMA

IL-12 appears to have activity in cutaneous T-cell lymphoma (CTCL). Ten patients with CTCL were treated in a phase-I study of twice weekly sc rhIL-12 (*see* Table 3) *(91)*. Dose levels ranged from 50 to 300 ng/kg, and intrapatient dose escalation was permitted after 4 wk of therapy. As a result, all patients received up to 100–300 ng/kg of IL-12. Treatment was generally well tolerated. The MTD was 300 ng/kg, with fatigue and transient elevations in liver function tests being the primary toxicities. Clinical responses varied depending on disease stage. All five patients with plaque like disease responded. Two had a CR, two a PR, and one a minor response. One of three patients with Sezary syndrome (T4 disease) one had a partial response, one withdrew, and one progressed. Two patients with rapidly progressive disease and T3/T4 lesions received intralesional instead of sc injections, with local but no systemic responses *(91)*. Biopsies obtained from skin lesions during regression showed a several-fold increase in the number of CD8+ cytotoxic T-cells.

A phase II study of 23 CTCL patients treated twice weekly with 300 ng/kg of sc rhIL-12 has completed enrollment and is pending publication at the time of this chapter. As in the phase-I trial, there was a high response rate among patients with early stage disease (Alain Rook M.D., personal communication). A second phase-II trial, based on the regimen developed by Gollob JA et al. *(83)* using sc rhIL-12 at 100 ng/kg with escalating doses of sc IL-2 from 0.5 MU/m^2 to 6.0 MU/m^2, is currently enrolling patients.

Several studies have evaluated the use of rhIL-12 in patients with Hodgkin's disease and non-Hodgkin's B-cell lymphoma (*see* Table 3). Subcutaneous rhIL-12 was administered with Rituximab in one phase-I study of patients with CD20 positive B-cell lymphoma *(92)*. Rituximab was given at 375 mg/m^2 weekly for 4 wk and up to 300 ng/kg of rhIL-12 sc was given twice weekly for up to 24 wk. The clinical response rate was 69% and appeared to be higher then what has been seen with Rituximab alone. Responses were seen in both aggressive and low grade lymphomas, including several patients with mantle cell lymphoma and several patients who had had bone marrow transplants. Both serum IP-10 and IFN-γ were show to increase dramatically, peaking 24 h after rhIL-12 administraion *(92)*.

In a second phase I trial, eight patients with non-Hodgkin's lymphoma, two with Hodgkin's disease and two with plasma cell myeloma were treated with iv rhIL-12 after autologous bone marrow transplant (Table 3) *(93)*. Treatment started on average 66 days after stem cell transplant and patients were given a single test dose followed by 2 wk rest and then daily infusions of rhIL-12 for days 1–5 of a 21-d cycle. The maximum tolerated dose of rhIL-12 was 100 ng/kg. Three patients experienced dose-limiting toxicity: one treated at 100 ng/kg had a grade-3 infection, and two of three patients treated at 250 ng/kg had grade-3 elevations of liver function tests, one of whom also had grade-3 diarrhea. Additionally, several patients treated at the MTD required dose reductions for transient leukopenia and neutropenia *(93)*. Five of 12 patients had stable disease for over 32 mo after starting rhIL-12 therapy; the other seven progressed.

Table 3
Select Published Clinical Trials of rhIL-12 in Lymphoma and Solid Tumors[a]

Author	Disease	Year	Phase	Number of patients	Regimen	Toxicity	Objective[a] responses	Comments
Rook, AH (91)	Cutaneous T-cell Lymphoma	1999	I	10	100–300 ng/kg SQ twice per week.	Fatigue LFT elevations	2 CR 3 PR	PR or CR in 4 of 5 patients with plaque like disease.
Ansell, SM (92)	Lymphoma, CD-20 positive	2002	I	43	Rituximab 375 mg/m² weekly 3 4 and IL-12 50–500 ng/kg SQ BIW 24 weeks	LFT elevations Hemolytic Anemia Nausea Fever	11 CR 18 PR	Difficult to determine relative contribution of IL-12 and Rituximab to response rate.
Robertson, MJ (93)	Lymphoma, post transplant	2002	I	12	30 to 250 ng/kg iv days 1–5 of 21 day cycle with test dose.	LFT elevations Leukopenia, Neutropenia, Thrombocytopenia, Diarrhea	None	Modest IFN-γ response but IL-12 induced lymphocyte proliferation.
Pluda, JM (96)	Kaposi's Sarcoma	1999	I	9	100–500 ng/kg SQ BIW	Hepatotoxicity Leukopenia	4 PR	Responses seen at 300 and 500 ng/kg
Walder, S (97)	Cervical Cancer	2004	II	34	250 ng/kg iv d 1–5 of 21-day cycle with test dose.	LFT elevations Leukopenia, Anemia, Fever	1 PR	Stopped early for lack of response.
Lenzi R, 2002 (99)	Peritoneal Tumors	2002	I	29	Escalation to MTD of 300 ng/kg ip	LFT elevations Fever, Abdominal pain, Nausea, Diarrhea	2 CR	CRs surgically confirmed.
Parihar, R (100)	Her2-Overexpressing Malignancies	2001	I	7	Herceptin given with 4 mg/kg load and then 2 mg/kg with 30–500 ng/kg of IL-12 given iv BIW starting week 3 of Herceptin	Fever Chills, Hypotension	1 CR	CR in patient with breast cancer.

[a]CR, complete response; PR, partial response.

The immune response to rhIL-12 of bone marrow transplant patients in this study differed from what has been seen in other studies. The IFN-γ response was modest compared to other studies, with a mean serum IFN-γ level 24 h after the first dose of 100 ng/kg rhIL-12 of 104 pg/mL compared to 679 pg/mL in similarly treated patients in earlier studies. It was hypothesized that a lack of IL-18 may have been responsible for the poor IFN-γ response; however, IL-18 was detectable in all patients in this study before therapy and rose several fold during the first cycle of rhIL-12, indicating this was not the case. When PBMC from study patients isolated before rhIL-12 therapy were exposed in vitro to rhIL-12 or rhIL-12 and IL-2, they showed significantly less IFN-γ production than healthy controls, indicating this may be an effect specific to the post-transplant lymphocyte population *(93)*. Although IFN-γ production was modest, lymphocyte proliferation was more pronounced *(94)*. After a transient decrease, lymphocyte counts increased progressively during treatment with rhIL-12. This effect had not been seen in prior trials of rhIL-12 in patients with solid tumors, except for the expansion of CD8+CD18[Bright] T-cells seen by Gollob et al. *(22)*, nor was it seen in patients with relapsed lymphoma treated with sc rhIL-12 for prolonged periods of time. The effect was dose dependent and occurred in all lymphocyte subpopulations *(94)*.

4.3.2. KAPOSI SARCOMA

AIDS associated Kaposi Sarcoma (KS) may be sensitive to both the anti-angiogenic and immune mediated effects of rhIL-12 (Table 3). Cell mediated immunity is compromised in HIV disease and PBMC from HIV infected patients have been shown to have impaired IL-12 production *(95)*. The ability of rhIL-12 to combine an augmented Th1 immune response with the anti-angiogenic effects of IFN-γ and IP-10 may make it a potent therapy for a highly vascular opportunistic malignancy like KS occurring in an immunocompromised host. Preliminary results of a phase I trial using biweekly sc rhIL-12 in HIV patients with KS were promising. Four of 9 patients treated with 300 ng/kg or 500 ng/kg had a PR, with several additional patients having stable disease *(96)*. Further work with rhIL-12 in KS is ongoing.

4.3.3. OTHER SOLID TUMORS

Several trials have evaluated the effectiveness of rhIL-12 against gynecologic malignancies (Table 3). EGOG E1E96 was a phase II trial that enrolled 34 patients with advanced cervical cancer *(97)*. The role of HPV infection in cervical cancer and the ability of an immune response to HPV to cause regression in dysplastic cervical lesions made advanced cervical cancer a reasonable target for immune modulation. Patients were treated with iv rhIL-12 at 250 ng/kg on days 1 through 5 of a 21-d cycle with a test dose on day -13. There were few grade-3 or grade-4 toxicities, and some evidence of an immune response against HPV as measured by in vitro lymphocyte proliferation in response to HPV antigens. However, there was only one clinical response out of the first 29 evaluable patients, and the trial was closed early *(97)*. A second phase II trial using the same dosing regimen enrolled 28 patients with advanced ovarian cancer. Again, the regimen was well tolerated, but with minimal clinical activity *(98)*.

Inraperitoneal (ip) administration of rhIL-12 may allow for greater efficacy against peritoneal solid tumors (Table 3). In a phase-I trial of 29 patients with mesothelioma or ovarian, Müllerian, or gastrointestinal cancer with peritoneal involvement, rhIL-12 was given as weekly ip injections *(99)*. The MTD was 300/ng/kg, and the side effect profile was similar to that seen with iv rhIL-12. Fever and fatigue were common, and the elevation of liver function tests was dose limiting. Terminal phase clearance of rhIL-12 from the peritoneum was prolonged, over 18 h, and peritoneal concentrations of rhIL-12 were 10–50-fold higher then contemporaneous serum concentrations. Peritoneal IFN-γ levels rose to over 175 pg/mL, peaking 36–48 h after injection of 300 ng/kg of rhIL-12. Maximum serum IFN-γ level stayed under 100 pg/mL. Two of the 29 patients had a surgically confirmed complete responses, and eight patients had stable disease *(99)*. A phase-II study of intraperitoneal rhIL-12 is currently enrolling patients.

Additional ongoing research includes a trial of rhIL-12 in Her-2/*neu* overexpressing tumors. A phase-I trial of Trastuzumab and rhIL-12 in Her-2/*neu* overexpressing tumors has been completed and is pending publication (Table 3). An interim analysis was presented at the 2001 meeting of the American Society of Clinical Oncology *(100)*. Patients were treated with weekly Trastuzumab, 2 mg/kg, and biweekly infusions of rhIL-12 at up to 500 ng/kg. There were no grade-3 or -4 toxicities after enrollment of the first seven patients, and one patient with breast cancer had a complete response *(100)*. A phase-I trial combining Paclitaxel, Trastuzumab and rhIL-12 is currently enrolling patients (William Carson, M.D., personal communication).

5. CONCLUSIONS

Since its discovery in 1989, significant progress has been made in understanding the role of IL-12 in the immune response and its potential antitumor effects, but no clear role for IL-12 in cancer therapy has been established. The tight regulation of IL-12 and of IL-12 responsiveness and the rapid dampening of IL-12 induced IFN-γ production has resulted in significant challenges to the successful application of rhIL-12 in cancer therapy. Toxicity from excessive IFN-γ production during the early phase of rhIL-12 treatment can be severe, and the consistent induction of IFN-γ with repeated IL-12 administration has been difficult to achieve. In the few trials where the IFN-γ response was sustained, clinical activity remained modest. However, a potential role for IL-12 exists in several malignancies including KS and CTCL, and several ongoing clinical trials are further evaluating that potential. Future trials further exploring the contribution of IL-12 with other cytokines and antineoplastic agents will help to determine whether rhIL-12 will find a place in the biologic therapy of cancer.

REFERENCES

1. Rosenberg SA, Lotze MT, Muul LM, et al. Observations on the systemic administration of autologous lymphokine-activated killer cells and recombinant interleukin-2 to patients with metastatic cancer. N Engl J Med 1985;313:1485–1492.
2. Kobayashi M, Fitz L, Ryan M, et al. Identification and purification of natural killer cell stimulatory factor (NKSF), a cytokine with multiple biologic effects on human lymphocytes. J Exp Med 1989;170:827–845.
3. Gubler U, Chua AO, Schoenhaut DS, et al. Coexpression of two distinct genes is required to generate secreted bioactive cytotoxic lymphocyte maturation factor. Proc Natl Acad Sci 1991;88:4143–4147.
4. Merberg DM, Wolf SF, Clark SC. Sequence similarity between NKSF and the IL-6/G-CSF family. Immunol Today 1992;13:77–78.
5. Gering DP, Cosman D. Homology of the p40 subunit of natural killer cell stimulatory factor (NKSF) with the extracellular domain of the interleukin-6 receptor. Cell 1991;66:9, 10.
6. D'Andrea A, Rengaraju M, Valiante NM, et al. Production of natural killer cell stimulatory factor (interleukin 12) by peripheral blood mononuclear cells. J Exp Med 1992;176:1387–1398.

7. Chua A, Chizzonite R, Desai BB, et al. Expression cloning of a human IL-12 receptor component. A new member of the cytokine receptor superfamily with strong homology to gp130. J Immunol 1994;153:128–136.

8. Presky DH, Minetti LJ, Gillessen S, et al. Analysis of the multiple interactions between IL-12 and the high affinity IL-12 receptor complex. J Immunol 1998;160:2174–2179.

9. van de Vosse E, Lichtenauer-Kaligis EG, van Dissel JT, Ottenhoff TH. Genetic variations in the interleukin-12/interleukin-23 receptor (beta1) chain, and implications for IL-12 and IL-23 receptor structure and function. Immunogenetics 2003;54:817–829.

10. Presky DH, Yang H, Minetti LJ, et al. A functional interleukin 12 receptor complex is composed of two beta-type cytokine receptor subunits. Proc Natl Acad Sci 1996;93:14,002–14,007.

11. Rogge L, Barberis-Maino L, Biffi M, et al. Selective expression of an interleukin-12 receptor component by human T helper 1 cells. J Exp Med 1997;185:825–831.

12. Galbiati F, Rogge L, Guery JC, Smiroldo S, Adorini L. Regulation of the IL-12 receptor beta2 subunit by soluble antigen and IL-12 in vivo. Eur J Immunol 1998;28:209–-220.

13. Trinchieri G, Scott P. Interleukin-12: basic principles and clinical applications. Curr Top Microbiol Immunol 1999;238:57-78.

14. Bacon CM, McVicar DW, Ortaldo JR, Rees RC, O'Shea JJ, Johnston JA. Interleukin 12 (IL-12) induces tyrosine phosphorylation of JAK2 and TYK2: differential use of Janus family tyrosine kinases by IL-2 and IL-12. J Exp Med 1995;181:399–404.

15. Visconti R, Gadina M, Chiariello M, et al. Importance of the MKK6/p38 pathway for interleukin-12-induced STAT4 serine phosphorylation and transcriptional activity. Blood 2000;96:1844–1852.

16. Jacobson NG, Szabo SJ, Weber-Nordt RM, et al. Interleukin 12 signaling in T helper type 1 (Th1) cells involves tyrosine phosphorylation of signal transducer and activator of transcription (Stat)3 and Stat4. J Exp Med 1995;181:1755–1762.

17. Morinobu A, Gadina M, Strober W, et al. STAT4 serine phosphorylation is critical for IL-12-induced IFN-gamma production but not for cell proliferation. Proc Natl Acad Sci 2002;99:12,281–12,286.

18. Zhang S, Kaplan MH. The p38 mitogen-activated protein kinase is required for IL-12-induced IFN-gamma expression. J Immunol 2000;165:1374–1380.

19. Gollob JA, Schnipper CP, Murphy EA, Ritz J, Frank DA. The functional synergy between IL-12 and IL-2 involves p38 mitogen-activated protein kinase and is associated with the augmentation of STAT serine phosphorylation. J Immunol 1999;162:4472–4481.

20. Thierfelder WE, van Deursen JM, Yamamoto K, et al. Requirement for Stat4 in interleukin-12-mediated responses of natural killer and T cells. Nature 1996;382:171–174.

21. Kaplan MH, Sun YL, Hoey T, Grusby MJ. Impaired IL-12 responses and enhanced development of Th2 cells in Stat4-deficient mice. Nature 1996;382:174–177.

22. Gollob JA, Schnipper CP, Orsini E, et al. Characterization of a novel subset of CD8(+) T cells that expands in patients receiving interleukin-12. J Clin Invest 1998;102:561–575.

23. Gollob JA, Veenstra KG, Jyonouchi H, et al. Impairment of STAT activation by IL-12 in a patient with atypical mycobacterial and staphylococcal infections. J Immunol 2000;165:4120–4126.

24. Heufler C, Koch F, Stanzl U, et al. Interleukin-12 is produced by dendritic cells and mediates T helper 1 development as well as interferon-gamma production by T helper 1 cells. Eur J Immunol 1996;26:659–668.

25. Bertagnolli MM, Lin BY, Young D, Herrmann SH. IL-12 augments antigen-dependent proliferation of activated T lymphocytes. J Immunol 1992;149:3778–3783.

26. Robertson MJ, Cameron C, Atkins MB, et al. Immunological effects of interleukin 12 administered by bolus intravenous injection to patients with cancer. Clin Cancer Res 1999;5:9–16.

27. Jelinek DF, Braaten JK. Role of IL-12 in human B lymphocyte proliferation and differentiation. J Immunol 1995;154:1606–1613.

28. Collison K, Saleh S, Parhar R, et al. Evidence for IL-12-activated Ca2+ and tyrosine signaling pathways in human neutrophils. J Immunol 1998;161:3737–3745.

29. Bacsó Z, Bene L, Damjanovich L, Damjanovich S. INF-gamma rearranges membrane topography of MHC-I and ICAM-1 in colon carcinoma cells. Biochem Biophys Res Commun 2002;290:635–640.

30. Reiner NE, Ng W, Ma T, McMaster WR. Kinetics of gamma interferon binding and induction of major histocompatibility complex class II mRNA in Leishmania-infected macrophages. Proc Natl Acad Sci 1988;85:4330–4334.

31. Kamijo R, Harada H, Matsuyama T, et al. Requirement for transcription factor IRF-1 in NO synthase induction in macrophages. Science 1994;263:1612–1615.

32. Carnaud C, Lee D, Donnars O, et al. Cutting edge: Cross-talk between cells of the innate immune system: NKT cells rapidly activate NK cells. J Immunol 1999;163:4647–4650.

33. Street SE, Cretney E, Smyth MJ. Perforin and interferon-gamma activities independently control tumor initiation, growth, and metastasis. Blood 2001;97:192–197.

34. Gollob JA, Li J, Reinherz EL, Ritz J. CD2 regulates responsiveness of activated T cells to interleukin 12. J Exp Med 1995;182:721–731.

35. Park WR, Park CS, Tomura M, et al. CD28 costimulation is required not only to induce IL-12 receptor but also to render janus kinases/STAT4 responsive to IL-12 stimulation in TCR-triggered T cells. Eur J Immunol 2001;31:1456–1464.

36. O'Sullivan BJ, Thomas R. CD40 ligation conditions dendritic cell antigen-presenting function through sustained activation of NF-kappaB. J Immunol 2002;168:5491–5468.

37. Avice MN, Demeure CE, Delespesse G, Rubio M, Armant M, Sarfati M. IL-15 promotes IL-12 production by human monocytes via T cell-dependent contact and may contribute to IL-12-mediated IFN-gamma secretion by CD4+ T cells in the absence of TCR ligation. J Immunol 1998;16:3408–3415.

38. Carson WE, Giri JG, Lindemann MJ, et al. Interleukin (IL) 15 is a novel cytokine that activates human natural killer cells via components of the IL-2 receptor. J Exp Med 1994;180:1395–1403.

39. Ahn HJ, Maruo S, Tomura M, et al. A mechanism underlying synergy between IL-12 and IFN-gamma-inducing factor in enhanced production of IFN-gamma. J Immunol 1997;159:2125–2131.

40. Couglin CM, Salhany KE, Wysocka M, et al. Interleukin-12 and interleukin-18 synergistically induce murine tumor regression which involves inhibition of angiogenesis. J Clin Invest 1998;101:1441–1452.

41. Grohmann U, Belladonna ML, Bianchi R, et al. IL-12 acts directly on DC to promote nuclear localization of NF-kappaB and primes DC for IL-12 production. Immunity 1998;9:315–323.

42. Skeen MJ, Miller MA, Shinnick TM, Ziegler HK. Regulation of murine macrophage IL-12 production. Activation of macrophages in vivo, restimulation in vitro, and modulation by other cytokines. J Immunol 1996;156:1196–1206.

43. Veenstra KG, Jonak ZL, Trulli S, Gollob JA. IL-12 induces monocyte IL-18 binding protein expression via IFN-gamma. J Immunol 2002;168:2282–2287.

44. Daftarian PM, Kumar A, Kryworuchko M, Diaz-Mitoma F. IL-10 production is enhanced in human T cells by IL-12 and IL-6 and in monocytes by tumor necrosis factor-alpha. J Immunol 1996;157:12–20.

45. Zhou L, Nazarian AA, Smale ST. Interleukin-10 inhibits interleukin-12 p40 gene transcription by targeting a late event in the activation pathway. Mol Cell Biol 2004;24:2385–2396.

46. Oppmann B, Lesley R, Blom B, et al. Novel p19 protein engages IL-12p40 to form a cytokine, IL-23, with biological activities similar as well as distinct from IL-12. Immunity 2000;13:715–725.

47. Brombacher F, Kastelein RA, Alber G. Novel IL-12 family members shed light on the orchestration of Th1 responses. Trends Immunol 2003;24:207–212.

48. Pflanz S, Timans JC, Cheung J, et al. IL-27, a heterodimeric cytokine composed of EBI3 and p28 protein, induces proliferation of naive CD4(+) T cells. Immunity 2002;16:779–790.

49. Pflanz S, Hibbert L, Mattson J, et al. WSX-1 and glycoprotein 130 constitute a signal-transducing receptor for IL-27. J Immunol 2004;172:2225–2231.

50. Lucas S, Ghilardi N, Li J, de Sauvage FJ. IL-27 regulates IL-12 responsiveness of naive CD4+ T cells through Stat1-dependent and -independent mechanisms. Proc Natl Acad Sci 2003;100:15047–15052.

51. Brunda MJ, Luistro L, Warrier RR, et al. Antitumor and antimetastatic activity of interleukin 12 against murine tumors. J Exp Med 1993;178:1223–1230.

52. Cavallo F, Di Carlo E, Butera M, et al. Immune events associated with the cure of established tumors and spontaneous metastases by local and systemic interleukin 12. Cancer Res 1999;59:414–421.

53. Zilocchi C, Stoppacciaro A, Chiodoni C, Parenza M, Terrazzini N, Colombo MP. Interferon gamma-independent rejection of interleukin 12-transduced carcinoma cells requires CD4+ T cells and Granulocyte/Macrophage colony-stimulating factor. J Exp Med 1998;188:133–143.

54. Mortarini R, Borri A, Tragni G, et al. Peripheral burst of tumor-specific cytotoxic T lymphocytes and infiltration of metastatic lesions by memory CD8+ T cells in melanoma patients receiving interleukin 12. Cancer Res 2000;60:3559–3568.

55. Cui J, Shin T, Kawano T, et al. Requirement for Valpha14 NKT cells in IL-12-mediated rejection of tumors. Science 1997;278:1623–1626.

56. Karnbach C, Daws MR, Niemi EC, Nakamura MC. Immune rejection of a large sarcoma following cyclophosphamide and IL-12 treatment requires both NK and NK T cells and is associated with the induction of a novel NK T cell population. J Immunol 2001;167:2569–2576.

57. Park SH, Kyin T, Bendelac A, Carnaud C. The contribution of NKT cells, NK cells, and other gamma-chain-dependent non-T non-B cells to IL-12-mediated rejection of tumors. J Immunol 2003;170: 1197–1201.

58. Kodama T, Takeda K, Shimozato O, Hayakawa Y, Atsuta M, Kobayashi K, Ito M, Yagita H, Okumura K. Perforin-dependent NK cell cytotoxicity is sufficient for anti-metastatic effect of IL-12. Eur J Immunol 1999 Apr;29(4):1390–1396.

59. Chen L, Chen D, Block E, O'Donnell M, Kufe DW, Clinton SK. Eradication of murine bladder carcinoma by intratumor injection of a bicistronic adenoviral vector carrying cDNAs for the IL-12 heterodimer and its inhibition by the IL-12 p40 subunit homodimer. J Immunol 1997;159:351–359.

60. Lauw FN, Dekkers PE, te Velde AA, et al. Interleukin-12 induces sustained activation of multiple host inflammatory mediator systems in chimpanzees. J Infect Dis 1999;179:646–652.

61. Nastala CL, Edington HD, McKinney TG, et al. Recombinant IL-12 administration induces tumor regression in association with IFN-gamma production. J Immunol 1994;153:1697–1706.

62. Propper DJ, Chao D, Braybrooke JP, et al. Low-dose IFN-gamma induces tumor MHC expression in metastatic malignant melanoma. Clin Cancer Res 2003;9:84–92.

63. Shankaran V, Ikeda H, Bruce AT, et al. IFNgamma and lymphocytes prevent primary tumour development and shape tumour immunogenicity. Nature 2001;410:1107–1111.

64. Luster AD, Ravetch JV. Genomic characterization of a gamma-interferon-inducible gene (IP-10) and identification of an interferon-inducible hypersensitive site. Mol Cell Biol 1987;7:3723–3731.

65. Liao F, Rabin RL, Yannelli JR, Koniaris LG, Vanguri P, Farber JM. Human Mig chemokine: biochemical and functional characterization. J Exp Med 1995;182:1301–1314.

66. Cole KE, Strick CA, Paradis TJ, et al. Interferon-inducible T cell alpha chemoattractant (I-TAC): a novel non-ELR CXC chemokine with potent activity on activated T cells through selective high affinity binding to CXCR3. J Exp Med 1998;187:2009–2021.

67. Garcia-Lopez MA, Sanchez-Madrid F, Rodriguez-Frade JM, et al. CXCR3 chemokine receptor distribution in normal and inflamed tissues: expression on activated lymphocytes, endothelial cells, and dendritic cells. Lab Invest 2001;81:409–418.

68. Luster AD, Leder P. IP-10, a -C-X-C- chemokine, elicits a potent thymus-dependent antitumor response in vivo. J Exp Med 1993;178:1057–1065.

69. Tannenbaum CS, Tubbs R, Armstrong D, Finke JH, Bukowski RM, Hamilton TA. The CXC chemokines IP-10 and Mig are necessary for IL-12-mediated regression of the mouse RENCA tumor. J Immunol 1998;161:927–932.

70. Sgadari C, Farber JM, Angiolillo AL, et al. Mig, the monokine induced by interferon-gamma, promotes tumor necrosis in vivo. Blood 1997;89:2635–2643.

71. Sgadari C, Angiolillo AL, Cherney BW, et al. Interferon-inducible protein-10 identified as a mediator of tumor necrosis in vivo. Proc Natl Acad Sci 1996;93:13,791–13,796.

72. Angiolillo AL, Sgadari C, Taub DD, et al. Human interferon-inducible protein 10 is a potent inhibitor of angiogenesis in vivo. J Exp Med 1995;182:155–162.

73. Sgadari C, Angiolillo AL, Tosato G. Inhibition of angiogenesis by interleukin-12 is mediated by the interferon-inducible protein 10. Blood 1996;87:3877–3882.

74. Coughlin CM, Salhany KE, Gee MS, et al. Tumor cell responses to IFNgamma affect tumorigenicity and response to IL-12 therapy and antiangiogenesis. Immunity 1998;:25–34.

75. Carson WE, Interferon-alpha-induced activation of signal transducer and activator of transcription proteins in malignant melanoma. Clin Cancer Res 1998;4:2219–2228.

76. Chin YE, Kitagawa M, Su WC, You ZH, Iwamoto Y, Fu XY. Cell growth arrest and induction of cyclin-dependent kinase inhibitor p21 WAF1/CIP1 mediated by STAT1. Science 1996;272:719–722.

77. Chin YE, Kitagawa M, Kuida K, Flavell RA, Fu XY. Activation of the STAT signaling pathway can cause expression of caspase 1 and apoptosis. Mol Cell Biol 1997;17:5328–5337.

78. Atkins MB, Robertson MJ, Gordon M, et al. Phase I evaluation of intravenous recombinant human interleukin 12 in patients with advanced malignancies. Clin Cancer Res 1997;3:409@NL:417.

79. Phan GQ, Attia P, Steinberg SM, White DE, Rosenberg SA. Factors associated with response to high-dose interleukin-2 in patients with metastatic melanoma. J Clin Oncol 2001;19:3477–3482.

80. Allione A, Bernabei P, Bosticardo M, Ariotti S, Forni G, Novelli F. Nitric oxide suppresses human T lymphocyte proliferation through IFN-gamma-dependent and IFN-gamma-independent induction of apoptosis. J Immunol 1999;163:4182–4191.

81. Leonard JP, Sherman ML, Fisher GL, et al. Effects of single-dose interleukin-12 exposure on interleukin-12-associated toxicity and interferon-gamma production. Blood 1997 Oct 1;90(7):2541–2548.

82. Gollob JA, Mier JW, Veenstra K, et al. Phase I trial of twice-weekly intravenous interleukin 12 in patients with metastatic renal cell cancer or malignant melanoma: Ability to maintain IFN-gamma induction is associated with clinical response. Clin Cancer Res 2000;6:1678–1692.

83. Gollob JA, Veenstra KG, Parker RA, et al. Phase I trial of concurrent twice-weekly recombinant human interleukin-12 plus low-dose IL-2 in patients with melanoma or renal cell carcinoma. J Clin Oncol 2003;21:2564–2573.

84. Bajetta E, Del Vecchio M, Mortarini R, et al. Pilot study of subcutaneous recombinant human interleukin 12 in metastatic melanoma. Clin Cancer Res 1998;4:75–85.

85. Portielje JE, Kruit WH, Schuler M, et al. Phase I study of subcutaneously administered recombinant human interleukin 12 in patients with advanced renal cell cancer. Clin Cancer Res 1999;5:3983–3989.

86. Portielje JE, Lamers CH, Kruit WH, et al. Repeated administrations of interleukin (IL)-12 are associated with persistently elevated plasma levels of IL-10 and declining IFN-gamma, tumor necrosis factor-alpha, IL-6, and IL-8 responses. Clin Cancer Res 2003;9:76–83.

87. Ohno R, Yamaguchi Y, Toge T, et al. A dose-escalation and pharmacokinetic study of subcutaneously administered recombinant human interleukin 12 and its biological effects in Japanese patients with advanced malignancies. Clin Cancer Res 2000;6:2661–2669.

88. Motzer RJ, Rakhit A, Schwartz LH, et al. Phase I trial of subcutaneous recombinant human interleukin-12 in patients with advanced renal cell carcinoma. Clin Cancer Res 1998;4:1183–1191.

89. Motzer RJ, Rakhit A, Thompson JA, et al. Randomized multicenter phase II trial of subcutaneous recombinant human interleukin-12 versus interferon-alpha 2a for patients with advanced renal cell carcinoma. J Interferon Cytokine Res 2001;21:257–263.

90. Hutson TH, Mekhail T, Molto L, et al. Phase I Trial of Subcutaneously Administered rHuIL-12 and rHuIFN-a2b in Patients with Metastatic Renal Cell Carcinoma or Malignant Melanoma. 2001 ASCO Annual Meetings; Abstract No: 1030.

91. Rook AH, Wood GS, Yoo EK, et al. Interleukin-12 therapy of cutaneous T-cell lymphoma induces lesion regression and cytotoxic T-cell responses. Blood 1999;94:902–908.

92. Ansell SM, Witzig TE, Kurtin PJ, et al. Phase 1 study of interleukin-12 in combination with rituximab in patients with B-cell non-Hodgkin lymphoma. Blood 2002;99:67–74.

93. Robertson MJ, Pelloso D, Abonour R, et al. Interleukin 12 immunotherapy after autologous stem cell transplantation for hematological malignancies. Clin Cancer Res 2002;8:3383–3393.

94. Pelloso D, Cyran K, Timmons L, Williams BT, Robertson MJ. Immunological consequences of interleukin 12 administration after autologous stem cell transplantation. Clin Cancer Res 2004;10: 1935–1942.

95. Marshall JD, Chehimi J, Gri G, Kostman JR, Montaner LJ, Trinchieri G. The interleukin-12-mediated pathway of immune events is dysfunctional in human immunodeficiency virus-infected individuals. Blood 1999;94:1003–1011.

96. Pluda JM, Wyvill K, Little R, et al. A Pilot/Dose-Finding Study of Interleukin 12 (IL-12) Administered to Patients (pts) with AIDS-Associated Kaposi's Sarcoma (KS) (Meeting abstract). 1999 ASCO Annual Meeting; Abstract No. 2111.

97. Wadler S, Levy D, Frederickson HL, et al. Eastern Cooperative Oncology Group. A phase II trial of interleukin-12 in patients with advanced cervical cancer: clinical and immunologic correlates. Eastern Cooperative Oncology Group study E1E96. Gynecol Oncol 2004;92:957–964.

98. Hurteau JA, Blessing JA, DeCesare SL, Creasman WT. Evaluation of recombinant human interleukin-12 in patients with recurrent or refractory ovarian cancer: a gynecologic oncology group study. Gynecol Oncol 2001;82:7–10.

99. Lenzi R, Rosenblum M, Verschraegen C, et al. Phase I study of intraperitoneal recombinant human interleukin 12 in patients with Mullerian carcinoma, gastrointestinal primary malignancies, and mesothelioma. Clin Cancer Res 2002;8:3686–3695.

100. Parihar R, Nadella P, Jensen R, Dierksheide J, Shapiro C, Carson W. A Phase I Trial of Herceptin and Interleukin-12 in Patients with HER2-Overexpressing Malignancies. 2001 ASCO Annual Meeting; Abstract No: 1031.

19 The Type I Interferon System With Emphasis on Its Role in Malignancies

Interferons Are More Than "Antivirals"

Stergios J. Moschos, Gregory B. Lesinski, William E. Carson, III, and John M. Kirkwood

CONTENTS

1. INTRODUCTION

Interferon-$\alpha2$ (IFN-$\alpha2$) has been tested extensively in human clinical trials and has proven to confer a survival benefit to patients with melanoma, renal cell carcinoma (RCC), chronic myelogenous leukemia (CML), hemangioma and various other malignancies. To date, the precise molecular determinants that differentiate responders from non-responders have not been defined. A majority of the current knowledge about IFN-$\alpha2$ has been derived from its role as an endogenously-produced antiviral compound. Importantly, new information on the activity of exogenously administered IFN-α is beginning to emerge as a result of its widespread use for tumor immunotherapy. This chapter will focus on the biology of IFN-α and its effects on downstream signaling events within the tumor cell and host immune effectors. We will highlight both endogenous and exogenous

From: *Cancer Drug Discovery and Development,*
Cytokines in the Genesis and Treatment of Cancer
Edited by: M. A. Caligiuri and M. T. Lotze © Humana Press Inc., Totowa, NJ

IFNα2, because information from each might provide insight into the mechanism of action of IFNα as an immunotherapeutic agent. Continued research on the basic biology of the IFN system could potentially lead to a greater understanding of its antitumor activity and greater clinical benefit while reducing its toxic side effects.

2. HISTORIC BACKGROUND

The biologic phenomenon known as "interference" was first described by Alick Isaacs and Jean Lindenmann in 1957 *(1)*. Interference was defined as a protective effect against viral infection imparted to cells that had previously been infected by another virus. The concept was rigorously examined because of its public health ramifications, during the era of the first-generation polio vaccines and the search for an "antiviral penicillin." In their research examining the molecular mechanism of this phenomenon, Isaacs and Lindenmann discovered IFN *(1,2)*. Early attempts by Derek Burke, a biochemist from Isaacs's laboratory, to purify and produce IFN in great quantities for research and clinical applications had been disappointing *(3)*; IFN research was hampered for more than two decades due to crude protein fractions, less than one percent of which consisted of actual IFN. Until the 1960s, IFN was thought to be a single molecule, rather than a family of distinct structurally related proteins *(4)*. Interest in IFN beyond the field of virology occurred in the early 1960s when its cytostatic, antitumor and immunomodulatory properties were discovered *(5,6)*. IFN research was further advanced by the landmark work on its purification to homogeneity in solution in sufficient amounts for its physicochemical characterization *(7)* as well as by cloning of the first IFN gene *(8)*. As a result of an exciting competition between the pharmaceutical industry and academic research, IFN was one of the first natural proteins to become available for the clinical treatment of malignancies *(9)*.

3. BIOLOGY OF INTERFERONS

Human IFNs represent a complex family of heterogenous proteins which uniformly protect cells from viral infection and induce major histocompatibility complex (MHC) class I antigen expression. IFNs have been traditionally classified based on the mechanism of their production and the cell-surface receptor complex they use (Table 1). Type I IFNs are generally produced and secreted by almost any cell in the body in response to viral infection or double strand-RNAs (ds-RNA). Type I IFN genes are clustered on human chromosome 9p21 *(10)* and exert their effects via a common receptor, IFN-αβR. The IFN gene family consists of 13 IFN-α members, named from the peaks obtained on chromatography for their isolation, and a single member of each of IFN-β, IFN-κ, IFN-ω and IFN-ε *(11–13)*. All of the IFN-α subtypes seem to have comparable biologic activities. The precise evolutionary explanation for this redundancy remains a mystery but may reflect the advantages of providing the host with alternative defense pathways. Translocations involving 9p21-22 bands are frequently found in hematologic malignancies, whereas 9p21 deletion and/or loss of heterozygosity of nearby genes (i.e., the cell cycle protein p16) are frequently found in many cancers in vivo and in neoplastic cell lines (i.e., renal, bladder, and pancreatic cancer, glioblastoma, neuroblastoma, melanoma, acute lymphoblastic leukemia (ALL)) (reviewed in ref. *14*) (Table 2). Interestingly, a recently described cytokine, limitin, acts via the type I IFN receptor, shares sequence homology with type I IFNs *(15)* and exerts similar antiproliferative,

Table 1
Classification of Interferons (IFNs)

Interferon	type	Chromosome locus	Source	Subtypes	Receptor
I	α	9p21	Leukocytes	13	IFN-αβR
	β		Fibroblasts	1	
				1	
				1	
				1	
	ε		Brain, lung kidney, Small intestine		
	κ		Keratinocytes		
	ω	9p21	Leukocytes		
I/IL-10	λ	19q13		3	IFN-λR
II	γ	12q24	T-cells, NK cells	1	IFN-γR

Table 2
Cytogenetic and Genetic Information Regarding IFNs[a]

Chromosome locus	Gene	Chromosome aberration	Malignancy
9p21-p22	IFN-α	Del 9p22	ALL
			L-L
			neuroblastoma
	IFN-β	t(8;9)	ALL
			NHL
12q24.1	IFN-γ	Breakpoint after Radiatiotherapy	
21q22	IFN-α/β R	t(8;21)	AML M2
	IFN-γ R2	21q	AML
			CML

[a]Abbreviations: ALL, acute lymphoblastic leukemia; L-L, lymphoblastic leukemia; NHL, non-hodgkin's lymphoma; AML, acute myelogenous leukemia; CML, chronic myelogenous leukemia.

immunomodulatory, and antiviral effects with IFN-α/β *(16)* but does not influence myeloid and erythroid progenitors *(17)*. Although a number of IFN species naturally occur, IFNα and IFNβ are the most common subtypes used in the clinical treatment of malignancy.

In contrast, the type II IFN family consists of a sole member, IFN-γ, encoded by a gene located in chromosome 12q24. IFN-γ is produced by T-lymphocytes and natural killer (NK) cells in response to antigens and mitogens and exerts its effect via a specific receptor, namely IFN-γR. Recently, a new family of cytokines structurally related to the type I IFNs and the interleukin-10 (IL-10) family was described *(18,19)*. These cytokines, termed IFN-λ1, IFN-λ2, and IFN-λ3, have a significant sequence similarity with IFN-α. Their genes are clustered on chromosome 19q13 and exert their effects via a distinct receptor, IFN-λR.

4. THE TYPE I INTERFERON SYSTEM RESPONDS
TO "DANGER" SIGNALS

Two general systems of immunity have evolved to recognize and respond to "non-self" and preserve the integrity of the organism: (1) the phylogenetically older innate or natural immunity, and (2) the more recently evolved adaptive or specific immunity *(20)*. The major difference between these two systems lies in the means by which "danger" signals are perceived. *Innate immunity* "inflexibly" senses either specific pathogen-associated molecular, nonprotein patterns normally not expressed by host tissues or endogenous molecules released from "stressed" cells. For example, in bacterial and viral infections molecular patterns are recognized by a limited number of host cells' recognition structures, termed pattern recognition receptors (PARs). Among the PARs are Toll-like receptors (TLRs), CD14, complement receptors (CR1/CD35), β2-integrins (CD11/CD18) and C-type lectins *(21)*. Innate immunity has proven importance in tumor immunosurveillance. If "cellular stress" is induced in cancer cells leading to necrotic cell death, upregulation of heat shock proteins (hsp) which chaperone tumor associated antigens to immune cells may occur *(22)* (Section 7 B). In contrast, *specific immunity* is almost infinitely adaptable, mediated by receptors on lymphocytes that predominantly recognize peptide-MHC complexes. This system provides a broad range of immune responses against molecular structures other than carbohydrates.

Endogenously produced type I IFNs provide an important link between innate and specific immunity by regulating the function of immune cells in both arms of the immune response. They are constitutively expressed at a low level, which is important for immunosurveillance and cell growth *(23,24)*. Upon exposure to "danger" stimuli type I IFNs are produced in vast amounts. Although all cells can produce type I IFN under appropriate stimulation, the capacity to secrete type I IFNs in detectable amounts in peripheral blood appears to be restricted to specialized cells. These cells were termed "plasmacytoid T-cells" and were originally identified in T-cell dependent areas of lymph nodes in patients with infectious diseases as well as the peripheral blood. More precise immunophenotypic characterization recently revealed that these cells represent an innate effector cell that migrates from peripheral blood to lymph nodes during infection or to the primary tumor site *(25)*. It functions as a professional IFN-producing cell at the precursor stages and as a professional antigen-presenting dendritic cell upon terminal differentiation *(26–28)*. Therefore these cells may play a crucial role in linking the innate and adaptive immune systems, acting as early sensors of "danger" signals and "sounding the alarm."

Binding to several but not all pattern-recognition receptors results in upregulated production of endogenous type I IFNs. Of these, TLRs are the major receptors for various pathogen-associated molecular patterns in the innate immune system (reviewed in ref. *29*). TLRs comprise a family of 10 members (TLR 1-10), are phylogenetically conserved proteins structurally related to the Drosophila Toll protein and are expressed on antigen presenting cells (APCs), including macrophages and dendritic cells (Table 3). TLRs are type I transmembrane proteins characterized by an extracellular domain composed of leucine-rich repeats and an intracytoplasmic domain conserved in members of the interleukin-1 receptor (IL-1R) family (Toll/IL-1R or TIR domain) (Fig. 1). The TLR expression profile on APCs varies, accounting for the induction of different sets of proinflammatory cytokines in response to the respective TLR ligands from invading

Table 3
Classification of Toll-like Receptors (TLR)

TLR	Ligands		APC expression			TLR adaptor molecules other than MyD88	Cytokine gene induction
	Exogenous	Endogenous	IPCs	Myeloid DCs precursors	Immature myeloid DCs		
1	Lipopeptides		Low	High	High	TIRAP	?
2	Lipopeptides peptidoglycan lipotechoic acid glycolipids GSLs	HSP70	No	High	High	TIRAP	IL-12 IL-6 TNF-α
3	ds-RNA		No	No	High	TICAM-1/TRIF	IFNα/β, IL-6, TNF-α
4	LPS taxol viral proteins	HSP60, HSP70β-Defensin fibrinogen fibronectin heparan sulfate, hyaluronic acid	No	High	Low	TIRAP TICAM-1/TRIF	IL-12 IL-6 TNF-α IFN-α/β
5	Flagellin		No	High	Low	?	?
6	Lipopeptides		Low	Low	Low	TIRAP	?
7	Synthetic compounds		High	Low/no	Low/no	?	IFN-α
8	?		No	High	Low	?	
9	CpG DNA		High	No	No	?	IFN-α/β
10	?		Low	No	Low	?	

343

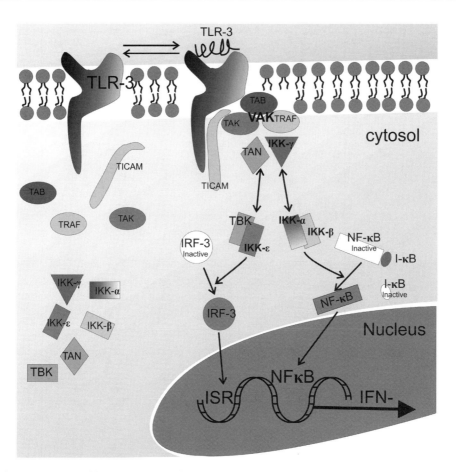

Fig. 1. An example of how "nonself" stimuli (e.g., double-strand RNA) are "sensed" via Toll-like receptors (TLR) and lead to activation of interferon (IFN) gene expression. Activation of the TLR-3 results in sequential recruitment of "adapter" molecules (i.e., TICAM-1) and "assembly" of the virus-activated kinase (VAK) complex consisting of kinases (TRAF6, TAB2, TAK1) that activate two three-protein complexes (TANK1-TBK1-IKKε and IKKα-IKKβ-IKKγ). These complexes activate the IFN regulatory factor-3 (IRF-3) and nuclear factor kappa B (NF-κB) which activate the IFN-β gene expression by interacting with positive regulatory elements in its promoter, such as the IFN-stimulated responsive and NF-κB response elements (ISRE and NF-κBre) Abbreviations: →, activated; TANK, TRAF family member associated NF-κB activator; TBK, TANK binding kinase; IKK, inhibitor of IκB kinase.

pathogens *(30)*. Their ligands are both endogenous and exogenous molecular pattern molecules. Upon stimulation, TLRs activate transcription factors, such as NF-κB, AP-1 and IRFs, leading to production of inflammatory cytokines, up-regulation of costimulatory molecules *(31)* and chemokine receptors *(32)* and suppression of regulatory T-cells *(33)* (Fig. 1). For example, TLR-3 is highly specific for type I IFN production by interferon-producing cells (IPCs) and monocytes may explain the "burst" of type I IFN production during viral infection. In contrast, the role of endogenous type I IFN production in tumor immunosurveillance *(23)* may be linked to endogenous TLR-4 ligands, such as hsps or β-defensins, which are released by damaged cells undergoing necrotic death. These ligands have been reported to be effective stimuli for the maturation of DCs and their ability to trigger a type 1 polarized immune response in vivo.

Furthermore, these ligands have the ability to chaperone tumor associated antigens to APCs *(22,34–36)*.

Other pattern recognition receptors may affect type I IFN gene expression. Thus, β2-integrins, such as the leukocyte function-associated antigen-1 (LFA-1, or CD11a/CD18) which mediates both antigen-dependent and antigen-independent cellular adhesion, are important for IFN-α production by IPCs *(37)*. Similarly, lectins *(38)* and the $F_c\gamma$ receptor II ($F_c\gamma$RII, CD32) *(39)* are potent inducers of IFN-α production via complex internalization. Blood dendritic cell antigen-2 (BDCA-2), another type II Ctype lectin, that is presumably involved in internalization processing and presentation, is uniquely expressed in IPCs and potently inhibits IFN-α/β expression *(40)*. Also, histamine type 2 receptors similarly mediate inhibition of IFN-α production by IPCs which along with modulation of other inflammatory cytokine production (i.e., ↓ TNF-α, ↓ IL-12p70, ↑/→ IL-10) may partially account for the polarization of naïve T-cells towards a T_{h2} phenotype *(41)*.

In summary, cellular damage, apoptosis, and pathogen associated molecular patterns bind to specific receptors, and lead to the production of endogenous type I IFN and other inflammatory cytokines. The resulting cytokine profile induces changes that prime the immune system to more efficiently prepare for an adaptive immune response.

5. REGULATION OF TYPE I INTERFERON GENES

Transcriptional regulation of type I IFN genes has been studied extensively in the prototype response to viral infection and is mediated via a complex mechanism involving interaction among specific transcription factors, chromatin and chromatin-remodeling complexes. For both IFN-α and IFN-β genes, transcription is mediated via 5′-flanking *cis*-acting regulatory sequences that show some degree of homology with each other (reviewed in ref. *42*). The regulatory sequences consist of repeated hex nucleotide consensus motifs (AA(A/G)(T/G)GA), termed virus responsive elements (VREs), which function cooperatively and contribute to gene expression, presumably by interacting with *trans*-acting regulatory factor(s). Interestingly, the IFN-β gene promoter contains another *cis*-element which is absent in the IFN-α1 gene, the binding site for the transcription factor NF-κB/H2TF1, which maximally induces the IFN-β gene transcription.

In the search for *trans*-acting factors involved in virus-induced activation of IFN gene transcription, a growing family of transcription factors, termed IFN regulatory factors (IRFs), was discovered (reviewed in ref. *43*). These factors bind to VREs and enhance or suppress IFN gene expression. Their expression may be constitutive or may be induced in response to stimuli. In addition, the expression of some VREs is ubiquitous, whereas others are confined to specific cell types (Table 4).

Viral infection has been the prototype to study the regulation of type I IFN gene transcription. Both IRF-1 and IRF-2 are constitutively expressed at low levels intracellularly, but IRF-1 has a much shorter half-life than IRF-2. In the absence of external stimuli, the effect of accumulation of IRF-2 and the histone deacetylation *(23)* result in a trancriptionally silent state of type I IFN genes thereby allowing a low-level of endogenous type I IFN production (Fig. 2). This spontaneous IFNα/β production, though yet unexplained, may have physiologic significance by ensuring a rapid and effective response of the host to effectively induce IFNα/β genes, "reving up the engine" to promptly adapt to environmental changes, such as viral infection *(24)*.

Table 4
Name Classification of IFN Regulatory Factors (IRF)

IRF_S	Regulation	Tissues expressed	Action	Comments
1	Upregulated upon viral infection and IFN stimulation	Ubiquitous	Antiviral. –bacterial response MHC class I/II expression/ Th1 response/ NK cell development-function cell cycle arrest/apoptosis inhibits cell transformation	T½, ~30 min transactivated by Ser phosphorylation interacts with NF-κB to form enhanceosome on IFN gene promoter
2		Ubiquitous	Transcriptional attenuator (including IFN-α/β gene) overexpression causes oncogenic transformation	T½, ~8 hours transactivated by Ser phosphorylation undergoes proteolytic processing and is converted as activator of strong repressor
3	Constitutive, not upregulated upon viral infection of IFNs	Ubiquitous	Critical for early and late phase of IFN-α/β gene expression	Transactivated by Ser phosphorylation IRF-3 associates with p300/CBP both form homo- or hetero-dimers affecting selective IFN-α gene subtypes
7	Dependent on IFN-α/β signaling	Ubiquitous	Critical for early phase of IFN-β gene expression	
4	Not induced by IFNs	Restricted to T- and	Overexpression causes	Interacts with PU.1
5	Induced upon IFN-α/β stimulation	B-cell lineages	Leukemogenesis	
6				
8	Induced by IFN-γ only	Restricted to myeloid and lymphoid lineages	Induces certain IFN-γ responsive genes/represses certain IFN-α/β genes tumor suppressor for CML	Trans modulated by Tyr of Ser phosphorylation associates with IRF-1/IRF-2
9	Induced by IFNs	Ubiquitous		

A **Inactivated state**

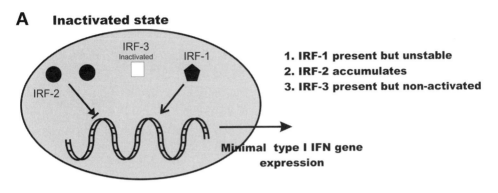

1. **IRF-1 present but unstable**
2. **IRF-2 accumulates**
3. **IRF-3 present but non-activated**

B **Viral infection-early phase**

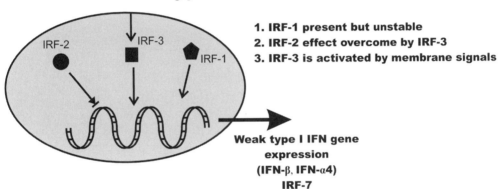

1. **IRF-1 present but unstable**
2. **IRF-2 effect overcome by IRF-3**
3. **IRF-3 is activated by membrane signals**

C **Viral infection-late phase**

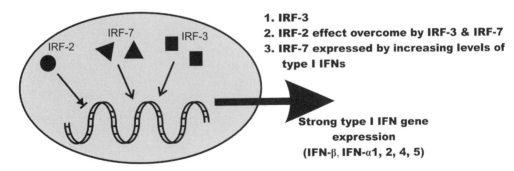

1. **IRF-3**
2. **IRF-2 effect overcome by IRF-3 & IRF-7**
3. **IRF-7 expressed by increasing levels of type I IFNs**

Fig. 2. Type I interferon (IFN) gene regulation has been most extensively studied in the viral infection model and is under the influence of positive (→, IRF-1, IRF-3, IRF-7) and negative regulators (→I, IRF-2). In the absence of external stimuli ("inactivated state", **A**) there is always a low grade of type I IFN gene expression. In the early phase **(B)**, membrane pattern recognition receptors (e.g. Toll-like receptors) activate, among others, IRF-3, a factor which is constitutively expressed, though inactive. A limited expression of type I IFN species is expressed along with type I IFN gene enhancers (IRF-7). At later stages **(C)** massive amounts of broader species type I IFNs are produced. Abbreviations: IRF, interferon regulatory factors.

The exact mechanism of gene regulation of different IFN-α subtypes is under investigation but it seems that intracellular levels of IRFs, such as IRF-3, -5, and -7, influence the formation of homo-/heterodimers of IRFs which have different affinities for IFN-α and IFN-β promoters. IRF-1 and IRF-2, the first two members of this family, were shown to bind the IFN-β gene promoter but with different effects (i.e. IRF-1 activates whereas IRF-2 "silences" transcription) *(44,45)*.

In the early phase of viral infection the constitutively expressed IRF-3 is activated by phosphorylation, resulting in weak and efficient activation of IFN-α4 and IFN-β genes, respectively, induction of IRF-7 and IRF-1 gene expression and further increase of IFNα/β proteins. In the late phase of viral induction both IRF-3 and IRF-7 amplify the induction of IFN-β and certain other IFN-α genes *(46)*. The exact mechanism of gene regulation of different IFN-α subtypes is under investigation but it seems that intracellular levels of each IRF influences the formation of specific homo-/hetero-dimers, which have different affinity for different IFN-α promoters. Also different cell types and inducing agents may affect the constitutive expression levels of different IRFs *(47,48)*.

6. INTERFERON-α/β SIGNALING

6.1. The Type I Interferon Receptor

IFN-α and IFN-β were originally thought to exert their effects via distinct receptors, however in 1994 a universal receptor for type I IFNs was described *(49)*. The type I IFN receptor is a heterodimer comprised of two transmembrane subunit receptor chains designated IFNAR-1 (or α subunit) and IFNAR-2 (or β subunit) *(50)*. Although congenital inactivating mutations for the type I IFN receptor have not been described in human families *(51)*, targeted gene inactivation ("knockout") of the type I IFN receptor in mice results in accelerated tumor development after inoculation of mice with diverse tumor cell lines *(52)*, alluding to the role of endogenous type I IFNs in tumor surveillance *(23)*. The genes for the type I IFN receptor subunits are colocalized in chromosome 21q22 and phylogenetically may have stemmed from a common ancestor gene within the immunoglobulin superfamily *(53)*.

A number of factors contribute to the transcriptional regulation of IFNA-R. The IFNA-R gene expression follows a diurnal rhythm related to cell cycle distribution, namely being higher during the S phase and the mid-morning hours *(54)* which may in part account for the circadian dependence of antitumor activity of all IFNs *(55)*. Hydroxyurea, an inhibitor of DNA synthesis and cell proliferation causing accumulation of leukemic cells in the early S phase, also increases IFN-α receptor expression *(56)* which may explain earlier reports about the stronger antiproliferative effect of IFN-α in nonproliferating cells compared to exponentially growing cells *(57)*. Similarly, recombinant IFN-γ was shown to upregulate both IFNAR-1 and IFNAR-2 genes *(58)* which could be the basis for the synergistic action of type I and type II IFNs in innate and adaptive immunity. Also, 9-*cis*-retinoic acid causes upregulation of IFNAR expression both at the mRNA and the protein level in a human hepatoma cell line *(59)*, which may provide the basis to explain the synergistic effects of retinoids and type I IFNs in a variety of neoplastic diseases *(60)*.

A number of studies have shown that the expression of the IFNAR-2 subunit is associated with treatment response in a variety of diseases *(61,62)*. IFNAR-2 is expressed in all leukocyte subsets and is higher in monocytes and granulocytes than in lymphocytes; in the latter IFNAR-2 expression is higher in natural killer (NK) cells than any other lymphocyte subset *(63)*. In several tumors both the pretreatment level of IFNAR-2 *(64)* and its downregulation by IFN-α therapy is associated with clinical response and favorable outcome *(65)*. Therefore, IFNAR-2 expression may be used as a clinical surrogate marker for response to IFN-α.

6.2. Signaling through the IFN-α/β receptor

Binding of type I IFNs to their common receptor involves initial binding to IFNAR-2$_c$ subunit and subsequent recruitment of the α subunit (Fig. 3). This results in dimerization, creating the high affinity site essential for activation. The β$_L$ subunit is the binding subunit, and the α subunit is necessary to form high-affinity receptors. The βs subunit, though nonfunctional, based on current knowledge, could potentially form a complex with the α- and β$_L$ subunits after their dimerization *(60)*. Type II cytokine receptors, like the IFNα/β receptor, lack intrinsic tyrosine (Tyr) kinase activity; this is counteracted by their noncovalent association of Janus kinases (JAKs) (reviewed in ref. 66).

JAKs are considered the "transcellular doorway" through which cytokine-mediated signals must pass. They exert their effect by activating signal-transducer-and-activator-of-transcription proteins (STATs) via Tyr phosphorylation (Fig. 3). Interestingly, the activated JAK protein kinases do not have specificity for a particular STAT substrate and it appears that the initial specificity for most STAT activation is determined by specific interactions between STATs and receptors *(67)*. Thus, within the cytoplasmic domain of each of the IFNAR subunits two JAKs and two STATs are directly preassociated: Tyk-2 *(68)* and STAT-3 *(69)* for the α subunit, JAK-1 *(70)* and STAT-2 *(71)*, for the β subunit. Other indirect preassociations involve: (1) IRF-9, a member of the IFN regulatory factor of proteins (Table 4), with STAT-2 *(72)*, (2) STAT-1 with the β subunit via the receptor for activated protein kinase C (RACK1) protein *(73)*, (3) STAT-5 with Tyk-2 *(74)* and (4) insulin receptor substrate (IRS) protein-1 and -2 with Tyk-2 *(75)*.

Binding of type I IFNs to their receptor induces dimerization of the two receptor subunits and Tyr phosphorylation of JAK-1 and Tyk-2 *(76)* (Fig. 3). Once Tyk-2 is activated, it can then cross-phosphorylate JAK-1. The phosphorylated IFNA-R subunits provide a docking site for STAT2 via its SH2 domain *(77)*, whereby STAT-1 is recruited to the receptor complex by the RACK1 adapter protein *(78)*. Here STAT-1 associates with STAT-2 and IRF-9 to form the IFN-stimulated gene factor 3 (ISGF3) *(79)*. The ISGF3 complex then translocates to the nucleus to drive the expression of IFN-α responsive genes. Within the ISGF3 complex, STAT-2 provides the essential transcriptional activation domain *(80)* whereas STAT-1 and IRF-9 contribute primarily to the selectivity and stability of DNA binding *(81)*. Independent of IRF-9, activated STATs may also form heterodimers (1-2) or homodimers (STAT—1-1, 3-3, 5-5). These alternative STAT protein complexes can induce the expression of specific genes *(82)* via binding to palindromic consensus sequences termed γ-activated sequences (GAS). Interestingly, different dimers preferentially interact with individual sequence patterns *(83)*. The STAT-2 component of ISGF3 can also interact with CREB-binding protein (CBP)/p300 transcription factor *(84)*, the ATP-dependent chromatin-remodeling factor BRG1 (Brahma-related gene 1) *(85)*, and the histone acetylase protein GCN5 *(86)* to activate several IFN-α regulated genes. Similar to STAT-2, activated Tyk-2 activates STAT-3 *(87)*

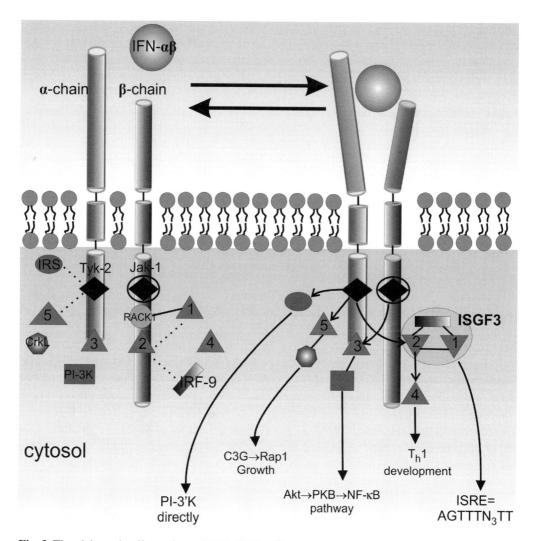

Fig. 3. The pleiotropic effects of type I IFNs (IFN-α/β) can be explained by activation of multiple signaling pathways beyond the JAK/STAT pathway. In the resting state (left hand) several direct (———; Tyk-2, JAK-1, RACK1, STAT-2, and STAT-3) and indirect associations (.......; STAT-1, STAT-3, STAT-5, IRF-9, IRS-1/2) are formed with the type I IFN receptor subunits (see text). Many other molecules–components of signaling transduction pathways (e.g, CrkL, PI-3'K, STAT-4) are activated/associated with the type I IFNR complex only after its activation (right hand). Upon activation, type I IFNR subunits dimerize, their preassociated JAKs are mutually activated, and several phosphorylated sites on subunits provide docking sites for STATs and subsequent events (see text). Abbreviations: →, activation; IRS, insulin receptor substrate; PI-3'K, phosphatidylinositol 3-kinase; Rap, receptor for activated protein kinase C; ISGF3, IFN stimulated gene factor 3; ISRE, IFN stimulated response element; naked numbers indicate type of STATs (e.g., 1 is STAT-1, 2 is STAT-2 etc.).

and IRS-1/-2 *(75,88,89)* which independently mediate recruitment and activation of the regulatory subunit (p85) of phosphatidylinositol 3-kinase (PI3'-kinase). Activated STAT-2 may also recruit and phosphorylate STAT-4 *(90)*. This event is important for the upregulation of IFN-γ gene in T-lymphocytes and T helper (T_h1) development *(91)*.

Binding of type I IFN to its receptor can result in signal transduction through a number of STAT-independent pathways (Fig. 3). These pathways either cooperate with JAK/STAT pathways by fully activating STATs via serine (Ser) phosphorylation or induce gene transcription via STAT-independent mechanisms. For example, activation of PI 3′-kinase, PKC-δ and STAT5 has been observed following stimulation of cells with type I IFNs. These STAT-independent signaling events may play a role in mediating growth inhibition or augmenting phosphorylation of specific STAT proteins (92–96).

Ligand binding to the type I IFN receptor may account for signaling "cross-talk" induced by other cytokines. This is mediated by the association of the IFNAR-1 subunit with subunits belonging to other cytokine receptors. Thus, subthreshold IFN-α/β signaling is important to maintain the IFNAR-1 subunit in a phosphorylated form, thereby providing sites for the IFN-γ activated STAT-1 to undergo efficient dimerization via association of the β subunit of the IFN-γ receptor (IFNGR-2) with the IFNAR-1 subunit (97). Similar to IFN-γ signaling, IL-6 signaling is adequate only in the presence of constitutively activated IFNAR-1 subunit which provides sites for efficient dimerization of STAT-1 and STAT-3 via possible association of the IFNAR-1 and the common cytokine subunit gp130 (98). The importance of the involvement of STAT-1 in cytokine signaling cross-talk was shown in mice with gene targeted inactivation of STAT-1 (99). These mice exhibit increased frequency in developing spontaneous tumors (100) along with susceptibility to mycobacterial and viral infections as was shown in humans with genetic STAT-1 deficiency (101).

A major challenge in the study of IFNAR signaling is to identify the molecular mechanisms underlying the functional differences in expression profiles among type I IFNs which signal through a sole receptor. Although there are several unresolved structural, kinetic and thermodynamic issues, it appears that: (a) the degree of binding affinity of the receptor-ligand complex does not correlate with the ultimate function (i.e. antiproliferation, antiviral activity), and (b) although the structural differences among complexes of IFNAR-2 with different type I IFNs are probably minor, only the distribution of binding energy on the same set of residues is different (60). Moreover, a region in the β subunit is important for IFN-β signaling (102) and IFN-β but not IFN-α treatment selectively associates the α and β_L subunits of the IFNAR (103) implying that such differences in signaling among the type I IFNs rely on induction of specific conformational changes made by each ligand.

It has become apparent that the Jak/STAT signaling pathway may represent a molecular target that could be modulated to increase IFN-responsiveness. For example, priming of both human peripheral blood mononuclear cells and melanoma cell lines with IFN-γ has been shown to upregulate ISGF3 components. The resulting cells displayed an augmented response to subsequent treatment with IFN-α (104,105). Recent studies have also shown that IL-12 pretreatments could lead to an increase in endogenous IFN-γ production, resulting in upregulated expression of key signaling intermediates (STAT-1, STAT-2, IRF-9) within both tumor cells and host immune effectors (106). Importantly, upregulation of these signaling components ultimately led to protection of mice against lethal challenge with B16 melanoma tumors, and increased in vitro sensitivity to lower doses of IFNα. These data underscore the importance of the Jak/STAT signaling pathway in IFNα responsiveness, and suggest that it could be an effective therapeutic target for enhancing the antitumor activity of IFNα. This hypothesis is currently being tested in a Cancer and Leukemia Group B (CALGB)-sponsored Phase II clinical trial of IL12 and IFN-α in patients with metastatic melanoma (CALGB 50001).

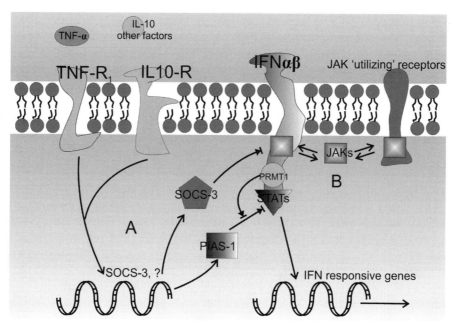

Fig 4. Mechanisms of downregulation of type I interferon (IFN) signaling. **(A)** Suppressors of cytokine signaling (SOCS-1, -3) and the protein inhibitor of activated STAT-1 (PIAS-1) inactivate JAKs and STATs, respectively. For the SOCS-3, specifically, the mechanism involves upregulation of SOCS-3 gene expression by tumor necrosis factor-alpha (TNF-α) and IL-10 signaling pathways. The regulation of PIAS-1 gene expression in IFN-α/β signaling is unknown but it has been shown that its effect on inactivation of STAT-1 is blocked by the protein arginine methyl-transferase PRMT1 which interacts with the α chain of the type I IFN receptor and activates STAT-1 by arginine methylation. **(B)** "Cross competition" between cytokine receptors (e.g., IL-12 receptor) and type I IFN receptor for limited amounts of JAK proteins. Abbreviations: → I, inactivation; TNF R1, TNF-α receptor type.

6.3. Downregulation of IFN-α/β Signaling

Although great progress has been made towards an understanding of the molecular mechanisms responsible for the activation of JAK/STAT signaling pathways, few studies have examined the downregulation of IFN-α/β signaling. Treatment of Jurkat cells with increasing physiologic doses of IFN-β resulted in a dose-dependent loss of IFNAR-1 from the cell surface membrane and increasing nonphosphorylated STAT-1 *(107)*. Also, the available Tyk-2 for interaction with IFNAR may be restricted under conditions when other cytokine receptors which use Tyk2 for signaling become activated concurrently (i.e., IL-12) *(108)*. Inactivation of the JAKs or STATs by other proteins is the dominant mechanism for the transient nature of IFN-α/β signaling. A family of molecules, termed *s*uppressors of *c*ytokine *s*ignaling (SOCS), are intracellular proteins several of which have shown to regulate the responses of immune cells to cytokines (reviewed in ref. *109*). SOCSs can directly interact with JAKs thereby inhibiting their catalytic activity and directing associated proteins, such as JAKs or receptors, for ubiquitin-mediated proteasomal degradation (Fig. 4). SOCS-1 and SOCS-3 inhibit IFN signaling (both type I and II) by interacting with Tyk2 and block nuclear translocation of STAT-1 *(110)*. Furthermore, high expression of SOCS-1 and SOCS-3 has been proposed as a mechanism of resistance to IFN-α treatment in CML *(111,112)*. Both tumor necrosis factor-α (TNF-α) and IL-10 inhibit IFN-α signaling by inducing expression of SOCS-3 mRNA *(113,114)*.

Similar to JAK inactivation, the regulation of STAT action is mediated by a diverse group of proteins (reviewed in ref. *115*). Thus, STAT-1 activation is terminated by protein tyrosine phosphatases (PTPases) which dephosphorylate STAT-1 resulting in rapid export back to the cytoplasm *(116)*. Also, the protein inhibitor of activated STAT-1 (PIAS-1), member of the PIAS family of proteins, binds and inhibits activated STAT-1 *(117)* and is an important downregulator of type I IFN immune response *(118)* (Fig. 4); the PIAS-1—STAT-1 interaction may be prevented by methylation of the arginine (Arg) residue-31 of STAT-1 protein during IFNAR-1 activation *(119)*. Increased knowledge regarding the negative regulatory aspects of JAK/STAT signal transduction could lead to novel therapeutic targets, and a greater understanding of individual responsiveness to IFN-α immunotherapy.

7. INTERFERON-α/β ACTION; NON-IMMUNE MEDIATED MECHANISMS

7.1. Antiproliferative Effects of Type I IFNs

Type I IFNs have well established antiproliferative activity potentially accounting for their therapeutic effects in malignancy *(120)* and their detrimental actions during IFN-α2b therapy, such as bone marrow suppression. The downstream targets of IFN's antiproliferative action are a growing list of molecules, including cell-cycle regulatory proteins (reviewed in ref. *121*). All phases of the cell cycle are susceptible to IFN-inducible arrest, and different cell types are targeted at different stages. IFN-α may interfere with the growth promoting effects of other cytokines and can upregulate expression of the cyclin dependent kinase inhibitors (CKI) p15, p19 and p21 *(122–124)*. In contrast, IFN does not upregulate the p27 protein *(125)* which interacts with cyclin dependent kinases (cdk) cdk2 and cdk4; the end result is inhibition of G1 cell cycle progression. Conversely, IFN-α downregulates cyclin D3 (major component of the cyclin D-associated cdk4 and cdk6 kinase) and cdc25A mRNA (phosphatase regulating the activity of cdk2-cyclin kinases) *(126)* causing a G_o-like state. The net result is that the retinoblastoma protein pRb, which controls entry into S phase of the cell cycle, remains activated either by interference with its phosphorylation by cdks or by inactivation by CKIs. The activation of pRb, along with the suppression of *c-myc (127)* and E2F-1 (a subunit of E2F) *(128)* mRNA expression complements cell cycle arrest blocking entry into S phase.

IFN-α upregulates a growing number of IFN-inducible genes, termed hemopoietic interferon-inducible nuclear proteins with a 200 amino acid repeat (HIN-200) which block cell growth via mechanisms that are sometimes cell-cycle dependent (reviewed in ref. *129*). The best studied example is p202 which interacts with a number of transcription factors, including the p53-binding protein 1 (p53bp), NF-κB, AP-1 (*c-fos/c-Jun*), cmyc and E2F resulting in loss of their transcriptional regulatory activities *(130–134)*. The end result is tumor suppressor activity in a variety of cancers *(135–137)*. p204, which has predominantly nucleolar localization, inhibits ribosomal RNA (rRNA) transcription by binding to the upstream binding protein (UBF), a component of the RNA polymerase I multiprotein complex, and inhibiting UBF's binding to the ribosomal DNA (rDNA) promoter *(138)*. Another HIN-200 member, IFI 16, interacts directly with p53 increasing its transcriptional activation *(139)*.

A mechanism for limiting the number of cell divisions in normal cells is the loss of telomeric sequences at each cell division ultimately activating the cellular senescence program. Once telomeres have been truncated below a critical threshold cell death occurs *(140)*. The activation of the RNA-dependent DNA polymerase, termed telomerase, results in replication of telomeric sequences, and upregulation of the catalytic subunit, hEST2, ultimately leading to the immortalization of cancer cells *(141)*. IFN-α inhibits telomerase expression in cancer cells redirecting their mitotic status to replicative senescence possibly via downregulation of the *c-myc* proto-oncogene *(142)*.

7.2. At the Interface Between Cell Stress, Damage, Apoptosis, and Survival

Type I IFNs have dual and unpredictable effect on cell survival. Recent studies have used oligonucleotide arrays to examine gene expression in melanoma cell lines following stimulation with type I IFN. Interestingly, a number of genes were identified as IFN-induced that have a pro-apoptotic effect *(143)*. Type I IFNs are generally considered nonapoptotic but may render cells apoptosis-prone when they act in concert with other proapoptotic mediators, such as TNF-α *(144)*. The net result is dependent on the cell type, its differentiation state, the type of extracellular stimuli and the activation state of other pathways regulating apoptosis. These data provide a rationale for the administration of IFN-α in combination with other cytotoxic agents.

The double stranded RNA (dsRNA)-activated protein kinase PKR is a ubiquitously expressed enzyme initially characterized as a translational inhibitor during antiviral response *(145)*. Although IFNs induce increased expression of PKR *(146)*, the newly synthesized protein is inactive. Activation of PKR prototypically occurs after binding to dsRNA *(147)*, but it can also be activated by a variety of other nonviral, diverse stimuli *(148–150)* via stress-activated protein kinases *(151,152)*. Conversely, small interfering RNAs (siRNAs), potent reagents for directed post-transcriptional gene silencing, may upregulate IFN-β response via PKR activation *(153)*. Therefore, activated PKR is an important mediator of cellular stress responses by modulating the action of multiple substrates involved in growth control, survival and apoptosis, including upregulation of the endogenous type I IFN signaling.

Thus, type I IFNs have both PKR-dependent and -independent effects on cell stress. Type I IFNs may protect cells from oxidative stress by upregulating antioxidant enzymes *(154)*. The effect of IFN-γ in upregulation of hsp expression is more established *(155)*; however type I IFNs selectively upregulate hsp96, a major component of the endoplasmic reticulum, and an accessory to antigen presentation by MHC class I molecules *(156)*. Activated PKR during cell stress increases hsp70 by stabilization of its mRNA *(157)*. Hsps are potent and abundant intracellular agents that under normal conditions interact with the entire intracellular content (including but not limited to invading pathogens) by assisting in protein folding, and overseeing interaction with other proteins and/or degradation. During cellular stress leading to necrotic cell death, hsp-peptide complexes are released from cells and are sensed by surface receptors on antigen presenting cells thereby making the host aware there is a nonspecific loss of physical integrity. This initiates a series of events associated with innate immunity, including peptide representation (reviewed in ref. *158*). The role of hsps as adjuvants to tumor antigen peptides has recently been demonstrated by successful induction of in vivo immune response to a variety of malignancies suggesting an alternative approach to immunotherapy of tumors *(159)*. In summary, type I IFNs play a major role in cellular stress by upregulating components of the host's "danger signal system."

Type I IFNs exert a pro-apoptotic effect via interactions with several downstream effectors. These may include upregulation of the activating ligands of the death receptor-mediated apoptotic machinery, such as the Fas ligand (**FasL**) *(160)* and the Tumor necrosis factor-related apoptosis-inducing ligand (TRAIL) *(161,162)*, direct activation of *caspases* from both the intrinsic and extrinsic pathway in a PKR independent fashion *(163)*, or suppression of inhibitors of apoptosis, such as the *X*-linked *i*nhibitor of *ap*optosis (XIAP) associated factor-1 *(164)*. Activated PKR inhibits eukaryotic initiation factor 2 (eIF2α) and subsequent translational initiation, thereby inhibiting protein synthesis, growth inhibition and apoptosis *(165)*. Activated PKR directly activates caspases, components of the apoptotic cascade *(166,167)* or indirectly activates other transcription factors which are involved in apoptotic signaling (reviewed in ref. *168*). The 2'—5' oligoadenylate (2-5A) is another IFN-inducible enzyme during antiviral response which activates the 2'—5' A-dependent RNase L ribonuclease leading to cleavage of single-stranded RNA and inhibition of protein synthesis *(169)*. In several malignancies degradation of RNA by RNase L is an important mechanism of tumor control *(170–172)*. Activated or overexpressed RNase L induces apoptosis by activating mitochondrial caspases *(173)* and mutations in RNase L gene have been identified in familial cases of hereditary prostate cancer *(174)*. Members of the regulators of IFN-induced death (RID) family of proteins, such as the RID-2/IHPK2 (inositol hexakisphosphated kinase), may induce cell death possibly by forming diphosphoinositol pentakiphosphate (InsP5PP) from inositol hexakisphosphate (IP6), facilitating assembly of the death-inducing signaling complex (DISC) *(175,176)*. *Phospholipid scramblase*, one of the most strongly inducible IFN-responsive genes, has an important role in apoptosis by promoting transbilayer movement ("flipping") of phosphatidylserine to the outer leaf of the cell membrane in response to injury or apoptosis thereby serving as a surface marker for recruited phagocytes to recognize and eliminate apoptotic bodies *(177)*. In several murine models the surface expression of phosphatidylserine affects tumorigenic potential by limiting cell growth and promoting apoptotic cell death *(178)*.

Type I IFNs also have a significant, though ambivalent effect, on NF-κB, an important transcription factor for cell survival and cell proliferation (reviewed in ref. *179*), which has been shown to be constitutively expressed in a variety of tumor cell lines *(180)*. Thus, the IFNA-R1→STAT-3→PI-3K→Akt→IκB kinase pathway leading to activation of the anti-apoptotic NF-κB has been described in Daudi cells *(93)* in accordance with the survival effect of type I IFNs in T- *(181)* and B-lymphocytes (182). In contrast, IFN-α either directly *(144,183,184)* or via IFN-inducible proteins *(132)* suppresses NF-κB activation in a variety of cancer cell lines in keeping with its tumor suppressive effect *(185)*. In conclusion, the effects of type I IFN on apoptosis vary and thus should be individually investigated for every cell type.

7.3. Effect on Cell Differentiation

In accordance with their antiproliferative and growth inhibitory role, type I IFNs have a well established effect on differentiation of normal cells *(186–188)*. Intuitively, there is a link between the processes of terminal differentiation and cell cycle progression because a cell that cannot arrest will not be able to differentiate. This process is normally mediated by a group of "differentiation genes" encoding a wide variety of proteins, including nuclear transcription factors (Hox, engrailed, and PAX), secreted factors (Wnt, TGFβ) and cell surface receptors (Wnt) *(189–192)*. Each of these genes is regulated in an opposite manner by at least two sets of genes, "differentiation suppressor genes" (Id family, *c-myc*, cyclins), and tumor suppressor genes (p53, pRb, p21$^{cip/Waf1}$) *(193)*. Type I IFNs allow the differentiation program to occur by favoring the expression of proteins causing cell cycle arrest, and subsequent exit from the cell cycle *(132,194)*. More specifically, type I IFNs activate the two cell-cyle proteins most closely linked to differentiation, namely pRb and p21$^{cip/Waf1}$. The retinoblastoma protein pRb relieves the cell from the action of Id-2, a member of the Id family of proteins which inhibit differentiation by sequestering basic helix-loop-helix (bHLH) transcription factors *(195)*.

Similar to normal cells, type I IFNs may induce differentiation in a variety of cancer cell types either alone *(196–198)* or in combination with other differentiation inducing agents *(199–202)*. This "tumor reprogramming" is partially mediated by modulating the expression of cell adhesion molecules (CAMs), which play an important role in determining the overall tissue architecture by binding cells to each other and to the internal cytoskeleton (homotypic homophylic interactions; reviewed in ref. *203*). For example, the expression of cadherins, negatively correlated with cancer aggressiveness *(204–206)*, is upregulated by IFN-α in different malignancies *(207–209)* and normal cells *(210)*. Other CAMs may promote cell adhesion and prevention of metastasis via heterotypic (i.e. between different cells)-heterophylic (i.e. between different CAMs) interactions. Normal levels of L-selectin (CD62L), a carbohydrate binding protein which mediates adhesion of leukocytes to endothelial cells (heterotypic heterophylic interactions), are restored in early hemopoietic progenitor (CD34$^+$) cells of CML patients treated with IFN-α *(211)*. Also, β_1 integrin-mediated cell adhesion is optimized via mechanisms involving increased protein expression *(212,213)*. Finally, IFN-α may prevent or promote tumor cell metastasis via integrin-mediated mechanisms *(214,215)*.

The role of type I IFNs alone or with other differentiation agents in the terminal differentiation of melanoma cells has been extensively studied. Treatment of melanoma cells with IFN-β alone or with the antileukemic compound mezerein (MEZ) results in irreversible growth arrest, altered cellular morphology, modifications in antigenic phenotype, and increased melanogenesis *(202)*. The repertoire of genes modulated during growth arrest and terminal differentiation includes genes involved in the cytoskeleton (vimentin, fibronectin), cytokine signaling and response (IL-8, ISGF-3), RNA processing (heterogenous nuclear ribonucleoprotein, core protein A1) and genes from the *mda* family (*mda*-1 to 7) *(216)*. These encode for proteins causing cell cycle arrest (*mda*-6, p21$^{Cip-1/sdi-1}$), growth suppression/apoptosis (*mda*-5, *mda*-7), or differentiation (*mda*-5, *mda*-9). The role of *mda*-1 remains to be elucidated *(217–219)*.

7.4. Effect on Angiogenesis

Tumor angiogenesis is the result of an imbalance in pro and anti-angiogenic molecules (reviewed in ref. *220*). Type I IFNs can potentially restore this imbalance by a variety of mechanisms including reduced expression of several pro-angiogenic mediators, such as the vascular endothelial growth factor (VEGF) *(221)*, basic fibroblast growth factor (bFGF) *(222,223)*, IL-8 *(224,225)* and leptin *(226)*. In fact, reduction of serum IL-8 levels but not of serum VEGF or bFGF during adjuvant IFN-α2b therapy for resected AJCC stage III and IV melanoma was noted in a small (*n* = 22) study *(227)*. IFNα also downregulates matrix metalloproteinase-2 and -9 *(207)*, enzymes involved in the degradation of the extracellular matrix and basal membranes, and upregulates various IFN-inducible chemokines, such as Mig and IP-10 *(228)*, which attract lymphocytes into tumors and elicits a type 1 T helper (T$_h$1) (response *[229]*, reviewed in ref. *230*). In addition, IFN-α affects the production of free radical producing enzymes, namely cyclooxygenase-1 -2 *(231)* and nitric oxide synthase II *(232–234)* which have a anti-angiogenic effect at certain levels and exert direct effects on endothelial cells causing growth arrest, pro-angiogenic factor starvation-mediated apoptosis *(232)*, and blockade of endothelial cell migration *(235)*.

In summary, type I IFNs are of the most potent angiogenic inhibitors known. Further understanding of their effect may be gained by defining the optimal dose and schedule (not always the maximally tolerated dose) (reviewed in ref. *236*) and by combining them with other angiogenic inhibitors, such as thalidomide and tamoxifen, for a synergistic, anti-angiogenic effect *(237,238)*.

8. INTERFERON-α/β ACTION; IMMUNE MEDIATED MECHANISMS

8.1. Introduction

There is increasing evidence that endogenously produced IFNs play a vital role in innate resistance to a wide variety of infectious agents and tumors. Constitutive low-grade production of IFN occurs in almost all nucleated cells in the body with a probable preventative intent (reviewed in refs. *23,24*). IFN can also be produced *en masse* by the specialized plasmacytoid dendritic cells during infection. This mechanism of production establishes a connection between innate and adaptive immunity affecting cellular components in both arms of the immune response (antigen presenting cells and lymphocytes (reviewed in ref. *239*). Exogenously administered IFN likely functions by manipulating the normal homeostasis of the innate immune system. High systemic concentrations of IFN stimulate more potent cytotoxic activity by immune effectors, expression of costimulatory molecules and activation markers, and upregulation of MHC Class I expression. The following portion of the chapter highlights the biologic effects of IFNs on immune effectors and recent work investigating the mechanism of action of exogenous IFN-α.

8.2. Role of Type I IFNs Acting on and Deriving From Antigen Presenting Cells

Dendritic cells are the fundamental "third party" for the two other components of the immune system, namely antigens and lymphocytes, to establish immunity (reviewed in ref. *240*). They arise, upon different signals, from many different progenitor cells of myeloid or lymphoid origin leading to heterogenous DC subpopulations *(241)*. In their immature state they are located in most tissues where they constantly "sample" their microenvirorment by capturing and processing antigens and displaying them in large amounts on their surface in a MHC-peptide fashion. The presence of exogenous antigens, direct stress and signals from necrotic cells activate DCs but not healthy or apoptotic cells *(34)*. Upon activation they mature by upregulating co-stimulatory molecules and migrating to lymphoid organs where they present antigens to lymphocytes resulting in their activation.

Type I IFNs have an important role at all stages of DC and monocyte/macrophage differentiation, maturation and function. Thus, type I IFNs upregulate expression of several TLRs on macrophages optimizing their antigen presenting function *(242)*. Vice versa, TLRs induce type I IFN production in DC subsets *(243)* and macrophages by induction of several genes during macrophage activation, such as chemokines (IP-10, MCP-5) and free radicals (NO) *(244)*. Type I IFNs have differential effects on the two major subsets of immature DCs, namely the myeloid CD11c$^+$ DCs (pDC$_1$) and the lymphoid CD11c$^-$ DC (pDC$_2$) *(245)*. Type I IFNs act as maturation factors for pDC$_1$s by upregulating class I and class II MHC (HLA-A, -B, -C, -DR) and costimulatory molecules (CD80, CD83 and CD86); and by downregulating CD1a and CD11b lineage markers *(186,246)*. In addition, type I IFNs serve as differentiation-inhibiting factors for pDC$_2$s by blocking the maturation effect of IL-3. Type I IFNs applied in vitro at an earlier timepoint of the differentiation process of CD14$^+$ monocytes, progenitor cells for pDC$_1$s, have an inhibitory effect, leading to decreased cell viability *(247)*. The effect of type I IFNs is enhanced during ongoing differentiation by both increased expression by maturing DCs in an autocrine fashion *(248)* and upregulation of the IFNR1 on their surface *(249)*. These effects are synergistic with other cytokines, such as TNF-α, IFN-γ, IL-4, granulocyte-monocyte colony stimulating factor (GM-CSF) and prostaglandin E$_2$ (PGE$_2$) *(250)*. Therefore, the origin of DC precursors (lymphoid vs myeloid), the stage of their differentiation (early vs late), and the type and sequence in which DCs encounter cytokines may all differentially affect DC maturation and function.

Type I IFNs switch the expression of several molecules via DC mediating mechanisms thereby affecting APCs or other effector cell function. Thus, IFN-α induces different sets of chemokines and their receptors on APCs affecting their maturation- trafficking pattern. More specifically, type I IFNs upregulate the chemokine receptor CCR7, its natural ligand, MIP-3β, and the T$_{h1}$ chemokine, IP-10, on the maturing antigen-loaded pDC$_1$s thereby facilitating their migration to the T-cell zone paracortical area of draining lymph nodes to encounter CCR7 expressing specific T-cells *(251)*. Mycobacterium tuberculosis (MTB) infected DCs produce type I IFNs which act in an autocrine/paracrine fashion to induce the expression of the chemokine CXL10 which may recruit NK, T$_{h1}$ and T$_{c1}$ cells to the site of infection; the cells then can directly destroy MTB infected cells and produce IFN-γ, stimulating macrophage activation *(252)*. They also upregulate the expression of CCR1 and CCR3 chemokine receptors on monocyte-derived cell subsets *(253)*. Adjuvant treatment in stage III melanoma with intravenous adjuvant IFN-α upregulated expression of transport proteins associated with antigen processing (TAP1 and TAP2) and proteasome activator 28 in peripheral blood mononuclear cells *(254)*. In addition, type I IFNs also have a major effect on B-cell function and survival via effects on APCs. IFN-α upregulates the B-lymphocyte stimulator protein (BLyS) and the proliferation-inducing ligand (APRIL) which both activate a CD40-like pathway enhancing B-cell survival and promoting isotype class switch DNA recombination to C$_γ$, C$_α$ and even C$_ε$ in IgD$^+$ and/IgM$^+$ B-cells *(255)*.

Lymphoid DCs (pDC2s) are the major producers of type I IFN. The DC-derived type I IFNs act in an autocrine manner for further type I IFN production or induction of other DC-derived cytokines, such as IL-15, which have an activation and survival effect on DCs *(248,256,257)*. These IFN producing cells may be inefficient stimulators of naïve T-cells but may potently expand nonpolarized antigen-primed IL-2-secreting T-cells towards a Th1 polarized phenotype *(258)*. However, DC–derived type I IFNs also have immunomodulatory effects that "shape" innate and adaptive immune responses. The paradox of suppression of IL-12 production from myeloid DCs (pDC$_1$s) *(259)* may represent another mechanism of crossregulation between DC subsets and reflect the delicate balance among different innate cellular responses (type I IFN-mediated strong NK cell IFN-γ secretion vs IL-12-mediated activation of CD4$^+$ cells and T-lymphocyte cytotoxicity) *(260)*.

8.3. Role on NK Cells and Other Lymphocyte Subsets

Further evidence that type I IFNs are an important link between innate and adaptive immunity is their effect on lymphocytes. Induction of NK cell-mediated proliferation and cytotoxicity were the earliest described immunologic effects of type I IFNs *(261–263)*. Type I IFNs also induce polyclonal activation of CD8$^+$ cells during viral infections *(264)*, and may also mount potent antitumoral cell-mediated cytotoxicity *(265,266)*. The mechanism of this activation is thought to be by the activation of a multitude of STATs (1, 3, 4, 5a, 5b) which lead to upregulation of the α chain of IL-2R (CD25), *cmyc* and *pim-1* oncogenes *(267)*, MHC class I molecules in both the tumor and the lymphocytes *(268)*, and probably anti-apoptotic genes *(264)*. Further IFN-α production from DCs may occur via complex DC T-cell interaction resulting in full activation of naïve T-cells *(269)*.

In patients with metastatic melanoma response to IFN-α was associated with an increase in the number of tumor infiltrating CD4$^+$ cells, an overall marker of favorable survival, possibly by reversing the tumor-induced immunosuppressive environment *(270)*. Type I IFNs influence CD4$^+$ cell differentiations towards a T$_h$1 response by antagonizing the suppressive effect of IL-4 on IFN-γ secreting CD4$^+$ cells *(271)*, suppressing IL-5 production by CD4$^+$ cells *(272)* and upregulating the β$_2$ chain of IL-12 receptor *(273)* in a STAT-4 dependent fashion *(274)*. This T$_h$1 cell polarization is also reflected in the type I IFN-induced differential lymphocyte traffic control pattern with upregulation of L-selectin (lymph nodes), cutaneous lymphocyte-associated antigen (CLA) (skin) *(275)* and the chemokine receptor CCR5 indirectly *(276)*. Thus, locally produced type I IFN may contribute to the influx of T$_h$1 rather than T$_h$2 lymphocytes at the inflammatory site, such as skin or lymph nodes. In keeping with their antiproliferative effect in cells, type I IFNs exert an antiproliferative effect on lymphocytes via interaction of IFNAR1 with components of T-cell receptor signaling, such as CD45, ZAP-70 and Lck *(277)*. This effect may be partially overcome by mitogenic stimuli depending on the activation state of lymphocytes *(278)*. This restriction of rapid lymphocyte proliferation during activation may slow the process of activation-induced cell death *(181,182)*. This anti-apoptotic effect of type I IFNs is NF-κB-dependent and has well been described in Daudi cells *(93)*.

Despite the well established boosting effect of type I IFNs on lymphocyte function, they also exert multiple immunomodulatory effects, namely they affect both B- and T-cell lymphopoiesis by inducing several immunohistochemical changes in thymic tissue *(279)* and they directly suppress the IL-7-mediated early stages of lymphocyte development *(280)*. Type I IFNs mediate early activation of lymphocyte response during viral infections via a common intracellular mechanism that is predominantly STAT-1 dependent *(279,281)*. This may result in suppression of lymphocyte mediated IFN-γ production seen during early stages of viral infections. During later stages of lymphocyte activation unknown mechanisms regulating STAT-1 activation allow type I IFN stimulation of IFN-γ expression *(280)*.

IFNα likely contributes to the formation and maintenance of immunologic memory. Adenoviral–IFNA-α-engineered DCs delivered into intracranial tumors in mice enhanced antitumor efficacy of prior vaccination with an ovalbumin-derived MHC class II-restricted epitope *(282)*. Administration of high dose IFNα following vaccination leads to immunologic recall of gp100-specific CD8$^+$ T-cells *(283)*. This finding has important implications for the maintenance of memory T-lymphocytes, and suggests that IFN-α may potentially be useful in cancer vaccines to assist in overcoming immunologic tolerance to tumor antigens.

8.4. The Relationship Between Signal Transduction Within Host Immune Effectors and the Response to Exogenous IFN-α

It has been well established that many antiviral effects of IFNα are mediated through STAT-1. However, in the setting of tumor immunotherapy, the precise molecular targets responsible for mediating the activity of IFNα have not been identified. Interestingly, recent studies in a murine model of malignant melanoma have provided evidence supporting the role of STAT-1 within host NK cells in mediating the antitumor effects of IFN-α *(284)*. These data point to a critical role for immunomodulatory effects of exogenously administered IFN-α in the setting of melanoma. Altered immune function has been routinely reported for tumor-bearing animals and cancer patients. Some of the observed defects include diminished levels of lymphocyte cytotoxic activity and proliferation *(285,286)*, altered delayed type hypersensitivity, impaired production of T$_{h1}$ cytokines, and reduced NK cell activity *(287,288)*. Alterations in specific signal transduction molecules have also been reported in tumor infiltrating and peripheral lymphocytes *(289)*. For example, defects in the T-cell receptor zeta chain (TCRζ), p56(lck) kinase, ZAP-70 expression and NF-κB activation have been correlated with stage of disease and prognosis in patients with melanoma and renal cell carcinoma *(290,291)*. Therefore, it is also likely that inherent defects in signaling within host immune effectors could influence responsiveness to exogenous IFN-α. In fact, a recent study has demonstrated that basal levels of phosphorylated STAT-1 (P-STAT1) were significantly lower in peripheral blood mononuclear cells (PBMCs) of melanoma patients when compared to levels in PBMCs from normal, healthy donors *(292)*. These data suggest that altered signaling and perhaps downstream expression of IFN-α-responsive genes might be altered in immune effectors of patients with malignancy.

9. FUTURE DIRECTIONS AND CHALLENGES

IFN-α and other cytokine-based therapeutics have emerged as a promising strategy for the treatment of cancer. A major advantage is that they represent a broad-based treatment strategy that can be used across groups of patients, regardless of HLA-haplotype and in a variety of disease settings. Unfortunately, the greatest setback to optimizing their usage is a lack of knowledge of the specific mechanisms leading to efficacy or toxicity in subsets of patients. These challenges underscore the need to devise improvements and design combinations rationally, and then to apply this therapy in patients with the highest likelihood of responding to therapy *(293)*.

Future research is in place to gain a better understanding of the molecular mechanisms and cellular compartments that mediate the activity of exogenously administered IFN-α. We are hopeful that advances in technology, and improved understanding of both tumor cells and the host immune system will uncover surrogate markers of IFN-α-responsiveness or toxicity. These challenges represent an important avenue of research, and may lead to new therapeutic combinations of immunomodulatory strategies to combat human malignancies.

REFERENCES

1. Isaacs, A. and J. Lindenmann, Virus interference I: The interferon. Proc R Soc Lond Ser B, 1957. 147: p. 258–67.
2. Isaacs, A., J. Lindenmann, and R.C. Valentine, Virus interference, II: Some properties of interferon. Proc R Soc Lond, 1957. 147B: p. 268–73.
3. Burke, D.C. and A. Isaacs, Some factors affecting the production of interferon. Br J Exp Pathol, 1958. 39: p. 452–58.
4. Gresser, I., Production of inteferon by suspensions of human leukocytes. Proc Soc Exp Biol Med, 1961. 108: p. 799–803.
5. Gresser, I. and C. Bourali, Exogenous interferon and inducers of interferon in the treatment Balb-c mice inoculated with RC19 tumour cells. Nature, 1969. 223(208): p. 844–5.
6. Paucker, K., K. Cantell, and W. Henle, Quantitative studies on viral interference in suspended L cells, III: Effect of interfering viruses and interferon on the growth rate of cells. Virology, 1962. 17: p. 324–34.
7. Rubinstein, M., et al., Human leukocyte interferon purified to homogeneity. Science, 1978. 202(4374): p. 1289–90.
8. Taniguchi, T., Y. Fujii-Kuriyama, and M. Muramatsu, Construction and identification of a bacterial plasmid containing the human fibroblast interferon gene sequences. Proc Japan Acad, 1979. 55B: p. 464–69.
9. Hall, S.S., The cloning of interferon and other mistakes, In: A Commotion in the Blood. 1997, Henry Holt and Company, Inc: New York, NY. p. 178–208.
10. Owerbach, D., et al., Leukocyte and fibroblast interferon genes are located on human chromosome 9. Proc Natl Acad Sci USA, 1981. 78(5): p. 3123–7.
11. Allen, G. and M.O. Diaz, Nomenclature of the human interferon proteins. J Interferon Cytokine Res, 1996. 16(2): p. 181–4.
12. Conklin, D.C., et al., Interferon-e. U.S. Patent 6329175, 2002.
13. LaFleur, D.W., et al., Interferon-kappa, a novel type I interferon expressed in human keratinocytes. J Biol Chem, 2001. 276(43): p. 39765–71.
14. Haus, O., The genes of interferons and interferon-related factors: Localization and relationships with chromosome aberrations in cancer. Arch Immunol Ther Exp (Warsz), 2000. 48(2): p. 95–100.
15. Oritani, K., et al., Limitin: An interferon-like cytokine that preferentially influences B-lymphocyte precursors. Nat Med, 2000. 6(6): p. 659–66.
16. Takahashi, I., et al., A new IFN-like cytokine, limitin, modulates the immune response without influencing thymocyte development. J Immunol, 2001. 167(6): p. 3156–63.
17. Oritani, K., P.W. Kincade, and Y. Tomiyama, Limitin: An interferon-like cytokine without myeloerythroid suppressive properties. J Mol Med, 2001. 79(4): p. 168–74.
18. Kotenko, S.V., et al., IFN-lambdas mediate antiviral protection through a distinct class II cytokine receptor complex. Nat Immunol, 2003. 4(1): p. 69–77.
19. Sheppard, P., et al., IL-28, IL-29 and their class II cytokine receptor IL-28R. Nat Immunol, 2003. 4(1): p. 63–8.
20. Fearon, D.T. and R.M. Locksley, The instructive role of innate immunity in the acquired immune response. Science, 1996. 272(5258): p. 50–3.
21. Medzhitov, R. and C.A. Biron, Innate immunity. Curr Opin Immunol, 2003. 15(1): p. 2–4.
22. Melcher, A., et al., Tumor immunogenicity is determined by the mechanism of cell death via induction of heat shock protein expression. Nat Med, 1998. 4(5): p. 581–7.
23. Gresser, I. and F. Belardelli, Endogenous type I interferons as a defense against tumors. Cytokine Growth Factor Rev, 2002. 13(2): p. 111–8.
24. Taniguchi, T. and A. Takaoka, A weak signal for strong responses: Interferon-alpha/beta revisited. Nat Rev Mol Cell Biol, 2001. 2(5): p. 378–86.
25. Siegal, F.P., et al., The nature of the principal type 1 interferon-producing cells in human blood. Science, 1999. 284(5421): p. 1835–7.
26. Cella, M., et al., Plasmacytoid monocytes migrate to inflamed lymph nodes and produce large amounts of type I interferon. Nat Med, 1999. 5(8): p. 919–23.
27. Zou, W., et al., Stromal-derived factor-1 in human tumors recruits and alters the function of plasmacytoid precursor dendritic cells. Nat Med, 2001. 7(12): p. 1339–46.
28. Vermi, W., et al., Recruitment of immature plasmacytoid dendritic cells (plasmacytoid monocytes) and myeloid dendritic cells in primary cutaneous melanomas. J Pathol, 2003. 200(2): p. 255–68.

29. Takeda, K., T. Kaisho, and S. Akira, Toll-like receptors. Annu Rev Immunol, 2003. 21: p. 335–76.
30. Kadowaki, N., et al., Subsets of human dendritic cell precursors express different toll-like receptors and respond to different microbial antigens. J Exp Med, 2001. 194(6): p. 863–9.
31. Akira, S., K. Takeda, and T. Kaisho, Toll-like receptors: Critical proteins linking innate and acquired immunity. Nat Immunol, 2001. 2(8): p. 675–80.
32. Fan, J. and A.B. Malik, Toll-like receptor-4 (TLR4) signaling augments chemokine-induced neutrophil migration by modulating cell surface expression of chemokine receptors. Nat Med, 2003. 9(3): p. 315–21.
33. Pasare, C. and R. Medzhitov, Toll pathway-dependent blockade of CD4+CD25+ T cell-mediated suppression by dendritic cells. Science, 2003. 299(5609): p. 1033–6.
34. Gallucci, S., M. Lolkema, and P. Matzinger, Natural adjuvants: Endogenous activators of dendritic cells. Nat Med, 1999. 5(11): p. 1249–55.
35. Asea, A., et al., Novel signal transduction pathway utilized by extracellular HSP70: role of toll-like receptor (TLR) 2 and TLR4. J Biol Chem, 2002. 277(17): p. 15028–34.
36. Biragyn, A., et al., Toll-like receptor 4-dependent activation of dendritic cells by beta-defensin 2. Science, 2002. 298(5595): p. 1025–9.
37. Cederblad, B., K. Sandberg, and G.V. Alm, The leukocyte function-associated antigen-1 (LFA-1) is involved in the interferon-alpha response induced by herpes simplex virus in blood leukocytes. J Interferon Res, 1993. 13(3): p. 203–8.
38. Zeng, J., P. Fournier, and V. Schirrmacher, Stimulation of human natural interferon-alpha response via paramyxovirus hemagglutinin lectin-cell interaction. J Mol Med, 2002. 80(7): p. 443–51.
39. Palmer, P., et al., Antibody-dependent induction of type I interferons by poliovirus in human mononuclear blood cells requires the type II fcgamma receptor (CD32). Virology, 2000. 278(1): p. 86–94.
40. Dzionek, A., et al., Plasmacytoid dendritic cells: from specific surface markers to specific cellular functions(1). Hum Immunol, 2002. 63(12): p. 1133–48.
41. Mazzoni, A., et al., Cutting edge: Histamine inhibits IFN-alpha release from plasmacytoid dendritic cells. J Immunol, 2003. 170(5): p. 2269–73.
42. Tanaka, N. and T. Taniguchi, Cytokine gene regulation: Regulatory cis-elements and DNA binding factors involved in the interferon system. Adv Immunol, 1992. 52: p. 263–81.
43. Taniguchi, T., et al., IRF family of transcription factors as regulators of host defense. Annu Rev Immunol, 2001. 19: p. 623–55.
44. Fujita, T., et al., Evidence for a nuclear factor(s), IRF-1, mediating induction and silencing properties to human IFN-beta gene regulatory elements. Embo J, 1988. 7(11): p. 3397–405.
45. Harada, H., et al., Structurally similar but functionally distinct factors, IRF-1 and IRF-2, bind to the same regulatory elements of IFN and IFN-inducible genes. Cell, 1989. 58(4): p. 729–39.
46. Sato, M., et al., Distinct and essential roles of transcription factors IRF-3 and IRF-7 in response to viruses for IFN-alpha/beta gene induction. Immunity, 2000. 13(4): p. 539–48.
47. Au, W.C. and P.M. Pitha, Recruitment of multiple interferon regulatory factors and histone acetyltransferase to the transcriptionally active interferon a promoters. J Biol Chem, 2001. 276(45): p. 41629–37.
48. Barnes, B.J., P.A. Moore, and P.M. Pitha, Virus-specific activation of a novel interferon regulatory factor, IRF-5, results in the induction of distinct interferon alpha genes. J Biol Chem, 2001. 276(26): p. 23382–90.
49. Novick, D., B. Cohen, and M. Rubinstein, The human interferon alpha/beta receptor: Characterization and molecular cloning. Cell, 1994. 77(3): p. 391–400.
50. Lundgren, E. and J.A. Langer, Nomenclature of interferon receptors and interferon-delta. J Interferon Cytokine Res, 1997. 17(7): p. 431–2.
51. Jouanguy, E., et al., A human IFNGR1 small deletion hotspot associated with dominant susceptibility to mycobacterial infection. Nat Genet, 1999. 21(4): p. 370–8.
52. Picaud, S., et al., Enhanced tumor development in mice lacking a functional type I interferon receptor. J Interferon Cytokine Res, 2002. 22(4): p. 457–62.
53. Lutfalla, G., et al., The structure of the human interferon alpha/beta receptor gene. J Biol Chem, 1992. 267(4): p. 2802–9.
54. Takane, H., et al., Relationship between diurnal rhythm of cell cycle and interferon receptor expression in implanted-tumor cells. Life Sci, 2001. 68(12): p. 1449–55.
55. Koren, S., E.B. Whorton, Jr., and W.R. Fleischmann, Jr., Circadian dependence of interferon antitumor activity in mice. J Natl Cancer Inst, 1993. 85(23): p. 1927–32.

56. Tamura, T., et al., Upregulation of interferon-alpha receptor expression in hydroxyurea-treated leukemia cell lines. J Investig Med, 1997. 45(4): p. 160–7.

57. Horoszewicz, J.S., S.S. Leong, and W.A. Carter, Noncycling tumor cells are sensitive targets for the antiproliferative activity of human interferon. Science, 1979. 206(4422): p. 1091–3.

58. Mizukoshi, E., et al., Upregulation of type I interferon receptor by IFN-gamma. J Interferon Cytokine Res, 1999. 19(9): p. 1019–23.

59. Hamamoto, S., et al., 9-cis retinoic acid enhances the antiviral effect of interferon on hepatitis C virus replication through increased expression of type I interferon receptor. J Lab Clin Med, 2003. 141(1): p. 58–66.

60. Moore, D.M., et al., Retinoic acid and interferon in human cancer: Mechanistic and clinical studies. Semin Hematol, 1994. 31(4 Suppl 5): p. 31–7.

61. Barthe, C., et al., Expression of interferon-alpha (IFN-alpha) receptor 2c at diagnosis is associated with cytogenetic response in IFN-alpha-treated chronic myeloid leukemia. Blood, 2001. 97(11): p. 3568–73.

62. Fukuda, R., et al., Effectiveness of interferon-alpha therapy in chronic hepatitis C is associated with the amount of interferon-alpha receptor mRNA in the liver. J Hepatol, 1997. 26(3): p. 455–61.

63. Tochizawa, S., et al., A flow cytometric method for determination of the interferon receptor IFNAR2 subunit in peripheral blood leukocyte subsets. J Pharmacol Toxicol Methods, 2004. 50(1): p. 59–66.

64. Wagner, T.C., et al., Interferon receptor expression regulates the antiproliferative effects of interferons on cancer cells and solid tumors. Int J Cancer, 2004. 111(1): p. 32–42.

65. Ito, K., et al., Initial expression of interferon alpha receptor 2 (IFNAR2) on CD34-positive cells and its down-regulation correlate with clinical response to interferon therapy in chronic myelogenous leukemia. Eur J Haematol, 2004. 73(3): p. 191–205.

66. Duhe, R.J. and W.L. Farrar, Structural and mechanistic aspects of Janus kinases: How the two-faced god wields a double-edged sword. J Interferon Cytokine Res, 1998. 18(1): p. 1–15.

67. Stahl, N., et al., Choice of STATs and other substrates specified by modular tyrosine-based motifs in cytokine receptors. Science, 1995. 267(5202): p. 1349–53.

68. Colamonici, O.R., et al., p135tyk2, an interferon-alpha-activated tyrosine kinase, is physically associated with an interferon-alpha receptor. J Biol Chem, 1994. 269(5): p. 3518–22.

69. Yang, C.H., et al., Direct association of STAT3 with the IFNAR-1 chain of the human type I interferon receptor. J Biol Chem, 1996. 271(14): p. 8057–61.

70. Domanski, P., et al., A region of the beta subunit of the interferon alpha receptor different from box 1 interacts with Jak1 and is sufficient to activate the Jak-Stat pathway and induce an antiviral state. J Biol Chem, 1997. 272(42): p. 26388–93.

71. Nadeau, O.W., et al., The proximal tyrosines of the cytoplasmic domain of the beta chain of the type I interferon receptor are essential for signal transducer and activator of transcription (Stat) 2 activation. Evidence that two Stat2 sites are required to reach a threshold of interferon alpha-induced Stat2 tyrosine phosphorylation that allows normal formation of interferon-stimulated gene factor 3. J Biol Chem, 1999. 274(7): p. 4045–52.

72. Lau, J.F., J.P. Parisien, and C.M. Horvath, Interferon regulatory factor subcellular localization is determined by a bipartite nuclear localization signal in the DNA-binding domain and interaction with cytoplasmic retention factors. Proc Natl Acad Sci USA, 2000. 97(13): p. 7278–83.

73. Usacheva, A., et al., The WD motif-containing protein receptor for activated protein kinase C (RACK1) is required for recruitment and activation of signal transducer and activator of transcription 1 through the type I interferon receptor. J Biol Chem, 2001. 276(25): p. 22948–53.

74. Fish, E.N., et al., Activation of a CrkL-stat5 signaling complex by type I interferons. J Biol Chem, 1999. 274(2): p. 571–3.

75. Platanias, L.C., et al., The type I interferon receptor mediates tyrosine phosphorylation of insulin receptor substrate 2. J Biol Chem, 1996. 271(1): p. 278–82.

76. Gauzzi, M.C., et al., Interferon-alpha-dependent activation of Tyk2 requires phosphorylation of positive regulatory tyrosines by another kinase. J Biol Chem, 1996. 271(34): p. 20494–500.

77. Russell-Harde, D., et al., Role of the intracellular domain of the human type I interferon receptor 2 chain (IFNAR2c) in interferon signaling. Expression of IFNAR2c truncation mutants in U5A cells. J Biol Chem, 2000. 275(31): p. 23981–5.

78. Krishnan, K., R. Pine, and J.J. Krolewski, Kinase-deficient forms of Jak1 and Tyk2 inhibit interferon alpha signaling in a dominant manner. Eur J Biochem, 1997. 247(1): p. 298–305.

79. Fu, X.Y., et al., ISGF3, the transcriptional activator induced by interferon alpha, consists of multiple interacting polypeptide chains. Proc Natl Acad Sci USA, 1990. 87(21): p. 8555–9.

80. Qureshi, S.A., et al., Function of Stat2 protein in transcriptional activation by alpha interferon. Mol Cell Biol, 1996. 16(1): p. 288–93.
81. Bluyssen, A.R., J.E. Durbin, and D.E. Levy, ISGF3 gamma p48, a specificity switch for interferon activated transcription factors. Cytokine Growth Factor Rev, 1996. 7(1): p. 11–7.
82. Li, X., et al., Formation of STAT1-STAT2 heterodimers and their role in the activation of IRF-1 gene transcription by interferon-alpha. J Biol Chem, 1996. 271(10): p. 5790–4.
83. Ghislain, J.J., et al., The interferon-inducible Stat2:Stat1 heterodimer preferentially binds in vitro to a consensus element found in the promoters of a subset of interferon-stimulated genes. J Interferon Cytokine Res, 2001. 21(6): p. 379–88.
84. Bhattacharya, S., et al., Cooperation of Stat2 and p300/CBP in signalling induced by interferon-alpha. Nature, 1996. 383(6598): p. 344–7.
85. Huang, M., et al., Chromatin-remodelling factor BRG1 selectively activates a subset of interferon-alpha-inducible genes. Nat Cell Biol, 2002. 4(10): p. 774–81.
86. Paulson, M., et al., IFN-Stimulated transcription through a TBP-free acetyltransferase complex escapes viral shutoff. Nat Cell Biol, 2002. 4(2): p. 140–7.
87. Rani, M.R., et al., Catalytically active TYK2 is essential for interferon-beta-mediated phosphorylation of STAT3 and interferon-alpha receptor-1 (IFNAR-1) but not for activation of phosphoinositol 3-kinase. J Biol Chem, 1999. 274(45): p. 32507–11.
88. Uddin, S., et al., Interferon-dependent activation of the serine kinase PI 3'-kinase requires engagement of the IRS pathway but not the Stat pathway. Biochem Biophys Res Commun, 2000. 270(1): p. 158–62.
89. Uddin, S., et al., Interferon-alpha engages the insulin receptor substrate-1 to associate with the phosphatidylinositol 3'-kinase. J Biol Chem, 1995. 270(27): p. 15938–41.
90. Farrar, J.D., et al., Selective loss of type I interferon-induced STAT4 activation caused by a minisatellite insertion in mouse Stat2. Nat Immunol, 2000. 1(1): p. 65–9.
91. Nguyen, K.B., et al., Critical role for STAT4 activation by type 1 interferons in the interferon-gamma response to viral infection. Science, 2002. 297(5589): p. 2063–6.
92. Pfeffer, L.M., et al., STAT3 as an adapter to couple phosphatidylinositol 3-kinase to the IFNAR1 chain of the type I interferon receptor. Science, 1997. 276(5317): p. 1418–20.
93. Yang, C.H., et al., Interferon alpha /beta promotes cell survival by activating nuclear factor kappa B through phosphatidylinositol 3-kinase and Akt. J Biol Chem, 2001. 276(17): p. 13756–61.
94. Uddin, S., et al., The Rac1/p38 mitogen-activated protein kinase pathway is required for interferon alpha-dependent transcriptional activation but not serine phosphorylation of Stat proteins. J Biol Chem, 2000. 275(36): p. 27634–40.
95. Uddin, S., et al., Protein kinase C-delta (PKC-delta) is activated by type I interferons and mediates phosphorylation of Stat1 on serine 727. J Biol Chem, 2002. 277(17): p. 14408–16.
96. Lekmine, F., et al., The CrkL adapter protein is required for type I interferon-dependent gene transcription and activation of the small G-protein Rap1. Biochem Biophys Res Commun, 2002. 291(4): p. 744–50.
97. Takaoka, A., et al., Cross talk between interferon-gamma and -alpha/beta signaling components in caveolar membrane domains. Science, 2000. 288(5475): p. 2357–60.
98. Mitani, Y., et al., Cross talk of the interferon-alpha/beta signalling complex with gp130 for effective interleukin-6 signalling. Genes Cells, 2001. 6(7): p. 631–40.
99. Durbin, J.E., et al., Targeted disruption of the mouse Stat1 gene results in compromised innate immunity to viral disease. Cell, 1996. 84(3): p. 443–50.
100. Kaplan, D.H., et al., Demonstration of an interferon gamma-dependent tumor surveillance system in immunocompetent mice. Proc Natl Acad Sci USA, 1998. 95(13): p. 7556–61.
101. Dupuis, S., et al., Impaired response to interferon-alpha/beta and lethal viral disease in human STAT1 deficiency. Nat Genet, 2003. 33(3): p. 388–91.
102. Domanski, P., et al., Differential use of the betaL subunit of the type I interferon (IFN) receptor determines signaling specificity for IFNalpha2 and IFNbeta. J Biol Chem, 1998. 273(6): p. 3144–7.
103. Platanias, L.C., et al., Differences in interferon alpha and beta signaling. Interferon beta selectively induces the interaction of the alpha and betaL subunits of the type I interferon receptor. J Biol Chem, 1996. 271(39): p. 23630–3.
104. Wong, L.H., et al., IFN-gamma priming up-regulates IFN-stimulated gene factor 3 (ISGF3) components, augmenting responsiveness of IFN-resistant melanoma cells to type I IFNs. J Immunol, 1998. 160(11): p. 5475–84.

105. Lehtonen, A., S. Matikainen, and I. Julkunen, Interferons up-regulate STAT1, STAT2, and IRF family transcription factor gene expression in human peripheral blood mononuclear cells and macrophages. J Immunol, 1997. 159(2): p. 794–803.

106. Lesinski, G.B., et al., IL-12 pretreatments enhance IFN-alpha-induced Janus kinase-STAT signaling and potentiate the antitumor effects of IFN-alpha in a murine model of malignant melanoma. J Immunol, 2004. 172(12): p. 7368–76.

107. Dupont, S.A., et al., Mechanisms for regulation of cellular responsiveness to human IFN-beta1a. J Interferon Cytokine Res, 2002. 22(4): p. 491–501.

108. Dondi, E., et al., Down-modulation of type 1 interferon responses by receptor cross-competition for a shared Jak kinase. J Biol Chem, 2001. 276(50): p. 47004–12.

109. Alexander, W.S., Suppressors of cytokine signalling (SOCS) in the immune system. Nat Rev Immunol, 2002. 2(6): p. 410–6.

110. Song, M.M. and K. Shuai, The suppressor of cytokine signaling (SOCS) 1 and SOCS3 but not SOCS2 proteins inhibit interferon-mediated antiviral and antiproliferative activities. J Biol Chem, 1998. 273(52): p. 35056–62.

111. Roman-Gomez, J., et al., The suppressor of cytokine signaling-1 is constitutively expressed in chronic myeloid leukemia and correlates with poor cytogenetic response to interferon-alpha. Haematologica, 2004. 89(1): p. 42–8.

112. Sakai, I., et al., Constitutive expression of SOCS3 confers resistance to IFN-alpha in chronic myelogenous leukemia cells. Blood, 2002. 100(8): p. 2926–31.

113. Hong, F., V.A. Nguyen, and B. Gao, Tumor necrosis factor alpha attenuates interferon alpha signaling in the liver: involvement of SOCS3 and SHP2 and implication in resistance to interferon therapy. Faseb J, 2001. 15(9): p. 1595–7.

114. Ito, S., et al., Interleukin-10 inhibits expression of both interferon alpha- and interferon gamma-induced genes by suppressing tyrosine phosphorylation of STAT1. Blood, 1999. 93(5): p. 1456–63.

115. Shuai, K., Modulation of STAT signaling by STAT-interacting proteins. Oncogene, 2000. 19(21): p. 2638–44.

116. ten Hoeve, J., et al., Identification of a nuclear Stat1 protein tyrosine phosphatase. Mol Cell Biol, 2002. 22(16): p. 5662–8.

117. Liu, B., et al., Inhibition of Stat1-mediated gene activation by PIAS1. Proc Natl Acad Sci USA, 1998. 95(18): p. 10626–31.

118. Liu, B., et al., PIAS1 selectively inhibits interferon-inducible genes and is important in innate immunity. Nat Immunol, 2004. 5(9): p. 891–8.

119. Mowen, K.A., et al., Arginine methylation of STAT1 modulates IFNalpha/beta-induced transcription. Cell, 2001. 104(5): p. 731–41.

120. Donskov, F., et al., In vivo assessment of the antiproliferative properties of interferon-alpha during immunotherapy: Ki-67 (MIB-1) in patients with metastatic renal cell carcinoma. Br J Cancer, 2004. 90(3): p. 626–31.

121. Sangfelt, O., S. Erickson, and D. Grander, Mechanisms of interferon-induced cell cycle arrest. Front Biosci, 2000. 5: p. D479–87.

122. Matsuoka, M., K. Tani, and S. Asano, Interferon-alpha-induced G1 phase arrest through up-regulated expression of CDK inhibitors, p19Ink4D and p21Cip1 in mouse macrophages. Oncogene, 1998. 16(16): p. 2075–86.

123. Sangfelt, O., et al., Molecular mechanisms underlying interferon-alpha-induced G0/G1 arrest: CKI-mediated regulation of G1 Cdk-complexes and activation of pocket proteins. Oncogene, 1999. 18(18): p. 2798–810.

124. Sangfelt, O., et al., Induction of Cip/Kip and Ink4 cyclin dependent kinase inhibitors by interferon-alpha in hematopoietic cell lines. Oncogene, 1997. 14(4): p. 415–23.

125. Mandal, M., et al., Interferon-induces expression of cyclin-dependent kinase-inhibitors p21WAF1 and p27Kip1 that prevent activation of cyclin-dependent kinase by CDK-activating kinase (CAK). Oncogene, 1998. 16(2): p. 217–25.

126. Tiefenbrun, N., et al., Alpha interferon suppresses the cyclin D3 and cdc25A genes, leading to a reversible G0-like arrest. Mol Cell Biol, 1996. 16(7): p. 3934–44.

127. Einat, M., D. Resnitzky, and A. Kimchi, Close link between reduction of c-myc expression by interferon and, G0/G1 arrest. Nature, 1985. 313(6003): p. 597–600.

128. Iwase, S., et al., Modulation of E2F activity is linked to interferon-induced growth suppression of hematopoietic cells. J Biol Chem, 1997. 272(19): p. 12406–14.

129. Landolfo, S., et al., The Ifi 200 genes: An emerging family of IFN-inducible genes. Biochimie, 1998. 80(8-9): p. 721–8.

130. Choubey, D., et al., Inhibition of E2F-mediated transcription by p202. Embo J, 1996. 15(20): p. 5668–78.

131. Datta, B., et al., p202, an interferon-inducible modulator of transcription, inhibits transcriptional activation by the p53 tumor suppressor protein, and a segment from the p53-binding protein 1 that binds to p202 overcomes this inhibition. J Biol Chem, 1996. 271(44): p. 27544–55.

132. Ma, X.Y., et al., The Interferon-inducible p202a protein modulates NF-kB activity by inhibiting the binding to DNA of p50/p65 heterodimers and p65 homodimers, while enhancng the binding of p50 homodimers. J Biol Chem, 2003. 3: p. 3.

133. Min, W., S. Ghosh, and P. Lengyel, The interferon-inducible p202 protein as a modulator of transcription: Inhibition of NF-kappa B, c-Fos, and c-Jun activities. Mol Cell Biol, 1996. 16(1): p. 359–68.

134. Wang, H., et al., The interferon- and differentiation-inducible p202a protein inhibits the transcriptional activity of c-Myc by blocking its association with Max. J Biol Chem, 2000. 275(35): p. 27377–85.

135. Wen, Y., et al., p202, an interferon-inducible protein, mediates multiple antitumor activities in human pancreatic cancer xenograft models. Cancer Res, 2001. 61(19): p. 7142–7.

136. Wen, Y., et al., Tumor suppression and sensitization to tumor necrosis factor alpha-induced apoptosis by an interferon-inducible protein, p202, in breast cancer cells. Cancer Res, 2000. 60(1): p. 42–6.

137. Yan, D.H., et al., Reduced growth rate and transformation phenotype of the prostate cancer cells by an interferon-inducible protein, p202. Oncogene, 1999. 18(3): p. 807–11.

138. Liu, C.J., H. Wang, and P. Lengyel, The interferon-inducible nucleolar p204 protein binds the ribosomal RNA-specific UBF1 transcription factor and inhibits ribosomal RNA transcription. Embo J, 1999. 18(10): p. 2845–54.

139. Johnstone, R.W., et al., Functional interaction between p53 and the interferon-inducible nucleoprotein IFI 16. Oncogene, 2000. 19(52): p. 6033–42.

140. Greider, C.W., Telomeres, telomerase and senescence. Bioessays, 1990. 12(8): p. 363–9.

141. Meyerson, M., et al., hEST2, the putative human telomerase catalytic subunit gene, is up-regulated in tumor cells and during immortalization. Cell, 1997. 90(4): p. 785–95.

142. Xu, D., et al., Interferon alpha down-regulates telomerase reverse transcriptase and telomerase activity in human malignant and nonmalignant hematopoietic cells. Blood, 2000. 96(13): p. 4313–8.

143. Der, S.D., et al., Identification of genes differentially regulated by interferon alpha, beta, or gamma using oligonucleotide arrays. Proc Natl Acad Sci USA, 1998. 95(26): p. 15623–8.

144. Manna, S.K., A. Mukhopadhyay, and B.B. Aggarwal, IFN-alpha suppresses activation of nuclear transcription factors NF-kappa B and activator protein 1 and potentiates TNF-induced apoptosis. J Immunol, 2000. 165(9): p. 4927–34.

145. Roberts, W.K., et al., Interferon-mediated protein kinase and low-molecular-weight inhibitor of protein synthesis. Nature, 1976. 264(5585): p. 477–80.

146. Meurs, E., et al., Molecular cloning and characterization of the human double-stranded RNA-activated protein kinase induced by interferon. Cell, 1990. 62(2): p. 379–90.

147. Maran, A. and M.B. Mathews, Characterization of the double-stranded RNA implicated in the inhibition of protein synthesis in cells infected with a mutant adenovirus defective for VA RNA. Virology, 1988. 164(1): p. 106–13.

148. Srivastava, S.P., M.V. Davies, and R.J. Kaufman, Calcium depletion from the endoplasmic reticulum activates the double-stranded RNA-dependent protein kinase (PKR) to inhibit protein synthesis. J Biol Chem, 1995. 270(28): p. 16619–24.

149. Ruvolo, P.P., et al., Ceramide regulates protein synthesis by a novel mechanism involving the cellular PKR activator RAX. J Biol Chem, 2001. 276(15): p. 11754–8.

150. Vorburger, S.A., et al., Role for the double-stranded RNA activated protein kinase PKR in E2F-1-induced apoptosis. Oncogene, 2002. 21(41): p. 6278–88.

151. Ito, T., M. Yang, and W.S. May, RAX, a cellular activator for double-stranded RNA-dependent protein kinase during stress signaling. J Biol Chem, 1999. 274(22): p. 15427–32.

152. Patel, C.V., et al., PACT, a stress-modulated cellular activator of interferon-induced double-stranded RNA-activated protein kinase, PKR. J Biol Chem, 2000. 275(48): p. 37993–8.

153. Sledz, C.A., et al., Activation of the interferon system by short-interfering RNAs. Nat Cell Biol, 2003. 5(9): p. 834–9.

154. Lu, G., et al., Interferon-alpha enhances biological defense activities against oxidative stress in cultured rat hepatocytes and hepatic stellate cells. J Med Invest, 2002. 49(3-4): p. 172–81.

155. Stephanou, A., et al., Signal transducer and activator of transcription-1 and heat shock factor-1 inter-
     act and activate the transcription of the Hsp-70 and Hsp-90beta gene promoters. J Biol Chem, 1999.
     274(3): p. 1723–8.
156. Anderson, S.L., et al., The endoplasmic reticular heat shock protein gp96 is transcriptionally upreg-
     ulated in interferon-treated cells. J Exp Med, 1994. 180(4): p. 1565–9.
157. Zhao, M., et al., Double-stranded RNA-dependent protein kinase (pkr) is essential for thermotoler-
     ance, accumulation of HSP70, and stabilization of ARE-containing HSP70 mRNA during stress. J
     Biol Chem, 2002. 277(46): p. 44539–47.
158. Srivastava, P., Interaction of heat shock proteins with peptides and antigen presenting cells:
     Chaperoning of the innate and adaptive immune responses. Annu Rev Immunol, 2002. 20: p. 395–425.
159. Tamura, Y., et al., Immunotherapy of tumors with autologous tumor-derived heat shock protein prepa-
     rations. Science, 1997. 278(5335): p. 117–20.
160. Kirou, K.A., et al., Induction of Fas ligand-mediated apoptosis by interferon-alpha. Clin Immunol,
     2000. 95(3): p. 218–26.
161. Chawla-Sarkar, M., et al., IFN-beta pretreatment sensitizes human melanoma cells to TRAIL/Apo2
     ligand-induced apoptosis. J Immunol, 2002. 169(2): p. 847–55.
162. Kayagaki, N., et al., Type I interferons (IFNs) regulate tumor necrosis factor-related apoptosis-induc-
     ing ligand (TRAIL) expression on human T cells: A novel mechanism for the antitumor effects of
     type I IFNs. J Exp Med, 1999. 189(9): p. 1451–60.
163. Thyrell, L., et al., Mechanisms of Interferon-alpha induced apoptosis in malignant cells. Oncogene,
     2002. 21(8): p. 1251–62.
164. Leaman, D.W., et al., Identification of X-linked inhibitor of apoptosis-associated factor-1 as an inter-
     feron-stimulated gene that augments TRAIL Apo2L-induced apoptosis. J Biol Chem, 2002. 277(32):
     p. 28504–11.
165. Levin, D. and I.M. London, Regulation of protein synthesis: Activation by double-stranded RNA of
     a protein kinase that phosphorylates eukaryotic initiation factor 2. Proc Natl Acad Sci USA, 1978.
     75(3): p. 1121–5.
166. Gil, J., M.A. Garcia, and M. Esteban, Caspase 9 activation by the dsRNA-dependent protein kinase,
     PKR: Molecular mechanism and relevance. FEBS Lett, 2002. 529(2-3): p. 249–55.
167. Gil, J. and M. Esteban, The interferon-induced protein kinase (PKR), triggers apoptosis through
     FADD-mediated activation of caspase 8 in a manner independent of Fas and TNF-alpha receptors.
     Oncogene, 2000. 19(32): p. 3665–74.
168. Gil, J. and M. Esteban, Induction of apoptosis by the dsRNA-dependent protein kinase (PKR):
     Mechanism of action. Apoptosis, 2000. 5(2): p. 107–14.
169. Floyd-Smith, G., E. Slattery, and P. Lengyel, Interferon action: RNA cleavage pattern of a (2'-
     5')oligoadenylate—dependent endonuclease. Science, 1981. 212(4498): p. 1030–2.
170. Koga, S., et al., Treatment of bladder cancer cells in vitro and in vivo with 2-5A antisense telomerase
     RNA. Gene Ther, 2001. 8(8): p. 654–8.
171. Maran, A., et al., 2',5'-Oligoadenylate-antisense chimeras cause RNase L to selectively degrade
     bcr/abl mRNA in chronic myelogenous leukemia cells. Blood, 1998. 92(11): p. 4336–43.
172. Kushner, D.M., et al., 2-5A antisense directed against telomerase RNA produces apoptosis in ovarian
     cancer cells. Gynecol Oncol, 2000. 76(2): p. 183–92.
173. Rusch, L., A. Zhou, and R.H. Silverman, Caspase-dependent apoptosis by 2',5'-oligoadenylate acti-
     vation of RNase L is enhanced by IFN-beta. J Interferon Cytokine Res, 2000. 20(12): p. 1091–100.
174. Carpten, J., et al., Germline mutations in the ribonuclease L gene in families showing linkage with
     HPC1. Nat Genet, 2002. 30(2): p. 181–4.
175. Hanakahi, L.A., et al., Binding of inositol phosphate to DNA-PK and stimulation of double-strand
     break repair. Cell, 2000. 102(6): p. 721–9.
176. Morrison, B.H., et al., Inositol hexakisphosphate kinase 2 mediates growth suppressive and apoptotic
     effects of interferon-beta in ovarian carcinoma cells. J Biol Chem, 2001. 276(27): p. 24965–70.
177. Zhou, Q., et al., Transcriptional control of the human plasma membrane phospholipid scramblase 1
     gene is mediated by interferon-alpha. Blood, 2000. 95(8): p. 2593–9.
178. Silverman, R.H., et al., Suppression of ovarian carcinoma cell growth in vivo by the interferon-
     inducible plasma membrane protein, phospholipid scramblase 1. Cancer Res, 2002. 62(2):
     p. 397–402.
179. Karin, M. and A. Lin, NF-kappaB at the crossroads of life and death. Nat Immunol, 2002. 3(3):
     p. 221–7.

180. Bours, V., et al., The NF-kappa B transcription factor and cancer: High expression of NF-kappa B- and I kappa B-related proteins in tumor cell lines. Biochem Pharmacol, 1994. 47(1): p. 145–9.

181. Marrack, P., J. Kappler, and T. Mitchell, Type I interferons keep activated T cells alive. J Exp Med, 1999. 189(3): p. 521–30.

182. Su, L. and M. David, Inhibition of B cell receptor-mediated apoptosis by IFN. J Immunol, 1999. 162(11): p. 6317–21.

183. Shigeno, M., et al., Interferon-alpha sensitizes human hepatoma cells to TRAIL-induced apoptosis through DR5 upregulation and NF-kappa B inactivation. Oncogene, 2003. 22(11): p. 1653–62.

184. Suk, K., et al., IFNalpha sensitizes ME-180 human cervical cancer cells to TNFalpha-induced apoptosis by inhibiting cytoprotective NF-kappaB activation. FEBS Lett, 2001. 495(1-2): p. 66–70.

185. Bharti, A.C. and B.B. Aggarwal, Nuclear factor-kappa B and cancer: its role in prevention and therapy. Biochem Pharmacol, 2002. 64(5-6): p. 883–8.

186. Radvanyi, L.G., et al., Low levels of interferon-alpha induce CD86 (B7.2) expression and accelerates dendritic cell maturation from human peripheral blood mononuclear cells. Scand J Immunol, 1999. 50(5): p. 499–.

187. Oreffo, R.O., et al., Effects of interferon alpha on human osteoprogenitor cell growth and differentiation in vitro. J Cell Biochem, 1999. 74(3): p. 372–85.

188. Niikura, T., R. Hirata, and S.C. Weil, A novel interferon-inducible gene expressed during myeloid differentiation. Blood Cells Mol Dis, 1997. 23(3): p. 337–49.

189. Taipale, J. and P.A. Beachy, The Hedgehog and Wnt signalling pathways in cancer. Nature, 2001. 411(6835): p. 349–54.

190. Mansouri, A., M. Hallonet, and P. Gruss, Pax genes and their roles in cell differentiation and development. Curr Opin Cell Biol, 1996. 8(6): p. 851–7.

191. Hidalgo, A., Growth and patterning from the engrailed interface. Int J Dev Biol, 1998. 42(3 Spec No): p. 317–24.

192. Magli, M.C., C. Largman, and H.J. Lawrence, Effects of HOX homeobox genes in blood cell differentiation. J Cell Physiol, 1997. 173(2): p. 168–77.

193. Hasskarl, J. and K. Munger, Id proteins—tumor markers or oncogenes? Cancer Biol Ther, 2002. 1(2): p. 91–6.

194. Subramaniam, P.S., et al., Type I interferon induction of the Cdk-inhibitor p21WAF1 is accompanied by ordered G1 arrest, differentiation and apoptosis of the Daudi B-cell line. Oncogene, 1998. 16(14): p. 1885–90.

195. Iavarone, A., et al., The helix-loop-helix protein Id-2 enhances cell proliferation and binds to the retinoblastoma protein. Genes Dev, 1994. 8(11): p. 1270–84.

196. Thulasi, R., et al., Alpha 2a-interferon-induced differentiation of human alveolar rhabdomyosarcoma cells: Correlation with down-regulation of the insulin-like growth factor type I receptor. Cell Growth Differ, 1996. 7(4): p. 531–41.

197. Lokshin, A., J.E. Mayotte, and M.L. Levitt, Mechanism of interferon beta-induced squamous differentiation and programmed cell death in human non-small-cell lung cancer cell lines. J Natl Cancer Inst, 1995. 87(3): p. 206–12.

198. Vedantham, S., H. Gamliel, and H.M. Golomb, Mechanism of interferon action in hairy cell leukemia: A model of effective cancer biotherapy. Cancer Res, 1992. 52(5): p. 1056–66.

199. Cinatl, J., Jr., et al., Induction of differentiation and suppression of malignant phenotype of human neuroblastoma BE(2)-C cells by valproic acid: Enhancement by combination with interferon-alpha. Int J Oncol, 2002. 20(1): p. 97–106.

200. Yokoyama, M., et al., Retinoic acid and interferon-alpha effects on cell growth and differentiation in cervical carcinoma cell lines. Obstet Gynecol, 2001. 98(2): p. 332–40.

201. Lam, P.K., et al., In vitro inhibition of head and neck cancer-cell growth by human recombinant interferon-alpha and 13-cis retinoic acid. Br J Biomed Sci, 2001. 58(4): p. 226–9.

202. Fisher, P.B. and S. Grant, Effects of interferon on differentiation of normal and tumor cells. Pharmacol Ther, 1985. 27(2): p. 143–66.

203. Gumbiner, B.M., Cell adhesion: The molecular basis of tissue architecture and morphogenesis. Cell, 1996. 84(3): p. 345–57.

204. Doki, Y., et al., Correlation between E-cadherin expression and invasiveness in vitro in a human esophageal cancer cell line. Cancer Res, 1993. 53(14): p. 3421–6.

205. Oka, H., et al., Expression of E-cadherin cell adhesion molecules in human breast cancer tissues and its relationship to metastasis. Cancer Res, 1993. 53(7): p. 1696–701.

206. Roman-Gomez, J., et al., Cadherin-13, a mediator of calcium-dependent cell-cell adhesion, is silenced by methylation in chronic myeloid leukemia and correlates with pretreatment risk profile and cytogenetic response to interferon alfa. J Clin Oncol, 2003. 21(8): p. 1472–9.

207. Slaton, J.W., et al., Treatment with low-dose interferon-alpha restores the balance between matrix metalloproteinase-9 and E-cadherin expression in human transitional cell carcinoma of the bladder. Clin Cancer Res, 2001. 7(9): p. 2840–53.

208. Masuda, T., et al., Up-regulation of E-cadherin and I-catenin in human hepatocellular carcinoma cell lines by sodium butyrate and interferon-alpha. In Vitro Cell Dev Biol Anim, 2000. 36(6): p. 387–94.

209. Matarrese, P., et al., Antiproliferative activity of interferon alpha and retinoic acid in SiHa carcinoma cells: The role of cell adhesion. Int J Cancer, 1998. 76(4): p. 531–40.

210. Lechner, J., et al., Effects of interferon alpha-2b on barrier function and junctional complexes of renal proximal tubular LLC-PK1 cells. Kidney Int, 1999. 55(6): p. 2178–91.

211. Martin-Henao, G.A., et al., L-selectin expression is low on CD34+ cells from patients with chronic myeloid leukemia and interferon-a up-regulates this expression. Haematologica, 2000. 85(2): p. 139–46.

212. Tenaud, I., et al., Modulation in vitro of keratinocyte integrins by interferon-alpha and interferon-gamma. Int J Dermatol, 2002. 41(12): p. 836–40.

213. Bhatia, R., et al., Interferon-alpha restores normal adhesion of chronic myelogenous leukemia hematopoietic progenitors to bone marrow stroma by correcting impaired beta 1 integrin receptor function. J Clin Invest, 1994. 94(1): p. 384–91.

214. Maemura, M., et al., Effects of interferon-alpha on cellular proliferation and adhesion of breast carcinoma cells. Oncol Rep, 1999. 6(3): p. 557–61.

215. Dao, T., et al., Natural human interferon-alpha inhibits the adhesion of a human carcinoma cell line to human vascular endothelium. J Interferon Cytokine Res, 1995. 15(10): p. 869–76.

216. Jiang, H. and P.B. Fisher, Use of a sensitive and efficient subtraction hybridization protocol for the identification of genes differentially regulated during the induction of differentiation in human melanoma cells. Mol Cell Differ, 1993. 1: p. 285–299.

217. Su, Z.Z., et al., Melanoma differentiation associated gene-7, mda-7/IL-24, selectively induces growth suppression, apoptosis and radiosensitization in malignant gliomas in a p53-independent manner. Oncogene, 2003. 22(8): p. 1164–80.

218. Kang, D.C., et al., mda-5: An interferon-inducible putative RNA helicase with double-stranded RNA-dependent ATPase activity and melanoma growth-suppressive properties. Proc Natl Acad Sci USA, 2002. 99(2): p. 637–42.

219. Lin, J.J., H. Jiang, and P.B. Fisher, Melanoma differentiation associated gene-9, mda-9, is a human gamma interferon responsive gene. Gene, 1998. 207(2): p. 105–10.

220. Carmeliet, P. and R.K. Jain, Angiogenesis in cancer and other diseases. Nature, 2000. 407(6801): p. 249–57.

221. von Marschall, Z., et al., Effects of interferon alpha on vascular endothelial growth factor gene transcription and tumor angiogenesis. J Natl Cancer Inst, 2003. 95(6): p. 437–48.

222. Singh, R.K., et al., Interferons alpha and beta down-regulate the expression of basic fibroblast growth factor in human carcinomas. Proc Natl Acad Sci USA, 1995. 92(10): p. 4562–6.

223. Dinney, C.P., et al., Inhibition of basic fibroblast growth factor expression, angiogenesis, and growth of human bladder carcinoma in mice by systemic interferon-alpha administration. Cancer Res, 1998. 58(4): p. 808–14.

224. Oliveira, I.C., et al., Downregulation of interleukin 8 gene expression in human fibroblasts: Unique mechanism of transcriptional inhibition by interferon. Proc Natl Acad Sci USA, 1992. 89(19): p. 9049–53.

225. Singh, R.K., et al., Interferon-beta prevents the upregulation of interleukin-8 expression in human melanoma cells. J Interferon Cytokine Res, 1996. 16(8): p. 577–84.

226. Kaser, S., et al., Interferon-alpha suppresses leptin levels: Studies in interferon-alpha treated patients with hepatitis C virus infection and murine adipocytes. Eur Cytokine Netw, 2002. 13(2): p. 225–9.

227. Dreau, D., et al., Angiogenic and immune parameters during recombinant interferon-alpha2b adjuvant treatment in patients with melanoma. Oncol Res, 2000. 12(5): p. 241–51.

228. Li, S., et al., Regression of tumors by IFN-alpha electroporation gene therapy and analysis of the responsible genes by cDNA array. Gene Ther, 2002. 9(6): p. 390–7.

229. Strasly, M., et al., IL-12 inhibition of endothelial cell functions and angiogenesis depends on lymphocyte-endothelial cell cross-talk. J Immunol, 2001. 166(6): p. 3890–9.

230. Naldini, A., et al., Regulation of angiogenesis by Th1- and Th2-type cytokines. Curr Pharm Des, 2003. 9(7): p. 511–9.
231. Bostrom, P.J., et al., Interferon-alpha inhibits cyclooxygenase-1 and stimulates cyclooxygenase-2 expression in bladder cancer cells in vitro. Urol Res, 2001. 29(1): p. 20–4.
232. Izawa, J.I., et al., Inhibition of tumorigenicity and metastasis of human bladder cancer growing in athymic mice by interferon-beta gene therapy results partially from various antiangiogenic effects including endothelial cell apoptosis. Clin Cancer Res, 2002. 8(4): p. 1258–70.
233. Wang, B., et al., Genetic disruption of host nitric oxide synthase II gene impairs melanoma-induced angiogenesis and suppresses pleural effusion. Int J Cancer, 2001. 91(5): p. 607–11.
234. Wang, B., et al., Intact nitric oxide synthase II gene is required for interferon-beta-mediated suppression of growth and metastasis of pancreatic adenocarcinoma. Cancer Res, 2001. 61(1): p. 71–5.
235. Brouty-Boye, D. and B.R. Zetter, Inhibition of cell motility by interferon. Science, 1980. 208(4443): p. 516–8.
236. Lindner, D.J., Interferons as antiangiogenic agents. Curr Oncol Rep, 2002. 4(6): p. 510–4.
237. Bauer, J.A., et al., IFN-alpha2b and Thalidomide Synergistically Inhibit Tumor-Induced Angiogenesis. J Interferon Cytokine Res, 2003. 23(1): p. 3–10.
238. Lindner, D.J. and E.C. Borden, Effects of tamoxifen and interferon-beta or the combination on tumor-induced angiogenesis. Int J Cancer, 1997. 71(3): p. 456–61.
239. Belardelli, F. and M. Ferrantini, Cytokines as a link between innate and adaptive antitumor immunity. Trends Immunol, 2002. 23(4): p. 201–8.
240. Banchereau, J. and R.M. Steinman, Dendritic cells and the control of immunity. Nature, 1998. 392(6673): p. 245–52.
241. Ahn, J.H., et al., Identification of the genes differentially expressed in human dendritic cell subsets by cDNA subtraction and microarray analysis. Blood, 2002. 100(5): p. 1742–54.
242. Miettinen, M., et al., IFNs activate toll-like receptor gene expression in viral infections. Genes Immun, 2001. 2(6): p. 349–55.
243. Ito, T., et al., Interferon-alpha and interleukin-12 are induced differentially by Toll-like receptor 7 ligands in human blood dendritic cell subsets. J Exp Med, 2002. 195(11): p. 1507–12.
244. Toshchakov, V., et al., TLR4, but not TLR2, mediates IFN-beta-induced STAT1alpha/beta-dependent gene expression in macrophages. Nat Immunol, 2002. 3(4): p. 392–8.
245. Ito, T., et al., Differential regulation of human blood dendritic cell subsets by IFNs. J Immunol, 2001. 166(5): p. 2961–9.
246. Luft, T., et al., Type I IFNs enhance the terminal differentiation of dendritic cells. J Immunol, 1998. 161(4): p. 1947–53.
247. McRae, B.L., et al., Interferon-alpha and -beta inhibit the in vitro differentiation of immunocompetent human dendritic cells from CD14(+) precursors. Blood, 2000. 96(1): p. 210–7.
248. Montoya, M., et al., Type I interferons produced by dendritic cells promote their phenotypic and functional activation. Blood, 2002. 99(9): p. 3263–71.
249. Eantuzzi, L., et al., Post-translational up-regulation of the cell surface-associated alpha component of the human type I interferon receptor during differentiation of peripheral blood monocytes: Role in the biological response to type I interferon. Eur J Immunol, 1997. 27(5): p. 1075–81.
250. Luft, T., et al., IFN-alpha enhances CD40 ligand-mediated activation of immature monocyte-derived dendritic cells. Int Immunol, 2002. 14(4): p. 367–80.
251. Parlato, S., et al., Expression of CCR-7, MIP-3beta, and Th-1 chemokines in type I IFN-induced monocyte-derived dendritic cells: Importance for the rapid acquisition of potent migratory and functional activities. Blood, 2001. 98(10): p. 3022–9.
252. Lande, R., et al., IFN-alpha beta released by Mycobacterium tuberculosis-infected human dendritic cells induces the expression of CXCL10: Selective recruitment of NK and activated T cells. J Immunol, 2003. 170(3): p. 1174–82.
253. Zella, D., et al., Recombinant IFN-alpha (2b) increases the expression of apoptosis receptor CD95 and chemokine receptors CCR1 and CCR3 in monocytoid cells. J Immunol, 1999. 163(6): p. 3169–75.
254. Abuzahra, F., et al., Adjuvant interferon alfa treatment for patients with malignant melanoma stimulates transporter proteins associated with antigen processing and proteasome activator 28. Lancet Oncol, 2004. 5(4): p. 250.
255. Litinskiy, M.B., et al., DCs induce CD40-independent immunoglobulin class switching through BLyS and APRIL. Nat Immunol, 2002. 3(9): p. 822–9.

256. Mattei, F., et al., IL-15 is expressed by dendritic cells in response to type I IFN, double-stranded RNA, or lipopolysaccharide and promotes dendritic cell activation. J Immunol, 2001. 167(3): p. 1179–87.

257. Tourkova, I.L., et al., Increased function and survival of IL-15-transduced human dendritic cells are mediated by up-regulation of IL-15Ralpha and Bcl-2. J Leukoc Biol, 2002. 72(5): p. 1037–45.

258. Krug, A., et al., Interferon-producing cells fail to induce proliferation of naive T cells but can promote expansion and T helper 1 differentiation of antigen-experienced unpolarized T cells. J Exp Med, 2003. 197(7): p. 899–906.

259. McRae, B.L., et al., Type I IFNs inhibit human dendritic cell IL-12 production and Th1 cell development. J Immunol, 1998. 160(9): p. 4298–304.

260. Dalod, M., et al., Interferon alpha/beta and interleukin 12 responses to viral infections: Pathways regulating dendritic cell cytokine expression in vivo. J Exp Med, 2002. 195(4): p. 517–28.

261. Ortaldo, J.R., et al., Effects of recombinant and hybrid recombinant human leukocyte interferons on cytotoxic activity of natural killer cells. J Biol Chem, 1983. 258(24): p. 15011–5.

262. Biron, C.A., G. Sonnenfeld, and R.M. Welsh, Interferon induces natural killer cell blastogenesis in vivo. J Leukoc Biol, 1984. 35(1): p. 31–7.

263. Carballido, J.A., et al., Interferon-alpha-2b enhances the natural killer activity of patients with transitional cell carcinoma of the bladder. Cancer, 1993. 72(5): p. 1743–8.

264. Tough, D.F., P. Borrow, and J. Sprent, Induction of bystander T cell proliferation by viruses and type I interferon in vivo. Science, 1996. 272(5270): p. 1947–50.

265. Palmer, K.J., et al., Interferon-alpha (IFN-alpha) stimulates anti-melanoma cytotoxic T lymphocyte (CTL) generation in mixed lymphocyte tumour cultures (MLTC). Clin Exp Immunol, 2000. 119(3): p. 412–8.

266. Steitz, J., et al., Depletion of CD25(+) CD4(+) T cells and treatment with tyrosinase-related protein 2-transduced dendritic cells enhance the interferon alpha-induced, CD8(+) T-cell-dependent immune defense of B16 melanoma. Cancer Res, 2001. 61(24): p. 8643–6.

267. Matikainen, S., et al., Interferon-alpha activates multiple STAT proteins and upregulates proliferation-associated IL-2Ralpha, c-myc, and pim-1 genes in human T cells. Blood, 1999. 93(6): p. 1980–91.

268. Giacomini, P., et al., Class I major histocompatibility complex enhancement by recombinant leukocyte interferon in the peripheral blood mononuclear cells and plasma of melanoma patients. Cancer Res, 1991. 51(2): p. 652–6.

269. Foster, G.R., et al., Human T cells elicit IFN-alpha secretion from dendritic cells following cell to cell interactions. Eur J Immunol, 2000. 30(11): p. 3228–35.

270. Hakansson, A., et al., Effect of IFN-alpha on tumor-infiltrating mononuclear cells and regressive changes in metastatic malignant melanoma. J Interferon Cytokine Res, 1998. 18(1): p. 33–9.

271. Brinkmann, V., et al., Interferon alpha increases the frequency of interferon gamma-producing human CD4+ T cells. J Exp Med, 1993. 178(5): p. 1655–63.

272. Schandene, L., et al., Recombinant interferon-alpha selectively inhibits the production of interleukin-5 by human CD4+ T cells. J Clin Invest, 1996. 97(2): p. 309–15.

273. Rogge, L., et al., Selective expression of an interleukin-12 receptor component by human T helper 1 cells. J Exp Med, 1997. 185(5): p. 825–31.

274. Rogge, L., et al., The role of Stat4 in species-specific regulation of Th cell development by type I IFNs. J Immunol, 1998. 161(12): p. 6567–74.

275. McRae, B.L., L.J. Picker, and G.A. van Seventer, Human recombinant interferon-beta influences T helper subset differentiation by regulating cytokine secretion pattern and expression of homing receptors. Eur J Immunol, 1997. 27(10): p. 2650–6.

276. Yang, Y.F., et al., IFN-alpha acts on T-cell receptor-triggered human peripheral leukocytes to up-regulate CCR5 expression on CD4+ and CD8+ T cells. J Clin Immunol, 2001. 21(6): p. 402–9.

277. Petricoin, E.F., 3rd, et al., Antiproliferative action of interferon-alpha requires components of T-cell-receptor signalling. Nature, 1997. 390(6660): p. 629-32.

278. Dondi, E., et al., Down-modulation of responses to type I IFN upon T cell activation. J Immunol, 2003. 170(2): p. 749–56.

279. Lee, C.K., et al., Distinct requirements for IFNs and STAT1 in NK cell function. J Immunol, 2000. 165(7): p. 3571–7.

280. Lin, Q., C. Dong, and M.D. Cooper, Impairment of T and B cell development by treatment with a type I interferon. J Exp Med, 1998. 187(1): p. 79–87.

281. Beadling, C., et al., Activation of JAK kinases and STAT proteins by interleukin-2 and interferon alpha, but not the T cell antigen receptor, in human T lymphocytes. EMBO J, 1994. 13(23): p. 5605–15.

282. Okada, H., et al., Delivery of interferon-alpha transfected dendritic cells into central nervous system tumors enhances the antitumor efficacy of peripheral peptide-based vaccines. Cancer Res, 2004. 64(16): p. 5830–8.

283. Astsaturov, I., et al., Amplification of virus-induced antimelanoma T-cell reactivity by high-dose interferon-alpha2b: Implications for cancer vaccines. Clin Cancer Res, 2003. 9(12): p. 4347–55.

284. Lesinski, G.B., et al., The antitumor effects of IFN-alpha are abrogated in a STAT1-deficient mouse. J Clin Invest, 2003. 112(2): p. 170–80.

285. Alexander, J.P., et al., T-cells infiltrating renal cell carcinoma display a poor proliferative response even though they can produce interleukin 2 and express interleukin 2 receptors. Cancer Res, 1993. 53(6): p. 1380–7.

286. Miescher, S., et al., Proliferative and cytolytic potentials of purified human tumor-infiltrating T lymphocytes. Impaired response to mitogen-driven stimulation despite T-cell receptor expression. Int J Cancer, 1988. 42(5): p. 659–66.

287. Healy, C.G., et al., Impaired expression and function of signal-transducing zeta chains in peripheral T cells and natural killer cells in patients with prostate cancer. Cytometry, 1998. 32(2): p. 109–19.

288. Sato, M., et al., Impaired production of Th1 cytokines and increased frequency of Th2 subsets in PBMC from advanced cancer patients. Anticancer Res, 1998. 18(5D): p. 3951–5.

289. Matsuda, M., et al., Alterations in the signal-transducing molecules of T cells and NK cells in colorectal tumor-infiltrating, gut mucosal and peripheral lymphocytes: Correlation with the stage of the disease. Int J Cancer, 1995. 61(6): p. 765-72.

290. Rabinowich, H., et al., Expression and activity of signaling molecules in T lymphocytes obtained from patients with metastatic melanoma before and after interleukin 2 therapy. Clin Cancer Res, 1996. 2(8): p. 1263–74.

291. Zea, A.H., et al., Alterations in T cell receptor and signal transduction molecules in melanoma patients. Clin Cancer Res, 1995. 1(11): p. 1327–35.

292. Lesinski, G.B., et al., Multiparametric flow cytometric analysis of inter-patient variation in STAT1 phosphorylation following interferon Alfa immunotherapy. J Natl Cancer Inst, 2004. 96(17): p. 1331–42.

293. Tagliaferri, P., et al., New pharmacokinetic and pharmacodynamic tools for interferon-alpha (IFN-alpha) treatment of human cancer. Cancer Immunol Immunother, 2004. 54(1): p. 1–10.

20 Combination Cytokine Therapy

Seth M. Cohen and Howard L. Kaufman

1. INTRODUCTION

Cytokines represent a diverse group of small, soluble polypeptides that are involved in regulating a wide range of physiologic processes, including inflammation, tissue repair, and immunity. The expanding role of cytokines in these processes and the identification of over 100 putative cytokine family members have made it difficult to easily classify cytokines based on structure or function. In addition, many cytokines exhibit a variety of biologic activities and these effects may be dependent on the concentration, timing, and duration of target cell exposure to a given cytokine, as well as the influence of other cytokine and growth factors in the local microenvironment. In fact, much of the early characterization of cytokines was based on simple in vitro experiments, which have failed to accurately predict the activity of cytokines in vivo. More recent investigation using targeted knockout mice and analysis of cytokine signaling pathways is leading to new insights into the biology of many cytokines. This is perhaps best exemplified by interleukin-2 (IL-2), originally described as a T-cell growth factor and defined by its ability to induce T-cell proliferation in vitro. Such *ex vivo* studies predicted that IL-2 would function to promote cellular immunity through expansion of naïve T-cell populations in vivo. The availability of IL-2 and IL-2 receptor knockout mice, however, demonstrated that in the absence of IL-2 signaling T-cell proliferation was increased, significant lymphadenopathy occurred, and animals succumb to aggressive autoimmune disease. This unexpected result suggests that IL-2 may actually function in vivo, not as a T-cell stimulant, but rather as a regulatory cytokine maintaining peripheral tolerance through balancing effector and regulatory T-cell pools *(1)*.

From: *Cancer Drug Discovery and Development,*
Cytokines in the Genesis and Treatment of Cancer
Edited by: M. A. Caligiuri and M. T. Lotze © Humana Press Inc., Totowa, NJ

The cytokines were initially described as soluble factors released by immune cells with a biologic effect on the cells releasing the cytokine, also referred to as an autocrine effect. Today it is clear that whereas cytokines may have a local role at the site of their synthesis and release, the effects can mediate interactions between cells and tissues at distant sites, also referred to as a paracrine effect. The complexity of the cytokine network is inherent in the fact that different cells can produce the same cytokine, many cytokines have similar or overlapping activities, cytokine receptor expression is often tightly regulated and can bind more than one cytokine, and the effects of any individual cytokine must be considered within the context of other cytokines, growth factors, and the status of cellular differentiation at the time of exposure. Thus, cytokines differ from hormones in several key respects, most notably that cytokines rarely have a single cell of origin and exert biologic effects on a wider array of target cells. Despite this current view of cytokine biology, many cytokines were named for the cells from which they were first identified or for other functional activities that were known before the factors were recognized as a cytokine. For example, cytokines released by leukocytes were initially referred to as interleukins, those from monocytes as monokines, and so on. The ability to interfere with viral replication led to the term "interferons" for these cytokines and TNF was named for its ability to induce necrosis in transplantable murine tumors. A relatively new class of cytokines was termed "chemokines" for their ability to induce chemotaxis of immune cells, although these molecules are now known to mediate a host of other biologic effects.

Although cytokines are diverse in structure and function, the cytokine receptors appear to be more conserved and share a higher degree of sequence homology allowing them to be grouped into distinct families. The type-1 cytokine receptors generally form multimeric complexes with a single chain binding to soluble cytokine and another chain inducing cellular signaling. The extracellular component of the type-1 cytokine receptor is notable for a highly conserved 200-amino-acid sequence with four positionally conserved cysteine residues providing structural integrity to the receptor. The intracellular component of the type-1 receptor is unusual in that it lacks intrinsic tyrosine kinase activity. The type-2 cytokine receptors also form multimeric complexes with conserved extracellular domains. In contrast to the type-1 receptors, type-2 receptors contain intracellular domains with binding sites for Janus kinases and STAT proteins. Table 1 lists some of the cytokines that are specific for each receptor. By convention the α subunit of the cytokine receptor is the chain that binds cytokine and other designations are used for those chains that are involved in cellular signaling. Many of the cytokine receptors exist in soluble form through proteolytic cleavage of the membrane bound receptor complex. The tumor necrosis factor α (TNF-α) and chemokine receptors differ from the typical cytokine receptors.

The clinical utility of cytokines as single-agent therapy in human disease has been well documented and represents one of the most successful applications of immunotherapy. Interferon-α (IFN-α) is approved for the treatment of some forms of hepatitis, chronic myelogenous and hairy cell leukemia, Kaposi's sarcoma, and as adjuvant therapy for stage III malignant melanoma. IFN-β has shown effectiveness in multiple sclerosis. High-dose IL-2 has become the standard treatment for metastatic renal cell carcinoma and melanoma. A major obstacle to wide acceptance of single agent cytokine therapy has been the disappointing low response rates in many advanced malignancies and the often significant toxicity associated with effective treatment regimens. Our improved understanding of the signaling pathways for specific cytokines coupled with better

Table 1
Cytokine Receptor Usage[a]

Type-1 cytokine receptor	Type-2 cytokine receptor	TNF-receptor family	Chemokine receptors
IL-2 (β subunit)	INF-α	TNF	CCR1-10
IL-3	INF-β	CD40	CXCR1-5, DARC
IL-4	INF-γ	Fas	XCR
IL-5	IL-10	CD30	CX3CR1
IL-6		CD27	
IL-7		NGFR	
IL-9			
IL-11			
IL-12			
EPO			
GM-CSF			
G-CSF			
LIF			
CNTF			

[a]CCR, CC chemokine receptor; CNTF, ciliary neurotrophic factor; CXCR, CXC chemokines receptor; CX3CR, CX3C chemokines receptor; G-CSF, granulocyte colony stimulating factor; GM-CSF, granulocyte-macrophage colony stimulating factor; EPO, erythropoietin; IL, interleukin; IFN, interferon; LIF, leukemia inhibitory factor; NGFR, nerve growth factor receptor; TNF, tumor necrosis factor; XCR, XCR chemokines receptor.

knowledge of the complex biologic effects of cytokine networks has renewed interest in the potential for combining cytokine agents as an approach to patients with a variety of cancers. The potential for two cytokines to act synergistically has been demonstrated in vitro and in animal models, producing effects both qualitatively and quantitatively different than either agent alone (2,3). There is now a more solid scientific basis on which to select specific combinations of cytokines for clinical investigation. This chapter will summarize some of the more well-established combination regimens that have been tested in patients and suggest areas for future research using novel combination cytokine therapy for the treatment of cancer.

2. INTERFERON COMBINATIONS

The interferons comprise a family of closely related factors secreted by cells in response to viral infection, reviewed extensively in Chapter 19. The type I interferons include three classes in humans, including about 20 species of IFN-α, a single IFN-β, and a single IFN-ω. In contrast to the many different type I interferons, IFN-γ is the only type II interferon. There is strong preclinical data suggesting that IFN-γ plays a pivotal role in tumor immunosurveillance and rejection although the relevance of this for human cancers is not well defined. Despite the importance of IFN-γ in these animal models, most of the beneficial effects of interferons for human cancer have focused on IFN-α2b. The mechanism of antitumor activity is not fully established and may be multi-factorial. There is evidence that IFN-α2b has direct effects on tumor cells, characterized as inhibition of cell proliferation, up-regulation of surface HLA complexes and increased expression of certain tumor antigens. In addition, IFN-α2b promotes immune recognition of tumor cells through enhanced dendritic cell antigen processing and presentation. When administered at low doses, IFN-α2b may also have anti-angiogenic effects which can contribute to tumor rejection.

The interferon's have been among the most widely studied cytokines in a variety of combinations with early, largely in vitro, evidence for synergy between specific interferon family members and with other cytokines. The IFN receptors are members of the type-2 cytokine receptor family and so much of the recent effort has concentrated on using IFN-α2b with other cytokines that target TNF-related or type-1 cytokine receptors. Since IFN-α was first purified in 1978 a large number of clinical trials have been conducted with intriguing results in selected cases. To date, however, there have been no randomized studies supporting the superiority of any combination interferon cytokine regimen for cancer.

2.1. Interferon-α (IFN-α) and Interferon-γ (IFN-γ)

Several early studies in the late 1970's suggested potential synergy between IFN-α and IFN-γ in vitro (2). A randomized phase II trial of IFN-α with or without IFN-γ, as well as a nonrandomized study of combination therapy, in patients with untreated chronic myelogenous leukemia (CML) demonstrated no clinical benefit to the combination. Furthermore, severe life-threatening and even fatal toxicity was seen in a small minority of patients (4,5).

In light of the effective management of patients with carcinoid tumors using single-agent IFN-α, 12 patients with liver metastases with documented biochemical or radiographic progression were treated with a combination of IFN-α and IFN-γ (6). Toxicity typical of interferons was seen, comparable to what might be expected with single-agent therapy. At 6 months, there was one biochemical response, and whereas half the patients had subjective improvements in symptoms, no objective radiographic responses were noted.

In preclinical experiments using intralesional injections of IFN-α and IFN-γ complete regression of human breast cancer cell xenografts in nude mice was observed, whereas lesser responses were seen when either agent was given alone (7). These investigators pursued a clinical trial of combination IFN treatment in patients with cutaneous recurrent breast cancer (7). Five of seven lesions treated with the combination regressed compared to responses in 5 of 11 recurrences treated with IFN-α alone. Characterization of cellular responses within injected lesions treated with the combination therapy included inhibition of mitotic activity, increased expression of antigens on tumor cells, activation of macrophages and dendritic cells, T-cell infiltration, and activation of endothelium with increased expression of HLA-DR and ICAM-1.

After observing synergistic effects of IFN-α, IFN-γ, and 5-fluorouracil (5-FU) against a colon carcinoma cell line, investigators at the National Cancer Institute performed a pilot trial of this combination in patients with advanced cancer for whom 5-FU was a reasonable treatment option, including patients with colorectal, pancreatic, gastric, esophageal, and liver cancer (8). Fifty-three patients were treated with escalating doses of IFN-γ once the tolerability of IFN-α, 5-FU, and leucovorin was confirmed. Objective clinical responses were seen in more than 40% of the colorectal cancer patients, and, because IFN-α and IFN-γ seemed to have opposite effects on 5-FU clearance, the total chemotherapy dose did not seem to be responsible for these encouraging results.

Finally, on the basis of several phase-II studies showing conflicting but ultimately encouraging results for the combination of IFN-α and IFN–γ in the treatment of renal cell carcinoma, the European Organization for the Research and Treatment of Cancer (EORTC) Genitourinary Group performed a randomized phase-III study comparing single-agent IFN-α therapy to combination treatment *(9–11)*. A planned interim analysis revealed a lower response rate (4% vs 13%) for the combination arm, despite equivalent dose intensity for the IFN-α. This disappointing result was confirmed in another randomized phase-II trial performed by the Eastern Cooperative Oncology Group (ECOG) *(12)*.

2.2. IFN-α and Tumor Necrosis Factor-α (TNF-α)

TNF-α has been widely studied for its antitumor activity with little evidence of direct therapeutic benefit as a single agent. Because TNF-α and IFN-α exert their effects through separate receptors, the potential for synergistic effects have led to numerous clinical investigations. Kramer et al. published a phase-I study of local intratumoral TNF-α and systemic IFN-α2b in patients with locally advanced prostate cancer after preclinical data suggested synergistic inhibition in the growth of both androgen-dependent and independent prostate cancer cell lines *(13,14)*. Ten patients were treated with the combination and nine achieved a statistically significant reduction in prostatic volume. Serum prostate specific antigen (PSA) levels dropped by 18–87%, reaching nadir values at 7 weeks, but no objective clinical responses were seen in patients with metastatic disease. The regimen was quite tolerable with toxicity primarily confined to flulike syndrome and mild nausea. The authors concluded that the administration of the combination regimen was feasible and might be relevant for those patients with locally advanced, hormone-refractory prostate tumors not amenable to surgical resection. Follow-up clinical trials comparing this regimen with radiation or hormonal manipulation have not yet been completed.

2.3. IFN-γ and TNF-α

Two Phase-I studies were conducted combining TNF-α and IFN-γ. Smith et al. evaluated the maximally tolerated dose (MTD) of each agent given intramuscularly (IM) every other day for 20 days in 36 patients with a variety of pretreated solid tumors *(15)*. Toxicities included fatigue, anorexia, and chills; a small minority of patients developed asymptomatic transaminitis or microscopic hematuria. Minimal efficacy was seen at the established MTD, although a single patient with melanoma had a mixed response and another patient with mesothelioma transiently cleared his ascites of neoplastic cells. Schiller et al. performed a similar study using these same cytokines given intravenously three times a week in 24 patients with advanced cancer *(16)*. Dose-limiting toxicities comprised orthostatic hypotension and constitutional symptoms, resulting in a MTD that was similar to the previously reported study. Biologic correlates of response were evaluated in a select cohort of patients treated at the defined MTD, revealing several markers of enhanced immune function including increased serum IL-2 receptor levels and neopterin secretion. Retrospective analyses comparing these results with prior phase-I studies of each agent alone, however, did not reveal a benefit to combination therapy. No clinical responses were noted.

These agents were also studied in combination with melphalan as part of a hyperthermic isolated limb perfusion (HILP) protocol in patients with melanoma *(17)*. Higher response rates were seen than with melphalan alone but no data regarding DLT were pursued. These results were confirmed in subsequent clinical trials by other groups *(18)*. The efficacy of this combination was also documented in patients with nonmelanoma skin cancers of the limbs in a multicenter phase-II clinical trial, producing a 60% complete response rate and an 80% limb salvage rate *(19)*.

2.4. IFN-γ and Granulocyte-Macrophage Colony-Stimulating Factor (GM-CSF)

Irradiated hepatoma cells transduced by viral vectors encoding GM-CSF combined with systemic IFN-γ administration showed reduced tumor formation in murine models *(20)*. As a result, Reinisch et al. performed a pilot study of these two agents in patients with advanced, inoperable liver cancer *(21)*. Thrice-weekly GM-CSF and biweekly IFN-γ was administered subcutaneously to 15 patients. No serious toxicities were noted, but only one partial response was seen; parameters compatible with immunogenic response were seen in all treated patients but did not correlate with clinical outcome. Interestingly, the median survival of those patients with inducible HLA-DR on hepatoma cells was significantly increased relative to HLA-DR-negative cases as well as a separate control group, suggesting that perhaps, for a select group of liver cancer patients, this combination might be worthwhile.

2.5. IFN-α and GM-CSF

Several groups have pursued combinations with IFN-α and GM-CSF in patients with cancer. In a trial of renal cell carcinoma patients, Lummen et al. treated 21 patients with GM-CSF at seven different dose levels between 15 and 300 μg in combination with IFN-α at a fixed dose of 10×10^6 IU thrice weekly for 12 wk *(22)*. The MTD of GM-CSF was 150 μg, with the major dose limiting toxicity being grade 3 constitutional symptoms. Fifteen patients were evaluable for response, with two exhibiting complete regression of lung metastases; no partial responses were reported. A dose-response relationship could not be identified. In another clinical trial, O'Donnell et al. treated 15 patients with IFN-α three-times weekly and daily GM-CSF, at similar dose levels *(23)*. In this trial, treatment was well-tolerated, but only 13% of patients responded and none had complete regression.

The combination of IFN-α and GM-CSF has also been reported in patients with gastrointestinal cancers. This has been based, in part, by previous observations that GM-CSF ameliorated 5-FU-related diarrhea and allowed for greater chemotherapy dose intensity *(8)*. Furthermore, there is considerable evidence that IFN-α induces enhanced cytotoxicity of 5-FU in vitro *(8,24)*. Thirty-one patients with no previous treatment for metastatic disease received IFN-α (5 MU/m^2 sc days 1–7), 5-FU (370 mg/m^2 IV days 2–6), Leucovorin (500 mg/m^2 IV days 2–6), and GM-CSF (250 μg/m^2 sc days 7–18), every 3 wk. Objective clinical response rate was 21%, perhaps slightly higher than in unselected patients treated with 5-FU and leucovorin alone. Toxicity appeared to be improved in the hematologic categories but at the expense of increased nausea, vomiting, and fatigue.

A number of groups have evaluated the use of GM-CSF to prevent cytopenias caused by IFN-α and zidovudine in the treatment of Kaposi's sarcoma (KS). Krown et al. treated 17 HIV patients with extensive KS using zidovudine at standard doses, escalating doses of IFN-α (5, 10, or 20 MU), and titrated GM-CSF to maintain the absolute neutrophil count between 1 and 5×10^9 cells/L *(25)*. Forty-one percent of patients had objective clinical responses. The MTD of IFN-α was 20 MU, with fever and constitutional symptoms constituting the dose limiting toxicity; neutropenia was not a limiting factor in dose escalation or maintenance therapy.

3. INTERLEUKIN COMBINATIONS

Interleukins are a broad group of cytokines initially identified from leukocytes and thought to play a major role in immune activation and expansion of specific effector cell populations. Today it is recognized that interleukins are members of the wider class of cytokine molecules and exhibit an array of biologic functions that collectively help regulate normal immune cell homeostasis. The best characterized interleukin is IL-2, which was first identified as a T-cell growth factor in the late 1970s. The ability of IL-2 to expand T-cells in vitro revolutionized cellular immunology. IL-2 was also used to support T-cell survival following adoptive therapy in patients with cancer. These early studies in the 1980s resulted in subsequent trials of single agent IL-2 and durable objective responses were observed in patients with metastatic renal cell carcinoma and malignant melanoma (*see* Chapter 17). Although overall objective responses were generally less than 20%, most complete responders were eventually cured of disease. Single agent IL-2 was approved for the treatment of renal cell carcinoma in 1992 and for metastatic melanoma in 1998. Although the high-dose regimens have been associated with considerable toxicity, thus far lower doses of IL-2 have not been associated with acceptable clinical responses. Management of toxicity is usually possible in experienced centers with staff trained in the administration of high-dose IL-2.

Under normal physiologic conditions, IL-2 is produced predominantly by activated T-cells and binds to the high affinity IL-2 receptor (IL-2R). The IL-2R is a classical type-1 cytokine receptor composed of three distinct subunits, which all contribute to IL-2 binding. The IL-2Rα chain is highly expressed on activated T-lymphocytes as well as the regulatory T-cell population, where IL-2 may be critical for maintaining the growth and inhibitory function of the regulatory pool. The IL-2Rβ chain contributes to IL-2 mediated signaling and is also expressed on natural killer (NK), NKT, and CD8+ memory T-cells. The IL-2 γc chain is also involved in signaling and can be found in a variety of other hematopoietic cells. The IL-2β chain is also part of the IL-15R complex, although these two receptor complexes result in different functional consequences, explained in part by differential expression patterns on individual cells. Similarly, the IL-2Rγc is also expressed by the receptors for IL-4, IL-7, IL-9, IL-15, and IL-21.

The significant clinical effects of high-dose IL-2 in melanoma and renal cell carcinoma patients, coupled with a large volume of preclinical studies demonstrating therapeutic benefits with combination cytokine therapy including IL-2 has lead investigators to undertake similar clinical studies. In some cases treatment regimens have included concurrent cytotoxic chemotherapy although randomized clinical trials in melanoma have not yielded any evidence of a survival advantage for such an approach. We will review some of the more intriguing combinations that have been reported.

3.1. IL-2 and TNF-α

The rationale for combining IL-2 and TNF-α was based on early murine studies showing that this combination synergistically supported the generation of lymphokine-activated killer cells (LAK) *(26)*. The cytokine combination was tested in patients with advanced nonsmall-cell lung cancer *(26)*. A low dose daily IL-2 infusion was combined with daily TNF-α IM injections given at escalating doses. The reported toxicity included fever, local injection site reactions, asthenia, and cytopenias, with the dose limiting toxicity of thrombocytopenia. Twelve patients were evaluable and one partial response with three minor responses was observed. All treated patients demonstrated biologic responses, including enhanced LAK activity in vitro.

These same agents were evaluated in parallel phase-I studies using similar doses except that IL-2 was given by continuous infusion *(27)*. Eleven of 15 patients developed grade 3 or 4 toxicity, predominantly of pulmonary or cardiac origin. Although no objective responses were seen, the median survival for these previously-untreated patients was more than 11 months, with one patient surviving more than 30 months despite the presence of metastatic disease, suggesting an improvement over standard chemotherapy.

The sequential administration of IL-2 and TNF-α was further evaluated in 15 patients with advanced solid tumors *(28)*—in total, 46 cycles of therapy comprising IV TNF-α followed by escalating doses of daily IL-2 infusions. Major toxicities were comparable to that seen with IL-2 alone in previous studies. NK and LAK activity was not enhanced by the addition of TNF-α, but two objective clinical responses were seen, both in patients with malignant melanoma.

3.2. IL-2 and IFN-β

IFN-β has exhibited synergistic activity with IL-2 in terms of increasing IL2R expression and stimulating NK cell activity *(29)*. Several groups studied this combination in the phase-II setting *(29–31)*. Krigel et al. treated 24 patients with renal cell cancer with 5×10^6 Cetus U/m^2 IL-2 and 6×10^6 U/m^2 IFN-β intravenously 3 times per week *(29)*. A 27% overall response rate was seen, including two responses lasting nearly 2 years at the time of publication. LAK and NK activity were significantly increased in responders compared to nonresponders (88 lytic units (LU) vs 4 LU and 288 LU vs 100 LU, respectively), suggesting a correlation between clinical response and in vitro immunologic effect.

The Cancer and Leukemia Group B (CALGB) randomized patients with refractory non-Hodgkin's lymphoma to IL-2 with or without IFN-β at nearly the same dosages as above *(30)*. Toxicity in this study was severe with more than a third of patients experiencing grade-4 toxicity, primarily cytopenias and cardiac events, and two patients died of treatment-related causes. The response rate was 17% with 1 complete response in each arm, and no differences were observed among the groups. However, median survival was improved in the combination arm (33% vs 7%) at 18 months.

The same cytokine combination and dosage was evaluated by ECOG in patients with advanced lung cancer *(31)*. Although only a 4% clinical response rate was observed, the median survival was 33 weeks. This was viewed as favorable to results with chemotherapy, although the authors could not conclude that the combination was superior to IL-2 alone. To date, these results have not been confirmed in phase-III trials.

3.3. IL-2 and Interleukin-12 (IL-12)

IL-12 has been shown to be active in a variety of murine tumor models and is thought to mediate tumor regression in a IFN-γ-dependent manner *(32,33)*. Gollob et al. treated 28 patients with advanced solid tumors with IL-12 given intravenously two times per week in combination with subcutaneous low-dose IL-2 *(34)*. Toxicities were primarily constitutional and felt to be related to the IL-2. At the MTD, IL-2 significantly augmented IFN-γ production by IL-12, leading to a threefold expansion of NK cells. One partial clinical response and two minor pathologic responses, all in patients with melanoma, were seen.

3.4. IL-2 and GM-CSF

A logical combination is IL-2 and GM-CSF because GM-CSF promotes dendritic cell mobilization and antigen presentation, whereas IL-2 helps expand recently primed T-cells. This particular cytokine combination increased proliferation of cytotoxic T-lymphocytes and enhanced expansion of $CD25^+$ T-cells to a greater degree that either cytokine alone *(35)*. In a phase-I study, Schiller et al. treated 34 patients with advanced solid tumors with increasing doses of GM-CSF (2.5, 5, or 10 mcg/kg sc daily for 12 d) before or concurrently with IL-2 (1.5 or 3 $MU/m^2/d$ by continuous infusion for 4 d) *(36)*. Grade 3 and 4 toxicities comprised hypotension, thrombocytopenia, hepatitis, nephrotoxicity, gastrointestinal bleeding, arrhythmia, constitutional symptoms, and two patients suffered reversible neurotoxicity. CD25 expression increased in the treated groups, but LAK activity was lower in the concurrently treated patients compared with those treated sequentially. Objective clinical responses in lung metastases were observed in four of eight patients with renal cell carcinoma, although no objective responses were seen at the primary tumor site.

Following the phase-I trial, a phase-II study in renal cell carcinoma was initiated. Twenty patients were treated with GM-CSF (100 μg/d sc for 2 wk) and IL-2 (11×10^6 IU sc 4 days per wk for 4 wk) *(37)*. Treatment was well tolerated with toxicity primarily confined to low-grade constitutional symptoms. Although there were no objective clinical responses, three patients had stable disease. Smith et al. performed a randomized study of low-dose intravenous IL-2 (72,000 U/kg IV every 8 h for 5 d), with or without concurrent GM-CSF (125 or 250 μg/m^2/d sc for 7 d), in patients with renal cell cancer or melanoma *(38)*. Although GM-CSF did not increase the toxicity of the IL-2 and serum soluble IL-2R levels were significantly increased in the combination arm (at the higher dose of GM-CSF), no clinical responses were seen.

Using a modified treatment design, O'Day et al. treated 33 patients with metastatic melanoma who had achieved a partial response or stable disease on induction biochemotherapy, with chronic low-dose IL-2 (1 MU/m^2 sc daily) and GM-CSF (125 μg/m^2 sc daily) and intermittent pulses of high-dose decrescendo IL-2 (54 MU/m^2 by CIV for 2 d of 7 of 12 cycles) over the course of one year *(39)*. Fifteen percent achieved a complete response and 12% maintained SD for at least 6 mo. Overall survival was 18.5 mo, comparing favorably to a group of historical controls (overall survival of 9.3 mo), suggesting a clinical benefit to such a strategy. The treatment was well-tolerated in the ambulatory setting without grade 3 or 4 toxicities.

Another group of investigators focused on using this combination of cytokines to alter the local tumor microenvironment. They injected intralesional GM-CSF (150ng/lesion) and perilesional IL-2 (3 MU sc for 5 d every 3 wk) in elderly patients with advanced, pretreated melanoma *(40)*. Among 16 patients, 2 had minor clinical responses and 2 had partial responses, whereas 56% had stable disease for at least 3 mo. One patient had grade-3 fever and arthralgias, but, otherwise, therapy was well tolerated. No immunological correlates were noted.

3.5. Interleukin-4 (IL-4) and GM-CSF

IL-4 is secreted by a variety of cells, including T-cells, eosinophils, basophils, mast cells, NK cells and some antigen-presenting cells (APCs). IL-4 functions to promote germinal center formation, B-cell development and differentiation, and Th2 type immune responses. An important role for IL-4 in combination with GM-CSF has been well established for inducing the maturation of monocytes into dendritic cells both in vitro and in vivo *(41,42)*. Therefore, Roth et al. treated a group of patients with advanced solid tumors with GM-CSF (2.5 µg/kg/d sc) alone or in combination with IL-4 (0.5–6.0 µg/kg/d sc) in a pilot study. Combined treatment did increase APC activity in terms of enhanced CD11c and HLA-DR expression, increased endocytic activity, and the ability to stimulate T-cells in a mixed leukocyte reaction, but only one clinical response was noted among 21 patients. In this trial, no significant toxicity was described. The same group performed a phase-I study of this combination in 21 patients treated with a fixed dose of GM-CSF and escalating doses of IL-4 *(43)*. The IL-4 MTD was 6 µg/kg/d, which resulted in grade-3 dyspnea, headache, and thrombocytopenia. Similar to the first trial, HLA-DR expression was increased at this dose level, but only one patient had an objective clinical response and three patients had stable disease. The authors concluded that perhaps this combination will be of value in the vaccine setting to expand dendritic cells in vivo.

3.6. Interleukin-6 (IL-6) and GM-CSF

IL-6 is another pleiotropic cytokine first isolated as a B-cell stimulatory factor capable of inducing B-cell differentiation. IL-6 is a pivotal cytokine in regulating immune responses and inflammation. The overproduction of IL-6 has been implicated in the pathology of several inflammatory diseases, including rheumatoid arthritis, Crohn disease, juvenile idiopathic arthritis and others. A phase-I trial of the combination of IL-6 and GM-CSF in patients with advanced renal cell carcinoma was conducted after demonstrating minimal therapeutic activity with each agent alone *(44)*. Thirteen patients, most previously treated with IL-2 or IFN-α, received GM-CSF at 3.0 µg/kg/d subcutaneously, as well as escalating doses of IL-6 (1.0, 5.0, or 10.0 µg.kg/d) on days 1–14. The dose limiting toxicities were thrombocytosis and hyperbilirubinemia, but the most common toxicities were constitutional in nature. Unfortunately, no objective clinical responses were seen.

In an attempt to take advantage of the hematopoietic stimulatory nature of IL-6, several studies were designed to add the combination of IL-6 and GM-CSF following chemotherapy. Hochster et al. examined this combination, vs placebo and GM-CSF, after standard paclitaxel and carboplatin in patients with ovarian cancer *(45)*. IL-6 treated patients exhibited a statistically improved time to platelet recovery in the first cycle only. No increase in the dose intensity of chemotherapy was permitted. Similarly discouraging results were seen in children after treatment with ifosfamide, carboplatin, and etoposide as salvage therapy for recurrent solid tumors. Although time to platelet recovery was reduced in a statistically significant fashion, limited clinical benefit and profound constitutional toxicity was reported *(46)*.

3.7. IL-2 and IL-4

IL-4 has been shown to increase tumor-specific cytotoxic T-cells in patients with melanoma when combined with IL-2, and enhanced LAK/NK cell activity of peripheral T-cells isolated from patients with cancer following IL-2 therapy in vitro *(47,48)*. Sosman et al. treated 17 patients with solid tumors using IL-4 (40–600 µg/m^2/d CIV for 7 d), followed by IL-2 (11.2 MIU/m^2/d CIV for 4 d) and a second course of IL-4 in a phase-I trial *(49)*. Dose limiting toxicity, which occurred at the highest dose of IL-4, comprised capillary leak syndrome. A marked increase in eosinophil number and NK/LAK fractions were seen after the second course of IL-4, and one minor, albeit durable, clinical response was noted. A follow-up study revealed evidence of eosinophil activation by the combination, which was thought to be relevant to the clinical effects of IL-4 *(50)*.

Another group administered this combination simultaneously (IL-2 at 9×10^6 IU/m^2 sc daily for 5 d, and IL-4 at 100–400 µg/m^2 sc daily for 5 d) in 15 patients with advanced cancers *(51)*. Although constitutional toxicity was most common and of low-grade, grade-3 and -4 toxicities were seen at the 300 µg/m^2 level (MTD was not calculated owing to withdrawal of the drug by the manufacturer). Statistically significant increases in several T-cell subsets were seen including cytotoxic T-cells and NK cells, but not B-cells. One patient with renal cell carcinoma had a partial response. Olencki et al. evaluated 39 patients with refractory cancers treated with the combination of IL-2 and IL-4 as well *(52)*. IL-2 was given in escalating doses (3, 12, and 48×10^6 IU/m^2 IV three times per week) concurrent with IL-4, again in escalating doses (4, 120, and 400 µg/m^2 sc three times per week). The MTD was not reached owing to insufficient IL-4 availability, but was at least 48×10^6 IU/m^2 for IL-2 and 120 µg/m^2 for IL-4; toxicity was comparable to that seen with IL-2 alone. NK cell activity was enhanced, but LAK activity was not. Serial biopsies from four of the six patients' tumors revealed increasing class-I and -II MHC expression, increased T-cell infiltrates, or both during therapy, but no radiographic responses were documented.

3.8. IL-2 and Erythropoietin

Preclinical data suggests that vascular endothelial growth factor (VEGF) predicts resistance to IL-2 in patients with renal cell carcinoma. Further, anemia-related hypoxia has been shown to negatively influence prognosis by stimulating VEGF production. Thus, investigators studied that combination of erythropoietin and IL-2 in a phase-II clinical trial of metastatic renal cell carcinoma *(53,54)*. Fourteen consecutive patients progressing after initial therapy with low-dose subcutaneous IL-2 were treated with continued IL-2 (3 MU sc twice daily for 4 wk) and erythropoietin (10,000u sc three times per week). VEGF levels increased significantly less in the combination therapy cohort, and hemoglobin values increased as expected. Among 12 evaluable patients there was one partial response and four patients with stabilization of metastatic disease.

4. INTERFERON AND INTERLEUKIN COMBINATIONS

The clinical success of single agent IFN-α and IL-2 and their availability as cancer therapeutics has prompted intense interest in the combination of these two cytokines. There have been innumerable studies evaluating this combination and these will be reviewed herein. Additional studies adding a third cytokine to this regimen have also been attempted and will be discussed briefly.

4.1. IL-2 and IFN-α

The combination of IL-2 and IFN-α builds on the potential to take advantage of the IFN-induced up-regulation of MHC class I and tumor-associated antigens on tumor cells in the context of IL-2-enhanced generation of cytotoxic T-cells and improved tumor cell killing. This synergy was noted in several animal tumor models and the combination has been pursued in the phase-I setting using a variety of cytokine doses, schedules, and routes of administration *(55–57)*.

A dose-finding study in 94 patients with metastatic cancer was conducted using IFN-α2b administered at a dose of 3–6 × 10^6 U/m^2 concomitant with IL-2, at 1–4.5 × 10^6 U/m^2 *(58)*. Doses were given intravenously as a bolus every 8 h, up to 15 doses, every 2 wk for 2 cycles. In 91 evaluable patients, a 27% overall clinical response rate was seen; 33% in patients with melanoma, 31% in patients with renal cell carcinoma, and 11% in those with colorectal cancer. There seemed to be a dose-response relationship, borne out with continued follow-up, although survival was not correlated with dose *(59)*. The toxicity profile included nausea, vomiting, diarrhea, cytokine-mediated hepatitis, hypotension, capillary leak syndrome necessitating six intubations, and hypotension, requiring pressor support in more than 25% of the cycles, comparable to what might be expected with high-dose IL-2 alone.

Huberman et al. treated 17 patients with solid tumors with a fixed dose of IFN-α (6 × 10^6 U/m^2/d IM 3 d/wk) and escalating doses of IL-2 (1–4 × 10^6 U/m^2/d by 2-h infusion 5 d/wk for 4 wk) *(60)*. One of 15 patients responded, but two out of five patients with melanoma exhibited tumor regression. Ratain et al. examined subcutaneous IL-2 (0.5–2.5 MU/m^2/d) and IFN-α (2.5–12.5 MU/m^2/d) in 33 patients with refractory cancers as well *(61)*. No clinical responses were seen in patients with diseases other than renal cell carcinoma where 4 out of 16 patients responded. A group from Genoa, Italy studied another IFN-α/IL-2 combination in 19 patients with sarcoma, renal cell carcinoma, or melanoma *(62)*. IL-2 was administered in escalating doses ranging from 1–3 MU/m^2 sc twice daily, 5 d/wk, whereas IFN-α was given at a fixed dose of 3 MU IM daily, 5 d/wk, in 3-wk cycles. Toxicity correlated with increasing IL-2 doses, but was manageable even at the highest level. Three of 19 patients responded, one of seven with melanoma and two of six with renal cell carcinoma. Budd et al. performed a dose-finding study using standard IFN-α (10 × 10^6 U/m^2 IM 3 d/wk) and IL-2 at doses ranging from 4–26 × 10^6 U/m^2 IV bolus three times weekly for 4 wk *(63)*. Fifty seven patients were treated, tolerating all but the highest dose level of IL-2. Nearly a third of patients with melanoma responded, including two complete clinical responses, but results were less encouraging in other tumor types.

Schiller et al. looked at immunological parameters in a small phase-IB randomized, crossover study of IL-2 (1.5–3 × 10^6 U/m^2/d by CI for 4 d, weekly for 3 wk) and IFN-α (0.5–5 × 10^6 U/m^2/d sc for 4 d, weekly for 3 wk) vs IL-2 alone *(64)*. No differences among the groups were seen in terms of biologic activity (i.e., LAK activity, monocytic HLA-DR and Fc receptor expression, or serum IL-2R expression) or clinical activity. Finally, Gause et al. studied an outpatient combination regimen comprising both IL-2 and IFN-α at doses of either 1.5 or 3 × 10^6 MU/m^2 sc 5 d/wk for 4-wk cycles (after an initial cycle of IL-2 alone) *(65)*. The MTD was 1.5 MU/m^2 of each cytokine owing to grade-3 fatigue. Twenty-four percent of patients with renal cell carcinoma responded (including four of eight previously treated patients); no other patients responded including those with melanoma.

Based on these phase-I studies, many phase-II studies were initiated in patients with both renal cell carcinoma *(66–108)* and melanoma *(109–125)*. Although the routes of administration, dosages, and schedules were quite variable, and in several cases, the cytokine combination was administered in conjunction with chemotherapeutic agents, encouraging response rates were seen in renal cell carcinoma, ranging from 0 to 48%, with complete response rates up to 17% (summarized in Table 2). This ultimately led

Table 2
Phase-II Studies of IFN-α and IL-2 in Renal Cell Cancer

Reference	N	ORR (%)	CRR (%)	Route of IFN	Route of IL2	Additional agents
Atzpodien et al. (66)	132	31	5	sc	sc	5FU
Vogelzang et al. (67)	42	12	2.4	sc	sc	
Atkins et al. (68)	28	11	0	IV	IV	
Stadler et al. (69)	47	17	2.1	sc	sc	Cis-retinoic acid
Tourani et al. (70)	62	19	1.6	sc	sc	5FU
Figlin et al. (71)	30	30	0	sc	CIV	
Facendola et al. (72)	50	18	12	sc	sc	
Ravaud et al. (73)	38	18	2.6	sc	sc	
Ravaud et al. (74)	111	1.8	0	sc	sc	
Jayson et al. (75)	60	0	0	sc	sc	
Naglieri et al. (76)	42	26	14.3	sc	sc	Megace
Mittelman et al. (77)	12	33	16.7	IM	CIV	
Canobbio et al. (78)	16	6	0	sc	sc	
Ellerhorst et al. (79)	52	31	7.7	sc	CIV	5FU
Bergmann et al. (80)	30	30	6.7	sc	IV	
Ravaud et al. (81)	66	8	3	sc	sc	
Ryan et al. (83)	41	14.6	2.4	sc	sc	Gemcitabine, 5FU
Buzio et al. (84)	50	12	2	IM	sc	
Elias et al. (85)	38	11	2.6	sc	CIV	5FU
Gez et al. (86)	62	29	6.4	sc	sc	5FU, vinblastine
Piga et al. (87)	20	15	5	IM	sc	
Rogers et al. (88)	33	9	0	sc	sc	
Fossa et al. (89)	16	18	0	sc	CIV	
Besana et al. (90)	17	35	5.9	sc	CIV	
Pectasides et al. (91)	31	38.7	12.9	sc	sc	Vinblastine
Lissoni et al. (92)	35	26	0	sc	sc	
Boccardo et al. (93)	22	9	0	IM	CIV	
Lummen et al. (94)	30	23	0	sc	sc	
Hofmockel et al. (95)	34	38	9	sc	sc	5FU
Clark et al. (96)	43	16	7	sc	dCIV	
Tourani et al. (98)	122	21	4.9	sc	sc	
Rathmell et al. (99)	20	0	0	sc	sc	5FU, leucovorin
Ravaud et al. (100)	35	5.7	0	sc	sc	5FU
Neri et al. (101)	15	26.7	6.7	IM	sc	Gemcitabine
Atzpodien et al. (102)	41	39.1	17.1	sc	sc	5FU
Clark et al. (103)	19	0	0	sc	sc	
Dutcher et al. (104)	50	18	4	sc	sc	5FU
Allen et al. (105)	55	31	5.4	sc	sc	5FU
Negrier et al. (106)	131	10.6	0	sc	sc	5FU
Van Herpen et al. (107)	51	11.8	0	sc	sc	5FU
Atzpodien et al. (108)	35	48.6	11.4	sc	sc	5FU

Abbreviations: N, number of patients; ORR, overall response rate; CRR, complete response rate; IL2, interleukin 2; IFN, interferon-alpha; sc, subcutaneous; IM, intramuscular; CIV, continuous infusion; dCIV, decrescendo infusion; IV, intravenous; 5FU, 5-flourouracil.

to a randomized phase-III clinical trial by the French Immunotherapy Study Group *(126)*. Four hundred twenty-five patients with metastatic renal cell carcinoma were randomized to either continuous infusion IL-2 (18×10^6 IU/m^2 for 5 d, for two induction cycles separated by 6 rest days, and four maintenance cycles separated by 3 wk), subcutaneous injections of IFN-α (18×10^6 IU three times per week for 23 wk), or both; in the combination arm, the IFN-α was reduced to 6×10^6 IU three times per week. Response rates were 6.5%, 7.5%, and 18.6% ($P < 0.01$) respectively. The subjects most likely to respond were those patients with only one organ site involved by metastatic disease and those patients undergoing combination cytokine treatment. After the 25-wk treatment period, the number of patients with complete responses in the IL-2, IFN-α, and combination treatment arms was 1, 2, and 5 respectively. Although there was a statistically significant difference in event-free survival at 1 yr (15%, 12%, and 20%, $P = 0.01$), no overall survival advantage was seen. With respect to toxicity, more grade-3 or -4 adverse events were noted in the two groups employing IL-2, but no difference was seen among the patients who received IL-2 alone compared with those undergoing combination therapy, except for fevers which were seen more frequently in the combination group.

Several additional phase-II studies of combination IL-2 and IFN-α in patients with melanoma have been reported (summarized in Table 3). Similar to the renal cell carcinoma trials, a variety of strategies have been employed, using variable doses, routes of administration, and schedules, and combining cytokines with chemotherapy and other agents. Overall response rates have ranged from 0 to 60%, with complete response rates of up to 24% *(109–125)*.

A randomized phase-III study comparing the combination of IL-2 and IFN-α to IL-2 alone was conducted *(127)*. Patients with advanced melanoma were stratified based on known prognostic factors, including the number and sites of metastatic lesions, and were randomized to IL-2 (6×10^6 U/m^2 every 8 h as tolerated up to a maximum of 14 doses on days 1–5 and 15–19) or IL-2 (4.5×10^6 U/m^2) plus IFN-α (3×10^6 U/m^2 IV using a similar schedule. Eighty-five patients were entered and served the basis for a published report at a planned interim analysis. Toxicity was not significantly different among the two arms, except for the presence of grade-4 transaminitis, which was more common in the combination therapy group. Other reasons for treatment withdrawal included oliguria, dyspnea, confusion, and hypotension, observed in both cohorts. Two treatment-related deaths were seen in the IL-2 alone arm and one in the combination arm. Although the number of IL-2 doses was equivalent among the groups, the dose intensity was 25% less in the combination arm as a result of the study design. No complete responses were seen in either arm; the partial response rate was not significantly different (5% vs 10%, $P = 0.30$). Median survival was also not significantly different (10.2 mo vs 9.7 mo). As a result of predefined early-stopping rules related to overall response rates, the trial was terminated. Although this study produced among the lowest response rates published for high-dose bolus IL-2, no justification for the continued use of the combination of IL-2 and IFN-α could be found.

Thus, a series of randomized clinical trials evaluating biochemotherapy regimens, which included and IL-2 and IFN-α combination were conducted in both the phase-II and -III setting *(128–132)*. Rosenberg et al. randomized 102 patients with metastatic

Table 3
Phase-II Studies of IFN-α and IL-2 in Melanoma

Reference	N	ORR (%)	CRR (%)	Route of IFN	Route of IL2	Additional agents
Whitehead et al. *(109)*	14	0	0	sc/IM	CIV	
Richards et al. *(110)*	42	57.1	23.8	sc	IV	BCNU, CDDP, DTIC
Khayat et al. *(111)*	39	53.8	12.8	sc	CIV	CDDP
Keilholz et al. (112)	27	18.5	3.7	sc	CIV	
	27	40.7	11.1	sc	dCIV	
Kruit et al. *(113)*	51	15.7	2	sc	CIV	
Eton et al. *(114)*	23	8.7	0	IM	CIV	
Atzopieden et al. *(115)*	40	35	7.5	sc	sc	Carboplatin, DTIC
	27	55.5	11	sc	sc	CDDP, DTIC, BCNU, tam
Proebstle et al. *(116)*	22	22.7	0	sc	CIV	CDDP, DTIC
Legha et al. *(117)*	40	32.5	5	sc	IV	CDDP, DTIC, vinblastine
	62	59.6	22.5	sc	IV	CDDP, DTIC, vinblastine (sequential)
Eton et al. *(118)*	21	0	0	sc	dCIV	
Richards et al. *(119)*	83	55.4	14.4	sc	IV	CDDP, DTIC, BCNU
McDermott et al. *(120)*	40	39.6	20	sc	CIV	CDDP, DTIC, vinblastine
Flaherty et al. *(121)*	44	36.4	11.4	sc	IV	CDDP, DTIC
	36	16.7	2.8	sc	sc	CDDP, DTIC
Donskov et al. *(122)*	42	9.5	0	sc	sc	Histamine dihydrochloride
Schmidt et al. *(123)*	41	4.9	0	sc	sc	Histamine dihydrochloride
Atkins et al. *(125)*	47	46.8	14.9	sc	CIV	CDDP, DTIC, temozolomide

N, number of patients; ORR, overall response rate; CRR, complete response rate; IL2, interleukin 2; IFN, interferon-alpha; sc, subcutaneous; IM, intramuscular; CIV, continuous infusion; dCIV, decrescendo infusion; IV, intravenous; CDDP, cisplatin; DTIC, dacarbazine; tam, tamoxifen; BCNU, carmustine.

melanoma to either chemotherapy alone, comprising cisplatin, dacarbazine, and tamoxifen, or a combination of high-dose IL-2, IFN-α, and the same chemotherapy regimen *(128)*. Although there was a trend towards improved overall response rates in the biochemotherapy arm (44% with three complete responses vs 27% with four complete responses, $P = 0.071$), there was an equivalent trend towards improved overall survival for those receiving chemotherapy alone (15.8 mo vs 10.7 mo, $P = 0.052$). Although there were no treatment-related deaths, the addition of immunotherapy clearly increased the toxicity profile.

The Dermatologic Cooperative Oncology Group studied the addition of bolus, infusional, and subcutaneous IL-2 to a combination of IFN-α and dacarbazine *(129)*. Nearly 300 patients were randomized to dacarbazine (850 mg/m^2 IV every 28 d) and IFN-α (3 MU/m^2 twice daily on day 1, once daily from days 2–5, and 5 MU/m^2 three times per week from week 2 to 4) or the same regimen plus IL-2 (4.5 MU/m^2 IV over 3 hours on day 3, 9 MU/m^2 over 24 h on day 3, and 4.5 MU/m^2 sc days 4–7). Response rates were not significantly different among the two treatment arms (18% vs 16%, $P = 0.87$) and no difference in overall survival was noted (median 11 mo in both arms). The addition of IL-2 was significantly more toxic, however, necessitating nearly twice as much treatment cessation owing to adverse events in the IL-2 containing group.

The Italian Melanoma Intergroup published a randomized study evaluating the addition of an outpatient regimen of IL-2 and IFN-α to chemotherapy *(132)*. One hundred seventy-six patients with metastatic melanoma were treated with cisplatin and dacarbazine with or without carmustine or the same chemotherapy regimen plus IL-2 (4.5 MU sc on days 3–5 and 8–12, every 3 wk) and IFN-α (3 MU IM days 3 and 5, and then thrice weekly). No differences in terms of toxicity, response rates, or survival were seen after nearly 2 yr follow-up.

Collectively, these clinical trials strongly suggest little survival benefit from IL-2/IFN-α combinations for renal cell carcinoma or melanoma with or without chemotherapy. These results should be interpreted cautiously as the optimal dose and timing of exposure to these cytokines may impact the outcome and little is firmly established in how best to optimize treatment, especially when combined with other agents, such as chemotherapy. Of note, the combination of IL-2 and IFN-α has also been piloted in a variety of other tumors, including non small-cell lung, breast, colorectal, and head and neck squamous cell cancers *(133–139)*. Unfortunately, encouraging results were only seen in a small cohort of patients with recurrent head and neck cancer, where 2 of 11 patients exhibited partial responses in the context of heavy pretreatment *(139)*, Thus, at the present time such combinations remain investigational.

4.2. IL-2, IFN-α and TNF-α

A three-drug combination of IL-2, IFN-α, and TNF-α was evaluated in a phase-I dose escalation study *(140)*. Eighteen patients with a variety of advanced solid tumors were treated with infusional IL-2, intramuscular or subcutaneous IFN-α, and intravenous TNF-α. Significant toxicities included cytopenias, arrhythmias, pulmonary edema, and weight loss, but the regimen was thought to be feasible in the ambulatory setting. One patient with melanoma had a partial response and three with renal cell carcinoma had stabilization of disease, whereas all others progressed or were not evaluable for response.

4.3. IFN-γ and IL-2

Based on preclinical data demonstrating that IFN-γ augmented antitumor effects of IL-2, possibly through up-regulation of the IL-2Rα subunit a clinical trial was performed *(141,142)*. A phase-I clinical trial combining escalating doses of IFN-γ with moderate doses of IL-2 was conducted in 41 patients with incurable solid tumors *(142)*. Dose limiting toxicity consisted of constitutional symptoms as expected, although one myocardial infarction occurred. Only two partial and two minor responses were seen, but clear evidence of treatment-related induction of NK and LAK activity was noted. Other phase-I studies involving outpatient regimens were reported by several groups, each with similar results *(143–145)*. Reddy et al. went on to add increasing doses of IFN-γ to high-dose bolus IL-2 in a cohort of patients with advanced cancer *(146)*. Although toxicity was tolerable and half the patients had increases in NK/LAK activity, only 1 of 20 patients had an objective clinical response. Nevertheless, phase-II studies were performed in patients with metastatic renal cell carcinoma. In two studies, response rates ranged from 11 to 21% with clear changes in the immunologic profile and augmentation of NK cell activity *(147,148)*. To date, no phase-III trials have been performed with this combination.

4.4. IFN-γ, IL-2 and GM-CSF

A single study administered IFN-γ, IL-2, and GM-CSF sequentially to 55 patients with metastatic renal cell cancer *(149)*. Toxicity was mild, with no grade 3 or higher effects noted. Five patients had documented radiographic responses, with one patient having complete regression of disease. Compared to previously reported trials of IFN-γ and IL-2, GM-CSF did not seem to improve efficacy.

4.5. IFN-α, IL-2, and GM-CSF

Several early phase studies were performed to evaluate the triple combination of IFN-α, IL-2, and GM-CSF, prefaced on the idea of reducing the toxicity related to high-dose bolus IL-2. Eleven patients with progressive metastatic renal cell carcinoma and seven DTIC-resistant ocular melanoma patients were treated with 5MU IFN-α, 1, 4, or 8 MIU/m^2 IL-2, and 2.5 or 5 µg/kg GM-CSF *(150)*. Dose limiting toxicity was hypotension and severe fever. Significant increases in immunologic parameters such as T-cell expansion and monocyte HLA-DR expression were noted. Interestingly, three of eight patients with renal cell carcinoma had complete responses, whereas one of seven patients with melanoma had a partial clinical response.

A small cohort of patients with renal cell carcinoma were treated with a complicated regimen of GM-CSF, low-dose IL-2 and IFN-α in the outpatient setting *(151)*. The regimen was well tolerated and led to increased numbers of peripheral blood mononuclear cells expressing costimulatory molecules after GM-CSF induction. Unfortunately, despite regression of lung metastases in several patients, none of the patients had confirmed objective responses. A phase-II study was ultimately undertaken with the same regimen in patients with progressive renal cell carcinoma *(152)*. This trial enrolled 59 patients and the main toxicities were flulike syndromes and transient hepatitis, requiring a reduction in the dose of IL-2 in several patients. The overall response rate was 19% with three complete responses and a median survival of 9.5 mo. Expansion and activation of T-cells seemed to correlate with clinical response. In sum, this regimen seems to be, in this small selected cohort, as effective as high-dose bolus IL-2 and less toxic, but it has yet to be compared in a prospectively, randomized clinical trial.

Two additional trials have combined this triple cytokine regimen with chemotherapy in the treatment of metastatic melanoma *(153,154)*. Groenewegen et al. treated 32 patients with an outpatient regimen comprising dacarbazine, followed by 10 d of sc GM-CSF and low-dose IL-2, followed in turn by 5 d of IFN-α *(154)*. No grade-3 or -4 toxicity was seen and 32% of all patients responded, with four complete clinical responses. Similar to the earlier studies, the numbers of activated T-cells were noted to increase over the course of therapy, but correlation with clinical response or survival was not evaluated. Vaughan et al. treated 19 patients with a regimen entailing cisplatin and DTIC for 3 d, followed by low-dose subcutaneous IL-2 and IFN-α with escalating doses of GM-CSF throughout the treatment period *(153)*. Interestingly, clinical responses correlated with increasing GM-CSF dose, which, in turn, was associated with increasing serum concentrations of TNF-α. Further clinical trials of this triple cytokine regimen with chemotherapy have not been performed to date.

5. FUTURE DIRECTIONS

The increasing number of cytokines and related agents as well as an improved understanding of the signaling pathways used by the cytokine network are leading to new and innovative combination therapies *(155,156)*. The optimal combination of cytokines and combinations with other types of therapeutic agents are only now being actively explored. Based on advances in basic immunology and preclinical studies in animal models, a more sophisticated and directed approach to manipulating immune responses can be envisioned for cancer and other diseases. Although murine studies can support specific combinations, only through well designed clinical trials in patients with cancer can we ultimately determine the best combination regimens. Further investigation is also needed to better define the dose, schedule, and route of administration for current and new cytokine combinations in patients. An important area for future investigation will be the combination of cytokines with other targeted therapeutics, such as tyrosine kinase inhibitors, epidermal growth factor inhibitors, and angiogenesis inhibitors *(157,158)*. The potential for synergistic activity of cytokines with targeted vaccines has also been supported by extensive preclinical experiments and numerous clinical trials are underway to study the effects of specific cytokines with a variety of vaccines strategies in patients with cancer.

6. CONCLUSIONS

Cytokines offer significant promise as cancer therapeutics based on the effects of single agent therapy in a number of human diseases. The potential for improved therapeutic effectiveness with combination cytokine therapy has been a well established paradigm in animal tumor models. The large number of cytokines and the redundancy inherent in the complex cytokine network have made logical selection of combination treatment strategies difficult. The increased knowledge of cytokine biology based on targeted knockout mice and new data on cytokine signaling pathways are providing new insights into how to optimize cytokine combinations as a therapeutic strategy. The concept has been tested using clinically available cytokine agents and has yielded important safety information and occasional clinical responses in selected populations. A major future goal will be to find appropriate combinations of cytokines, with synergy, and without competing toxicity profiles, that may harness the inherent power and specificity of the immune system as a means of preventing or treating cancer.

REFERENCES

1. Malek T, Bayer A. Tolerance, not immunity, crucially depends on IL-2. Nat Rev Immunol 2004;4(9):665–674.
2. Fleischman W, Georgiades J, Osborne L. Potentiation of interferon activity by mixed preparations of fibroblast and immune interferon. Infect Immun 1979;26:248–153.
3. Feinman R, Henriksen-DeStefano D, Tsujimoto M, Vilcek J. Tumor Necrosis Factor is an important mediator of tumor cell killing by human monocytes. Journal of Immunology 1987;138:635–640.

4. Kloke O, Wandl U, Moritz T, et al. A prospective randomized comparison of single-agent interferon (IFN)-alpha with the combination of IFN-alpha and low-dose IFN-gamma in chronic myelogenous leukemia. Eur J Haematol 1992;48:93–98.

5. Talpaz M, Kurzrock R, Kantarjian H, et al. A Phase II Study Alternating Alpha-2a-Interferon and Gamma-Interferon Therapy in Patients with Chronic Myelogenous Leukemia. Cancer 1991; 68:2125–2130.

6. Janson E, Kauppinen H-L, Oberg K. Combined Alpha- and Gamma-Interferon Therapy for Malignant Midgut Carcinoid Tumors. Acta Oncologica 1993;32(2):231–233.

7. Ozzello L, Habif D, De Rosa C, Cantell K. Cellular Events Accompanying Regression of Skin Recurrences of Breast Carcinomas Treated with Intralesional Injections of Natural Interferons alpha and gamma. Cancer Res 1992;52:4571–4581.

8. Grem J, McAtee N, Murphy R, et al. A Pilot Study of gamma-Interferon in Combination with Fluorouracil, Leucovorin, and alpha-2a-Interferon. Clin Cancer Res 1997;3:1125–1134.

9. Foon K, Doroshow J, Bonnem E, et al. A prospective randomized trial of alpha-2B-interferon/ gamma-interferon or the combination in advanced metastatic renal cell cancer. J Biolog Res Modifiers 1988;7(540–545).

10. De Mulder P, Oosteroff G, Bouffioux C, van OOsterom A, Vermeylen K, Sylvester R. EORTC (30885) randomised phase III study with recombinant interferon alpha and gamma in patients with advanced renal cell carcinoma. British Journal of Cancer 1995;71:371–375.

11. De Mulder P, Debruyne FMJ, Franssen M, et al. Phase I/II study of recombinant interferon alpha and gamma in advanced progressive renal cell carcinoma. Cancer Immunol Immunother 1990;31: 321–324.

12. Dutcher J, Fine J, Krigel R, et al. Stratification by Risk Factors Predicts Survival on the Active Treatment Arm in a Randomized Phase II Study of Interferon-gamma Plus/Minus Interferon-alpha in Advanced Renal Cell Carcinoma (E6890). Medical Oncology 2003;20(3):271–281.

13. Kramer G, Steiner GE, Sokol P, et al. Local Intratumoral Tumor Necrosis Factor-alpha and Systemic IFN-alpha 2b in Patients with Locally Advanced Prostate Cancer. Journal of Interferon and Cytokine Research 2001;21:475–484.

14. Van Mooreselaar RJ, Hendriks BT, Van Stratum P, Van Der Melde PH, Debruyne FMJ, Schalken JA. Synergistic antitumor effects of rat gamma interferon and human tumor necrosis factor alpha against androgen dependent and independent rat prostatic tumors. Cancer Res 1991;51:2329–2334.

15. Smith JW, Urba WJ, Clark JW, et al. Phase I Evaluation of Recombinant Tumor Necrosis Factor Given in Combination with Recombinant Interferon-gamma. Journal of Immunotherapy 1991;10: 355–362.

16. Schiller JH, Witt PL, Storer B, et al. Clinical and Biologic Effects of Combination Therapy with Gamma-Interferon and Tumor Necrosis Factor. Cancer 1992;69(2):562–571.

17. Lienard D, Lejeune F, Ewalenko I. In transit metastases of malignant melanoma treated by high dose rTNF-alpha in combination with interferon-gamma and melphalan in isolation perfusion. World Journal of Surgery 1992;16:234–240.

18. Fraker DL, Alexander HR, Andrich M, Rosenberg SA. Treatment of patients with melanoma of the extremity using hyperthermic isolated limb perfusion with melphalan, tumor necrosis factor, and interferon gamma: Results of a tumor necrosis factor dose-escalation study. J Clin Oncol 1996;14(2):479–489.

19. Olieman A, Lienard D, Eggermont A, et al. Hyperthermic isolated limb pefusion with tumor necrosis factor alpha, interferon gamma, and melphalan for locally advanced nonmelanoma skin tumors of the extremities. Arch Surg 1999;134:303–307.

20. Karpoff H, D'Angelica M, Blair S. Prevention of hepatic metastases in rats with herpes viral vaccines and gamma-interferon. J Clin Invest 1997;99:799–804.

21. Reinisch W, Holub M, Katz A, et al. Prospective Pilot Study of Recombinant Granulocyte-Macrophage Colony-Stimulating Factor and Interferon-gamma in Patients with Inoperable Hepatocellular Carcinoma. Journal of Immunotherapy 2002;25(6):489–499.

22. Lummen G, Sperling H, Luboldt H, Otto T, Rubben H. Granulocyte-Macrophage Colony-Stimulating Factor and Interferon-Alpha 2B in Patients with Advanced Renal Cell Carcinoma. Int Urology 1998;61:215–219.

23. O'Donnell R, Dea G, Meyers F. A Phase II Trial of Concomitant Interferon-alpha-2b and Granulocyte-Macrophage Colony-Stimulating Factor in Patients with Advanced Renal Cell Cancer. Journal of Immunotherapy 1995;17:58–61.

24. Shapiro J, Harold N, Takimoto C, et al. A Pilot Study of Interferon-alpha-2a, Fluoruracil, and Leucovorin Given with Granulocyte-Macrophage Colony Stimulating Factor in Advanced Gastrointestinal Adenocarcinoma. Clin Cancer Res 1999;5:2399–2408.

25. Krown S, Paredes J, Bundow D, Polsky B, Gold J, Flomenberg N. Interferon-alpha, Zidovudine, and Granulocyte-Macrophage Colony-Stimulating Factor: A Phase I AIDS Clinical Trials Group Study in Patients with Kaposi's Sarcoma Associated with AIDS. Journal of Clinical Oncology 1992; 10(8):1344–1351.

26. Yang S, Grimm E, Parkinson D, et al. Clinical and Immunomodulatory Effects of Combination Immunotherapy with Low-Dose Interleukin 2 and Tumor Necrosis Factor alpha in Patients with Advanced Non-Small Cell Lung Cancer: A Phase I Trial. Cancer Research 1991;51:3669–3676.

27. Schiller JH, Morgan-Ihrig C, Levitt M. Concomitant Aministration of Interleukin-2 Plus Tumor Necrosis Factor in Advanced Non-Small Cell Lung Cancer. American Journal of Clinical Oncology 1995;18(1):47–51.

28. Krigel R, Padavic-Schaller K, Toomey C, Comis R, Weiner L. Phase I study of sequentially administered recombinant tumor necrosis factor and recombinant interleukin-2. J Immunother 1995;17: 161–170.

29. Krigel R, Padavic-Schaller K, Rudolph A, Konrad M, Bradley E, Comis R. Renal cell carcinoma: Treatment with recombinant interleukin-2 plus beta-interferon. J Clin Oncol 1990;8(3):460–467.

30. Duggan D, Santarelli M, Zamkoff K, et al. A phase ii study of recombinant interleukin-2 with or without recombinant interferon-beta in non-Hodgkin's lymphoma. a study of the cancer and leukemia group B. J Immunother 1992;12:115–122.

31. Tester W, Kim K, Krigel R, et al. A randomized Phase II study of interleukin-2 with and without beta-interferon for patients with advanced non-small cell lung cancer. An Eastern Cooperative Oncology Group study (PZ586). Lung Cancer 1999;25:199–206.

32. Brunda M, Luistro L, Warrier T. Antitumor and antimetastatic activity of interleukin 12 against murine tumors. J Exp Med 1993;178:1223–1230.

33. Nastala C, Edington H, McKinney T. Recombinant IL-12 administration induces tumor regression in association with IFN-gamma production. J Immunol 1994;153:1697–1706.

34. Gollob J, Veenstra K, Parker R, et al. Phase I trial of concurrent twice-weekly recombinant human interleukin-12 plus low-dose il-2 in patients with melanoma or renal cell cancer. J Clin Oncol 2003;21(13):2564–2573.

35. Santoli D, Clark S, Kreider B, Maslin P, Rovera G. Amplification of IL-2-driven T cell proliferation by recombinant IL-3 and granulocyte-macrophage colony-stimulating factor. J Immunol 1988;141:519–526.

36. Schiller JH, Hank J, Khorsand M, et al. Clinical and immunological effects of granulocyte-macrophage colony-stimulating factor coadministered with interleukin-2: A phase IB study. Clin Cancer Res 1996;2:319–330.

37. Ryan C, Vogelzang N, Dumas M, Kuzel T, Stadler W. Granulocyte-macrophage-colony-stimulating factor in combination immunotherapy for patients with metastatic renal cell carcinoma. Cancer 2000; 88:1317–1324.

38. Smith JW, Kurt R, Baher A, et al. Immune effects of escalating doses of granulocyte-macrophage colony-stimulating factor added to a fixed, low-dose, inpatient interleukin-2 regimen: a randomized phase I trial in patients with metastatic melanoma and renal cell carcinoma. Journal of Immunotherapy 2003;26(2):130–138.

39. O'Day S, Boasberg P, Piro L, et al. Maintenance biotherapy for metastatic melanoma with interleukin-2 and granulocyte macrophage-colony stimulating factor improves survival for patients responding to induction concurrent biochemotherapy. Clin Cancer Res 2002;8:2775–2781.

40. Ridolfi L, Ridolfi R, Ascari-Raccagni A, et al. Intralesional GM-CSF followed by subcutaneous IL2 in metastatic melanoma. Journal of the European Academy of Dermatology and Venereology 2001; 15:218-23.

41. Kiertscher S, Roth M. Human CD14+ leukocytes acquire the phenotype and function of antigen-presenting dendritic cells when cultured in GM-CSF and IL-4. J Leukocyte Biol 1996;59:208–218.

42. Kiertscher S, Gitlitz B, Figlin R, Roth J. Granulocyte/macrophage-colony stimulating factor and interleukin-4 expand and activate type-1 dendritic cells (dc1) when administered in vivo to cancer patients. Int J Cancer 2003;107:256–261.

43. Gitlitz B, Figlin R, Kiertscher S, Moldawer N, Rosen F, Roth J. Phase I trial of granulocyte macrophage colony-stimulating factor and interleukin-4 as combined immunotherapy for patients with cancer. J Immunother 2003;26(2):171–178.

44. Tate J, Olencki T, Finke J, Kottke-Marchant K, Rybicki L, Bukowski R. Phase I trial of simultaneously administered GM-CSF and IL-6 in patients with renal-cell carcinoma: Clinical and laboratory effects. Ann Oncol 2001;12:655–659.

45. Hochster H, Speyer J, Mandeli J, et al. A phase II double-blind randomized study of the simultaneous administration of recombinant human interleukin-6 and recombinant human granulocyte colony-stimulating factor following paclitaxel and carboplatin chemotherapy in patients with advanced epithelial ovarian cancer. Gyn Onc 1999;72:292–297.

46. Bracho F, Krailo M, Shen V, et al. A phase I clinical, pharmacological, and biological trial of interleukin 6 plus granulocyte-colony stimulating factor after ifosfamide, carboplatin, and etoiposide in children with recurrent/refractory solid tumors: Enhanced hematological responses but a high incidence of grade III/IV constitutional toxicities. Clin Cancer Res 2001;7:58–67.

47. Kawakami Y, Rosenberg SA, Lotze M. Interleukin-4 promotes the growth of tumor-infiltrating lymphocytes cytotoxic form human autologous melanoma. Journal of Experimental Medicine 1988;168: 2183–2191.

48. Higuichi C, Thompson J, CG L. Induction of lymphokine-activated killer activity by interleukin-4 in human lymphocytes preactivated by interleukin-2 in vivo and in vitro. Cancer Res 1989;49: 6487–6492.

49. Sosman J, Fisher S, Kefer C, Fisher R, Ellis T. A phase I trial of continuous infusion interleukin-4 (IL-4) alone and following interleukin-2 (IL-2) in cancer patients. Annals of Oncology 1994;5: 447–452.

50. Sosman J, Bartemes K, Offord K, et al. Evidence for eosinophil activation in cancer patients receiving recombinant interleukin-4: Effects of interleukin-4 alone and following interleukin-2 administration. Clin Cancer Res 1995;1:805–812.

51. Whitehead R, Friedman K, Clark D, Pagani K, Rapp L. Phase I trial of simultaneous administration of interleukin-2 and interleukin-4 subcutaneously. Clin Cancer Res 1995;1:1145–1152.

52. Olencki T, Finke J, Tubbs R, et al. Immunomodulatory effects of interleukin-2 and interleukin-4 in patients with malignancy. J Immunother 1996;19(1):69–80.

53. Blay J, Pallardy M, Ravaud A. Serum VEGF is an independent prognostic factor in patients with metastatic renal cell carcinoma, treated with IL2 and/or IFN: Analysis of the Crecy trial. Proc Am Ass Clin Oncol 1997;18:1669 (abstract).

54. Lissoni P, Rovelli F, Baiocco N, Tangini G, Fumagalli L. A Phase II study of subcutaneous low-dose interleukin-2 plus erythropoietin in metastatic renal cell carcinoma progressing on interleukin-2 alone. Anticancer Res 2001;21:777–780.

55. Iogo M, Sakurai M, Tamura T. In vivo antitumor activity of multiple injections of recombinant interleukin 2, alone and in combination with three different types of recombinant interferon, on various syngeneic murine tumors. Cancer Res 1988;48:260–264.

56. Rosenberg SA, Schwartz S, Spiess P. Combination immunotherapy for cancer: Synergistic antitumor interactions of interleukin-2, alfa interferon, and tumor-infiltrating lymphocytes. J Natl Cancer Inst 1988;80:1393–1397.

57. Cameron R, McIntosh J, Rosenberg S. Synergistic antitumor effects of combination immunotherapy with recombinant interleukin-2and a recombinant hybrid alpha-interferon in the treatment of established murine hepatic metastases. Cancer Res 1988;48:5810–5817.

58. Rosenberg SA, Lotze M, Yang J, et al. Combination therapy with interleukin-2 and alpha-interferon for the treatment of patients with advanced cancer. J Clin Oncol 1989;7(12):1863–1874.

59. Marincola F, White D, Wise A, Rosenberg SA. Combination therapy with interferon alpha-2a and interleukin-2 for the treatment of metastatic cancer. J Clin Oncol 1995;13(5):1110–1122.

60. Huberman M, Bering H, Fallon B, et al. A phase I study of an outpatient regimen of recombinant human interleukin-2 and alpha-2a-interferon in patients with solid tumors. Cancer 1991;68:1708–1713.

61. Ratain M, Priest E, Janisch L, Vogelzang N. A phase I study of subcutaneous recombinant interleukin-2 and interferon alfa-2a. Cancer 1992;71:2371–2376.

62. Rosso R, Sertoli M, Queirolo P, et al. An outpatient phase I study of a subcutaneous interleukin-2 and intramuscular alpha-2a-interferon combination in advanced malignancies. Ann Oncol 1992;3: 559–563.

63. Budd G, Murthy S, Finke J, et al. Phase I trial of high-dose bolus interleukin-2 and interferon alfa-2a in patients with metastatic malignancy. J Clin Oncol 1992;10(5):804–809.

64. Schiller JH, Hank J, Storer B, et al. A direct comparison of immunological and clinical effects of interleukin 2 with a without interferon-alpha in humans. Cancer Res 1993;53:1286–1292.

65. Gause B, Sznol M, Kapp W, et al. Phase I study of subcutaneously administered interleukin-2 in combination with interferon alfa-2a in patients with advanced cancer. J Clin Oncol 1996;14(8):2234–2241.
66. Atzpodien J, Kirchner H, Jonas U, et al. Interleukin-2 and interferon alfa-2a-based immunochemotherapy in advanced renal cell carcinoma: A prospectively randomized trial of the german cooperative renal carcinoma chemoimmunotherapy group. J Clin Oncol 2004;22(7):1188–1194.
67. Vogelzang N, Lipton A, Figlin R. Subcutaneous interleukin-2 plus interferon alfa-2a in metastatic renal cancer: An outpatient multicenter trial. J Clin Oncol 1993;11(9):1809–1816.
68. Atkins M, Sparano J, Fisher R, et al. Randomized phase II trial of high-dose interleukin-2 either alone or in combination with interferon alfa-2b in advanced renal cell carcinoma. J Clin Oncol 1993; 11(4):661–670.
69. Stadler W, Kuzel T, Dumas M, Vogelzang N. Multicenter phase II trial of interleukin-2, interferon-alpha, and 13-cis-retinoic acid in patients with metastatic renal-cell carcinoma. J Clin Oncol 1998; 16(5):1820–1825.
70. Tourani J-M, Pfister C, Berdah J-F. Outpatient treatment with subcutaneous interleukin-2 and interferon alfa administration in combination with fluorouracil in patients with metastatic renal cell carcinoma: Results of a sequential nonrandomized phase II study. J Clin Oncol 1998;16(7):2505–2513.
71. Figlin R, Belldegrun A, Moldawer N, Zeffren J, deKernion J. Concomitant administration of recombinant human interleukin-2 and recombinant interferon alfa-2a: An active outpatient regimen in metastatic renal cell carcinoma. J Clin Oncol 1992;10(3):414–421.
72. Facendola G, Locatelli M, Pizzocaro G, et al. Subcutaneous administration of interleukin 2 and interferonj-alpha-2b in advanced renal cell carcinoma: A confirmatory study. Br J Cancer 1995;72(6): 1531–1535.
73. Ravaud A, Negrier S, Cany L, et al. Subcutaneous low-dose recombinant interleukin 2 and alpha-interferon in patients with metastatic renal cell carcinoma. Br J Cancer 1994;69:1111–1114.
74. Ravaud A, Audhuy B, Gomez F, et al. Subcutaneous interleukin-2, interferon alfa-2a, and continuous infusion of fluorouracil in metastatic renal cell carcinoma: A multicenter phase II trial. J Clin Oncol 1998;16(8):2728–2732.
75. Jayson G, Middleton M, Lee S, Ashcroft L, Thatcher N. A randomized phase II trial of interleukin 2 and interleukin 2-interferon alpha in advanced renal cancer. Br J Cancer 1998;78(3):366–369.
76. Naglieri E, Lopez M, Lelli G, et al. Interleukin-2, interferon-alpha, and medroxyprogesterone acetate in metastatic renal cell carcinoma. Anticancer Res 2002;22:3045–3052.
77. Mittelman A, Puccio C, Ahmed T, Zeffren J, Choudhury A, Arlin Z. A phase II trial of interleukin-2 by continuous infusion and interferon by intramuscular injection in patients with renal cell cancer. Cancer 1991;68:1699–1702.
78. Canobbio L, Curotto A, Cannata D, et al. Combination therapy with subcutaneous interleukin-2 and interferon-alpha in advanced renal cancer patients with poor prognostic factors. Anticancer Res 1996;16:541–544.
79. Ellerhorst J, Sella A, Amato R, et al. Phase II trial of 5-fluorouracil, interferon-alpha and conmtinuous infusion interleukin-2 for patients with metastatic renal cell carcinoma. Cancer 1997;80:128–132.
80. Bergmann L, Fenchel K, Weidmann E, et al. Daily alternating administration of high-dose alpha-2b-interferon and interleukin-2 bolus infusion in metastatic renal cell cancer. Cancer 1993;72(5): 1734–1742.
81. Ravaud A, Delva R, Gomez F, et al. Subcutaneous interleukin-2 and interferon alpha in the treatment of patients with metastatic renal cell carcinoma—less efficacy compared with intravenous interleukin-2 and interferon alpha. Cancer 2002;95:2324–2330.
82. Atzpodien J, Hoffmann R, Franzke M, Stief C, Wandert T, Reitz M. Thirteen-year, long-term efficacy of interferon 2alpha and interleukin 2-based home therapy in patients with advanced renal cell carcinoma. Cancer 2002;95:1045–1050.
83. Ryan C, Vogelzang N, Stadler W. A phase II trial of intravenous gemcitabine and 5-fluorouracil with subcutaneous interleukin-2 and interferon-alpha in patients with metastatic renal cell carcinoma. Cancer 2002;94:2602–2609.
84. Buzio C, Andrulli S, Santi R, et al. Long-term immunotherapy with low-dose interleukin-2 and interferon-alpha in the treatment of patients with advanced renal cell carcinoma. Cancer 2001;92: 2286–2296.
85. Elias L, Lew D, Figlin R, et al. Infusional interleukin-2 and 5-fluorouracil with subcutaneous interferon-alpha in the treatment of patients with advanced renal cell carcinoma. Cancer 2000;89: 597–603.

86. Gez E, Rubinov R, Gaitini D, et al. Interleukin-2, interferon-alpha, 5-fluorouracil, and vinblastine in the treatment of metastatic renal cell carcinoma. Cancer 2002;95:1644–1649.
87. Piga A, Giordani P, Quattrone A, et al. A phase II study of interferon alpha and low-dose interleukin-2 in advanced renal cell carcinoma. Cancer Immunol Immunother 1997;44:348–351.
88. Rogers E, Bredin H, Butler M, et al. Combined subcutaneous recombinant alpha-interferon and interleukin-2 in metastatic renal cell cancer: Results of the Multicentre All Ireland Immunotherapy Study Group. European Urol 2000;37:261–266.
89. Fossa S, Aune H, Baggerud E, Granerud T, Heilo A, Theodorsen L. Continuous intravenous interleukin-2 infusion and subcutaneous interferon-alpha in metastatic renal cell carcinoma. Eur J Cancer 1993;29A(9):1313–1315.
90. Besana C, Borri A, Bucci E, et al. Treatment of advanced renal cell cancer with sequential intravenous recombinant interleukin-2 and subcutaneous alpha-interferon. Eur J Cancer 1994;30A(9):1292–1298.
91. Pectasides D, Vartalitis J, Kostopoulou M, et al. An outpatient phase ii study of subcutaneous interleukin-2 and interferon-alpha-2b in combination with intravenous vinblastine in metastatic renal cell cancer. Oncology 1998;55:10–15.
92. Lissoni P, Barni S, Ardizzola A, et al. A randomized study of low-dose interleukin-2 subcutaneous immunotherapy versus interleukin-2 plus interferon-alpha as first-line threapy for metastatic renal cell carcinoma. Tumori 1993;79:397–400.
93. Boccardo F, Rubagotti A, Canobbio L, et al. Interleukin-2, interferon-alpha and interleukin-2 plus interferon-alpha in renal cell carcinoma. a randomized phase II trial. Tumori 1998;84:534–539.
94. Lummen G, Goepel M, Mollhoff S, Hinke A, Otto T, Rubben H. Phase II study of interferon-gamma versus interleukin-2 and interferon-alpha2B in metastatic renal cell carcinoma. J Urol 1996;155:455–458.
95. Hofmockel G, Langer W, Theiss M, Gruss A, Frohmuller H. Immunochemotheapy for metastatic renal cell carcinoma using a regimen of interleukin-2, interferon-alpha, and 5-fluorouracil. J Urol 1996;156:18–21.
96. Clark J, Kuzel T, Lsetingi T, et al. A multi-institutional phase II trial of a novel inpatient schedule of continuous interleukin-2 with interferon alpha-2b in advanced renal cell carcinoma: Major durable responses in a less highly selected patient population. Ann Oncol 2002;13:606–613.
97. Atzpodien J, Kuchler T, Wandert T, Reitz M. Rapid deterioration in quality of life during interleukin-2 and alpha-interferon-based home therapy of renal cell carcinoma is assocaited with a good outcome. Br J Cancer 2003;89:50–54.
98. Tourani J-M, Pfister C, Tubiana N, et al. Subcutaneous interleukin-2 and interferon alfa administration in patients with metastatic renal cell carcinoma: Final results of SCAPP III, a large, multicenter, phase II, nonrandomized study with sequential analysis design—The subcutaneous administration propeukin Program Cooperative Group. J Clin Oncol 2003;21(21):3987–3994.
99. Rathmell W, Malkowicz S, Holroyde C, Luginbuhl W, Vaughn D. Phase II trial of 5-fluorouracil and leucovorin in combination with interferon-alpha and interleukin-2 for advanced renal cell cancer. Am J Clin Oncol 2004;27:109–112.
100. Ravaud A, Trufflandier N, Ferriere J, et al. Subcutaneous interleukin-2, interferon-alpha-2b and 5-fluorouracil in metastatic renal cell carcinoma as second-line treatment after failure of previous immunotherapy: A phase II trial. Br J Cancer 2003;89:2213–2218.
101. Neri B, Doni L, Gemelli M, et al. Phase II trial of weekly intravenous gemcitabine administration with interferon and interleukin-2 immunotherapy for metastatic renal cell cancer. J Urol 2002;168:956–958.
102. Atzpodien J, Kirchner H, Illiger H, et al. IL-2 in combination with IFN-alpha and 5-FU versus tamoxifen in metastatic renal cell carcinoma: Long-term results of a controlled randomized clinical trial. Br J Cancer 2001;85(8):1130–1136.
103. Clark J, Gaynor E, Martone B, et al. Daily subcutaneous ultra-low-dose interleukin 2 with daily low-dose interferon-alpha in patients with advanced renal cell carcinoma. Clin Cancer Res 1999;5:2374–2380.
104. Dutcher J, Logan T, Gordon M, et al. Phase II trial of interleukin-2, interferon alpha, and 5-fluorouracil in metastatic renal cell cancer: A cytokine working group study. Clin Cancer Res 2000;6:3442–3450.
105. Allen M, Vaughan M, Webb A, et al. Protracted venous infusion 5-fluorouracil in combination with subcutaneous interleukin-2 and alpha-interferon in patients with metastatic renal cell cancer. Br J Cancer 2000;83(8):980–985.

106. Negrier S, Caty A, Lesimple T, et al. Treatment of patients with metastatic renal cell carcinoma with a combination of subcutaneous interleukin-2 and interferon alfa with or without fluorouracil. J Clin Oncol 2000;18(24):4009–4015.

107. van Herpen C, Jansen R, Kruit W, et al. Immunochemotherapy with interleukin-2, interferon-alpha and 5-fluorouracil for progressive metastatic renal cell carcinoma: A multicenter phase II study. Br J Cancer 2000;82(4):772–776.

108. Atzpodien J, Kirchner H, Hanninen E, Deckert M, Fenner M, Poliwada H. Interleukin-2 in combination with interferon-alpha and 5-fluorouracil for metastatic renal cell cancer. Eur J Cancer 1993;29A:S6–8.

109. Whitehead R, Figlin R, Citron M, et al. A phase II trial of concomitant human interleukin-2 and interferon-alpha-2a in patients with disseminated malignant melanoma. J Immunother 1993;13:117–121.

110. Richards J, Mehta N, Ramming K, Skosey P. Sequential chemoimmunotherapy in the treatment of metastatic melanoma. J Clin Oncol 1992;10(8):1338–1343.

111. Khayat D, Borel C, Tourani J-M, et al. Sequential chemoimmunotherapy with cisplatin, interleukin-2, and interferon alfa-2a for metastatic melanoma. J Clin Oncol 1993;11(11):2173–2180.

112. Keilholz U, Scheibenbogen C, Tilgen W, et al. Interferon-alpha and interleukin-2 in the treatment of metastatic melanoma. Cancer 1993;72:607–614.

113. Kruit W, Goey S, Calabresi F, et al. Final report of a phase II study of interleukin 2 and interferon alpha with metastatic melanoma. Br J Cancer 1995;71:1319–1321.

114. Eton O, Talpaz M, Lee K, Rothberg J, Brell J, Benjamin R. Phase II trial of recombinant human interleukin-2 and interferon-alpha-2a. Cancer 1995;77:893–899.

115. Atzpodien J, Hanninen E, Kirchner H, et al. Chemoimmunotherapy of advanced malignant melanoma: Sequential administration of subcutaneous interleukin-2 and interferon-alpha after intravenous dacarbazine and carboplatinor intravenous dacarbazine, cisplatin, carmustine, and tamoxifen. Eur J Cancer 1995;31A(6):876–881.

116. Proebstle T, Scheibenbogen C, Sterry W, Keilholz U. A phase ii study of dacarbazine, cisplatin, interferon-alpha and high-dose interleukin-2 in 'poor-risk' metastatic melanoma. Eur J Cancer 1996;32A(9):1530–1533.

117. Legha S, Ring S, Bedikian A, et al. Treatment of metastatic melanoma with combined chemotherapy containing cisplatin, vinblastine and dacarbazine (CVD) and biotherapy using interleukin-2 and interferon-alpha. Ann Oncol 1996;7(8):827–835.

118. Eton O, Buzaid A, Bedikian A, et al. A phase II study of "decrescendo" interleukin-2 plus interferon-alpha-2a in patients with progressive metastatic melanoma after chemotherapy. Cancer 1999;88:1703–1709.

119. Richards J, Gale D, Mehta N, Lestigni T. Combination of chemotherapy with interleukin-2 and interferon alfa for the treatment of metastatic melanoma. J Clin Oncol 1999;17(2):651–657.

120. McDermott D, Mier J, Lawrence D, et al. A phase II pilot trial of concurrent biochemotherapy with cisplatin, vinblastine, dacarbazine, interleukin 2, and interferon alpha-2B in patients with metastatic melanoma. Clin Cancer Res 2000;6:2201–2208.

121. Flaherty L, Atkins M, Sosman J, et al. Outpatient biochemotherapy with interleukin-2 and interferon alfa-2b in patients with metastatic malignant melanoma: Results of two phase II cytokine working group trials. J Clin Oncol 2001;19(13):3194–3202.

122. Donskov F, von der Maase H, Henriksson R, et al. Outpatient treatment with subcutaneous histamine dihydrochloride in combination with interleukin-2 and interferon-alpha in patients with metastatic renal cell carcinoma: Results of an open single-armed multicentre phase II study. Ann Oncol 2002;13:441–449.

123. Schmidt H, Larsen S, Bastholt L, Fode K, Rytter C, von der Maase H. A phase II study of outpatient subcutaneous histamine dihydrochloride, interleukin-2 and interferon-alpha in patients with metastatic melanoma. Ann Oncol 2002;13:1919–1924.

124. Hauschild A, Weichenthal M, Balda B, et al. Prospective randomized trial of interferon alfa-2b and interleukin-2 as adjuvant treatment for resected intermediate- and high-risk primary melanoma without clinically detectable node metastasis. J Clin Oncol 2003;21(15):2883–2888.

125. Atkins M, Gollob J, Sosman J, et al. A phase II pilot trial of concurrent biochemotherapy with cisplatin, vinblastine, temozolomide, interleukin 2, and IFN-alpha 2B in patients with metastatic melanoma. Clin Cancer Res 2002;8:3075–3081.

126. Negrier S, Escudier B, Lasset C, et al. Recombinant human interleukin-2, recombinant human interferon alfa-2a, or both in metastatic renal-cell carcinoma. New Engl J Med 1998;338:1272–1278.

127. Sparano J, Fisher R, Sunderland M, et al. Randomized phase III trial of treatment with high-dose interleukin-2 either alone or in combination with interferon alfa-2a in patients with advanced melanoma. J Clin Oncol 1993;11(10):1969–1977.

128. Rosenberg SA, Yang J, Schwartzentruber J, et al. Prospective randomized trial of the treatment of patients with metastatic melanoma using chemotherapy with cisplatin, dacarbazine, and tamoxifen alone or in combination with interleukin-2 and interferon alfa-2b. J Clin Oncol 1999;17(3):968–975.

129. Hauschild A, Garbe C, Stolz W, et al. Dacarbazine and interferon-alpha with or without interleukin-2 in metastatic melanoma: A randomized phase III multicentre trial of the Dermatologic Cooperative Oncology Group (DeCOG). Br J Cancer 2001;84(8):1036–1042.

130. Atzpodien J, Neuber K, Kamanabrou D, et al. Combination chemotherapy with or without s.c. IL-2 and IFN-alpha: Results of a prospectively randomized trial of the Cooperative Advanced Malignant Melanoma Chemoimmunotherapy Group (ACIMM). Br J Cancer 2002;86:179–184.

131. Dorval T, Negrier S, Chevreau C, et al. Randomized trial of treatment with cisplatin and interleukin-2 either alone or in combination with interferon-alpha-2a in patients with metastatic melanoma: A Federation Nationale des Centres de Lutte Contre le Cancer Multicenter, parallel study. Cancer 1998;85:1060–1066.

132. Ridolfi R, Chiarion-Sileni V, Guida M, et al. Cisplatin, dacarbazine with or without subcutaneous interleukin-2, and interferon alpha-2b in advanced melanoma outpatients: Results from an Italian multicenter phase III randomized clinical trial. J Clin Oncol 2002;20(6):1600–1607.

133. Tummarello D, Graziano F, Isidori P, et al. Consolidation biochemotherapy for patients with advanced nonsmall cell lung carcinoma responding to induction PVM (cisplatin, vinblastine, mitomycin-C) regimen. A phase II study. Cancer 1996;77:2251–2257.

134. Jansen R, Slingerland R, Hoo Goey S, Franks C, Bolhuis R, Stoter G. Interleukin-2 and interferon-alpha in the treatment of patients with advanced non-small-cell lung cancer. J Immunother 1992;12:70–73.

135. Atzpodien J, Kirchner H, Hanninen E, et al. Treatment of metastatic colorectal cancer patients with 5-fluorouracil in combination with recombinant subcutaneous human interleukin-2 and alpha-interferon. Oncology 1994;51:273–275.

136. Chang A, Cameron M, Sondak V, Geiger J, Vander Woude D. A phase II trial of interleukin-2 and interferon-alpha in the treatment of metastatic colorectal carcinoma. J Immunother 1996;18(4):253–262.

137. Walters R, Theriault R, Holmes F, Esparza L, Hortobagyi G. Phase II study of recombinant alpha-interferon and recombinant interleukin-2 metastatic breast cancer. J Immunother 1994;16:303–305.

138. Kimmick G, Ratain M, Berry D, Woolf S, Norton L, Muss H. Subcutaneously administered recombinant human interleukin-2 and interferon alfa-2a for advanced breast cancer: A phase II study of the Cancer and Leukemia Group B (CALGB 9041). Invest New Drugs 2004;22:83–89.

139. Urba S, Forastiere A, Wolf G, Amrein P. Intensive recombinant interleukin-2 and alpha-interferon therapy in patients with advanced head and neck squamous carcinoma. Cancer 1993;71:2326–2331.

140. Eskander E, Harvey H, Givant E, Lipton A. Phase I study combining tumor necrosis factor with interferon-alpha and interleukin-2. Am J Clin Oncol 1997;20(5):511–514.

141. Itoh K, Shiiba K. Generation of activated killer (AK) cells by recombinant interleukin-2 (rIL-2) in collaboration with interferon-gamma (IFN-gamma). J Immunol 1985;134:3124–3129.

142. Weiner L, Padavic-Schaller K, Kitson J, Watts P, Krigel R, Litwin S. Phase I evaluation of combination therapy with interleukin-2 and gamma-interferon. Cancer Res 1991;51:3910–3918.

143. Taylor C, Chase E, Whitehead R, et al. A Southwest Oncology Group phase I study of the sequential combination of recombinant interferon-gamma and recombinant interleukin-2 in patients with cancer. J Immunother 1992;11:176–183.

144. Margolin K, Doroshow J, Akman S, et al. Phase I study of interleukin-2 plus interferon-gamma. J Immunother 1992;11:50–55.

145. Baars J, Wagstaff J, Boven E, et al. Phase I study on the sequential administration of recombinant human interferon-gamma and recombinant human interleukin-2 in patients with metastatic solid tumors. J Natl Cancer Inst 1991;83(19):1408–1410.

146. Reddy S, Harwood R, Moore D, Grimm E, Murray J, Vadhan-Raj S. Recombinant interleukin-2 in combination with recombinant interferon-gamma in patients with advanced malignancy: A phase I study. J Immunother 1997;20(1):79–87.

147. Escudier B, Farace F, Angevin E, et al. Combination of interleukin-2 and gamma-interferon in metastatic renal cell carcinoma. Eur J Cancer 1993;29A(5):724–728.

148. Schmidinger M, Steger G, Wenzel C, et al. Sequential administration of interferon-gamma and inter-leukin-2 in metastatic renal cell carcinoma: Results of a phase II trial. Cancer Immunol Immunother 2000;49:395–400.

149. Schmidinger M, Steger G, Wenzel C, et al. Sequential administration of interferon-gamma, gm-csf, and interleukin-2 in patients with metastatic renal cell carcinoma: Results of a phase II trial. J Immunother 2001;24(3):257–262.

150. de Gast G, Klumpen H, Vyth-Dreese F, et al. Phase I Trial of combined immunotherapy with subcu-taneous granulocyte macrophage colony-stimulating factor, low-dose interleukin 2, and interferon alpha in progressive metastatic melanoma and renal cell carcinoma. Clin Cancer Res 2000;6: 1267–1272.

151. Westermann J, Reich G, Kopp J, Haus U, Dorken B, Pezzutto A. Granulocyte/macrophage-colony-stimulating-factor plus interleukin-2 plus interferon-alpha in the treatment of metastatic renal cell car-cinoma: A pilot study. Cancer Immunol Immunother 2001;49:613–620.

152. Verra N, Jansen R, Groenewegen G, et al. Immunotherapy with concurrent subcutaneous GM-CSF, low-dose IL2 and IFN-alpha in patients with progressive metastatic renal cell carcinoma. Br J Cancer 2003;88:1346–1351.

153. Vaughan M, Moore J, Riches P, et al. GM-CSF with biochemotherapy (cisplatin, DTIC, tamoxifen, IL-2 and interferon-alpha): A phase I trial in melanoma. Annals of Oncology 2000;11:1183–1189.

154. Groenewegen G, Bloem A, de Gast G. Phase I/II study of sequential chemoimmunotherapy (SCIT) for metastatic melanoma: Outpatient treatment with dacarbazine, granulocyte-macrophage colony-stimulating factor, low-dose interleukin-2, and interferon-alpha. Cancer Immunol Immunother 2002;51:630–636.

155. Takeda K, Tsutsui H, Yoshimoto T, et al. Defective NK cell activity and Th1 response in IL-18-defi-cient mice. Immunity 1998;8(3):383–390.

156. Moroz A, Eppolito C, Li Q, Tao J, Clegg C, Shrikant P. IL-21 enhances and sustains CD8+ T cell responses to achieve durable tumor immunity: Comparative evaluation of IL-2, IL-15, and IL-21. J Immunol 2004;173(2):900–909.

157. Maruyama S, Yagita A, Sukegawa Y. Significance of gefitinib combined with immunotherapy in tumor-bearing mice (in Japanese). Gan To Kagaku Ryoho 2003;30(11):1773–1775.

158. Rini B, Halabi S, Taylor J, Small E, RL S. Cancer and Leukemia Group B 90206: A randomized phase III trial of interferon-alpha or interferon-alpha plus anti-vascular endothelial growth factor anti-body (bevacizumab) in metastatic renal cell carcinoma. Clin Cancer Res 2004;10(8):2584–2586.

21 Novel Strategies for Cytokine Administration Via Targetting

Paul M. Sondel, Jackie A. Hank,
Mark R. Albertini, and Stephen D. Gillies

CONTENTS

1. IMMUNOCYTOKINES

Immunocytokines (IC) are fusion proteins that use genetic linkage to fuse cytokines with immunologically reactive monoclonal antibodies (mAb) or components thereof. The goal is to retain the functions of both the cytokine and the antibody components in a single bifunctional molecule. As such, the functions of the antibody (long circulating half life, antigen specific binding, complement activation, interaction with Fc Receptors (FcRs) to induce antibody dependent cytotoxicity [ADCC]) are retained. In addition, the functions of the cytokine that are linked to the antibody (such as IL-2, IL-12, or IL-7), are also retained. The goal is to allow the biologic activities of one component of the IC (the antibody) to be expanded by colocalizing it with the biologic function of the other component of the IC (the cytokine). A few distinct immunocytokines have been created by EMD-Lexigen *(1–3)*, and by others *(4–7)*. These have used antibodies with some degree of selectivity for molecules expressed predominantly by tumors, and have been linked to different cytokines. The first IC to be described resulted from linking IL-2 to the 14.18 mAb that recognizes the GD2 disialoganglioside. Testing of this agent, and its derivatives, has moved forward in parallel with preclinical and clinical testing of other ICs (including the huKS-IL-2 IC that recognizes the epithelial cell adhesion molecule, which is overexpressed on many epithelial carcinomas).The purpose of this chapter is to summarize the preclinical testing of ICs, and a recently completed Phase I study, with an emphasis on recent data with the hu14.18-IL-2 IC. We also present a brief summary of preclinical data utilizing newer ICs being developed for future clinical testing.

From: *Cancer Drug Discovery and Development,*
Cytokines in the Genesis and Treatment of Cancer
Edited by: M. A. Caligiuri and M. T. Lotze © Humana Press Inc., Totowa, NJ

2. THE HU14.18-IL-2 IC

The hu14.18-IL-2 IC has human IL-2 linked to the heavy chains of the intact humanized anti-GD2 antibody, hu14.18. This IC binds to the GD2 disialoganglioside, expressed on human melanoma (MEL) and neuroblastoma (NBL), stimulates cells bearing IL-2 receptors (IL-2Rs) and (FcRs), and mediates potent antitumor activity in mice. This antitumor activity of hu14.18-IL-2 is observed when this IC is used alone, or when it is combined with other therapies. We have now completed the initial phase I clinical trials of hu14.18-IL-2 in patients with MEL and NBL. These trials document that hu14.18-IL-2 is clinically safe and tolerated at doses that induce immunologic activation.

3. BACKGROUND

3.1. IL-2 as an Enhancer of In Vivo ADCC

IL-2 is an anticancer therapeutic that activates immune cells to mediate antitumor effects (8–10) Patients (Pts) receiving IL-2 show a dose dependent activation of NK cells, which appear to be involved in antitumor activity (11). One way to potentially improve the antitumor efficacy of activated NK cells is to direct their lytic activity more selectively towards tumor cells, using a tumor reactive monoclonal antibody (mAb), through the process of ADCC (12,13). FcR bearing NK cells can mediate augmented ADCC of tumor cells if they are first activated with IL-2 (14). Mice receiving IL-2 plus tumor specific mAb show improved antitumor effects compared to animals treated with either agent alone (12–15). Only intact mAb, not Fab fragments, have been shown to induce ADCC in vitro or mediate antitumor effects in vivo (13). These results suggest that direct effector cell-tumor cell contact is involved in the antitumor mechanism and that it may be possible, with in vivo activation of effector cells by IL-2, to improve clinical antitumor effects of mAb treatment. As such, clinical trials of tumor reactive mAb given with IL-2 as a means to induce ADCC in vivo are underway in the treatment of several types of malignancy, including lymphoma, colon cancer, breast cancer, MEL, and NBL (16–19).

In vitro and in vivo preclinical studies show that greater ADCC can be obtained with mAb linked to IL-2, than is obtained with the same amount of mAb and IL-2 infused simultaneously as separate molecules (1,20,21). A potential mechanism is for the IC molecule to localize to the tumor cell owing to its recognition by the mAb component of the IC molecule. This would allow the NK cells to be activated by the IL-2 component of the IC molecule, and then mediate ADCC via FcRs on the NK cell that use the Fc component of the IC molecule. T-cells may also be activated by the IL-2 localized to the tumor site.

3.2. Anti-GD2 mAb Therapy

The GD2 disialoganglioside is expressed on tumors of neuroectodermal origin including MEL and NBL (22,23), but not on normal tissues other than certain neurons and melanocytes. MEL and NBL express GD2 with relatively little heterogeneity within tumors, with higher density expression seen on NBL than MEL (24,25). The 3F8 and 14.18 mAbs were the originally described murine anti-GD2 mAbs (22,23). Clinical testing has been performed with the 3F8 mAb, the murine IgG2a class switch variant of 14.18 (designated 14.G2a), and with the human-mouse chimeric variant of 14.18 (designated ch14.18) in children with NBL and adults with MEL (26–33). GD2 is not lost from the cell surface when bound to anti-GD2 mAb. Furthermore, GD2 is found in low concentrations in serum and is bound within lipoprotein complexes, thereby masking the circulating GD2 from recognition by anti-GD2 mAb *(22,33,34)*. This may explain why circulating GD2 in most patients has not interfered with antibody targeting in vivo, which typically achieves a high tumor to normal-tissue ratio, in patient studies *(35,36)*. In vitro, anti-GD2 antibodies can mediate substantial ADCC and complement-dependent cytotoxicity (CDC) against GD2$^+$ tumor target cells *(37,38)*.

Dose limiting toxicities (DLT) caused by these anti-GD2 mAbs include fever, chills, anaphylactoid reactions, and nausea, all felt to result from cytokine activation owing to infusion of heterologous immunoglobulin. The most characteristic DLT for anti-GD2 mAbs is transient neuropathic pain, owing to the recognition of GD2 on peripheral pain fibers by the mAb *(39,40)*. This pain is controllable with appropriate analgesics, including administration of narcotics *(39–42)*. Clinical antitumor effects seen in phase-I and -II trials of these anti-GD2 mAbs include shrinkage of measurable MEL or NBL *(26–33)* as well as improvement in microscopic metastatic disease in bone marrows of children with NBL *(27,29,43)*.

3.3. Combination of Anti-GD2 mAb and ADCC Augmenting Cytokines

The 14.G2a, ch14.18 and 3F8 mAbs all mediate augmented ADCC with activated effector cells. Peripheral blood mononuclear cells (PBMCs) from patients treated with IL-2 in vivo mediate enhanced ADCC with these mAbs *(14,44)*. This suggested that anti-GD2 antibodies should be tested in subjects receiving in vivo IL-2 treatment. This approach was initiated simultaneously in our studies of 14.G2a plus IL-2 in NBL through the Children's Cancer Group (CCG), and of 14.G2a or ch14.18 plus IL-2 in adults with MEL at the University of Wisconsin Comprehensive Cancer Center (UWCCC) *(45,46)*. Analyses of blood samples from patients treated with 14.G2a plus IL-2 document that conditions are achieved in vivo to mediate ADCC *(47)*. A decrease of measurable tumor was observed in a few patients receiving 14.G2a or ch14.18 plus IL-2 (one PR and one CR in the NBL study, and one CR and one PR in the MEL study). To enhance neutrophil mediated ADCC, these anti-GD2 mAb have been combined with GM-CSF in phase I and phase II trials *(48,49)*. Improvement in microscopic marrow disease was noted frequently in patients receiving anti-GD2 plus GM-CSF *(49,50)*. Thus, COG has completed pilot studies of ch14.18 plus cytokines for refractory NBL patients following autologous stem cell transplant (ASCT) *(51,52)*. Based on acceptable toxicity and potentially improved disease free survival (DFS) (75% ±14% 5-yr DFS), compared to historical controls (~40% DFS) in these pilot studies *(52)*, COG is now conducting a randomized phase-III trial testing an immunotherapy regimen consisting of ch14.18 plus IL-2 plus GM-CSF for children with NBL in remission following ASCT *(53)*.

3.4. Creation of an IC That Links Anti-GD2 mAb to IL-2

ADCC depends upon the number and function of FcRs on the effector cells *(14,44,54)*. When NK cells with FcRs are activated and expanded with IL-2 in vivo, they mediate dramatically augmented ADCC *(14,44)*. However, we showed that up to 50% of the activated NK cells circulating in cancer patients following in vivo treatment with IL-2 do not have FcRs, in contrast to resting NK cells *(55)*. These FcR(-) activated NK cells are more lytic to tumor cells in direct assays not dependent on mAb and FcRs. We also showed that NK cells activated in vivo by IL-2 have augmented expression of the IL-2Rα *(56)* and

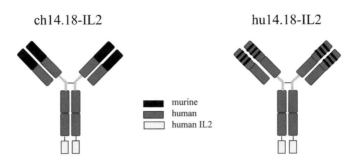

Fig. 1. The chimeric IC, ch14.18-IL2 links IL2 to each of the heavy chains of chimeric mAb The humanized IC,hu14.18-IL2, links IL2 to each of the heavy chains of humanized mAb.

demonstrate a dramatic in vitro response to IL-2 *(57)*. Furthermore, IL-2R-bearing T-cells that may not be able to specifically recognize these tumors (with their TCRs) should still be responsive to IL-2. It may be beneficial to activate these IL-2Rs with a molecule that will bridge the NK cells and T-cells to tumor cells to induce antitumor interactions, and to enhance the ability of the IL-2 activated FcR(-) cells to recognize tumor.

These are some of the proposed functions of the ch14.18-IL-2 IC (Fig. 1), which was constructed by fusing the human IL-2 gene to the ch14.18 IgG1 gene *(58)*. This IC uses the 14.18 anti-GD2 antibody-mediated recognition component to bind to tumor cells, the Fc component (which is still functional on this IC molecule) to bind to cells expressing FcRs, and the IL-2 component to activate cells expressing IL-2Rs. These interactions should result in effector cell binding to tumor followed by activation of the effector cell functions. Activation of effector cell mediated lysis can occur for both T-cells with IL-2Rs and NK cells *(58,59)*. The ch14.18-IL-2 IC induces anti-MEL activity in a murine SCID human-tumor-xenograft model *(60)*, and in conventional mice bearing syngeneic tumors transfected to express GD2 (i.e., the B78 MEL) *(61,62)*. In addition, anti-NBL activity is induced in conventional mice bearing a murine NBL that expresses GD2 and is recognized by ch14.18 (NXS2) *(20,21)*.

Ch14.18-IL-2 induces better antitumor effects against localized or metastatic NXS2 NBL than comparable amounts of ch14.18 mAb and IL-2 combination therapy (Table 1, top panel) *(20,21)*. Under these conditions, animals receiving the IC show no metastases. Similar results are obtained with the B78 MEL *(62)* (not shown). The in vivo destruction of NXS2 in animals receiving ch14.18-IL-2 is largely NK mediated *(20,21)*. In contrast, the ch14.18-IL-2 mediated antitumor effect against the B78 MEL is predominantly T-cell mediated *(62)*. This T-cell effect demonstrates epitope spread, as ch14.18-IL-2 enables C57Bl mice to destroy GD2⁻ B16 MEL cells only if they are a component of mixed tumors, created by co-injection with the GD2⁺ B78 MEL cells *(62)* (Table 1, bottom panel).Thus ch14.18-IL-2 induces potent antitumor effects in MEL or NBL bearing mice, and can function both as a T-cell inducing vaccine and as a potent activator of NK mediated ADCC. These preclinical data provided the rationale for initiation of clinical testing of a 14.18 based IC molecule as potential cancer therapy for NBL and MEL.

3.5. Clinical Implications: Melanoma

The incidence of melanoma continues to rise, with 55,100 newly diagnosed cases in the United States estimated for 2004 *(63)*. Forty eight percent of newly diagnosed patients present with features putting them at increased risk for recurrent disease (≥35% risk),

Table 1

Efficacy of ch14.18-IL-2 Exceeds ch14.18 Plus rIL-2

Treatment	Tumor	Number of tumor foci[a]
PBS	NXS2	>250, >250, >250, >250, 240, 115
rIL-2+ch14.18	NXS2	174, 134, 105, 102, 91, 83
ch14.18-IL-2[b]	NXS2	0, 0, 0, 0, 0, 0,
ch14.18-IL-2	B16	>500, >500, >500, >500, >500, 138, 97
PBS	B78 +B16	>500, >500, >500, >500, >500, >500, >500,>500
rIL-2+ch14.18	B78 + B16	>500, >500, >500, >500, 189, 179, 104
ch14.18-IL-2[c]	B78 + B16	0, 0, 2, 7, 9, 12, 21, 43

[a]Mets were scored for each of 6 mice on day 21, and were less in the IC group than the other 2 groups ($P < 0.001$) (21).

[b]IC group

[c]Mice with mixed tumors treated with IC had fewer mets than all other groups ($p < 0.002$) (62).

Top panel: Hepatic metastases (mets) were induced by injecting 10^6 NXS2 cells IV into AJ mice. On day 1 mice received PBS, 10 µg ch14.18 mAb + 30,000 IU rIL-2/d, or 10 µg of ch14.18-IL-2 daily, 6 × d.

Bottom panel: Pulmonary mets in C57Bl mice were induced by IV injection of 1×10^6 B16 cells (GD2–) alone, or combined with 5×10^6 B78 cells (GD2+). One week post-inoculation, 7 d of PBS, 8 µg ch14.18 + 24,000 IU rIL-2, or 8 µg ch14.18-IL-2 was initiated, and mets were scored 4 wk later.

and 13% of these patients are at high risk for recurrence (≥60% risk) (64). There will be an estimated 7,900 deaths in the United States from MEL this year. Remission can be accomplished surgically for most newly diagnosed high risk MEL pts and for most patients who develop a local or regional recurrence. To date, interferon (IFN) is the only treatment shown reproducibly to help delay or prevent recurrence following surgery in some high risk pts (65). Many other immunotherapies are now being tested for patients with metastatic or high risk *MEL(66–75)*. Some of these are technologically complex and may be difficult to deliver to several thousands of patients each year. Others are applicable only to patients with certain HLA types. Large phase III trials will be required to determine which of these can improve disease free survival (DFS) and overall survival for MEL pts. The ability to store a reagent in a standard hospital pharmacy, apply it to virtually all patients independent of HLA type, and induce both T and NK reactivity against neoplastic cells, would offer many clinical advantages. Hu14.18-IL-2 fulfills these criteria and thus phase II clinical testing in MEL is under way.

3.6. Clinical Implications: Neuroblastoma

Neuroblatoma (NBL) is the most common extracranial solid tumor of childhood, and nearly half of all newly diagnosed patients present with high risk features (76). Most patients with high risk NBL can achieve minimal residual disease (MRD) status with current standard therapy (combined chemo and radiotherapy, followed by ablative chemotherapy and autologous stem cell reinfusion, followed by *cis*-retinoic acid). Yet, despite the aggressive nature of this multimodality treatment, this combined approach is only curative for approx 30% of the high risk patients that begin this comprehensive regimen (77). Over the next 3 yr, the COG randomized trial of ch14.18 mAb plus IL-2 plus GM-CSF will determine whether an anti-GD2 based immunotherapy regimen, delivered to children in MRD status, can help prevent recurrence (53). Given the preclinical data in Table 1 it will be essential to complete phase II testing of hu14.18-IL-2 in patients with

NBL, including children with bulky disease and children with measurable, but relatively minimal/non bulky disease.

3.7. Clinical Implications: Other Malignancies

GD2 is expressed on neuroectodermally derived tumors. In addition to MEL and NBL, it is also expressed on tumors from many patients with small-cell lung cancer, osteosarcoma and soft tissue sarcomas (78,79). These GD2+ diseases account for approx 8% of all cancer deaths in the United States (63). Clinical results using hu14.18-IL-2 for melanoma and neuroblastoma should be translatable to all GD2+ diseases in the future.

3.8. Phase-I Testing of hu14.18-IL-2 in Melanoma
3.8.1. Preclinical Development and Study Design

The initial preclinical testing of an anti-GD2 IC had used the ch14.18-IL-2 reagent (46). However, because many patients receiving ch14.18 mAb developed high levels of neutralizing human antichimeric antibody (HACA) (80), our efforts switched to the clinical development of the hu14.18-IL-2 molecule (Fig. 1). The hu14.18-IL-2 IC contains only minimal murine amino acid sequences in the CDR-1,2, and three regions. As a nearly "pure" human protein it is predicted to be less likely to induce a neutralizing anti-IC response than ch14.18-IL-2.

Preclinical in vitro and murine data indicated that hu14.18-IL-2 was likely to be more effective in vivo clinically than ch14.18 (or hu14.18) mAb when administered to patients receiving IL-2; however, the regimen for administration needed to be designed. Although the halflife of murine or chimeric anti-GD2 IgG mAbs injected IV is normally 2–5 d (29,45), the halflife of the ch14.18-IL-2 in mice was only ~4 h (81). This was because the ch14.18-IL-2 IC (and the hu14.18-IL-2 IC) was sensitive to enzymatic cleavage by proteases in the mouse serum. When the IC was put into mouse serum at room temperature or at 37° C, the IL-2 component was cleaved from the hu14.18 component, leaving separate IL-2 and hu14.18 moieties. When the intact IC is injected IV into mice, the halflife of the intact IC is 4 h. The halflife of the human IL-2 linked to the IC is also 4 h (81). In contrast, the halflife of the hu14.18 mAb component of the IC is 27 h. This suggested that in vivo, the hu14.18-IL-2 IC circulates intact with a halflife of 4 h. The IL-2 component is cleaved after 4h and is then cleared rapidly. This is similar to recombinant IL-2, which is cleared rapidly after IV bolus injection (half life of <1 h) (82). The remaining hu14.18 IgG, no longer linked to the IL-2, is able to continue circulating for a longer halflife. This suggested that hu14.18-IL-2 IC should be given frequently (daily) to maintain both IL-2 and hu14.18 in vivo activity. Hu14.18-IL-2 was given to nonhuman primates in an FDA required toxicity study (Gillies et al., unpublished). It was given as an IV infusion daily for 5 d. Toxic effects were primarily related to IL-2, (hypotension and capillary leak) with an MTD in primates of 16 mg/m^2/d for 5 d. Toxicity seemed to worsen with subsequent days of treatment. At 48mg/m^2/d, monkeys developed anaphylaxis on day 5. This suggested that for shorter courses of treatment, the MTD might be higher. It also suggested that the antibody (Ab) response against the heterologous IC might be developing as early as 4–5 d after starting IC treatment and might be a factor in human studies. However, a weaker Ab response against the humanized IC was expected in humans compared to cynomolgous monkeys. To provide for a clear safety

Table 2
Adverse Events[a] Observed With hu14.18-IL-2: Grade 3 Adverse
Events Observed in Patients for All Courses of Therapy[b]

Dose (mg/m²)	N[c]	No. of courses[d]	BP	O₂	plt	Bili/ast	PO₄	GLU
0.8	3	5						
1.6	6	12				1	1	
3.2	6	7						2
4.8	6	11			1	1	4	
6.0	6	9		1	1		3	
7.5	6	8	2	1	2	1	3	1

[a]Adverse events graded 1–4 as per NCI Common Toxicity Criteria, Version 2.0.
[b]For each category of toxicity shown (BP, hypotension; O₂, hypoxia; plt, low platelets; Bili/AST; PO₄, low phosphate; GLU, high glucose), the number of patients showing grade 3 toxicity as their highest grade is shown for each dose level of hu14.18-IL-2.
[c]Total number of patients treated at each dose level.
[d]Total number of courses administered for all patients at the indicated dose level.

margin, the starting dose in this phase I trial *(83,84)* was 1/20 of the daily MTD in primates (0.8 mg/m²/d). Infusions were given for only 3 instead of 5 d to patients admitted to our inpatient General Clinical Research Center. Because the known neuropathic pain associated with anti-GD2 mAb was less intense when mAb is infused slowly, this trial gave hu14.18-IL-2 as a 4-h daily infusion.

3.9. Conduct of the Study

This phase I study treated 33 adults with refractory MEL. A detailed report of the clinical findings has recently been published *(84)*. The rapid dose acceleration design of Storer was initially planned to be used *(85)*. At the first dose level (0.8 mg/m²/d), fever beyond grade 1 was noted in the first pt. Thus three pts. were entered at that dose. All remaining dose levels had six patients entered per dose level. Grade 3 clinical and laboratory toxicities for all courses are shown in Table 2.

3.10. Dose Limiting Toxicities (DLTs)

Only DLTs for course 1 were used to define MTD. One of the first patients at 1.6 mg/m²/d had an elevated AST and one had grade 3 hypophosphatemia. Based on analyses of urine phosphate values in patients with hypophospatemia, we demonstrated that the hypophosphatemia was not owing to renal wastage of PO₄. This result is consistent with a cytokine induced flux of PO₄ from the extracellular to the intracellular compartment *(86)*. Thus asymptomatic, spontaneously resolving grade 3 PO₄ was not used as a criteria for DLT. Hu14.18-IL-2 was thus tolerated well at the 1.6-4.8 mg/m² dose levels. At 6.0 mg/m², 1 patient developed reversible hypoxia, requiring entry of three more patients at that dose level. At 7.5 mg/m², one patient developed reversible hypoxia and hypotension, and one developed a transiently elevated ALT/AST; both qualified as DLT. Thus, with two of six patients developing DLT at 7.5 mg/m², this dose level met study criteria for MTD.

3.11. Cause of Toxicities

Most clinical toxicities seen were similar to those previously reported for IL-2 and anti-GD2 mAb treatments *(45,46,51,52)*. All 33 patients had grade 2 fever. Most patients in the three highest dose levels had pelvic, abdominal, chest, or extremity pain that could be adequately controlled with intravenous morphine. This pain was similar to the pain reported for patients treated with ch14.18 *(46,51,52)*. The remaining toxicities were similar to those frequently seen with IL-2 given alone. In our previous clinical trial, the MTD of the ch14.18 mAb combined with systemic IL-2 was found to be 7.5 mg/m^2/d *(46)*. As the hu14.18-IL-2 is comprised of 17% IL-2 and 83% hu14.18, the amount of hu14.18 mAb in 7.5 mg of hu14.18-IL-2 is 6.3 mg. Thus the 7.5 mg/m^2/d MTD of the ch14.18 when combined with systemic IL-2 is similar to the amount of hu14.18 mAb (6.3 mg/m^2/d) present in the MTD determined here for the hu14.18-IL-2 molecule.

3.12. Antitumor Data

No patient showed improvement of measurable disease to qualify as a complete or partial response (CR or PR). Eight of the 33 patients maintained stable disease (SD) after two courses of therapy, and four of these eight patients continue with no evidence of progressive disease (1 with SD treated at 4.8 mg/m^2/day and three high-risk patients continue with no evidence of disease, treated at 0.8, 3.2, and 6.0 mg/m^2/day) for 30–62 mo since completing protocol therapy. Five of the 33 patients entered the study with no measurable disease following surgical resection of recurrences or metastases. Three of these five patients continue with no evidence of disease (41–74 mo) *(84)*. These findings are consistent with the hypothesis that clinical benefit from an immunotherapeutic intervention is more likely in patients with a low tumor burden.

3.13. Analyses of Specimens from 33 Patients in the Phase I MEL Trial

Serum specimens and PBMC specimens were obtained at serial time points from each patient for all courses of treatment and analyzed for pharmacokinetics (PK), multiple parameters of immune activation, and for the immunogenicity of the IC.

3:13.1. PK Assays

Serum samples from all 33 patients were obtained on days 1 and 3 at each of the following times: before the 4-h infusion, 0.5 h into and at the completion of the 4-h infusion, and then 0.5 h, 1 h, 2 h, 4 h, 12 h, and 20 h after completion of the 4-h infusion. These specimens were tested in an ELISA assay using an anti-id mAb(1A7) *(88,89)* to measure the intact hu14.18-IL-2 molecule (Fig. 2) *(90)*. A detailed listing of all results obtained for the Course-1/day 1 (C1D1) infusion is shown in Table 3. The peak serum levels and area under the curve (AUC) show a progressive increase with dose ($P < 0.001$) that is near linear after the first two doses. This is consistent with a nonspecific "sink effect" at low doses of this agent. When data from all 33 patients for these time points for C1D1 were evaluated, the half-life following the first 4-h infusion was found to be 3.7 ± 0.9 h. This is between the half-life of its two components (approx 45 min for IL-2 and 2–3 d for ch14.18 mAb), and comparable to that which was observed for the half-life of ch14.18-IL-2 in mice *(81)*. Separate assays for hu14.18 mAb were performed on these same serum specimens from select pts and showed PK curves similar to those for the hu14.18-IL-2 (Fig. 3). In other words, following the clearance of hu14.18-IL-2 from the serum of these pts, the

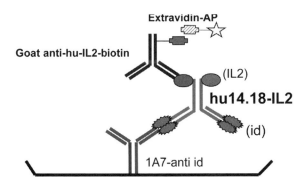

Fig. 2. ELISA assay that detects intact hu14.18-IL2 by capture to plate with the 1A7 anti-id mAb, and detection with goat anti-IL2 Ab.

Table 3

Pharmacokinetics in Phase I Testing of hu14.18-IL-2 in Patients With Melanoma

Dose (mg/m2)	N	Peak Conc. (ng/mL)[a,b]		Clearance (L/h)[c]		Halflife (h)		AUC (ng/mL × h)[a,d]	
		Mean	SD	Mean	SD	Mean	SD	Mean	SD
0.8	3	185	31	1.39	0.45	2.7	0.21	1138	248
1.6	6	696	390	0.67	0.16	3.5	1.10	5106	2540
3.2	6	1490	693	0.66	0.22	3.8	0.45	11448	4970
4.8	6	3965	2001	0.39	0.11	4.2	1.25	25529	6794
6.0	6	6339	1519	0.33	0.09	3.8	0.86	38944	12294
7.5	6	5514	2808	0.38	0.11	3.9	0.66	40870	18958

[a]Peak concentration, clearance, halflife and area under the curve (AUC) were obtained at course 1, day 1. Values shown are mean and standard deviation (SD) for all patients at each dose level.
[b–d]The peak concentration, clearance and AUC were all dose dependent ($P < 0.001$).

hu14.18mAb component could not be detected, which contrasts with data from mice *(81)* where residual ch14.18 mAb, cleaved of its IL-2 component, was found circulating with a halflife of 27 h.

We compared the peak hu14.18-IL-2 levels and AUC values for the 31 patients that received C1D3 treatment at the same dose they received on C1D1. The values for day 3 were significantly less than those for day 1 (Table 4). We hypothesize that this difference may reflect either: (a) The induction of a neutralizing anti-IC antibody in these patients (however, this C1D3 infusion begins only 48 h after the start of the C1D1 infusion, a time before the anticipated detection of any primary antibody response); (b) The activation of augmented expression of IL-2 receptors on IL-2 responsive cells that have been stimulated by the hu14.18-IL-2 infusions on days 1 and 2 (these may be clearing the IC more rapidly through IL-2R binding to the IC); (c) The activation of augmented FcR expression or function, in response to the first 2 d of IC infusion; (d) Some other physiologic change (such as a modification of extracellular fluid volume) following the first 2 d of IC treatment. Additional studies are needed to account for this change in PK for day 3 vs day 1, to measure its importance to antitumor activity, and to determine whether IC treatment regimens should be modified owing to this finding.

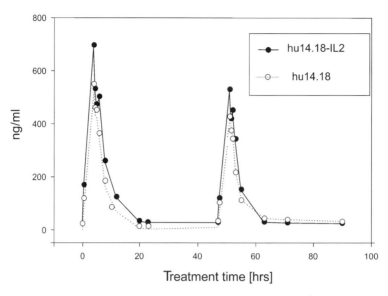

Fig. 3. ELISA assays from C1D1 and C1D3 sera from Pt #4 (1.6 mg/m^2/d) for hu14.18-IL2 (as in Fig. 2) and 14.18 (capture with 1A7 but detected with goat-anti-huIgG).

Table 4
Pharmacokinetics on Day 1 and Day 3 of Treatment

	Hu14.18-IL-2 Peak ng/mL		Hu14.18-IL-2 AUC ng/mL × h	
C1D1	3211		21188	
C1D3	2619	p<0.001	13362	P < 0.001

Table 5
Lymphocyte Cell Surface Phenotypes

	D1	D8	p
CD16	23%	30%	0.0003
CD56	18%	30%	0.001

3.13.2. Lymphocyte Numbers and Phenotype

Peripheral blood lymphopenia occurred on protocol days 2–4 ($P < 0.0001$), and this was followed by a rebound lymphocytosis on days 5–22 ($P < 0.0001$) in course 1 (Fig. 4). Both of these changes were dose-dependent ($P < 0.01$ and $P < 0.05$, respectively). Similar results were seen for course 2. In addition, lymphocyte counts on days 1, 5, 8, and 15 of course 2 were also significantly greater than those days' values during course 1, indicating that the effects of course 1 augment those of course 2 (not shown). Lymphocyte cell surface phenotype (percent positive PBMC by flow cytometry; Table 5) showed an expansion of CD16$^+$ and CD56$^+$ lymphocytes (NK cell markers) from d1 (pretreatment) to day 8. This increase was still present on day 29 of course 1 (not shown).

3.13.3. Soluble IL-2R$_\alpha$ (sIL-2R$_\alpha$) and C-Reactive Protein (CRP) Levels

SIL-2Rα levels *(91,92)* were obtained at 7 time points for each treatment course for all pts. The sIL-2Rα level was significantly increased over baseline ($P < 0.001$) for all

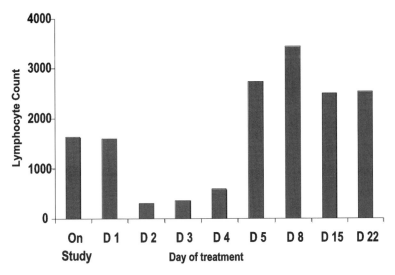

Fig. 4. Mean PBL count/mL for 31 pts completing course 1. Values from day 2 on are different from pretreatment ($p < 0/0001$).

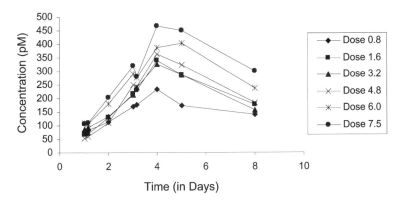

Fig. 5. sIL2Rα levels in sera from day 1 (prior to and at the end of 4 h hu14.18-IL2 infusion) and days 2, 3, 4, 5, and 8 for 31 patients completing course 1. All values from day 2 on are greater than baseline ($p < 0.0001$).

time points from days 2–8, during both course 1 (Fig. 5) and course 2 (not shown). SIL-2Rα levels peaked at day 4–5 and then declined. The increase in sIL-2Rα was found to be dose dependent ($P = 0.014$). sIL-2Rα values for course 2 were increased compared with corresponding values in course 1 for days 1–5 for patients receiving the same dose in both courses ($P < 0.02$). The pretreatment CRP value of 2.4 mg/dl increased to 14.9 after 2 doses of hu14.18-IL-2 ($P < 0.001$) and returned to normal after 3 wk (not shown).

3.13.4. NK AND ADCC ACTIVITY

The LA-N-5 NBL cell line that expresses GD2 and binds hu14.18-IL-2 was used to evaluate IL-2 activated NK function and ADCC on PBMC from 31 patients completing course 1 (Table 6). Cytotoxicity was evaluated in a standard 4-h *(51)* Cr release assay using three different effector to target (E:T) ratios. The targets were incubated in the presence of PBMC obtained from patients on day 1 (C1D1, before treatment) and

Table 6
Lytic Units LA-N-5 ± SD

	C1D1	C1D8	P
Medium	5.3 ± 2.2	9.7 ± 2.2	0.09
IL-2	11.9 ± 6.5	39.6 ± 6.6	0.006
Hu14.18-IL-2	173 ± 36	404 ± 37	0.003

Table 7
% Cytotoxicity on K562 ±SD

	C1D1	C1D8	C1D22
NK(medium)	11.1 ± 2.8	*19.7 ± 3.0	**22.6 ± 2.8
NK (IL-2)	22.2 ± 4.1	**48.8 ± 4.6	**40.7 ± 4.2

*$P < 0.05$
**$P < 0.01$

day 8. Lytic units/10^6 cells were measured in cultures containing medium alone, IL-2 or hu14.18-IL-2. There was a significant increase in killing mediated by lymphocytes collected on C1D8 when compared with C1D1 when IL-2 or hu14.18-IL-2 were added to the assay. Because the LA-N-5 target is relatively resistant to fresh NK cells, it is useful for measuring IL-2 augmented killing and ADCC. However, the weak killing of LA-N-5 mediated by fresh PBMC in medium (without supplemental IL-2 in vitro) was not significantly greater on d8 than on d1. For patients 19-33, standard NK assays were performed on days 1, 8, 15 and 22, using the NK susceptible K562 target cells (Table 7; E/T 60:1). A significant increase in NK lysis of K562 target cells, either in medium or IL-2, was seen on d8 and d22 vs d1.

3.13.5. Immune Function of IC Circulating in Patient Sera

Serum samples from selected patients were also evaluated to determine functional IL-2 activity of circulating IC and anti-GD2 binding ability of the mAb component of IC. The IL-2 responsive Tf1βcell line (93,94) demonstrated IL-2-induced proliferation with patient serum obtained during the first 4 h following the infusion of hu14.18-IL-2 (data not shown). Values returned to baseline with serum obtained by 20 h after this infusion. Serum samples collected at these same time-points were also examined by flow cytometry for the presence of intact hu14.18-IL-2 IC that retains its IL-2 component and its anti-GD2 antibody activity. Patient serum samples obtained 4–8 h following the hu14.18-IL-2 infusion contained hu14.18-IL-2 capable of binding to the M21 (GD2$^+$) cell line and delivering IL-2 to its surface as detected by flow cytometry using a PE labeled anti-IL-2 detection antibody (84) (data not shown).

3.13.6. Ex vivo ADCC

The same ADCC assay as shown in Table 6 was performed with PBMC from day 8; however, instead of adding hu14.18-IL-2 to the assay, serum obtained from the patient (before [pre] or after [4 h] hu14.18-IL-2 administration) was added. As shown in Fig. 6, PBMC obtained from patients on C2D8 mediated augmented killing of the LA-N-5 cell line in the presence of serum obtained following hu14.18-IL-2 administration, compared to that observed with serum obtained before infusion ($P < 0.05$). Thus the hu14.18-IL-2

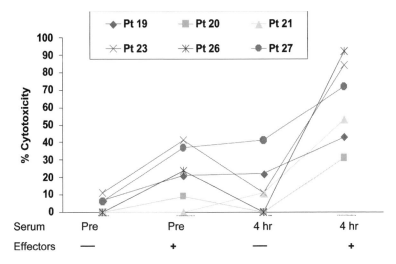

Fig. 6. LA-N-5 NBL were killed in a 4-h assay with serum obtained pretreatment or at the end of the 4-h hu14.18-IL2 infusion with or without PBMC effectors obtained on course 2 day 8.

circulating in patients after IV administration is able to facilitate ADCC with PBMCs activated in vivo by hu14.18-IL-2 from that same patient, suggesting that in vivo conditions were achieved to allow ADCC.

3.14. A Phase-I Study of hu14.18-IL-2 in Children With GD2+ Tumors (87)

This recently completed trial, was conducted by the Children's Oncology Group (87). Hu14.18-IL-2 was given as 4-h infusions for three consecutive days each month to 28 children with GD2+ tumors. This is the same as the administration schedule of hu14.18-IL-2 used for the adult melanoma study. Unlike the adult study, up to four courses (rather than 2) could be given for patients with stable disease. Interest in this study was great and required that COG establish a new "random selection assignment system" to fairly assign patients to spots in this study from the many patients attempting to become enrolled.

3.15. Mechanisms of Antitumor Efficacy and Escape in Tumor-Bearing Mice

Continued basic and preclinical studies have focused on mechanisms whereby IC treatment may be even more effective against established cancers.

3.15.1. Tumor Escape

Treatment of tumor-bearing mice with hu14.18-IL-2 can cause dramatic antitumor effects. Initial experiments involved mice with newly established tumors (20,21,61,62). However, current and future clinical application of this approach involves treating patients with clinically evident cancer that has already been diagnosed. Even high risk patients that have achieved remission as a result of surgery, radiotherapy, and/or chemotherapy are expected to have a substantially greater tumor load than mice injected 1–3 d earlier with IV or SQ tumor. Thus we have initiated 5 d of IC treatment at later times after IV injection of NXS2 tumor cells. Liver metastases were scored on d28 (Fig. 7). PBS-treated mice had >200 metastatic liver foci, whereas mice treated on day 9 showed 50–80 foci, and mice beginning treatment on day 5 had relatively few foci. These results indicate that the

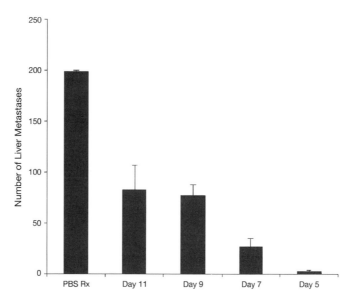

Fig. 7. Hu14.18-IL2 is more effective against minimal disease. hu14.18-IL2 (10 μg/d) for 5 d starting on days 5, 7, 9, or 11 following 5 3 10^5 NXS2 cells injected on day 0, and harvested on day 28.

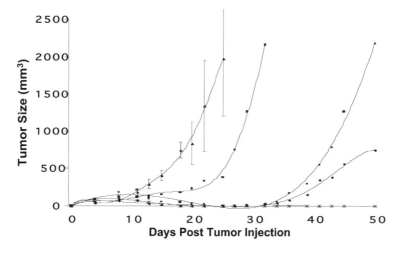

Fig. 8. Suboptimal hu14.18-IL2 induces transient resolution of NXS2 tumors. Eight mice were injected SQ with 2×10^6 tumor cells on day 0. Mice were treated with 5 mcg/d IC or PBS for 5 d starting on day 5. Data points represent mean ± SD of 4 PBS treated mice (triangles) and data from 4 individual IC treated mice (diamonds, circles, boxes, and stars).

hu14.18-IL-2 treatment is more effective when initiated early after establishment of metastases when there is a smaller tumor burden. Similar analyses looked at the ability of hu14.18-IL-2 to eradicate measurable SQ NXS2 tumors. Hu14.18-IL-2 injected IV starting on d9 caused most tumors to shrink, some to the point of nondetection. Nevertheless, most of these tumors recurred over the next 3 wk and were then fatal (Fig. 8). Thus these tumors initially respond to the immunotherapy, but then escape.

We have used this SQ NXS2 model to address the mechanisms of escape from hu14.18-IL-2 immunotherapy *(95)* to devise therapies that are more effective and prevent

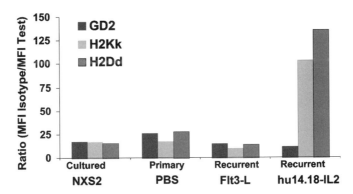

Fig. 9. MFI mean ratios for 5 NXS2 cultures, 5 SQ control NXS2 tumors (PBS) and 6–10 SQ tumors that recurred after FLT3-L or IC treatment. Compared to control tumors, tumors from hu14.18-IL2-treated mice had elevated MHC ($p < 0.001$) and decreased GD2 ($p < 0.02$), and MHC on Flt3-L

escape. First we confirmed that the partial control of NXS2 tumors in this model was NK mediated. We then found that NXS2 tumors that recurred following hu14.18-IL-2 treatment showed enhanced (>fivefold) MHC class I expression compared to NXS2 tumors from PBS-treated mice(Fig. 9). Enhanced MHC class I expression on NXS2 cells was associated with reduced susceptibility to both NK cell-mediated tumor cell lysis and ADCC in vitro (not shown) *(95)*. This is likely the result of Ly49 inhibitory receptors on the NK cells in response to the elevated MHC-I on the modulated NXS2 tumor cells. We have shown that ADCC induced by a separate IC (KS-IL-2) *(96)* is augmented by anti-Ly49 mAb that blocks the inhibitory interaction of the Ly49 receptor and the MHC-I molecule during the IC facilitated ADCC interaction *(97)*. The recurrent NXS2 tumors following hu14.18-IL-2 were not constitutive high MHC class I expressers, as their class I levels returned to near normal after culturing them for 1 wk (not shown) *(95)*. This result suggested that the immunotherapeutic effect of NK mediated ADCC using the IC caused a physiologic modulation of class I MHC in vivo on NXS2 cells that had survived the initial ADCC interactions. This result was then replicated in vitro. When NXS2 tumor cells were cultured with IL-2 activated splenocytes together with hu14.18-IL-2, most tumor cells died during the 5-day culture; however, some survived. Those NXS2 tumor cells that survived demonstrated enhanced levels of MHC class-I, which could be prevented if anti-IFN-γ antibody was added to the culture (Fig. 10). These results suggest that the ADCC process is associated with anti-IFN-γ release by the NK cells as they are destroying some of the NXS2 cells; however, residual NXS2 cells in the microenvironment that have not yet been destroyed by ADCC would be induced by the anti-IFN-γ to increase their MHC class-I and thereby escape from the *ADCC (95)* .

We next showed that recurrent NXS2 tumors that escaped from a T-cell mediated response (induced by Flt3-L) have decreased expression of MHC class I antigens (Fig. 9) *(95)* This decrease in MHC class-I should make these tumor cells more resistant to T-cell mediated destruction, as shown for many other T-cell resistant murine tumors *(98–100)*. Thus NXS2 cells may express either higher or lower levels of MHC class I to resist either NK cell (ie: 14.18-IL-2), or T-cell (i.e., Flt3-L)-mediated immunotherapy, respectively.These data support the following hypotheses: 1) Enhanced activation and targeting of tumor-reactive effector cells should be induced at a time of minimal tumor burden; 2) Enhanced

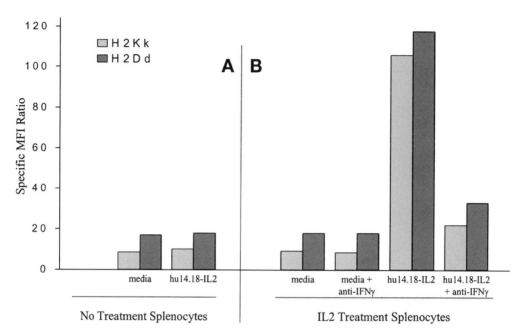

Fig. 10. MHC class I expression is increased on NXS2 cells when cocultured (5 d) with hu14.18-IL2 and splenocytes from IL2-treated mice. Anti-IFNg mAb (50 mcg/mL) on day 0 blocked this.

activation and targeting of tumor-reactive effector cells should be induced to an effective level and sustained as tolerated, to destroy tumor cells before they may be able to modulate their behavior and induce resistance mechanisms; 3) Activating and targeting of distinct populations of tumor-destructive effector cells (i.e., NK cells, T-cells, macrophages), either in parallel (simultaneously) or in series (consecutively) should allow the distinct destructive mechanisms of these effector cells to prevent resistance, as tumor cells that become resistant to one, may retain sensitivity to another *(95)*.

3.15.2. Combining hu14.18-IL-2 With Constant Infusion IL-2 As an Initial Step

We tested whether augmented activation of NK cells can help hu14.18-IL-2 to be more effective in destroying NXS2 in vivo *(101)* . In vivo administration of IL-2 induces a systemic activation of NK cells *(11,56)*. Furthermore, administration of IL-2 by constant infusion (c.i.) appears more potent at causing NK activation *(57,102–104)*. We thus delivered IL-2 to NXS2 tumor bearing mice by c.i. for 7d with Alzet SQ osmotic infusion pumps. The addition of this c.i. IL-2 treatment to a suboptimal hu14.18-IL-2 regimen started 9 d after injection of NXS2 tumors provided enhanced control of metastatic liver disease (Fig. 11). It also induced complete eradication of 9 d SQ NXS2 lesions in many treated animals. For example, in one experiment, IC started on d9 for mice with SQ tumors resulted in two of eight mice tumor-free, whereas eight of eight mice became and remained tumor-free after the combined IC plus IL-2 regimen (not shown) *(101)*. Animals showing long term eradication of their primary NXS2 tumors following combined IC plus IL-2 therapy demonstrated T-cell memory, able to protect against a rechallenge of NXS2 cells *(101)* (not shown).

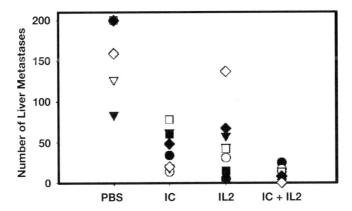

Fig. 11. Mice with 9-d hepatic metastases received IC, IL2, or both. Tumor foci were scored on day 28. Each symbol represents a mouse. Mice treated with IC + IL2 had fewer metastases than all three other groups (p < 0.05).

3.16. Preclinical Testing of Recently Created Immunocytokines

3.16.1. SPECIES-RELATED IL-2 BIOACTIVITY

Clinical testing of both hu14.18-IL-2 and huKS-IL-2 has provided important insights into the relative biologic activities of these molecules in mice and man and has prompted us to re-examine the IL-2 bioactivity in the two species. This has led to the observation that these IL-2 based immunocyokines are far more potent in man than they are in mice. For example, when human immune cells, e.g., human T-cell lines, bearing the high affinity IL-2R are used to measure bioactivity and the ICs are compared to human rIL-2, they are equally potent on a molar basis. In mice, both ICs are roughly threefold less active than human rIL-2. The situation is even more pronounced when mouse immune cells bearing only the intermediate affinity receptor are used, e.g., mouse NK cells, in which case the ICs are roughly 20-fold less active than human rIL-2 (unpublished results). This relative selectivity for the high affinity receptor bearing cells over those expressing only the intermediate receptor might be advantageous in improving the therapeutic index of IL-2 *(105)*. The basis of this approach is that, upon intravenous administration, the selective form of IL-2 would have a reduced ability to trigger responses in the vascular compartment in which most cells express only the intermediate affinity IL-2R. The same molecule would still maintain the ability to trigger cells bearing the high affinity IL-2R, such as T-cells encountering tumor cells or their antigens in the tumor microenvironment or in draining lymph nodes. A similar rationale has been proposed for selective activation using low dose, subcutaneous administration of rIL-2 *(106)*. This selectivity of IL-2 based ICs on T versus NK cells is better seen in mouse rather than human therapy. Therefore, we have taken multiple approaches that might improve the therapeutic index in man.

3.16.2. SUBCUTANEOUS DOSING

We have found that subcutaneous dosing of IL-2 based ICs greatly reduces the overall bioavailability in the blood by reducing the Cmax but sustains the overall duration at lower concentrations. Such an approach would favor the selective activation of high affinity IL-2R bearing cells while reducing the vascular toxicity. Although this effect is similar to that of rIL-2, the longer circulating half-life of ICs might increase the success of such an approach through the specific targeting of tumor cells. To improve this further, we have modified sequences in the junction between the antibody and IL-2 components that greatly improve the half-life and thus increase tumor targeting to an even greater extent. To avoid a potential increase in immunogenicity owing to subcutaneous dosing, we have taken an additional step in de-immunizing our IC molecules. This is achieved by removing helper T-cell epitopes capable of binding the class II MHC molecules and thus providing helper function for B-cell antibody production. Mutations are made that remove these potential epitopes in the antibody V regions as well as at the junction between the antibody H chain and IL-2 that might represent a neo-epitope. The first de-immunized, long-acting IC that we produced was derived from huKS-IL-2 and is called DI-2. Its circulating half-life in mice and monkeys is roughly 12 h (compared to 4 h for huKS-IL-2) following IV injection and shows reduced immunogenicity in monkeys. Preliminary efficacy studies in mouse tumor models show a potent antitumor effect when administered by the subcutaneous route and at doses that are far below those causing overt toxicity. It remains to be seen if the same reduction in toxicity and lack of immunogenicity will be seen in human clinical trials.

3.17. Targeting Hematologic Tumors

Most of our previous work with immunocytokines has focused on targeting solid tumors expressing either the ganglioside GD2 or the pan-carcinoma antigen, EpCAM. Clinically, however, antibodies have proven more effective against hematologic tumors. The best example is the anti-CD20 chimeric antibody, rituximab, for the treatment of non-Hodgkin's lymphoma. Recently we have constructed and tested an IL-2 based IC containing the V regions from the well-known anti-CD20 antibody, Leu16 (106). We have used the technology developed with DI-2 to increase its circulating half-life and have also de-immunized both the V regions and the fusion junction. Thus, both intravenous and subcutaneous administration of DI-Leu16-IL-2 could be considered for clinical trials. This IC has been tested in a SCID mouse model of disseminated Daudi lymphoma and has proven to be highly efficacious as a single agent, even when administered long after disease has been established and despite a complete lack of functional T-cells. It has also been found to be more efficacious than higher doses of an anti-CD20 antibody and rIL-2. We are currently testing DI-Leu16-IL-2 in a sygeneic model to test whether antitumor efficacy in immune competent animals leads to T-cell cross-priming and the development of a long term memory response. Clinical testing of this IC is planned for 2007.

3.17.1. Reduced-Toxicity IL-2 Based ICs

An additional approach we have taken to reduce the IL-2 related side effects of our ICs is to modify their IL-2R selectivity to an even greater extent than what we currently see in mice. As discussed above, the IL-2 based ICs containing wild-type human IL-2 are approximately sevenfold selective for the high affinity receptor, relative to free IL-2. We then screened several IL-2 mutants for far greater levels of selectivity and that would have the same pattern of selectivity for both mouse and human immune cells. One such mutant is D20T, in which the aspartic acid at position 20 that is known to interact with the beta chain of the IL-2R, has been mutated to threonine *(108)*. Interestingly, this mutation has little or no effect on the selectivity of receptor binding as a free molecule, but is >500-fold selective for the high affinity receptor when it is fused to the carboxyl terminus of an antibody H chain. Also, this selectivity is quite similar for both human and mouse IL-2 responsive cells and cell lines. A number of preclinical studies have demonstrated that this IC with the D20T mutation is far less toxic than the same IC with wild-type IL-2 using a short term (5 day) dosing scheme, and has nearly the same level of antitumor activity. These results support the hypothesis that selective activation of immune cells bearing only the high affinity IL-2R can result in antitumor responses. It remains to be determined whether this approach translates into an improved therapeutic index in man.

3.17.2. ICs Based on Other Cytokines

We and others have already described several ICs based on additional cytokines including TNFα and TNFβ, GM-CSF, IFNs, and IL-12 (reviewed in ref. *108*). Recently we have applied the same technology with many additional cytokines, especially those with a potential for antitumor immune stimulation. Most of these ICs have not yet shown the potency of IL-2 and IL-12 in preclinical models, at least when applied as monotherapies. Finally, we have recently reported on the combination of two potentially synergistic cytokines in a single molecule. One very potent molecule consists of a fusion of IL-12 and IL-2 that together are fused to a whole antibody targeting the pan-carcinoma antigen EpCAM *(109)*. Intratumoral injection of this multi-functional molecule caused regression of established tumors in mice and lead to potent systemic immunity rendering mice resistant to a lethal injection of the same tumor months after regression of the primary lesion. Futher exploration of this approach and in the use of combination therapies with traditional chemotherapy, targeted therapies, and other immune approaches is needed to fully understand what role ICs might play in future therapies of cancer.

4. SUMMARY

Preclinical testing demonstrates that enhanced antitumor efficacy can be obtained when tumor reactive antibodies are liked to immune-activating cytokines. This has now been demonstrated in several murine tumor models, utilizing different tumor reactive mAb and different cytokines. Efficacy in these models is most prominent when ICs are used in the MRD setting. Phase I and II clinical testing is proceeding for the lead compounds (hu14.18-IL-2 and huKS-IL-2). Laboratory developments are testing the benefits of combining ICs with chemotherapy, anti-angiogenic therapy *(110)* and other immunotherapies, while molecular modifications are being made in ICs to enhance efficacy while limiting toxicity.

ACKNOWLEDGMENTS

The authors thank their many colleagues at the UWCCC and EMO-Lexigen, and Dr. Ralph Reisfeld at the Scripps Research Institute for collaboration. Support is provided by NIH grants CA032685, RR03186, CA87025. The UW-CureKids Cancer Coalition, and the Midwest Athletes Against Childhood Cancer Fund.

REFERENCES

1. Reisfeld RA, Gillies SD. Antibody-interleukin-2 fusion proteins: A new approach to cancer therapy. J Clin Lab Anal 10:160–166, 1996.
2. Sondel PM, Gillies SD. Immunocytokines for Cancer Immunotherapy. *In:* Morse M, Clay TM, Lyerle HM eds. *Handbook of Cancer Vaccines.* Humana Press, Totowa NJ. pp:341–358, 2004.
3. Sondel PM, Hank JA, Gan J, Neal Z, Albertini MR. Preclinical and Clinical Development of Immunocytokines. Current Opinion in Investigational Drugs, 4:696–700, 2003.
4. Lustgarten J, Marks J, Sherman LA. Redirecting effector T-cells through their IL-2 receptors. J Immunol 162:359–365, 1999.
5. Lustgarten J. Anti-Her-2/neu-IL-2 or heregulin-IL-2 fusions proteins redirect non-tumor specific CTL to the tumor site for tumor eradication. Cancer Immunol Immunother. 52:751–760, 2003.
6. Helguera G. Morrison SL. Penichet ML. Antibody-cytokine fusion proteins: harnessing the combined power of cytokines and antibodies for cancer therapy. Clinical Immunol. 105:233–246, 2002.
7. Hornick JL. Khawli LA. Hu P. Sharifi J. Khanna C. Epstein AL. Pretreatment with a monoclonal antibody/interleukin-2 fusion protein directed against DNA enhances the delivery of therapeutic molecules to solid tumors. Clinl Cancer Res. 5:51–60, 1999.
8. Weinreich DM, Rosenberg SA. Response rates of patients with metastatic melanoma to high-dose intravenous interleukin-2 after prior exposure to alpha-interferon or low-dose interleukin-2. J Immunother 25:185–187, 2002.
9. Yang JC, Sherry RM, Steinberg SM, et al. Randomized study of high-dose and low-dose interleukin-2 in patients with metastatic renal cancer. J Clin Oncol 21:3127–3132, 2003.
10. Clark JI, Atkins MB, Urba WJ, et al. Adjuvant high-dose bolus interleukin-2 for patients with high-risk renal cell carcinoma: A cytokine working group randomized trial. J Clin Oncol 21:3133–3140, 2003.
11. Weil-Hillman G, Voss SD, Fisch P, et al. Natural killer cells activated by Interleukin-2 treatment *in vivo* respond to Interleukin-2 primarily through the p75 receptor and maintain the p55 (TAC) negative phenotype. Cancer Res 50:2683–2691, 1990.
12. Shiloni E, Eisenthal A, Sachs D, et al. Antibody-dependent cellular cytotoxicity mediated by murine lymphocytes activated in recombinant interleukin-2. J Immunol 138:1992–1998, 1987.
13. Bernstein N, Starnes C, Levy R. Specific enhancement of the therapeutic effect of anti-idiotype antibodies on a murine B cell lymphoma by IL-2. J Immunol 140:2839–2845, 1988.
14. Hank JA, Robinson RR, Surfus J, et al. Augmentation of antibody dependent cell mediated cytotoxicity following *in vivo* therapy with recombinant Interleukin-2. Cancer Res. 50:5234–5239, 1990.
15. Schultz KR, Peace DJ, Badger CC, et al. Monoclonal antibody therapy of murine lymphoma: Enhanced efficacy by concurrent administration of interleukin 2 or lymphokine-activated killer cells. Cancer Res 50:5421–5425, 1990.
16. Fleming GF, Meropol NJ, Rosner GL, et al. A phase I trial of escalating doses of trastuzumab combined with daily subcutaneous interleukin 2: report of cancer and leukemia group B 9661. Clin Cancer Res 8(12):3718–3727, 2001.
17. Bajorin DF, Chapman PB, Wong G, et al. Phase I evaluation of a combination of monoclonal antibody R24 and interleukin 2 in patients with metastatic melanoma. Cancer Res 50:7490–7495, 1990.
18. Friedberg JW, Neuberg D, Gribben JG, et al. Combination immunotherapy with rituximab and interleukin 2 in patients with relapsed or refractory follicular non-Hodgkin's lymphoma. Br J Haematol. 117:828–834, 2002.
19. Fiedler W, Kruger W, Laack E, Mende T, Vohwinkel G, Hossfeld DK. A clinical trial of edrecolomab, IL-2 and GM-CSF in patients with advanced Colon Cancer. Oncol Reports. 8:225–231, 2001
20. Lode HN, Xiang R, Varki NM, et al. Targeted interleukin-2 therapy of spontaneous neuroblastoma to bone marrow. J Nat Cancer Inst 89:1586–1591, 1997.
21. Lode Hn, Xiang R, Drier T, et al. Natural killer cell mediated eradication of neuroblastoma metastases to bone marrow by targeted IL-2 therapy. Blood 91:1706–1715, 1998.
22. Mujoo K, Cheresh D, Yang HM, et al. Disialoganglioside GD2 on human neuroblastoma: Target antigen for monoclonal antibody mediated cytolysis and suppression of tumor growth. Cancer Res 47:1098–1104, 1986.
23. Cheung NK, Saarinen UM, Neely JE, et al. Monoclonal antibodies to a glycolipid antigen on human neuroblastoma cells. Cancer Res 45:2642–2649, 1985.

24. Schulz G, Cheresh DA, Varki NM, et al. Detection of ganglioside GD2 in tumor tissues and sera of neuroblastoma patients. Cancer Res 44:5914–5920, 1984.
25. Kramer K, Gerald WL, Kushner BH, et al. Disialoganglioside G(D2) loss following monoclonal antibody therapy is rare in neuroblastoma. Clin Cancer Res 4:2135–2139, 1998.
26. Cheung NK, Lazarus H, Miraldi FD, et al. Ganglioside GD2 specific monoclonal antibody 3F8: a phase I study in patients with neuroblastoma and malignant melanoma. J Clin Oncol 5:1430–1440, 1987.
27. Cheung NK, Kushner BH, Cheung IY, et al. Anti-G(D2) antibody treatment of minimal residual stage 4 neuroblastoma diagnosed at more than 1 year of age. J Clin Oncol 16:3053–3060, 1998.
28. Handgretinger R, Baader P, Dopfer R, et al. A phase I study of neuroblastoma with the anti-ganglioside GD2 antibody 14.G2a. Cancer Immunol. Immunother. 35:199–204, 1992,
29. Yu A, Uttenreuther-Fischer M, Huang C-S, et al. Phase I trial of a human-mouse chimeric anti-disialoganglioside monoclonal antibody ch14.18 in patients with refractory neuroblastoma and osteosarcoma. J Clin Oncol 16:2169–2180, 1998.
30. Handgretinger R, Anderson K, Lang P, et al. A phase I study of human/mouse chimeric antiganglioside GD2 antibody ch 14.18 in patients with neuroblastoma. Eur J Cancer 31:261–267, 1995.
31. Murray JL, Cunningham JE, Brewer H, et al. Phase I trial of murine monoclonal antibody 14.G2a administered by prolonged intravenous infusion in subjects with neuroectodermal tumors. J Clin Oncol 12:814–1193, 1994.
32. Saleh MN, Khazaeli MB, Wheeler RH, et al. Phase I trial of the murine monoclonal anti-GD2 antibody 14.G2a in metastatic melanoma. Cancer Res 52:4342–4347, 1992.
33. Saleh MN, Khazaeli MB, Wheeler RH, et al. Phase I trial of the chimeric anti-GD2 monoclonal antibody ch14.18 in subjects with malignant melanoma. Human Antibodies and Hybridomas 3:19–24, 1992.
34. Yeh SD, Larson SM, Burch L, et al. Radioimmunodetection of neuroblastoma with iodine-131-3F8: Correlation with biopsy, iodine-131-metaiodobenzylguanidine (MIBG) and standard diagnostic modalities. J Nucl Med 32:769–776, 1991.
35. Larson SM, Divgi C, Sgouros G, et al. Monoclonal antibodies: Basic priciples - Radioisotope conjugates, In: DeVita VT, Hellman S, Rosenberg SA eds. *Biologic Therapy of Cancer - Principles and Practice*. Philadelphia, J.B. Lippincott Co., 2000, pp 396–412.
36. Reuland P, Geiger L, Thelen MH, et al. Follow-up in neuroblastoma: comparison of metaiodobenzylguanidine and a chimeric anti-GD2 antibody for detection of tumor relapse and therapy response. J PediatriHematol/Oncol. 23:437–442, 2001.
37. Barker E, Reisfeld RA. A mechanism for neutrophil-mediated lysis of human neuroblastoma cells. Cancer Res 53:362–367, 1993.
38. Munn DH, Cheung NKV. Interleukin-2 enhancement of monoclonal antibody-mediated cellular cytotoxicity against human melanoma. Cancer Res 47:6600, 1987.
39. Lammie GA, Cheung NKV, Gerald W, et al. Ganglioside GD2 expression in the human nervous system and in neuroblastomas - an immunohistochemical study. Int J Oncol 3:909–915, 1993.
40. Xiao W-h, Yu A, Sorkin LS. Electrophysiological characteristics of primary afferent fibers after systemic administration of anti-GD2 ganglioside antibody. Pain 69:145–151, 1997.
41. Svennerholm L, Bostrom K, Fredman P, et al. Gangliosides and allied glycosphingolipids in human peripheral nerve and spinal cord. Biochim Bioshys Acta 1214(2):115–123, 1994.
42. Yuki N, Yamada M, Tagawa Y, et al. Pathogenesis of the neurotoxicity caused by anti-GD2 antibody therapy. J Neurol Sci 149:127–130, 1997.
43. Simon T, Hero B, Faldum A, et al. Consolidation treatment with chimeric anti-GD2–antibody ch14.18 in children older than 1 year with metastatic neuroblastoma. J Clin Oncol. 22(17):3549–3557, 2004.
44. Sondel PM, Hank JA. Antibody directed, effector cell mediated, tumor destruction. Hematol/Oncol Clin North Am 15:4:703–721, 2001.
45. Frost JD, Ettinger LJ, Hank JA, et al. Phase I/IB trial of murine monoclonal anti-GD2 antibody 14.Ga plus IL-2 in children with refractory neuroblastoma: A report of the Children's Cancer Group. Cancer, 80:317–333, 1997.
46. Albertini MR, Hank JA, Schiller JH, et al. Phase IB trial of chimeric anti-GD2 antibody plus interleukin-2 for melanoma patients. Clin Cancer Res 3:1277–1288, 1997.
47. Hank J, Surfus J, Gan J, et al. Treatment of neuroblastoma patients with antiganglioside GD2 antibody plus Interleukin-2 induces antibody dependent cellular cytotoxicity against neuroblastoma detected *in vitro*. J Immunother 15:29–37, 1994.

48. Kushner BH, Kramer K, Cheung NKV. Phase II trial of the anti-G(D2) monoclonal antibody 3F8 and granulocyte-macrophage colony-stimulating factor for neuroblastoma. J Clin Oncol 19:4189–4194, 2001.

49. Yu AL, Uttenreuther MM, Kamps A, Batova A, Reisfeld RA. Combined use of a human- mouse chimeric anti-GD2 (ch14.18) and GM-CSF in the treatment of refractory neuroblastoma. Antibody Immunoconjugates, and Radiopharmaceuticals 8:12, 1995.

50. Cheung IY, Lo Piccolo MS, Kushner B, et al. Early molecular response in marrow is highly prognostic following treatment with anti-GD2 and GM-CSF. J Clin Oncol 21:3853–3858, 2003.

51. Ozkaynak MF, Seeger R, Bauer M, Sondel P, Blazer B, Reaman G. A Phase I study of ch14.18 with GM-CSF in children with neuroblastoma following autologous BMT. Children's Cancer Group Study, J Clin Oncol 18:4077–4085, 2000.

52. Gilman A, Sondel PM, Krailo M, et al. A pahse I study of ch14.18 with GM-CSF and IL-2 in children with neuroblastoma and other GD2 positive malignancies immediately post ABMT. CCG-0935A. Clinical Protocol, Open 1997–2002. (manuscript in preparation).

53. Yu A, Gilman A, Ozkaynak F, et al. COG ANBL0032. A Phase III trial of ch14.18 mAb plus IL-2 plus GM-CSF for children with high risk neuroblastoma following ASCT. COG protocol, open Dec. 2001. Available on COG website, and NCI-PDQ.

54. W.-K. Weng, R. Levy. Two Immunoglobulin G Fc receptor polymorphisms independently predict response to rituximab in patients with follicular lymphoma. J Clin Oncol 2003, 21:3940–3947.

55. Weil-Hillman G, Fisch P, Prieves AF, Sosman JA, Hank JA, Sondel PM. Lymphokine-activated killer activity indiced by *in vivo* interleukin-2 therapy: Predominant role for lymphocytes with increased expression of CD2 and Leu19 antigens but negative expression of CD16 antigens. Can Res 49: 3680–3688, 1989.

56. Voss SD, Robb RJ, Weil-Hillman G, et al. Increased expression of the interleukin-2 (IL-2) receptor beta chain (p70) on CD56+ natural killer cells after *in vivo* IL-2 therapy: p70 expression does not alone predict the level of intermediate affinity IL-2 binding. J Exp Med 172:1101–1114, 1990.

57. Sondel PM, Kohler PC, Hank JA, et al. Clinical and immunological effects of recombinant interleukin-2 given by repetitive weekly cycles to subjects with cancer. Cancer Res 48:2561–2567, 1988.

58. Gillies SD, Reilly EB, Lo K-M, Reisfled RA. Antibody-targeted interleukin 2 stimulates the T-cell killing of autologous tumor cells. Proc Natl Acad Sci (USA) 89:1428, 1992.

59. Hank JA, Surfus JE, Gan J, et al. Activation of human effector cells by a tumor reactive recombinant anti-ganglioside GD2/interleukin-2 immunocytokine (ch14.18-IL-2). Clin Cancer Res 2:1951–1959, 1996.

60. Sabzevari H, Gillies SD, Mueller BM, Pancook JD, Reisfeld RA. A recombinant antibody-interleukin 2 immunocytokine suppresses growth of hepatic human neuroblastoma metastases in severe combined immunodeficiency mice. Proc Natl Acad Sci (USA) 91:9626, 1994.

61. Becker JC, Pancook JD, Gillies SD, et al. T cell mediated eradiation of murine metastatic melanoma induced by targeted interleukin-2 therapy. J Exp Med 183:2361, 1996.

62. Becker JC, Varki N, Gillies SD, et al. An antibody-interleukin-2 fusion protein overcomes tumor heterogeneity by induction of a cellular immune response. Proc Natl Acad Sci USA 93:7826–7831. 1996.

63. American Cancer Society. *Cancer Facts and Figures*. ACS publications, Atlanta GA. 2004.

64. Balch CM, Buzaid AC, Soong SJ, et al. Final version of the American Joint Committee on Cancer Staging System for cutaneous melanoma. J. Clin. Oncol. 19:3635–3648, 2001.

65. Kirkwood JM, Ibrahim JG, Sosman JA, et al. High-dose interferon alfa-2b significantly prolongs relapse-free and overall survival compared with the GM2-KLH/QS-21 vaccine in patients with resected stage IIB-III melanoma: results of intergroup trial E1694/S9512/C509801. J Clin Oncol 19:2370–2380, 2001.

66. Chung MH, Gupta RK, Hsueh E, et al. Humoral immune response to a therapeutic polyvalent cancer vaccine after complete resection of thick primary melanoma and sentinel lymphadenectomy. J Clin Oncol 2003, 21:313–319.

67. Sosman JA, Unger JM, Liu PY, et al. Adjuvant immunotherapy of resected, intermediate-thickness, node- negative melanoma with an allogeneic tumor vaccine: impact of HLA class I antigen expression on outcome. J Clin Oncol 20:2067–2075, 2002.

68. Bystryn JC, Zeleniuch-Jacquotte A, Oratz R, Shapiro RL, Harris MN, Roses DF. Double-blind trial of a polyvalent, shed-antigen, melanoma vaccine. Clin Cancer Res 7:1882–1887, 2001.

69. Hersey P, Coates AS, McCarthy WH, Thompson JF, Sillar RW, McLeod R, Gill PG, Coventry BJ, McMullen A, Dillon H, et al.: Adjuvant immunotherapy of patients with high-risk melanoma using vaccinia viral lysates of melanoma: results of a randomized trial. J Clin Oncol 20:4181–4190, 2002.

70. Berd D. Autologous, hapten-modified vaccine as a treatment for human cancers. Vaccine 19: 2565–2570, 2001.

71. Chapman PB, Morrissey DM, Panageas KS, et al. Induction of antibodies against GM2 ganglioside by immunizing melanoma patients using GM2-KLH + QS21 vaccine: A dose-response study. Clin Cancer Res 6:874–879, 2000.

72. Wang F, Bade E, Kuniyoshi C, et al. Phase I trial of a MART-1 peptide vaccine with incomplete Freund's adjuvant for resected high-risk melanoma. Clin Cancer Res 5:2756–2765, 1999.

73. Slingluff CL, Jr., Petroni GR, Yamshchikov GV, et al. Clinical and immunologic results of a randomized phase II trial of vaccination using four melanoma peptides either administered in granulocyte-macrophage colony-stimulating factor in adjuvant or pulsed on dendritic cells. J Clin Oncol 21: 4016–4026, 2003.

74. Dudley ME, Wunderlich JR, Robbins PF, et al. Cancer regression and autoimmunity in patients after clonal repopulation with antitumor lymphocytes. Science 298(5594):850–854, 2002.

75. Soiffer R, Hodi FS, Haluska F, et al. Vaccination with irradiated, autologous melanoma cells engineered to secrete granulocyte-macrophage colony-stimulating factor by adenoviral-mediated gene transfer augments antitumor immunity in patients with metastatic melanoma. J Clin Oncol. 21(17): 3343–3350, 2003

76. Brodeur GM, Maris JM. Neuroblastoma. *In:* Principles and practice of pediatric Oncology. Eds. Pizzo PA, Poplack DG. Lippincott. Philadelphia. pp 895–938, 2002.

77. Matthay KK, Villablanca JG, Seeger RC, et al. Treatment of high-risk neuroblastoma with intensive chemotherapy, radiotherapy, autologous bone marrow transplantation, and 13-cis-retinoic acid. N Engl J Med 341: 1165–1173, 1999.

78. Chang HR. Cordon-Cardo C. Houghton AN. Cheung NK. Brennan MF. Expression of disialogangliosides GD2 and GD3 on human soft tissue sarcomas. Cancer 70(3):633–638, 1992.

79. Yoshida S, Kawaguchi H, Sato S, Ueda R, Furukawa K. An anti-GD2 monoclonal antibody enhances apoptotic effects of anti-cancer drugs against small cell lung cancer cells via JNK (c-Jun terminal kinase) activation. Jap J Cancer Res 93(7):816–824, 2002.

80. Albertini MR, Gan J, Jaeger P, et al. Systemic Interleukin-2 modulates the anti-idiotypic response to chimeric anti-GD2 antibody in patients with melanoma. J Immunother 19(4):278–295, 1996.

81. Kendra K, Gan J, Ricci M, et al. Pharmacokinetics and stability of the 14.18-IL-2 fusion protein in mice. Cancer Immunol Immunother 48:219–229, 1999.

82. Lotze M, Matory YL, Ettinghausen SE, et al. *In vivo* administration of IL-2. Half-life, immunologic effects, and expansion of PBL cells *in vivo* with recombinant IL-2. J Immunol 135: 2865–2875, 1985.

83. Albertini MR, Kendra K, King D, et al. Phase I/Ib trial of the hu14.18-IL-2 fusion protein in patients with GD2+ tumors. CTEP- UWCCC protocol #CO 98901. Amendment 7, approved 1/17/02. Available on NCI-PDQ website.2002.

84. King DM, Albertini MR, Schalch H, et al. PM. A phase I clinical trial of the immunocytokine EMD 273063 (hu14.18-IL-2) in patients with melanoma. J Clin Oncol, 22:4463–4473, 2004.

85. Storer B. Design and analysis of phase I clinical trials. Biometrics 45:925–937, 1989.

86. Webb DE, Austen HA, Belldegrun A, Vaughan E, Linehan WM, Rosenberg SA. Metabolic and renal effects of interleukin-2 immunotherapy for metastatic cancer. Clin Nephrol 30(3):141–145, 1988

87. Osenga KL, Hank JA, Albertini MR, et al. A Phase I clinical trial of hu 14.18.IL2 (EMD 273063) as a treatment for children with refractory or recurrent neuroblastoma and melanoma: a study of the Children's Oncology Group. Clin Cancer Res 12:1750–1759, 2006

88. Foon KA, Sen G, Hutchins L, et al. Antibody responses in melanoma patients immunized with an anti-idiotype antibody mimicking disialoganglioside GD2. Clin Cancer Res 4:1117–1124, 1998.

89. Batova A, Strother D, Castleberry RP, et al. Immune response to an anti-idiotype monoclonal antibody 1A7 as a tumor vaccine in children with high risk neuroblastoma. Proc Am Assoc Cancer Res 43:143, 2002.

90. Gan J, Kendra, K, Ricci M, Hank JA, Gillies SD, Sondel PM. Specific ELISA systems for quantitation of antibody-cytokine fusion proteins. Clin Diagn Immunol. 6(2):236–242, 1999.

91. Bogner MP, Voss SD, Bechhofer R, et al. Serum CD25 levels during Interleukin-2 therapy: Dose dependence and correlations with clinical toxicity and lymphocyte surface sCD25 expression. J Immunother 11:111–118, 1992.

92. Voss SD, Hank JA, Nobis C, Fisch P, Sosman JA, Sondel PM. Serum levels of the low-affinity Interleukin-2 receptor molecule (TAC) during IL-2 therapy reflect systemic lymphoid mass activation. Cancer Imm Immunother 29:261–269, 1989.

93. Farner NL, Voss SD, Leary TP, et al. Distinction between gamma c detection and function in YT lymphoid cells and in the granulocyte-macrophage colony-stimulating factor-responsive human myeloid cell line, Tf-1. Blood 86(12):4568–4578, 1995.

94. Hank JA, Surfus JE, Gan J, Ostendorf A, Gillies SD, Sondel PM. Determination of peak serum levels and immune response to the humanized anti-ganglioside antibody-Interleukin 2 immunocytokine. *In:* Eds. Buolamwini JK, Adjei AA. *Methods in Molecular Medicine- Novel Anticancer Drug Protocols.* Humana Press, Totowa NJ, 85:123–131, 2003.

95. Neal ZC, Imboden M, Rakhmilevich AL, et al. NXS2 murine neuroblastomas express increased levels of MHC class I antigens upon recurrence following NK-dependent immunotherapy. Cancer Immunol Immunother 53:41–52, 2003.

96. Connor J, Felder M, Hank JA, et al. Ex vivo evalution of anti-IpCAM immunocytokine hu kS-IL-2 in ovarian cancer. J Immunother 27:211–219, 2004.

97. Imboden M, Murphy KR, Rakhmilevich AL, et al. The level of MHC Class I expression on murine adenocarcinoma can change the antitumor effector mechanism of immunocytokine therapy. Cancer Res 61(4):1500–1507, 2001.

98. Algarra I, Cabrera T, Garrido F. The HLA crossroad in tumor immunology. Hum Immunol 61: 65, 2000.

99. Marincola FM, Wang E, Herlyn M, Seliger B, Ferrone S. Tumors as elusive targets of T-cell-based active immunotherapy. Trends in Immunol 24:335–342, 2003.

100. Yu Z, Restifo NP. Cancer vaccines: progress reveals new complexities. J Clin Invest 110: 289, 2002.

101. Neal ZC, Yang JC, Rakhmilevich AL, et al. Enhanced activity of hu14.18-IL-2 immunocytokine against the murine NXS2 neuroblastoma when combined with IL-2 therapy. Clin Cancer Res 10: 4839–4847, 2004.

102. Chang AE, Hyatt CL, Rosenberg SA. Systemic administration of recombinant human interleukin-2 in mice. J Biol Response Mod 3: 561–572, 1984.

103. Hank JA, Surfus J, Gan J, et al. Distinct clinical and laboratory activity of two recombinant interleukin-2 preparations. Clin Cancer Res 5: 281–289, 1999.

104. Sosman JA, Kohler PC, Hank JA, et al. Repetitive weekly cycles of interleukin-2. II. Clinical and immunologic effects of dose, schedule, and indomethacin. J Natl Cancer Inst 80:1451–1460, 1988.

105. Shanafelt AB, Lin Y, Shanafelt MC, et al. A T-cell-selective interleukin 2 mutein exhibits potent antitumor activity and is well tolerated in vivo. Nat Biotechnol 18:1197–1202. 2000.

106. Gillies SD, Lo KM, Burger C, Lan Y, Dahl T, Wong WK. Improved circulating half-life and efficacy of an antibody-interleukin 2 immunocytokine based on reduced intracellular proteolysis. Clin Cancer Res 8:210–216. 2002.

107. Gillies, SD, Lan, Y, Williams, S, et al. An anti-CD20-IL-2 immunocytokine is highly efficacious in a SCID mouse model of established human B lymphoma. Blood 105: 3972–3978, 2005.

108. Davis CB, Gillies SD. Immunocytokines: amplification of anti-cancer immunity. Cancer Immunol Immunother 52:297–308. 2003.

109. Gillies SD, Lan Y, Brunkhorst B, Wong WK, Li Y, Lo KM. Bi-functional cytokine fusion proteins for gene therapy and antibody-targeted treatment of cancer. Cancer Immunol Immunother 51:449–460, 2002.

110. Lode HN, Moehler T, Xiang R, Jonczyk A, Gillies SD, Cheresh DA, Reisfeld RA. Synergy between an antiangiogenic integrin av antagonist and an antibody–cytokine fusion protein eradicates spontaneous tumor metastases. PNAS 96: 1591–1596, 1999.

22 Cytokines and Cancer Vaccines

Hideho Okada and Michael T. Lotze

CONTENTS

INTRODUCTION
CANCER VACCINE IN COMBINATION WITH RECOMBINANT CYTOKINES
CYTOKINE GENE TRANSFECTED CANCER VACCINES
CLINICAL STUDIES OF CYTOKINE-GENE THERAPY FOR CANCERS
CONCLUSIONS
REFERENCES

1. INTRODUCTION

Since the late 1980s, tumor immunology has made truly revolutionary progress. Perhaps the two most significant contributing factors are the discovery of tumor antigens (TAs) and advances in cytokine-biotechnology. Molecular characterization of T-cell-epitopes within TAs led an evolution of tumor immunology from the rather empirical observation of tumor regressions into a sophisticated science established on a solid molecular basis *(1,2)*. In addition, the availability of recombinant cytokines and their cDNAs promoted our understanding of the role of cytokines in tumor immunosurveillance, and allowed us to examine the administration of cytokines to facilitate anti-tumor inflammatory response within the tumor microenvironment.

Cancer vaccines were designed to induce systemic immunity against nominally weak tumor antigens for which no or little response could be measured. In particular, in recent years, T-cell epitope-peptides within the TAs have been, or are being, used in clinical trials to induce or enhance the TA-specific cellular immune response of the host *(3–5)*. Regrettably, induction or enhancement of antitumor immune reactivity detected by various immunologic monitoring methods has not closely correlated with tumor regression *(6,7)*.

The rejection of tumors by an immune system activated by TA-specific vaccination is the final outcome of a series of events that initiate with an immune or inflammatory response at the site of vaccination to the execution of tumor cells within the tumor tissue. The phenotypic characteristics and activation status of the antigen-presenting cells (APCs) that accumulate at the vaccine site will determine their ability to initiate the activation and expansion of TA-specific T-cells within draining lymph nodes, which in turn

From: *Cancer Drug Discovery and Development,*
Cytokines in the Genesis and Treatment of Cancer
Edited by: M. A. Caligiuri and M. T. Lotze © Humana Press Inc., Totowa, NJ

may induce a systemically detectable immune response. Vaccine-induced effector cells are expected to traffic to the tumor site and exert their antitumor activity. However, by a variety of mechanisms that are often called as "immune-escape of the tumors," the tumor microenvironment is not always favorable for immune effector cells. Cytokines can influence the outcome of each stage of response within the tumor microenvironment. Delivery of pro-inflammatory cytokines at the site of vaccination may enhance induction of immune response by activating and maturing APCs. At the target tumor site, delivery of immunostimulatory cytokines may modulate the tumor microenvironment in such a way that the vaccine-induced effector cells can infiltrate and recognize the tumor cells more efficiently.

This chapter reviews recent progress in studies aimed to potentiate the efficacy of cancer vaccines by delivery of immuno-stimulatory cytokines using recombinant cytokines or cytokine gene therapy strategies. The main message from this chapter is that proper understanding and use of cytokines are necessary for achieving clinical anti-tumor effects employing various cancer vaccine strategies.

2. CANCER VACCINE IN COMBINATION WITH RECOMBINANT CYTOKINES

Cytokines function in either an autocrine or paracrine manner and tend to operate in cascades, regulating both the innate and adaptive immune systems. Although many cytokines are required to orchestrate a successful immune response, the list of recombinant cytokine proteins that are currently approved by the Food and Drug Administration for patients with cancer comprises only IL-2 and IFN-α. In addition to their standard use for cancer treatment, these cytokines have been shown to enhance the efficacy of antigen-specific cancer vaccines.

As discussed in the Introduction, the current paradox with the application of cancer vaccines include the discrepancy between the increased number of TA-specific T-cells that are capable of binding TAs and the lack of clinical response in the same patient. What are the key factors that create such a paradoxical puzzle of the coexistence of cancer cells and effector immune cells in the same host? Indeed, although immunization-induced T-cells are capable of binding antigen-epitope specific tetramers, they do not express perforin and are of small size, which is a phenotype compatible with a resting state (8). Thus, it remains undefined whether the activation status of circulating vaccine-induced antigen-specific CD8+ T-cells is adequate to induce tumor regression. In vitro stimulation of these cells in the presence of IL-2 restores expression of perforin, suggesting that circulating vaccine-elicited T-cells require additional boosting stimulation in vivo to exert their antitumor response (8). Spontaneous inflammatory reaction at the site of tumor probably is not sufficient to promote the full-activation of tumor-infiltrating T-cells. Therefore, the additional inflammatory stimulus brought to the tumor site by nonspecific immune stimulation, such as the systemic administration of IL-2, may shift the balance in favor of host defense, and response to therapy may occur (3).

The complex requirements for T-cell activation through TCR–HLA–epitope engagement render cellular immune responses heavily susceptible to changes in target molecule expression. This is a significant problem because tumor cells frequently display downregulated HLA expression (9). HLA–epitope complex loss from tumor cells has an obvious effect on their recognition by TA-specific T-cells, and indeed, HLA–epitope complex downregulation on tumor cell membranes correlates with decreased T-cell-triggering capability *(10)*.

Delivery of interferons (IFNs) may help to overcome the issue of downregulated HLA-epitope complexes. IFNs are a complex family of proteins that can be subdivided into at least five classes. IFN-α, β, δ, and κ belong to type-I class of IFNs *(11,12)*; whereas IFN-γ represents is a type-II IFN. Type I IFNs have a variety of functions including activation of APC, natural killer (NK) cells and cytotoxic T-lymphocytes (CTLs) generation and induction of memory *(13)*; and up-regulation HLA expression *(14)*. Currently, IFN-α is approved for treatment of patients with high-risk malignant melanomas *(15)*.

Astsaturov et al. examined whether addition of high doses of IFN-α (20 MU/m^2 × 20 doses) could improve the duration of specific T-cell responses and therapeutic effects of viral vaccines expressing a melanoma associated antigen gp100. In patients who had previously responded to vaccination, subsequent administration of high dose IFN-α recalled gp100-reactive T-cells with the ability to kill gp100-expressing tumor targets in vitro. Concomitant with the reappearance of these CTLs, tumor regression was observed in the two patients with clinically evident metastatic disease. Although data are still preliminary and toxicity associated with IFN-α is of concern, these data suggest that high-dose IFN-α may be an effective strategy to recall and maintain antitumor responses initiated by cancer vaccines *(16)*. IL-12 has also been used as an adjuvant with peptide vaccines in patients with resected stage III/IV melanoma and is able to boost the vaccine response *(17)*.

3. CYTOKINE GENE TRANSFECTED CANCER VACCINES

Recombinant cytokine proteins have been employed as biologic drugs for cancer, viral, and autoimmune targets. Unfortunately, systemic delivery of pharmacologic doses of proteins often results in severe side effects and toxicities *(18)*. Furthermore, recombinant proteins made by bacteria lack post-transcriptional modifications such as glycosylation. Their administration therefore can lead to reduced biologic activity, and induction of neutralizing antibodies. As these therapeutic proteins tend to have very short half-lives and are complex to manufacture and deliver, many investigators are evaluating the genetic delivery of cytokine genes. Physiologically, most cytokines are quite potent proteins acting at small quantities. Although they circulate systemically, they are generally produced at the precise site where they are needed. Their requisite biologic effect is mediated by high local concentration at the site of inflammatory response.

3.1. Cytokine Gene Therapy Using Gene-Transfected Tumor Cells

One of the early concepts of gene transfer to promote immunotherapy against cancer employed genetic modification of tumor cells with a cytokine gene either by ex vivo transfection of tumor cells or in vivo intratumoral injection of gene-vectors. The modulation of the tumor immune microenvironment with delivery of various cytokine genes induces an inflammatory process thereby enhancing immunogenicity of TA in vivo *(19)*. This interpretation fits well with the "danger" model postulated by Matzinger *(20)* and recently updated and expanded to include the notion of hydrophobicity of so called exogenous and endogenous danger signals *(21)*. This approach is used as a means of inducing systemic responses that can target residual primary, as well as, metastatic lesions. Therapeutic effects of cytokine gene transfer in a preclinical setting, i.e., those which are capable of allowing or inducing rejection of well established tumors, have now been demonstrated with cytokines including but not limited to IL-2 *(22–24)*, GM-CSF *(25,26)*, Type-I IFNs such as IFN-α *(27–29)*, IL-4 *(30)*, IL-12 *(31)*, IL-18 *(32)*, and IL-23 *(33)*.

The most effective cytokine for vaccination may differ depending upon the location and the type of the tumor because each organ has distinct immunologic environment. With this regard, we have compared various cytokines and delivery modes to find the most efficacious strategy of cytokine gene therapy against central nervous (CNS) tumors *(30)*, which often has been described as "immunologically privileged" tumors *(34)*. We generated rat 9L gliosarcoma cells stably transfected with retroviral vectors encoding IL-4, IL-12, GM-CSF, or IFN-α. To simulate direct and highly efficient cytokine gene delivery, 9L cells transfected with cytokine genes were implanted into the brain of syngeneic rats. Despite high levels of cytokine expression within the CNS tumor site, most animals died from the tumor outgrowth, whereas these same cell lines were rejected following subcutaneous (sc) injection. In the settings of treatment of nontransfected 9L tumor in the CNS, sc vaccination with IL-4 transfected 9L resulted in the most significant increase of long-term survival among the cytokines tested. Interestingly, for the treatment of sc 9L tumors, GM-CSF-, IL-4, and IFN-α transfected 9L were equally effective. These data indicate that peripheral immunization with IL-4 transfected tumors may have unique ability to induce effective immune response against CNS 9L tumors *(30)*.

As with other cytokines, IL-4 has pleiotropic effects on immune cells of multiple lineages (reviewed in refs. *35,36*). Among its various interesting biologic properties, IL-4, in combination with GM-CSF, promotes bone marrow precursors or monocytes to develop/convert into DCs, which are the most efficient APCs in vitro in both mice and humans *(37,38)*. The local production of IL-4 by genetically engineered tumor cells induces potent protective *(39,40)*, as well as, therapeutic immunity *(41,42)* in animal models. Interestingly, IL-4 transduced cancer cells display increased lesional infiltration by DCs, relative to other cytokines *(43)*, which may result in enhanced cross-presentation of tumor-associated antigens. IL-4 plays an important role in DC maturation *(44)* and promote enhanced IL-12p70 secretion from DCs *(45,46)*. Thus, under certain circumstances, this typical Th2-type cytokine may indirectly (through its effects on DCs) polarize helper T-cell responses toward the Th1-type *(45,46)*. Indeed, local delivery of IL-4 at an immunization site in a Leishmania major model results in augmented IL-12 production and Th1-type responses in vivo *(47)*, which contrasts with the Th-2 type response associated with systemic or prolonged recombinant (r)IL-4 delivery in the same disease model. In addition, in the analyses of underlying mechanisms of the anti-tumor immunity induced by IL-4 gene transfected tumors by us and others, remarkable levels of IFN-γ were induced in the splenocytes and lymph node cells, suggesting that this type of vaccine tends to induce Th-1 type responses in certain models *(48,49)*. Novel findings on cytokine biology provide us with insights regarding the most suitable cytokines and the location and timing of their administration for optimum induction of antitumor immune responses.

3.2. Cytokine Gene Therapy Using Gene-Transfected DCs

In addition to transfection of autologous tumor cells, recently, the ex vivo transfer of genes to immune cells has shown positive impacts on cancer immunotherapy. Particularly, DC based vaccination represents a promising approach against cancer as DCs play a pivotal role in mediating immune responses. Although DCs are known to secrete cytokines and chemokines that have critical roles for activating antigen-specific effector T-cells *(50,51)*, the tumor microenvironment inhibits expression of these endogenous cytokines such as IL-12, IL-23, and IFN-α *(52)*. It was reasoned, therefore, that forced expression of immunostimulatory cytokines by means of ectopic expression of transgenes would enhance the antigen-presenting function of DCs *(53)*. In contrast to cumbersome procedures necessary for ex vivo gene-transfection of tumor cells, DCs are efficiently transfected using viral vectors such as adenoviral vectors *(54–56)*; and thus, delivery of immunostimulatory cytokines via DCs has been extensively explored recent years. The other advantages of DCs as vehicles for adenoviral vector-based cytokine genes are: (1) to provide supplemental APCs to tumors where the function of endogenous APC may be suppressed *(57)*; (2) to deliver T-cell-stimulating cytokines not only the tumor site, but also to the draining lymph nodes (LNs) because DCs migrate to LNs, allowing for benefits of cytokine delivery to be manifest in both of these clinically important tissue compartments; and (3) that this approach will likely prove safer than injection into sensitive organs such as the CNS of high-titer recombinant adenoviruses for ultimate clinical translation of our findings *(58)*.

In terms of the relative efficacy, vaccinations with GM-CSF-transfected DC induced a higher level of antitumor response than GM-CSF-transfected tumor cells in a melanoma model that express human melanoma-associated gene (MAGE)-1 as the model antigen *(59)*. With the paradigm of subcutaneous injection of DCs that are pulsed with tumor antigens ex vivo, DCs transfected with a lymphocyte attracting chemokine lymphotactin displayed enhanced antitumor response *(60,61)*.

Cytokine-transfected DCs were also injected directly to the tumor tissues. IL-12 transfected DCs, when injected into tumor-nodules, induced potent antitumor immune responses that resulted in a complete eradication in various tumor models *(53,62)*. In these models, tumor antigens were acquired by DC in the tumor environment and transported to lymph nodes. Transgene-derived IL-12 appeared to promote DC-survival and induction of IFN-γ-producing CTL activity. In addition, IL-12 may activate DC themselves by nuclear translocation of NF-κB, which resulted in endogenous IL-12 production *(63)*. IL-12 production may also promote interaction between natural killer (NK) cells and DCs thereby enhancing the induction of type-1 adaptive immunity *(64)*. Delivery of IL-12 transfected DCs appears to trigger a concerted immunologic milieu; activated NK cell-mediated tumor cell-killing may facilitate the release of tumor antigen, which in turn can be engulfed by DCs. In the draining lymph nodes, DCs present tumor antigens and still express IL-12, thereby promoting an induction of type-1 adaptive T-cell responses.

Not only the immune system, but also IL-12-induced anti-angiogenic effect may also have contributed in the antitumor effect as IL-12 is known to induce IFN-γ and secondary inflammatory/anti-angiogenic chemokines such as interferon-inducible protein (IP)-10 and monokine induced by IFN-γ (MIG) *(65,66)*.

Another potent Th1-biasing cytokine IL-18 is known to activate antitumor response that is primarily mediated by NK cells *(67)*. The presence of NK cells and DC was essential for the induction of tumor-specific CTL activity by IL-18 in vitro *(68)*. In this system, NK cells played a critical role in the release of tumor antigens. Intratumoral injection of DCs adenovirally engineered to secrete both IL-12 and IL-18 resulted in enhanced antitumor response in comparison to single cytokine regimens. The IL-12/IL-18 combination regimen displayed the broadest repertoire of IFN-γ response to acid-eluted, tumor-derived peptides among all treatment cohorts. This enhancement of cross-presentation of tumor-associated

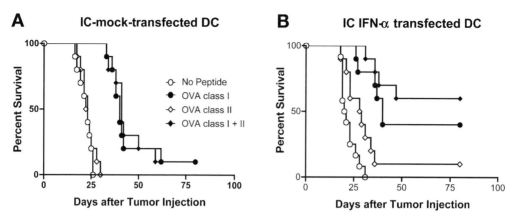

Fig. 1. Intratumoral injection of DC-IFN-α enhances the efficacy of vaccines with a mouse MHC class I K^b-restricted $OVA_{257-264}$ and a mouse MHC restricted $OVA_{265-280}$ "tumor" epitopes. C57BL/6 mice received two cycles of sc preimmunizations with either the K^b-restricted peptide epitope $OVA_{257-264}$ (SIINFEKL, closed circles), the I-A^b- restricted peptide epitope $OVA_{265-280}$ (TEWTSSNVMEERKIKV, open diamonds) or both epitopes (closed diamonds). Control animals received nonpulsed DC only (open circles). Animals received i.t. injection with mock-transfected DCs **(A)** or IFNα-transfected DCs **(B)**. $n = 10$ in all groups; Significance of differences (Logrank test): (A), $OVA_{257-264}$ vs no peptide: $P < 0.0001$; $OVA_{265-280}$ vs no peptide: $P = 0.5830$; $OVA_{257-264}$ plus $OVA_{265-280}$ vs no peptide: $P < 0.0001$; $OVA_{257-264}$ plus $OVA_{265-280}$ vs $OVA_{257-264}$: $P = 0.7330$; (B), $OVA_{257-264}$ vs. no peptide: $P < 0.0001$; $OVA_{265-280}$ vs no peptide: $P = 0.0174$; $OVA_{257-264}$ plus $OVA_{265-280}$ vs no peptide: $P < 0.0001$; $OVA_{257-264}$ plus $OVA_{265-280}$ vs. $OVA_{257-264}$: $P = 0.3458$. Okada H et al. Cancer Research (in press). Reprinted with permission by the American Association for Cancer Research.

epitopes might have resulted from the increased capacity of engineered DCs to kill tumor cells and to present immunogenic MHC/tumor peptide complexes to T-cells after intratumoral injection *(69)*. These results support the ability of combined cytokine gene transfer to enhance multiple effector functions mediated by intralesionally injected DCs that may concertedly promote cross-priming and the accelerated immune-mediated rejection of tumors *(69)*.

3.3. Modulation of Immunologic Microenvironment of CNS Tumors with Cytokine-Gene Transfected DCs and TA-Epitope Based Vaccines

Although we have demonstrated a potent efficacy of peripheral vaccination strategies against CNS tumors using CNS-tumor cells *(42)* or CNS-tumor-antigens *(70)*, the immunologic microenvironment of the CNS tumors is still believed to be suboptimal for the effective execution of antitumor effector response *(34)*.

We believe that systemic induction of TA-specific responses by peripheral vaccines should be followed by enhanced attraction of, and re-activation of vaccine-induced effector cells at the target CNS tumor site. Delivery of appropriate antigen presentation signals and stimulatory cytokines at the CNS tumor site may provide assistance to overcome tumor-derived immunosuppression.

Indeed, our data have indicated that injection of CNS tumors with DCs secreting IFN-α (DC-IFNα) remarkably enhanced the therapeutic effect of peripheral vaccinations with DCs loaded with TA-specific T-cell epitopes *(55)* (Fig. 1). The injected DC-IFNα migrated from the CNS tumor site to the draining cervical lymph nodes (CLNs), where they cross-primed tumor antigen-specific CTLs (Fig. 2). In this same setting,

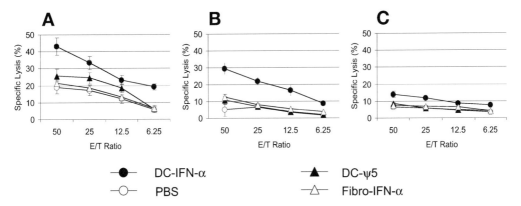

Fig. 2. Intratumoral injection of DC-IFNα enhances specific CTL reactivities in the cervical lymph nodes of animals that also received peripheral vaccines. Animals pre-immunized with either the K^b-restricted peptide epitope $OVA_{257-264}$ (**A**), the $I\text{-}A^b$- restricted peptide epitope $OVA_{265-280}$ (**B**) or adjuvant DC only (**C**) received i.c. injections of M05 tumors. On day 5 following the intracranial (i.c.) tumor challenge, animals also received either IFN-α transfected DC (closed circles), mock-transfected DC (closed triangles), syngeneic fibroblasts transfected with Ad-IFN-α (open triangles) or PBS (open circles). Animals were then sacrificed on day 15 following the i.c. tumor challenge (i.e., 10 d after the DC injection), and cervical lymph node (CLN) cells were in vitro stimulated with the K^b-restricted peptide epitope $OVA_{257-264}$ for 5 d. These cells were subjected to CTL assays using EL4 cells pulsed with $OVA_{257-264}$ as the target cells and nonpulsed EL4 cells as control cells. As the specific lysis values against nonpulsed EL4 cells were constantly below 8%, data were not included in the presented figures. Each value represents the average of triplicate determinations for each group. Statistical significance at effector vs target ratio 50:1 (Student's t-test); $P < 0.05$ for DC-IFN-α vs any other control group in panels A, B and C. Okada H et al. Cancer Research (*in press*). Reprinted with permission by the American Association for Cancer Research.

injections of mock-transfected DC or fibroblasts engineered to secrete IFN-α failed to demonstrate effective cross-priming or to provide therapeutic benefit, suggesting that DC-IFNα is a preferred modality for IFN-α gene therapy of CNS tumors.

This approach of "prime and boost" by the peripheral TA_vaccine plus intratumoral DC-IFN-α may lead to not only the enhancement of the magnitude of response against the antigen targeted by the peripheral vaccine, but also diversification of antigen repertoire for the response, thereby inhibiting the outgrowth of tumor cells that do not express the original target-antigen ("antigen-loss variant").

Taken together, use of DCs that are engineered to express cytokines, such as IFN-α, may be an effective cytokine gene therapy approach, particularly in combination with peripheral vaccines.

4. CLINICAL STUDIES OF CYTOKINE-GENE THERAPY FOR CANCERS

The National Institute of Health's Office of Biotechnology Activities (OBA) web site (http://www4.od.nih.gov/oba/rac/PROTOCOL.pdf) displays over 90 clinical trials with regard to cytokine gene transfer. The following section summarizes some of recent published studies (Table 1).

Trudel et al. conducted a phase-I clinical trial (*71*) primarily to test the safety and feasibility of adenovirus expressing IL-2 in prostate cancer. No dose-limiting toxicity was

Table 1
Published Clinical Studies of Cytokine Gene Therapy

Cytokine	Vector	Tumor type	Observation	Reference
IL-2	Adeno	Multiple Myeloma	Tolerated; no systemic immune or clinical response	85
IL-2	Adeno	Prostate Ca	Tolerated and PSA decreased	86
IL-2	Vero-IL2 cells	Melanoma	Phase II: tolerability and transient disease stabilization	87
IL-2	Cytokine-induced killer cells transfected with plasmid	Renal ca, colorectal ca and lymphoma	Systemic IFN-γ response, CR in 1 of 10 patients (lymphoma)	88
IL-4	Allogeneic melanoma transfected with retro	Melanoma	Increase of IFN-γ response in 7 of 11 patients	75
IL-4	Autologous fibroblasts transfected with retro	Glioma	A case report with a favorable clinical response	73
IL-12	Autologous tumor transfected with plasmid	Melanoma	DTH in 2 of 6 patients; positive CTL in 2 of 6 patients	87
IL-12	Autologous fibroblasts with retro	Any malignancy with accessible lesion	Local tumor response 4 of 9 patients; shrinkage of distant lesion in 1 of 9 patients	70d
IL-12	Adeno	GI cancers	Tolerated, 29% stable disease mainly with liver cancers.	70a
IFN-β	Cationic liposome	Glioma	PR in 2 of 4 and SD in 2 of 4 patients	89
IFN-γ	Autologous melanoma transfected with retro	Melanoma	Humoral immune response in 8 of 13 patients	70b
IFN-γ	Adeno	Melanoma	SD in 1 of 11 patients	74
GM-CSF	Autologous melanoma with retro	Melanoma	Metastatic lesions densely infiltrated with immune cells in 11 of 16 patients	25
GM-CSF	Autologous melanoma with adeno	Melanoma	Use of adenoviral vectors simplified vaccine manufacture	70c

observed up to 1×10^{10} PFU of virus injection. Pathology demonstrated in some cases an inflammatory response consisting predominantly of CD3+CD8+ T-lymphocytes with areas of tumor necrosis, accompanied by the decrease of prostate specific antigen (PSA) levels.

Based on our own studies discussed in Section 3., we initiated a phase I clinical study of vaccination with autologous glioma cells that are retrovirally transfected to express hIL-4 (UPCI-95-033) *(72)*. Although the study is still ongoing, some patients demonstrated temporary clinical and radiological improvement following vaccinations, with no evidence of allergic encephalitis *(73)*.

Although preparation of autologous gene transfected cells may be sometimes difficult due to the low-transfection efficacy, alternative strategy may be the use of allogeneic gene-transfected cells. Melanoma vaccines using HLA-A2+ allogeneic cell line transduced with IL-2 or IL-4 *(74)* demonstrated regression of skin nodules in some patients, but no changes were observed in other lesions. The side-effects were mild, including transient fever and erythema at the site of injection. Vaccination with allogeneic melanoma cells releasing IL-4 locally can expand a T-cell response against peptide Melan-A/MART-1(27–35) of autologous, untransduced tumor, although only in one of six patients' samples examined *(75)*.

Sangro et al. evaluated the feasibility and safety of intratumoral injection of an adenoviral vector encoding human IL-12 gene (Ad.IL-12) and secondarily, its biologic effect for the treatment of advanced digestive tumors *(76)*. Twenty-one patients (nine with primary liver, five with colorectal, and seven with pancreatic cancers) received injections of Ad.IL-12 in doses ranging from 2.5×10^{10} to 3×10^{12} viral particles. The treatment was well tolerated, and dose-limiting toxicity was not reached. In 4 of 10 assessable patients, a significant increase in tumor infiltration by effector immune cells was apparent. A partial objective remission of the injected tumor mass was observed in a patient with hepatocellular carcinoma. Stable disease was observed in 29% of patients, mainly those with primary liver cancer.

Khorana et al. treated patients with recurrent malignant melanoma with direct intratumoral injections of adenoviral IFN-γ *(77)*. Up to 1×10^{10} adenoviral IFN-γ particles were injected per injection per week for 3 wk. A maximum tolerated dose was not reached. Although no systemic immunologic activity was detected, one of 11 patients treated demonstrated stable disease.

In general, phase-I studies with intratumoral injection of adenoviral cytokine vectors have proven their safety. Immunogenicity of adenoviral vectors may have limited the transfection efficiency particularly in repeated injections *(78)*. Thus, as discussed in the previous section, injection of DCs ex vivo transfected with cytokine genes in combination with TA-specific vaccinations may be tested in clinical trials near future to improve the efficacy of the approach. Also, it is likely that the complexity of immune reactivity will preclude the use of a single cytokine to elicit or maintain long-term effective immune reactivity to human tumors. Therefore, further testing of cytokine gene therapy may be directed towards cytokine-combination strategies.

5. CONCLUSIONS

We have learned that the elimination of tumor cells by TA-specific vaccination is the final outcome of a series of events that initiate with an inflammatory response at the site of vaccination, antigen-presentation and expansion of functional TA-specific effector cells, which in turn traffic to and exert their antitumor activity at the target tumor sites. Various factors, including factors derived from tumors, appear to influence each of these steps. Priming with DC vaccine pulsed with TA-epitopes solely may not be sufficient to achieve the ultimate outcome because vaccine-induced TA-specific effectors have to be sufficiently activated systemically and at the site of the target tumors. Delivery of cytokines that are most suitable for the goal of each of immunologic steps may promote the efficacy of cancer vaccines. Such cytokines can be delivered either by the form of recombinant protein or gene vectors. With regard to the dose and mode of cytokine administration, although IL-2 and IFN-α have been established as standard therapy for certain cancers such as renal cell carcinoma and high risk melanoma, a major focus of future investigations should be directed towards local and sustained delivery of cytokines at the site where the function of the cytokine is expected to promote the immunologic milieu. Indeed, one of the major characteristics of most cytokines is that they regulate immunity at a local or regional level. Loco-regional delivery of cytokines particularly in the form of gene-therapy is expected to positively impact the efficacy of TA-specific vaccines.

Remaining issues after the discovery of TA-epitopes include heterogenicity of TA-profiles that may lead to outgrowth of antigen-loss variants. As discussed earlier, combinations of antigen-specific vaccines and cytokine delivery, especially by intratumoral injections of cytokine gene transfected DCs, appear to induce effective immune responses against diversified antigen-repertoire by facilitating a process called "antigen-spreading." We have come to the point to consider clinical trial designs that will examine the effect of the combination approaches of priming with the vaccine and boosting with local cytokine delivery.

In our efforts to further understand the inflammatory processes within the tumor immune microenvironment, we have recently recognized that high mobility group box 1 (HMGB1) is one of the critical molecules that promote a variety of molecular events in inflammation. Indeed this 30 kDa, highly conserved nuclear protein HMGB1 can be secreted (79) and itself promote the subsequent release of other cytokines (80) and enhance DC maturation (81,82), thereby promoting an immune response. Thus understanding how to deal with death within the tumor microenvironment will increasingly have to consider the modulatory effect of molecules released by dying tumor cells (83) which has been inferred from its increased presence in most tumor cells and our detection in culture supernatants of tumors following UV irradiation or NK mediated lysis [unpublished observations]. Taking into consideration the fact that many tumors arise in the setting of chronic inflammation (84) requires that we contemplate in earnest how to deal with death (83) in the tumor microenvironment and consider strategies how cytokines or other means to elicit tumor death can be effectively applied to future designs of effective cancer vaccines.

REFERENCES

Sun, Y., Jurgovsky, K., Moller, P., et al. Vaccination with IL-12 gene-modified autologous melanoma cells: preclinical results and a first clinical phase I study. Gene Ther. 1998;5:481-490.

1. Boon, T., Coulie, P.G., and van den Eynde, B. Tumor antigens recognized by T cells. Immunol. Today 1997;18:267–268.
2. Old, L.J. and Chen, Y.T. New paths in human cancer serology [comment]. J. Exp. Med. 1998;187: 1349–1354.
3. Rosenberg, S.A., Yang, J.C., Schwartzentruber, D.J., et al. Immunologic and therapeutic evaluation of a synthetic peptide vaccine for the treatment of patients with metastatic melanoma. Nature Med. 1998;4:321–327.

4. Marchand, M., Van, B.N., Weynants, P., et al. Tumor regressions observed in patients with metastatic melanoma treated with an antigenic peptide encoded by gene MAGE-3 and presented by HLA-A1. Int. J. Cancer 1999;80:219–230.

5. Jager, D., Jager, E., and Knuth, A. Vaccination for malignant melanoma: recent developments. Oncology 2001;60:1–7.

6. Nestle, F.O., Alijagic, S., Gilliet, M., et al. Vaccination of melanoma patients with peptide- or tumor lysate-pulsed dendritic cells. Nature Med. 1998;4:328–332.

7. Cormier, J.N., Salgaller, M.L., Prevette, T., et al. Enhancement of cellular immunity in melanoma patients immunized with a peptide from MART-1/Melan A. Cancer J. Sci. Am. 1997;3:37–44.

8. Monsurro, V., Nagorsen, D., Wang, E., et al. Functional heterogeneity of vaccine-induced CD8(+) T cells. J. Immunol 2002;168:5933–5942.

9. Ferrone, S. and Marincola, F.M. Loss of HLA class I antigens by melanoma cells: molecular mechanisms, functional significance and clinial relevance. Immunol. Today 1995;16:487–494.

10. Marincola, F.M., Jaffee, E.M., Hicklin, D.J., and Ferrone, S. Escape of human solid tumors from T-cell recognition: molecular mechanisms and functional significance. Adv. Immunol. 2000;74: 181–273.

11. Lefevre, F., Guillomot, M., D'Andrea, S., Battegay, S., and La Bonnardiere, C. Interferon-delta: the first member of a novel type I interferon family. Biochimie 1998;80:779–788.

12. Nardelli, B., Zaritskaya, L., Semenuk, M., et al. Regulatory effect of IFN-kappa, a novel type I IFN, on cytokine production by cells of the innate immune system. J Immunol 2002;169:4822–4830.

13. Hiroishi, K., Tuting, T., and Lotze, M.T. IFN-alpha-expressing tumor cells enhance generation and promote survival of tumor-specific CTLs. J. Immunol. 2000;164:567–572.

14. De Maeyer, E. and De Maeyer-Guignard, J. Interferons. In The Cytokine Handbook, A.Thomson, ed., 1998. London: Elsevier Science pp. 491–516.

15. Kirkwood, J.M. and Tarhini, A.A. Adjuvant high-dose interferon-alpha therapy for high-risk melanoma. Forum (Genova.) 2003;13:127–143.

16. Astsaturov, I., Petrella, T., Bagriacik, E.U., et al. Amplification of virus-induced antimelanoma T-cell reactivity by high-dose interferon-alpha2b: implications for cancer vaccines. Clin. Cancer Res. 2003;9:4347–4355.

17. Lee, P., Wang, F., Kuniyoshi, J., et al. Effects of interleukin-12 on the immune response to a multipeptide vaccine for resected metastatic melanoma. J. Clin. Oncol. 2001;19:3836–3847.

18. Kirkwood, J.M., Bender, C., Agarwala, S., et al. Mechanisms and management of toxicities associated with high-dose interferon alfa-2b therapy. J. Clin. Oncol. 2002;20: 3703–3718.

19. Pardoll, D.M. Paracrine cytokine adjuvants in cancer immunotherapy. Ann. Rev. Immunol. 1995;13: 399–415.

20. Matzinger, P. Tolerance, danger, and the extended family. Ann. Rev. Immunol. 1994;12:991–1045.

21. Seong, S.Y. and Matzinger, P. Hydrophobicity: an ancient damage-associated molecular pattern that initiates innate immune responses. Nat. Rev. Immunol. 2004;4:469–478.

22. Glick, R.P., Lichtor, T., de Zoeten, E., Deshmukh, P., and Cohen, E.P. Prolongation of survival of mice with glioma treated with semiallogeneic fibroblasts secreting interleukin-2. Neurosurg. 1999;45: 867–874.

23. Sampath, P., Hanes, J., Dimeco, F., et al. Paracrine immunotherapy with interleukin-2 and local chemotherapy is synergistic in the treatment of experimental brain tumors. Cancer Res. 1999;59:2107–2114.

24. Trudel, S., Trachtenberg, J., Toi, A., et al. A phase I trial of adenovector-mediated delivery of interleukin-2 (AdIL-2) in high-risk localized prostate cancer. Cancer Gene Ther. 2003;10:755–763.

25. Soiffer, R., Lynch, T., Mihm, M., et al. Vaccination with irradiated autologous melanoma cells engineered to secrete human granulocyte-macrophage colony-stimulating factor generates potent antitumor immunity in patients with metastatic melanoma. Proc. Natl. Acad. Sci. USA 1998;95:13141–13146.

26. Dranoff, G. GM-CSF-secreting melanoma vaccines. Oncogene 2003;22:3188–3192.

27. Horton, H.M., Anderson, D., Hernandez, P., Barnhart, K.M., Norman, J.A., and Parker, S.E. A gene therapy for cancer using intramuscular injection of plasmid DNA encoding interferon alpha. Proc Nat Acad Sci USA. 1999;96:1553–1558.

28. Hiroishi, K., Tuting, T., Tahara, H., and Lotze, M.T. Interferon-alpha gene therapy in combination with CD80 transduction reduces tumorigenicity and growth of established tumor in poorly immunogenic tumor models. Gene Ther. 1999;6:1988–1994.

29. Ferrantini, M., Giovarelli, M., Modesti, A., et al. IFN-alpha 1 gene expression into a metastatic murine adenocarcinoma (TS/A) results in CD8+ T cell-mediated tumor rejection and development of antitumor immunity. Comparative studies with IFN-gamma-producing TS/A cells. J. Immunol. 1994; 153:4604–4615.

30. Okada, H., Villa, L.A., Attanucci, J., et al. Cytokine Gene Therapy of Gliomas: Effective Induction of Therapeutic Immunity to Intracranial Tumors by Peripheral Immunization with Interleukin-4 Transduced Glioma Cells. Gene Ther. 2001;8:1157–1166.

31. Tahara, H., Zitvogel, L., Storkus, W.J., et al. Effective eradication of established murine tumors with IL-12 gene therapy using a polycistronic retroviral vector. J. Immunol. 1995;154:6466–6474.

32. Osaki, T., Hashimoto, W., Gambotto, A., et al. Potent antitumor effects mediated by local expression of the mature form of the interferon-gamma inducing factor, interleukin-18 (IL-18). Gene Ther. 1999;6:808–815.

33. Lo, C.H., Lee, S.C., Wu, P.Y., et al. Antitumor and antimetastatic activity of IL-23. J. Immunol 2003;171:600–607.

34. Walker, P.R., Calzascia, T., De Tribolet, N., and Dietrich, P.Y. T-cell immune responses in the brain and their relevance for cerebral malignancies. Brain Res. Rev. 2003;42:97–122.

35. Okada, H., Banchereau, J., and Lotze, M.T. Interleukin-4. In: A.W.Thomson and M.T.Lotze, eds. The Cytokine Handbook, 2003, London: Elsevier Science, pp. 227–262.

36. Okada, H. and Kuwashima, N. Gene therapy and biologic therapy with interleukin-4. Curr. Gene Ther. 2002;2:437–450.

37. Mayordomo, J.I., Zorina, T., Storkus, W.J., et al. Bone marrow-derived dendritic cells pulsed with synthetic tumour peptides elicit protective and therapeutic antitumor immunity. Nature Med. 1995;1:1297–1302.

38. Rosenzwajg, M., Camus, S., Guigon, M., and Gluckman, J.C. The influence of interleukin (IL)-4, IL-13, and Flt3 ligand on human dendritic cell differentiation from cord blood CD34+ progenitor cells. Exp. Hematol. 1998;26:63–72.

39. Tepper, R.I., Pattengale, P.K., and Leder, P. Murine interleukin-4 displays potent anti-tumor activity in vivo. Cell 1989;57:503–512.

40. Pericle, F., Giovarelli, M., Colombo, M.P., et al. An efficient Th2-type memory follows CD8+ lymphocyte-driven and eosinophil-mediated rejection of a spontaneous mouse mammary adenocarcinoma engineered to release IL-4. J. Immunol. 1994;153:5659–5673.

41. Golumbek, P.T., Lazenby, A.J., Levitsky, H.I., et al. Treatment of established renal cancer by tumor cells engineered to secrete interleukin-4. Science 1991;254:713–716.

42. Okada, H., Giezeman-Smits, KM., Tahara, H., et al. Effective cytokine gene therapy against an intracranial glioma using a retrovirally transduced IL-4 plus HSV-TK tumor vaccine. Gene Ther 1999;6:219–226.

43. Stoppacciaro, A., Paglia, P., Lombardi, L., Parmiani, G., Baroni, C., and Colombo, M.P. Genetic modification of a carcinoma with the IL-4 gene increases the influx of dendritic cells relative to other cytokines. Eur. J. Immunol. 1997;27:2375–2382.

44. Nestle, F.O., Filgueira, L., Nickoloff, B.J., and Burg, G. Human dermal dendritic cells process and present soluble protein antigens. J. Inv. Dermatol. 1998;110:762–766.

45. Kalinski, P., Smits, H.H., Schuitemaker, J.H., et al. IL-4 is a mediator of IL-12p70 induction by human Th2 cells: reversal of polarized Th2 phenotype by dendritic cells. J. Immunol. 200;165: 1877–1881.

46. Hockrein, H., O'Keeffe, M., Luft, T., et al. Interleukin (IL)-4 is a major regulatory cytokine governing bioactive IL-12 production by mouse and human dendritic cells. J. Exp. Med. 2000;192:823–833.

47. Biedermann, T., Zimmermann, S., Himmelrich, H., et al. IL-4 instructs TH1 responses and resistance to Leishmania major in susceptible BALB/c mice. Nat. Immunol. 2001;2:1054–1060.

48. Nishihori, H., Tsuji, H., Wang, H., et al. Participation of endogenously produced interferon gamma in interleukin 4-mediated tumor rejection. Human Gene Ther 2000;11:659–668.

49. Giezeman-Smits, KM., Okada, H., Brissette-Storkus, S.C., et al. Cytokine gene therapy of gliomas: Induction of reactive CD4+ T cells by interleukin-4 transfected 9L gliosarcoma is essential for protective immunity. Cancer Res. 2000;60:2449–2457.

50. Banchereau, J. and Steinman, R.M. Dendritic cells and the control of immunity. Nature 1998;392:245–252.

51. Nestle, F.O., Banchereau, J., and Hart, D. Dendritic cells: On the move from bench to bedside. Nat. Med 2001;7:761–765.

52. Hartmann, E., Wollenberg, B., Rothenfusser, S., et al. Identification and functional analysis of tumor-infiltrating plasmacytoid dendritic cells in head and neck cancer. Cancer Res 2003;63:6478–6487.

53. Nishioka, Y., Hirao, M., Robbins, P.D., Lotze, M.T., and Tahara, H. Induction of systemic and therapeutic antitumor immunity using intratumoral injection of dendritic cells genetically modified to express interleukin 12. Cancer Res. 1999;59:4035–4041.

54. Kim, S.H., Kim, S., Evans, C.H., Ghivizzani, S.C., Oligino, T., and Robbins, P.D. Effective treatment of established murine collagen-induced arthritis by systemic administration of dendritic cells genetically modified to express IL-4. J. Immunol. 2001;166:3499–3505.

55. Okada, H., Tsugawa, T., Sato, H., et al. Delivery of interferon- transfected DCs into central nervous system tumors enhances the anti-tumor efficacy of peripheral peptide-based vaccines. Cancer Res. 2004;64:5830–5838.

56. Rouard, H., Leon, A., Klonjkowski, B., et al. Adenoviral transduction of human 'clinical grade' immature dendritic cells enhances costimulatory molecule expression and T-cell stimulatory capacity. J. Immunol. Methods 2000;241:69–81.

57. Suter, T., Biollaz, G., Gatto, D., et al. The brain as an immune privileged site: dendritic cells of the central nervous system inhibit T cell activation. Eur. J. Immunol. 2003;33:2998–3006.

58. Dewey, R.A., Morrissey, G., Cowsill, C.M., et al. Chronic brain inflammation and persistent herpes simplex virus 1 thymidine kinase expression in survivors of syngeneic glioma treated by adenovirus-mediated gene therapy: implications for clinical trials. Nature Med. 1999;5:1256–1263.

59. Klein, C., Bueler, H., and Mulligan, R.C. Comparative analysis of genetically modified dendritic cells and tumor cells as therapeutic cancer vaccines. J. Exp. Med. 2000;191:1699–1708.

60. Cao, X., Zhang, W., He, L., et al. Lymphotactin gene-modified bone marrow dendritic cells act as more potent adjuvants for peptide delivery to induce specific antitumor immunity. J. Immunol. 1998;161:6238–6244.

61. Zhang, W., He, L., Yuan, Z., et al. Enhanced therapeutic efficacy of tumor RNA-pulsed dendritic cells after genetic modification with lymphotactin. Human Gene Ther 1999;10:1151–1161.

62. Melero, I., Duarte, M., Ruiz, J., et al. Intratumoral injection of bone-marrow derived dendritic cells engineered to produce interleukin-12 induces complete regression of established murine transplantable colon adenocarcinomas. Gene Ther. 1999;6:1779–1784.

63. Grohmann, U., Belladonna, M.L., Bianchi, R., et al. IL-12 acts directly on DC to promote nuclear localization of NF-kappaB and primes DC for IL-12 production. Immunity 1998;9:315–323.

64. Mailliard, R.B., Son, Y.I., Redlinger, R., et al. Dendritic cells mediate NK cell help for Th1 and CTL responses: two-signal requirement for the induction of NK cell helper function. J. Immunol 2003;171:2366–2373.

65. Farber, J.M. Mig and IP-10: CXC chemokines that target lymphocytes. J. Leukoc. Biol. 1997;61:246–257.

66. Tannenbaum, C.S., Tubbs, R., Armstrong, D., Finke, J.H., Bukowski, R.M., and Hamilton, T.A. The CXC chemokines IP-10 and Mig are necessary for IL-12-mediated regression of the mouse RENCA tumor. J. Immunol. 1998;161:927–932.

67. Osaki, T., Peron, J.M., Cai, Q., et al. IFN-gamma-inducing factor/IL-18 administration mediates IFN-gamma- and IL-12-independent antitumor effects. J. Immunol. 1998;160:1742–1749.

68. Tanaka, F., Hashimoto, W., Okamura, H., Robbins, P.D., Lotze, M.T., and Tahara, H. Rapid generation of potent and tumor-specific cytotoxic T lymphocytes by interleukin 18 using dendritic cells and natural killer cells. Cancer Research 2000;60:4838–4844.

69. Tatsumi, T., Huang, J., Gooding, W.E., et al. Intratumoral delivery of dendritic cells engineered to secrete both interleukin (IL)-12 and IL-18 effectively treats local and distant disease in association with broadly reactive Tc1-type immunity. Cancer Res. 2003;63:6378–6386.

70. Okada, H., Tahara, H., Shurin, M.R., et al. Bone marrow derived dendritic cells pulsed with a tumor specific peptide elicit effective anti-tumor immunity against intracranial neoplasms. Int. J. Cancer 1998;78:196–201.

70a. Sangro, B., Mazzolini, G., Ruiz, J., et al. Phase I trial of intratumoral injection of an adenovirus encoding interleukin-12 for advanced digestive tumors. J. Clin. Oncol. 2004;22:1389–1397.

70b. Abdel-Wahab, Z., Weltz, C., Hester, D., et al. A Phase I clinical trial of immunotherapy with interferon-gamma gene-modified autologous melanoma cells: monitoring the humoral immune response. Cancer 1997;80:401–412.

70c. Soiffer, R., Hodi, F.S., Haluska, F., et al. Vaccination with irradiated, autologous melanoma cells engineered to secrete granulocyte-macrophage colony-stimulating factor by adenoviral-mediated gene transfer augments antitumor immunity in patients with metastatic melanoma. J. Clin. Oncol. 2003;21:3343–3350.

70d. Kang, W.K., Park, C., Yoon, H.L., et al. Interleukin 12 gene therapy of cancer by peritumoral injection of transduced autologous fibroblasts: outcome of a phase I study. Hum. Gene Ther. 2001;12: 671–684.

71. Trudel, S., Trachtenberg, J., Toi, A., et al. A phase I trial of adenovector-mediated delivery of interleukin-2 (AdIL-2) in high-risk localized prostate cancer. Cancer Gene Ther. 2003;10:755–763.

72. Okada, H., Pollack, I.F., Lotze, M.T., et al. Gene therapy of malignant gliomas: a phase I study of IL4HSV-TK genemodified autologous tumor to elicit an immune response (clinical protocol). Human Gene Ther 2000;11:637–653.

73. Okada, H., Lieberman, F.S., Edington, H.D., et al. Autologous glioma cell vaccine admixed with interleukin-4 gene transfected fibroblasts in the treatment of recurrent glioblastoma: preliminary observations in a patient with a favorable response to therapy. J. Neurooncol. 2003;64:13–20.

74. Belli, F., Mascheroni, L., Gallino, G., et al. Active immunization of metastatic melanoma patients with IL-2 or IL-4 gene transfected, allogeneic melanoma cells. Adv. Exp. Med. Biol. 1998;451: 543–545.

75. Arienti, F., Belli, F., Napolitano, F., et al. Vaccination of melanoma patients with interleukin 4 gene-transduced allogeneic melanoma cells. Hum. Gene Ther. 1999;10:2907–2916.

76. Sangro, B., Mazzolini, G., Ruiz, J., et al. Phase I trial of intratumoral injection of an adenovirus encoding interleukin-12 for advanced digestive tumors. J. Clin. Oncol. 2004;22:1389–1397.

77. Khorana, A.A., Rosenblatt, J.D., Sahasrabudhe, D.M., et al. A phase I trial of immunotherapy with intratumoral adenovirus-interferon-gamma (TG1041) in patients with malignant melanoma. Cancer Gene Ther. 2003;10:251–259.

78. Ohmoto, Y., Wood, M.J., Charlton, H.M., Kajiwara, K., Perry, V.H., and Wood, K.J. Variation in the immune response to adenoviral vectors in the brain: influence of mouse strain, environmental conditions and priming. Gene Ther 1999;6:471–481.

79. Rendon-Mitchell, B., Ochani, M., Li, J., et al. IFN-gamma induces high mobility group box 1 protein release partly through a TNF-dependent mechanism. J. Immunol. 2003;170:3890–3897.

80. Li, J., Wang, H., Mason, J.M., et al. Recombinant HMGB1 with cytokine-stimulating activity. J. Immunol. Methods 2004;289:211–223.

81. Messmer, D., Yang, H., Telusma, G., et al. High mobility group box protein 1: an endogenous signal for dendritic cell maturation and Th1 polarization. J. Immunol. 2004;173: 307–313.

82. Rovere-Querini, P., Capobianco, A., Scaffidi, P., et al. HMGB1 is an endogenous immune adjuvant released by necrotic cells. EMBO Rep. 2004;5:825–830.

83. Lotze, M.T. and DeMarco, R.A. Dealing with death: HMGB1 as a novel target for cancer therapy. Curr. Opin. Investig. Drugs 2003;4:1405–1409.

84. Vakkila, J. and Lotze, M.T. Inflammation and necrosis promote tumour growth. Nat. Rev. Immunol. 2004;4:641–648.

85. Trudel, S., Li, Z., Dodgson, C., et al. Adenovector engineered interleukin-2 expressing autologous plasma cell vaccination after high-dose chemotherapy for multiple myeloma—a phase 1 study. Leukemia 2001;15:846–854.

86. Trudel, S., Trachtenberg, J., Toi, A., et al. A phase I trial of adenovector-mediated delivery of interleukin-2 (AdIL-2) in high-risk localized prostate cancer. Cancer Gene Ther. 2003;10:755–763.

87. Rochlitz, C., Dreno, B., Jantscheff, P., et al. Immunotherapy of metastatic melanoma by intratumoral injections of Vero cells producing human IL-2: phase II randomized study comparing two dose levels. Cancer Gene Ther. 2002;9:289–295.

88. Schmidt-Wolf, I.G., Finke, S., Trojaneck, B., et al. Phase I clinical study applying autologous immunological effector cells transfected with the interleukin-2 gene in patients with metastatic renal cancer, colorectal cancer and lymphoma. Br. J. Cancer 1999;81:1009–1016.

89. Yoshida, J., Mizuno, M., Fujii, M., et al. Human gene therapy for malignant gliomas (glioblastoma multiforme and anaplastic astrocytoma) by in vivo transduction with human interferon beta gene using cationic liposomes. Hum. Gene Ther. 2004;15:77–86.

23 Anticytokine Treatment

Miguel A. Villalona-Calero

1. INTRODUCTION

Much has been written regarding the use of pro-inflammatory cytokines in the treatment of cancer. This stems from their potential in the acute situation to induce death of diseased cells, as well as to destroy tumor blood vessels and activation of proteins involved in apoptosis. However, as discussed earlier, it is important to consider that several chronic inflammatory conditions lead to the development of the malignant phenotype. Examples include ulcerative colitis/Crohn disease, associated with colorectal carcinoma; Barrett's esophagus with esophageal cancer; schistosomiasis with bladder cancer; and *Helicobacter pylori* with gastric carcinoma/lymphoma. Stimulation of fibroblastic and tumor stroma growth, as well as induction of angiogenic and anti apoptotic factors have all been reported in the presence of chronic inflammation *(1,2)*. In addition, secretion of a pro-inflammatory chemokine, macrophage migration inhibitory factor (MIF) has been reported to result in suppression of p53 function *(3)*. This chapter will discuss the rationale for inhibiting pro-inflammatory cytokines and their potential use to treat cancer and its sequelae. Given the availability of agents to block TNF and IL-1, these proteins will be discussed in detail.

2. TUMOR NECROSIS FACTOR (TNF)

TNF is a cytotoxic cytokine secreted by macrophages in response to infection and tumor invasion *(4)*. Its oncogenic and anti-oncogenic properties have been detailed earlier in Chapter 7 and will not be reviewed here.

2.1. TNF Mechanism of Action

The mechanisms of TNF action were also detailed earlier in Chapter 7. TNF mediates activation of NF-κB through activation of a terminal kinase complex called IKK *(5–7)*. The IKK complex is composed of two catalytic subunits name IKKα and IKKβ

From: *Cancer Drug Discovery and Development,*
Cytokines in the Genesis and Treatment of Cancer
Edited by: M. A. Caligiuri and M. T. Lotze © Humana Press Inc., Totowa, NJ

and a smaller regulatory subunit named IKKγ *(8,9)*. Activated IKK phosphorylates two serine residues on the the I-κB proteins, targetting these proteins for degradation by the 26S proteasome complex *(10)*. Degradation of I-κB proteins unmasks the nuclear localization REL sequences of NF-κB, thus allowing NF-κB to freely translocate to the nucleus to activate gene expression.

2.2. NF-κB and Oncogenesis

A growing body of evidence strongly suggests that NF-κB plays a role in oncogenesis *(11)*. A potential transcriptional target of NF-κB that may contribute to NF-κB-associated cell growth is the c-myc proto-oncogene. The c-myc promoter contains two NF-κB binding sites, which are required for myc expression *(12)*. These sites have also been found to function as positive regulatory regions for the translocated c-myc gene in Burkitt's lymphoma *(13)*. A second growth-promoting transcriptional target of NF-κB is cyclin D1, which is a well characterized marker of transformation *(14)*. Additional evidence of the importance of NF-κB in carcinogenesis, and which may have therapeutic and preventative implications, stems from the observations of involvement of this transcription factor in the transcriptional control of the COX-2 and iNOS genes *(15–19)*. In addition to expression of these genes, more direct evidence that NF-κB is required in oncogenesis derives from studies where disruption of IκB by antisense expression leads to the cellular transformation of 3T3 fibroblasts *(20)*, and conversely, disruption of the p65 subunit of NF-κB causes tumor regression in animals *(21)*. Chronic activation of NF-κB has been reported in primary breast cancer *(22,23)* and oncogene-signaling pathways such as Ras, and Ras-dependent transformation have been found to require NF-κB activity *(24)*. Similarly, the chimeric oncoprotein Bcr-Abl implicated in acute lymphoblastic and chronic myelogenous leukemias also requires NF-κB to induce cellular transformation *(25)*, and Hodgkin's lymphoma cells depleted of NF-κB activity revealed strongly impaired tumor cell growth and viability *(26)*. In addition, recent evidence suggests NF-κB is constitutively activated in approx 67% of human pancreatic adenocarcinomas and in most human pancreatic tumor cell lines, but not in normal pancreatic tissues *(27)*. Interestingly, inhibition of NF-κB in both in vitro and in vivo studies has resulted in reversal of inducible chemoresistance and potentiation of anticancer drugs *(28–34)*. Consistent with these findings, NF-κB activation is associated with resistance to apoptosis in ductal pancreatic adenocarcinoma cells *(35)*, whereas inhibition of NF-κB sensitizes human pancreatic carcinoma cells to apoptosis induced by etoposide (VP-16) or doxorubicin *(36)*.

2.3. TNF and Cachexia

Part of the role that TNF may play in oncogenesis may be in cachexia. In differentiating C2C12 myocytes Guttridge et al. have shown that TNF-induced activation of NF-κB inhibits skeletal muscle differentiation *(37)*. In addition, NF-κB has been identified in human skeletal muscle biopsies *(38)*, suggesting in vivo relevance of NF-κB in muscle. This function may relate to the ability of NF-κB to induce muscle degeneration, because in an injury model, inhibitors of NF-κB were found to accelerate muscle regeneration *(39)*. In tumor models, numerous known inhibitors of NF-κB activity including proteasome inhibitors, antioxidants and IL-10, have been used to block cachexia *(40–42)*. More recently, direct inhibition of NF-κB activity with usage of DNA decoys was also shown to block cancer-induced cachexia in mice *(43)*.

2.4. TNF Blockade

The above offers a rationale for the study of blockade of TNF chronic activation as an strategy to enhance the efficacy of cancer therapy and to block cachexia. On this premise, our group at The Ohio State University is conducting three studies of TNF biologic blockade using soluble TNF receptor molecules (etanercept) as an adjunct to cancer chemotherapy treatment. Etanercept is a recombinant human TNF receptor (TNFR) that specifically binds and renders soluble TNF biologically inactive by blocking its interaction with cell surface TNF receptors *(44)*. This biologic activity has led to significant clinical responses in patients with rheumatoid arthritis and other inflammatory conditions in which TNF is implicated *(45,46)*. The working hypotheses for the clinical trials we are conducting is that TNF blockade should make chemotherapy more tolerable, should improve quality of life and should retard the time to tumor progression.

Preliminary results are available for the first trial, which evaluated TNF blockade to maintain dose intensity *(47)*. Because fatigue/asthenia is the most common toxicity of the chemotherapeutic agent docetaxel when it is administered on a weekly schedule *(48)*, and there is in vitro and in vivo evidence for induction of TNF-α gene expression after administration of the taxanes *(49–51)*, weekly docetaxel was administered in combination with etanercept in patients with refractory solid malignancies. A cycle was comprised of 6 weekly docetaxel treatments followed by 2 wk of rest. Subsequent cycles were initiated in the case of no disease progression and the absence of dose-limiting toxicities (DLT). The starting docetaxel dose was 43 mg/m^2 (maximal recommended dose of docetaxel in the weekly schedule). The dose of etanercept (25 mg subcutaneously twice a week) remained fixed throughout the study. A control group of 6 patients receiving docetaxel alone weekly for 6 wk every 8 wk at 43 mg/m^2 was also entered in the study to control for pharmacokinetics and biologic variations between patients receiving docetaxel alone and docetaxel and etanercept. Accrual to this group occurred by 1:1 randomization with the first dose group of docetaxel (43 mg/m^2) with etanercept until this cohort was filled.

A total of 24 courses (8-wk-long each) were administered; seven courses to patients receiving docetaxel alone and 17 to patients receiving the combination. Of 42 planned docetaxel doses in the docetaxel alone group, 10 doses (24%) were missed. Eleven of 102 planned doses (11%) (none within the first cycle) were missed in the docetaxel/etanercept group. Three patients, all in the docetaxel/etanercept arm, including two previously treated with chemotherapy, achieved partial antitumor responses and received at least three cycles (6 mo). Quality of life was assessed by using the patient self-reporting Fatigue Inventory System *(52)*. Total body disruption, a computation that can be derived from the questions in the Fatigue Inventory System, is described in Fig. 1 for the first 12 patients in the study.

The first cycle of treatment for both groups of patients is depicted in Fig. 1 on the left, whereas subsequent courses of treatment (patients receiving the combination) is depicted on the right.

Although the small number of patients and differences in previous treatments and quality of life at baseline precludes any differential analysis, it is of interest that patients which remained on the study receiving the combination did not have significant worsening in quality of life during subsequent courses, including a patient who has received eight courses (64 weeks) of treatment. NF-κB activation was measured in peripheral

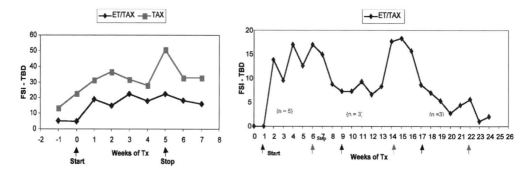

Fig. 1. Fatigue inventory system total body disruption (FSI-TBD) in patients receiving docetaxel (TAX) or the combination of docetaxel and etanercept (ET/TAX). Time intervals are weeks. The starting and stopping points of docetaxel weekly treatments is depicted by arrows.

blood mononuclear cells at different time points in both groups of patients ($n = 10$). Increases in NF-κB activation were observed in patients receiving docetaxel alone and not in patients receiving the combination. TNF–α, IL-1β, IL-6 and IFN-γ expression, measured in peripheral blood mononuclear cells by real-time RT-PCR were observed to decrease during treatment with docetaxel in combination with etanercept ($n = 5$ patients), whereas no effect was observed for the anti-inflammatory cytokine IL-10. Currently these data are available for only one patient in the docetaxel alone group. In this patient, an initial rise in the expression of pro-inflammatory cytokines was observed, followed by a return to baseline levels.

Based on the above and the rationale previously discussed in regards to cachexia, we are conducting a trial of etanercept in conjunction with standard chemotherapy in patients with advanced pancreatic cancer with the aim of increasing clinical benefit response, quality of life and the rate of progression-free survival at 6 mo. The influence of TNF blockade on pro-inflammatory cytokines in these patients is being studied. Lastly, we are also evaluating the effect of TNF blockade in combination with chemotherapy in tumor progression and recurrence in patients with advanced small-cell lung cancer.

In summary, blockade of chronic activation of TNF may evolve into a useful approach as an adjunct to chemotherapy treatment. Results of trials currently ongoing of etanercept as a single agent, evaluating its impact in fatigue and quality of life are eagerly awaited. In addition, therapeutic agents that are based on antibodies to the TNF receptor have demonstrated efficacy in chronic inflammatory conditions. The evaluation of these agents for anticancer properties in humans would be of considerable interest given the longer half-life of these compounds.

3. INTERLEUKIN 1 (IL-1)

IL-1 is a mediator of several acute and chronic inflammatory conditions. Intravenous administration in humans is associated with various clinical manifestations including fever, hypotension, headaches, myalgias, and stimulation of the hypothalamic-pituitary adrenal axis *(53)*. In the presence of infection IL-1 helps to recruit inflammatory cells and elevated levels are detected in the synovial fluid in patients with rheumatoid arthritis, where it is associated with joint cartilage degeneration and bone resorption *(54,55)*.

In addition, overexpression of IL-1 has been detected in the brains of patients with Alzheimer's disease, as well as in the vessel wall of aortic aneurisms and aortic occlusive disease *(56–58)*.

At the cellular level, IL-1 has been shown to regulate several genes involved in inflammatory and immune responses and at the same time to suppress the expression of housekeeping genes not necessary for the inflammatory response *(59)*. IL-1 α or β can increase the expression of the IL-1 family of genes and the expression of colony-stimulating and mesenchymal growth factor genes. Other inflammatory cytokines, as well as lymphocyte growth factors are upregulated by IL-1. In addition, IL-1 induces transcription or stabilize mRNA levels for the iNos, type 2 cyclooxygenase (Cox2) and type 2 phospholipase A2 (PLA2) genes *(59,60–62)*. The products of these genes, nitric oxide (NO), prostaglandins, leukotrienes, and platelet-activating factor are potent mediators of inflammation *(63)*. Intercellular cell adhesion molecule-1 (ICAM-1) and vascular cell adhesion molecule-1 (VCAM-1) expression on endothelial cells are also increased by IL-1 *(64–66)*.

Three IL-1 proteins have been characterized. Two are agonistic, IL-1α and IL-1β, and one is antagonistic, IL-1Ra. Both IL-1 α and β are produced as the precursor proteins, proIL-1α and proIL-1β. The proIL-1 forms are subsequently cleaved by specific cellular proteases, including the IL-1 converting enzyme (ICE). IL-1α typically remains intracellular or is expressed in the membrane and is thought to serve as an autocrine factor, whereas IL-1β is secreted from the cell and exerts its effect on other cells *(67)*.

The three members of the IL-1 family can bind to two different receptors, IL-1RI and IL-1RII. Binding of IL-1α or β to IL-RI leads to intracellular transduction, whereas no transduction is elicited upon binding to IL-1RII. Therefore, IL-RII serves as a decoy receptor to buffer excessive IL-1 concentrations *(68)*. In addition, IL-1 α/β and IL-Ra have different effects on IL-1R1. This appears to be owing to a lack of a second binding site to the receptor for IL-1Ra. This second binding site permits IL-1 α and β to produce the structural changes in their third IgG-like domain that are necessary for the docking of the IL-1R accesory protein (IL-1R-AcP). The complex of IL-1R-AcP/IL-1RI/IL-1β is essencial for signal transduction to occur *(69)*. The lack of signal transduction upon binding of IL-1Ra to the receptor, allows it to become a competitive antagonist to the functions elicited by IL-1 α and β and to maintain a tight control and equilibrium in this pathway.

3.1. Interleukin 1 and Cancer

In models of infection and inflammation IL-1 mediates induction of granulocyte colony stimulating factor (GCSF), granulocyte-macrophage colony stimulating factor (GM-CSF) and IL-3 (IL-3) *(70)*. IL-1 also exerts a protective effect in marrow cells after irradiation *(71,72)*. This effect is thought owing to protection of pluripotent stem cells, the myeloid stem cell and the early progenitor cells. Although the gene for IL-1β is not expressed in peripheral blood monuclear cells of healthy subjects *(73)*, spontaneous production of IL-1 has been detected in various leukemic cells, including acute myelogenous leukemia (AML) and chronic myelogenous leukemia (CML) cells *(74)*. Given the property of IL-1 to stimulate production of GCSF and GMCSF, IL-1 may constitute an autocrine growth factor sustaining and increasing cell proliferation. Indeed, specific blockade of IL-1 has been shown to result in a significant reduction in proliferation of AML cells *(75)*. Interestingly, cells from CML patients in chronic phase or lymphoid blast crisis do not express IL-1, whereas CML blasts do *(76)*.

Constitutive production of IL-1α and β has been detected in melanoma, hepatoblastoma, sarcoma, squamous and transitional carcinoma cells, as well as in ovarian carcinomas *(64,77–80)*. However, the addition of IL-1 to malignant cell cultures, including melanoma, glioma, meningioma, breast, cervical, thyroid, and ovarian carcinoma cells, can inhibit tumor cell growth *(81–86)*. The mechanisms for the growth inhibition are not clear, but induction of other cytokines and generation of NO are most likely required. *(87)*.

Evidence also exists for IL-1 to promote metastasis. IL-1 appears to prime animals for metastases following injection of tumor cells *(88,89)*. This has been thought to result from enhanced expression of adhesion molecules on endothelial and malignant cells, which would facilitate the passage of malignant cells into the circulation *(90,91)*. Furthermore, mice solely deficient in IL-1 exhibit dramatically impaired tumor blood vessel growth after injection of several different cancer cell lines, suggesting IL-1 is essential for angiogenesis and cancer invasiveness *(92)*.

3.2. Interleukin 1 Blockade

Similar to TNF there is rationale to support IL-1 use as an anticancer agent and rationale to support that IL-1 blockade can be use to treat cancer. These two concepts are not necessarily mutually exclusive, because in the acute situation, generation of other cytokines and NO radicals may help to deter proliferation. However, under chronic conditions, IL-1 may serve as an autocrine or paracrine stimulator of cancer proliferation, invasion and metastases.

Different strategies can be considered to accomplish IL-1 blockade *(53)*. Nonselective interventions include corticosteroids, dietary omega-3 fatty acids, methotrexate, nonsteroidal anti-inflammatory agents and other cytokines (e.g., interferon, IL-4, IL-13, IL-10 and transforming growth factor-β). Selective interventions include antibodies to IL-1 or to IL-1R-AcP, soluble IL-1 decoy receptor, IL-1Ra, and inhibition of IL-1β converting enzymes (ICE).

To date, no clinical trials have been reported with antibodies to IL-1 α or β or to IL-1R-AcP and although soluble IL-1 receptor has been administered to healthy volunteers, simultaneuous inhibition of the antagonistic IL-1Ra by binding to the receptor has limited the utility of this approach *(93)*. Given the multiplicity of actions of ICE, a high degree of specificity for the cleavage sites of proIL-1β would be required for an ICE inhibitor to be practical for clinical use.

Most clinical trials featuring IL-1 blockade have been conducted using IL-1Ra (anakinra). In early trials, IL-1Ra appeared to produce some benefit in patients with acute sepsis and graft vs host disease *(94–96)*. Unfortunately, randomized trials failed to support this advantage for the sepsis situation *(97)*. However, in rheumatoid arthritis, IL-1Ra administered daily subcutaneously is able, as a single agent, to produce clinical responses and to produce benefit in joint space narrowing *(98)*. The benefit was even higher when administered in conjunction with methotrexate *(99)*.

3.3. IL-1 and TNF Synergism

IL-1 induces the activation of several transcription factors. Notably IL-1 induces translocation of NF-kB and AP-1, as well as activation of p38 MAP Kinase *(100–103)*. These factors play a considerable role in carcinogenesis and in cancer resistance to chemotherapy treatment. Because a similar profile has been established for TNF, this would suggest that these proteins may collaborate at the cellular level. In fact, there is very consistent in vivo and in vitro evidence for synergistic interaction between TNF and IL-1 *(59,104–109)*. Interestingly, production of IL-6 and cachexia in mice with sarcoma has been observed to be under the control of IL-1 and TNFα *(110)*. Although IL-1 has been observed to downregulate and to stimulate shedding of the TNF receptor, this effect is confined to the p55 TNF receptor *(111,112)*. This TNF receptor in particular, is the TNF receptor associated with the activation of intracellular signals leading to programmed cell death.

The above would support the hypothesis that TNF blockade in combination with IL-1 inhibition could result in a higher therapeutic effect as compared to a single intervention. Indeed, in vivo models have shown a synergistic effect for the inhibitory combination in preventing cartilage destruction *(113)*, as well as in reducing joint inflammation, loss of bone mineral density and body weight *(114)*. Furthermore, a combination of soluble tumor necrosis factor receptors plus interleukin-1 receptor antagonist decreased sepsis mortality in an animal model of intestinal perforation, as compared to single agent treatment *(115)*.

No data have been generated to date on the use of interleukin-1 blockade as a therapeutic strategy in patients with malignancies and very preliminary data exist in the use of the combination of IL-1 and TNF blockade in humans. Serious infections were noted in 7% of 58 patients treated with the combination of anakinra and etanercept, including two patients with neutrophil counts below $1000/mm^3$ *(53,116)*. Although these risks are considerable for the treatment of chronic inflammatory diseases, this toxicity could be acceptable for an otherwise effective approach in patients with advanced malignancies.

In summary, there is sufficient evidence to support a rationale for the use of anticytokine treatment in the treatment of patients with cancer and to improve their quality of life. Given the interplay between the different cytokines, it is likely that a combinatory approach will be necessary to see substantial effects. Safety and efficacy clinical trials to test this concept are warranted.

REFERENCES

1. O'Byrne KJ, Dalgleish AG. Chronic immune activation and inflammation as the cause of malignancy. Br J Cancer. 85: 473–483, 2001.
2. Shacter E, Weitzman SA. Chronic inflammation and cancer. Oncology 16: 217–226, 229, 2002
3. Hudson JD, Shoaibi MA, Maestro R, Carnero A, Hannon GJ, Beach DH. A proinflammatory cytokine inhibits p53 tumor suppressor activityJ.Exp Med 190: 1375.1999
4. Smith CA, Farrah T, Goodwin RG. The TNF receptor superfamily of cellular and viral proteins: Activation, costimulation and death. Cell 1994: 75:959.
5. Chen, Z.J., Parent L, Maniatis T. Site-specific phosphorylation of IκBalpha by a novel ubiquitination-dependent protein kinase activity. Cell 84:853–862, 1996.
6. Regnier, CH, Song HY, Gao X, Goeddel DV, Cao Z, Rothe M. Identification and characterization of an IκB kinase. Cell 90:373–383, 1997.
7. DiDonato JA, Hayakawa M, Rothwarf DM, Zandi E, Karin M. A cytokine-responsive IκB kinase that activates the transcription factor NF-κB. Nature 388:548–554, 1997.
8. Mercurio F, Zhu H, Murray BW, et al. IKK-1 and IKK-2: cytokine-activated IκB kinases essential for NF-κB activation. Science 278:860–866, 1997..
9. Yamaoka S, Courtois G, Bessia C, et al. Complementation cloning of NEMO, a component of the IκB kinase complex essential for NF-κB activation. Cell. 93:1231–1240, 1998.
10. Karin M, Ben-Neriah Y. Phosphorylation meets ubiquitination: The control of NF-κB activity. Ann Rev Immun 18:621–663, 2000.
11. Gilmore TD, Koedood M, Piffat KA, White DW. Rel/NF- κB/IκB proteins and cancer. Oncogene 13:1367–1378, 1996.

12. La Rosa FA, Pierce JW, Sonenshein GE. Differential regulation of the c-myc oncogene promoter by the NF-κ B rel family of transcription factors. Mol Cell Biol 14:1039–1044, 1994.

13. Ji L, Arcinas M, Boxer LM. NF-κB sites function as positive regulators of expression of the translocated c-myc allele in Burkitt's lymphoma. Mol Cell Biol 14:7967–7974, 1994.

14. Hinz M, Krappmann D, Eichten A, Heder A, Scheidereit C, Strauss M. NF-κB function in growth control: Regulation of cyclin D1 expression and G0/G1-to-S-phase transition. Mol Cell Biol 19:2690-2698, 1999.

15. Newton R, Kuitert LM, Bergmann M, Adcock IM, Barnes PJ. Evidence for involvement of NF-κB in the transcriptional control of COX-2 gene expression by IL-1beta. Biochem Biophys Res Commun Aug 8;237(1):28–32, 1997.

16. Jobin C, Morteau O, Han DS, Balfour Sartor R. Specific NF-κB blockade selectively inhibits tumour necrosis factor-alpha-induced COX-2 but not constitutive COX-1 gene expression in HT-29 cells. Immunology Dec;95(4):537–43, 1998.

17. Newton R, Stevens DA, Hart LA, Lindsay M, Adcock IM, Barnes PJ. Superinduction of COX-2 mRNA by cycloheximide and interleukin-1beta involves increased transcription and correlates with increased NF-κB and JNK activation. FEBS Lett. 24;418(1, 2):135–138, 1997.

18. Surh YJ, Chun KS, Cha HH, et al. Molecular mechanisms underlying chemopreventive activities of anti-inflammatory phytochemicals: Down-regulation of COX-2 and iNOS through suppression of NF-κ B activation. Mutat Res 2001 Sep 1;480–481:243–268. Review.

19. Adcock IM, Newton R, Barnes PJ. NF-κ B involvement in IL-1 beta- induction of GM- CSF and COX-2: Inhibition by glucocorticoids does not require I-κ B. Biochem Soc Trans May;25(2):154S, 1997.

20. Higgins KA, Perez JR, Coleman TA, et al. Antisense inhibition of the p65 subunit of NF-κ B blocks tumorigenicity and causes tumor regression. Proc Nat Acad of Sci USA 90:9901–9905, 1993.

21. Beauparlant P, Kwan I, Bitar R, et al. Disruption of I κ B alpha regulation by antisense RNA expression leads to malignant transformation. Oncogene 9:3189–3197, 1994.

22. Cogswell PC, Guttridge DC, Funkhouser WK, Baldwin Jr AS. Selective activation of NF-κ B subunits in human breast cancer: Potential roles for NF-κ B2/p52 and for Bcl-3. Oncogene 19: 1123–1131, 2000.

23. Dejardin E, Bonizzi G, Bellahcene A, Castronovo V, Merville MP, Bours V. Highly-expressed p100/p52 (NFKB2) sequesters other NF-κ B-related proteins in the cytoplasm of human breast cancer cells. Oncogene 11:1835–1841, 1995.

24. Finco TS, Westwick JK, Norris JL, Beg AA, Der CJ, Baldwin Jr AS. Oncogenic Ha-Ras-induced signaling activates NF-κB transcriptional activity, which is required for cellular transformation. J Biol Chem 272:24113–24116, 1997.

25. Reuther JY, Reuther GW, Cortez D, Pendergast AM, Baldwin Jr AS. A requirement for NF-kB activation in Bcr-Abl-mediated transformation. Genes & Dev 12:968–981, 1997.

26. Bargou RC, Emmerich F, Krappmann D, et al. Constitutive nuclear factor-κB-RelA activation is required for proliferation and survival of Hodgkin's disease tumor cells. J Clin Invest 100:2961-2969, 1997.

27. Wang W, Abbruzzese JL, Evans DB, Larry L, Cleary KR, Chiao PJ. The nuclear factor-κ B RelA transcription factor is constitutively activated in human pancreatic adenocarcinoma cells. Clin Cancer Res, 5: 119–127, 1999.

28. Bentires-Alj M, Merville MP, Bours V. NF- κ B and chemoresistance: Could NF- κ B be an antitumor target? Drug Resist Updat 2(4):274-276, 1999.

29. Cusack JC, Liu R, Baldwin AS. NF- κ B and chemoresistance: Potentiation of cancer drugs via inhibition of NF- κ B. Drug Resist Updat 2(4):271–273, 1999.

30. Weldon CB, Burow ME, Rolfe KW, Clayton JL, Jaffe BM, Beckman BS. NF-κ B-mediated chemoresistance in breast cancer cells. Surgery 130(2):143–50, 2001.

31. Cheng Q, Lee HH, Li Y, Parks TP, Cheng G. Upregulation of Bcl-x and Bfl-1 as a potential mechanism of chemoresistance, which can be overcome by NF-κB inhibition. Oncogene 5;19(42): 4936–4940, 2000.

32. Wang CY, Cusack JC Jr, Liu R, Baldwin AS Jr. Control of inducible chemoresistance: Enhanced antitumor therapy through increased apoptosis by inhibition of NF-κB. Nat Med;5 :412–417, 1999.

33. Cusack JC, Liu R, Baldwin AS. Inducible chemoresistance to 7-ethyl-10-[4-(1-piperidino)-1-piperidino]-carbonyloxycamptothecin (CPT-11) in colorectal cancer cells and a xenograft model is overcome by inhibition of nuclear factor-κB activation. Cancer Res 60: 2323–2330, 2000.

34. Cusack JC, Liu R, Houston M, et al. Enhanced chemosensitivity to CPT-11 with proteosome inhibitor PS-341: Implications for systemic nuclear factor-κB inhibition. Cancer Res 61: 3535–3540, 2001.

35. Trauzold A, Wermann H, Arlt A, et al. CD95 and TRAIL receptor-mediated activation of protein kinase C and NF-κB contributes to apoptosis resistance in ductal pancreatic adenocarcinoma cells. Oncogene 20: 4258–4269, 2001.

36. Arlt A, Vorndamm J, Breitenbroich M, et al. Inhibition of NF-κB sensitizes human pancreatic carcinoma cells to apoptosis induced by etoposide (VP-16) or doxorubicin. Oncogene 20: 859–868, 2001.

37. Guttridge D, Mayo M, Madrid L, Wang C, Baldwin A. NF-κB-induced loss of MyoD messenger RNA: Possible role in muscle decay and cachexia. Science 289: 2363-2365, 2000.

38. Baghdiguian S, Martin M, Richard I, et al. Calpain 3 deficiency is associated with myonuclear apoptosis and profound perturbation of the IκB alpha/NF-κB pathway in limb-girdle muscular dystrophy type 2A. Nat Med 5:503–511, 1999.

39. Thaloor D, Miller KJ, Gephart J, Mitchell PO, Pavlath GK. Systemic administration of the NF-κB inhibitor curcumin stimulates muscle regeneration after traumatic injury. Amer J Physiol 277:C320–329, 1999.

40. Lazarus DD, Destree A.T., Mazzola L.M., et al. A new model of cancer cachexia: Contribution of the ubiquitin-proteasome pathway. Amer J Physiol 277:E332–341, 1999.

41. Buck M, Chojkier M. Muscle wasting and dedifferentiation induced by oxidative stress in a murine model of cachexia is prevented by inhibitors of nitric oxide synthesis and antioxidants. EMBO J 15:1753–1765, 1996.

42. Fujiki F, Mukaida N, Hirose K, et al. Prevention of adenocarcinoma colon 26-induced cachexia by interleukin 10 gene transfer. Cancer Res 57:94—99, 1997.

43. Kawamura I, Morishita R, Tomita N, et al. Intratumoral injection of oligonucleotides to the NF κB binding site inhibits cachexia in a mouse tumor model. Gene Ther 6:91–97, 1999.

44. Mohler KM, Torrance DS, Smith CA, et al. Soluble tumor necrosis factor (TNF) receptors are effective therapeutic agents in lethal endotoxemia and function simultaneously as both TNF carriers and TNF antagonists. J Immunol 151: 1548-1561, 1993.

45. Moreland L, Baumgartner S, Schiff M, et al. Treatment of rheumatoid arthritis with a recombinant human tumor necrosis factor receptor (p75)-Fc fusion protein. NEJM 337: 141–147, 1997.

46. Lovell D, Giannini E, Reiff A, et al. Etanercept in children with poliarticular juvenile rheumatoid arthritis. NEJM 342: 763–769, 2000

47. Monk JP, Phillips G, Waite R, et al. Tumor necrosis alpha blockade improves tolerability of dose intensive chemotherapy J Clin Oncol. 24(12):1852–1859, 2006.

48. Hainsworth J, Burris H, Erland J, et al. Phase I trial of docetaxel administered by weekly infusion in patients with advanced refractory cancer. J Clin Oncol, 16 (6): 2164–2168, 1998.

49. Bogdan C, Ding A. Taxol, a microtubule-stabilizing antineoplastic agent, induces expression of tumor necrosis factor α and interleukin-1 in macrophages. J Leukocyte Biol 52: 119–121, 1992.

50. Ding A, Porteu F, Sanchez E, et al. Shared actions of endotoxin and taxol on TNF receptors and TNF release. Science 248:370–372, 1990.

51. Sawada N, Ishikawa T, Fukase Y, et al. Induction of thymidine phosphorylase activity and enhancement of capecitabine efficacy by taxol/taxotere in human cancer xenografts. Clin Cancer Res 4: 1013–1019, 1998.

52. Hann DM, Jacobsen PB, Azzarello LM, et al. Measurement of fatigue in cancer patients: Development and validation of the Fatigue Symptom Inventory. Qual Life Res May; 7(4): 301–310, 1998.

53. Hallegua DS, Weisman MH. Potential uses of interleukin 1 receptor antagonists in human diseases. Ann Rheum Dis 61: 960–967, 2002.

54. Eastgate JA, Symons JA, Wood NC, et al. Correlation of plasma interleukin 1 levels with disease activity in rheumatoid arthritis. Lancet 2: 706–708, 1988.

55. Kahle P, Saal JG, Schaudt K, et al. Determinations of cytokines in synovial fluids: correlation with diagnosis and histomorphological characteristics of synovial fluid. Ann Rheum Dis 51: 731–734, 1992.

56. Sheng JG, Mrak RE, Griffin WST. Interleukin 1 expression in brain regions in Alzheimer disease: Correlation with neuritic plaque distribution. Neuropathol Appl Neurobiol 21: 290–301, 1995.

57. Pearce WH, Sweis I, Yao JS, et al. Interleukin-1β and tumor necrosis factor-α release in normal and diseased human infrarenal aortas. J Vasc Sur 16:784–789, 1992.

58. Vasilakos JP, Carroll RT, Emmerling MR, et al. Interleukin-1 beta dissociates beta-amyloid precursor protein and beta-amyloid peptide secretion. FEBS lett 354: 289, 1994.

59. Dinarello C. Biologic basis for interleukin-1 in disease. Blood 87: 2095–2147, 1996.

60. Kunz D, Muhl H, Walker G, Pfeilschifter J. Two distinct signaling pathways trigger the expression of inducible nitric oxide synthase in rat mesangial cells. Proc Natl Acad Sci USA 91: 5387, 1994.

61. Adams V, Nehrhoff B, Spate U, et al. Induction of iNOS expression in skeletal muscle by IL-1 beta and NFKappaB activation: An in vitro and in vivo study. Cardiovasc Res 54: 95–104, 2002.

62. Gronich J, Konieczkowski M, Gelb MH, et al. Interleukin-1α causes a rapid activation of cytosolic phospholipase A2 by phosphorylation in rat mesangial cells. J Clin Invest 93: 1224–1233, 1994.

63. Szabo C, Wu C-C, Gross SS, et al. Interleukin-1 contributes to the induction of nitric oxide synthase by endotoxin in vivo. Eur J Pharmacol 150: 157, 1993.

64. Alexandra AB, Jackson AM, Esuvaranathan K, et al. Autocrine regulation of ICAM-1 expression on bladder cancer cell lines: Evidence for the role of IL-1α. Immunol Lett 40: 117, 1994.

65. Watanabe Y, Morita M, Ikematsu N, Akaike T. Tumor necrosis factor alpha and interleukin-1 beta but not interferon gamma induce vascular cell adhesion molecule-1 expression on primary cultured murine hepatocytes. Biochem Biophys Res Commun 209: 335–342, 1995.

66. Pang G. Couch L, Batey R, et al. GM-CSF, IL-1 alpha, IL-1 beta, IL-6, IL-8, IL-10, ICAM-1 and VCAM-1 gene expression and cytokine production in human duodenal fibroblasts stimulated with lipopolysaccharide, IL-1 alpha and TNF-alpha. Clin Exp Immunol 96: 437–443, 1994.

67. Mora M, Carinci V, Bensi G, et al. Differential expression of the human I-1 alpha and beta genes. Prog Clin Biol Res 349:205, 1990.

68. Sims JE, Giri JG, Dower SK. The two interleukin-1 receptors play different roles in IL-1 activities. Clin Immunol Immunopathol 72: 9–14, 1994.

69. Greenfeder SA, Nunes P, Kwee L, et al. Molecular cloning and characterization of a second subunit of the interleukin-1 receptor complex. J Biol Chem 270: 13,757–13,765, 1995.

70. Neta R, Sztein MB, Oppenheim JJ, et al. The in vivo effects of interleukin-1. Bone marrow cells are induced to cycle after administration of interleukin-1. J immunol 139: 1861, 1987.

71. Zucali JR, Moreb J, Gibbons W, et al. Radioprotection of hematopoietic stem cells by interleukin-1. Exp Hematol 22: 130, 1994.

72. Neta R, Oppenheim JJ, Wang J-M, et al. Synergy of IL-1 and stem cell factor in radioprotection in mice is associated with IL-1 up-regulation of mRNA and protein expression for c-kit on bone marrow cells. J Immunol 153: 1536, 1994.

73. Mileno MD, Margolis NH, Clark BD, et al. Coagulation of whole blood stimulates interleukin-1β gene expression: Absence of gene transcripts in anticoagulated blood. J Infect Dis 172: 308, 1995.

74. Kurrzock R, Kantarjian H, Wetzler M, et al. Ubiquitous expression of cytokines in diverse leukemia of lymphoid and myeloid lineage. Exp Hematol 21: 80, 1993.

75. Stosic-Grujicic S, Basara N, Milenkovic P, Dinarello CA. Modulation of acute myeloblastic leukemia (AML) cell proliferation and blast colony formation by antisense oligomer of IL-1 beta converting enzyme (ICE) and IL-1 receptor antagonist (IL-1ra). J Chemother 7: 67, 1995.

76. Wetzler M, Kurrzock R, Lowe DG, et al. Alterations in one marrow adherent layer growth factor expression: A novel mechanism of chronic myelogenous leukemia progression. Blood 78: 2400, 1991.

77. Burger RA, Grosen EA, Ioli GR, et al. Host-tumor interaction in ovarian cancer. Spontaneous release of tumor necrosis factor and interleukin-1 inhibitors by purified cell populations from human ovarian carcinoma in vitro. Gynecol Oncol 55: 294, 1994.

78. Castelli C, Sensi M, Lupetti R, et al. Expression of interleukin 1-α, interleukin-6 and tumor necrosis factor genes in human melanoma clones is associated with that of mutated N-RAS oncogene. Cancer Res 54: 4785, 1994.

79. Tyler DS, Francis GM Fredeick M, et al. Interleukin-1 production in tumor clls of human melanoma surgical specimens. Lymphokine Cytokine Res 15: 331, 1995.

80. Von Schweinitz D, Hadam MR, Welte K, et al. Production of interleukin-1β and interleukin-6 in hepatoblastoma. Int J Cancer 53: 728, 1993.

81. Onozaki K, Matsushima K, Aggarwal BB, Oppenheim JJ. Human interleukin-1 is a cytocidal factor for several human tumor cell lines. J Immunol 135: 3962, 1985.

82. Lachman LB, Dinarello CA, Llansa ND, Fidler IJ. Natural and recombinant human interleukin 1-β is cytotoxic for human melanoma cells. J Immunol 136: 3098, 1986.

83. Herzog TJ, Collin JL. Comparison of the cytostatic and cytolytic activity of tumor necrosis factor α and interleukin-1 α in human cell lines. Cytokine 4: 214, 1992.

84. Kilian PL, Kaffka KL, Lipman JM, et al. Antiproliferative effect of interleukin-1 on human ovarian carcinoma cell line (NIH:OVCAR-3). Cancer Res 51: 1823, 1991.

85. Hanauske AR, Degen D, Marshall MH, et al. Effects of recombinant interleukin-1α on clonogenic growth of primary human tumors in vitro. J Immunother 11: 155, 1992.

86. Braunschweiger PG, Basrur VS, Santos O, et al. Synergistic antitumor activity of cisplatin and interleukin-1 in sensitive and resistant solid tumors. Cancer Res 53: 1091, 1993.

87. Hirose K, Longo DL, Oppenheim JJ, Matsushima K. Overexpression of mitocondrial manganese superoxide dismutase promotes the survival of tumor cells exposed to interleukin-1, tumor necrosis factor, selected anticancer drugs and ionizing radiation. FASEB J 7: 361, 1993.

88. Giavazzi R, Garofolo A, Bani NR, et al. IL-1 induced augmentation of experimental metastases from a human melanoma in nude mice. Cancer Res 50: 4771, 1990.

89. Bani MR, Garofalo A, Scanziani E, Giavazzi R. Effect of interleukin-1-beta on metastasis formation in different tumor systems. J Natl Cancer Inst 83: 119, 1991.

90. Bevilacqua MP, Nelson RM. Endothelial-leukocyte adhesions molecules in inflammation and metastasis. Thromb Haemost 70:152, 1993.

91. Lauri D, Needham L, Martin-Padura I, Dejan E. Tumor cell adhesion to endothelial cells: Endothelial leukocyte adhesion molecule-1 as an inducible adhesive receptor specific for colon carcinoma. J Natl Cancer Inst 83: 1321, 1991.

92. Voronov E, Shouval D, Krelin Y, et al. IL-1 is required for tumor invasiveness and angiogenesis. Proc Natl Acad Sci USA 100: 2645–2650, 2003.

93. Preas HL, Reda D, Tropea M, et al. Effects of recombinant soluble type 1 interleukin-1 receptor on human inflammatory responses to endotoxin. Blood 88: 2465–2472, 1996.

94. Granowitz EV, Porat R, Mier JW, et al. Hematologic and immunomodulatory effects of an interleukin-1 receptor antagonist coinfusion during low dose endotoxemia in healthy humans. Blood 82: 2985–2990, 1993.

95. Fisher CJ, Slotman GJ, Opal SM, et al. Initial evaluation of human recombinant interleukin-1 receptor antagonist in the treatment of sepsis syndrome: A randomized open-label, placebo-controlled multicenter trial. Crit Care Med 22:12–21, 1994.

96. Antin JH, Weinstein HJ, Guinan EC, et al. Recombinant human interleukin-1 receptor antagonist in the treatment of steroid-resistant graft-versus-host disease. Blood 84: 1342–1348, 1994.

97. Fisher CJ, Dhainaut JF, Opal SM et al. Recombinant human interleukin-1 receptor antagonist in the treatment of patients with sepsis syndrome: Results from a randomized double-blind, placebo-controlled trial. JAMA 271; 1836–1843, 1994.

98. Bresnihan B, Alvaro-Gracia JM, Cobby M, et al. Treatment of rheumatoid arthritis with recombinant human interleukin-1 receptor antagonist. Arthritis Rheum 41: 2196–2204, 1998.

99. Cohen S, Hurd E, Cush JJ, et al. Treatment with interleukin-1 receptor antagonist in combination with methotrexate (MTX): Results of a twenty-four-week, multicenter randomized, randomized, double-blind, placebo controlled trial. Arthitis Rheum 46: 614–624, 2002.

100. Bird TA, Downey H, Virca GD. Interleukin-1 regulates casein kinase II- mediated phosphorylation of the p65 subunit of NFkB. Cytokine 7: 603, 1995.

101. Arlt A, Vorndamm J, Muerkoster S, et al. Autocrine prduction of interleukin 1β confers constitutive nuclear factor κB activity and chemoresistance in pancreatic carcinoma cell lines. Cancer Res 62: 910–916, 2002.

102. Muegge K, Vila M, Gusella GL, et al. IL-1 induction of the c-jun promoter. Proc Natl Acad Sci USA 90: 7054–7058, 1993.

103. Guesdon F, Freshney N, Waller RJ, et al. Interleukin 1 and tumor necrosis factor stimulate two novel protein kinases that phosphorylate the heat shock protein hsp27 and beta-casein. J Biol Chem 268: 4236, 1993.

104. LeGrand A, Fermor B, Fink C, et al. Interleukin-1, tumor necrosis alpha, and interleukin-17 synergistically up-regulate nitric oxide and prostaglandin E2 production in explants of human osteoarthritic knee menisci. Arthritis Rheum 44: 2078–2083, 2001.

105. McGee DW, Bamberg T, Vitkis SJ, McGhee JR. A synergistic relationship between TNF-alpha, IL-1 beta, and TGF-beta 1 on IL-6 secretion by the IEC-6 intestinal epithelial cell line. Immunology 86: 6–11, 1995.

106. Henderson B, Pettipher ER. Arthritogenic actions of recombinat IL-1 and tumor necrosis factor alpha in the rabbit: Evidence for synergistic interactions between cytokines in vivo. Clin Exp Immunol 75: 306–310, 1989.

107. Last-Barney K, Homon CA, Faanes RB, Merluzzi VJ. Synergistic and overlapping activities of tumor necrosis factor-alpha and IL-1. J Immunol 141: 527–530, 1988.

108. Wankowicz Z, Megyeri P, Issekutz A. Synergy between tumour necrosis factor alpha and interleukin-1 in the induction of polymorphonuclear lekocyte migration during inflammation. J Leukoc Biol 43: 349–356, 1988.

109. Stashenko P, Dewhirst FE, Peros WJ, et al. Synergistic interactions between interleukin-1, tumor necrosis factor, and lymphotoxin in bone resorption. J Immunol 138: 1464–1468, 1987.

110. Evans R, Fong M, Fuller J, et al. Tumor cell IL-6 gene expression is regulated by IL-1α/β and TNFα. Proposed feedback mechanisms induced by the interaction of tumor cells and macrophages. J Leukoc Biol 52: 463, 1992.

111. Holtman H, Wallach D. Down regulation of the receptors for tumor necrosis factor by interleukin 1 and 4 beta-phorbol-12-myristate-13-acetate. J Immunol 139: 1161, 1987.

112. Brakebusch C, Varfolomeev EE, Batkin M, Wallach D. Structural requirements for inducible shedding of the p55 tumor necrosis factor receptor. J Biol Chem 269: 32,488, 1994.

113. Zwerina J, Hayer S, Tohidast-Akrad M, et al. Single and combined inhibition of tumor necrosis factor, interleukin-1, and RANKL pathways in tumor necrosis factor-induced arthritis: Effects on synovial inflammation, bone erosion, and cartilage destruction. Arthritis Rheum 50: 277–290, 2004.

114. Feige U, Hu YL, Gasser J, et al. Anti-interleukin-1 and anti-tumor necrosis factor-alpha synergistically inhibit adjuvant arthritis in Lewis rats. Cell Mol Life Sci. 57: 1457–1470, 2000.

115. Remick DG, Call DR, Ebong SJ, et al. Combination immunotherapy with soluble tumor necrosis factor receptors plus interleukin 1 receptor antagonist decreases sepsis mortality. Crit Care Med 29: 473–481, 2001.

116. Schiff M, Bulpitt K, Weaver A, et al. Safety of combination therapy with anakinra and etanercept in patients with rheumatoid arthritis. Arthritis Rheum 44(suppl): S79, 2001.

24 Cytokines in the Supportive Care of Cancer

John A. Glaspy

CONTENTS

1. INTRODUCTION

The last 15 years have witnessed a transformation in our ability to manage the debilitating symptoms associated with cancer and its treatment and thereby to optimize functional status and the quality of patients' lives while providing the best possible anticancer therapy. Like a proactive, patient-centered approach to the effective treatment of pain, the development of highly efficacious anti-emetic regimens and the introduction of bisphosphonates for hypercalcemia and the prevention of skeletal events in patients with lytic bone metastases, the advent of biotechnology provided us with therapeutic proteins that have decreased infection and transfusion risk. The latter have dramatically improved hematopoietic cell support for patients undergoing myeloablative chemotherapy, and improved energy levels in patients suffering the frequent and debilitating fatigue associated with cancer and its treatment. The landscape of oncology practice today differs radically from that just 20 years ago with these advances in supportive care allowing patients to spend more of their time outside hospital engaged in meaningful activity. This chapter will review the role of therapy with cloned human glycoprotein ligands with hematopoietic activity in the modern supportive care of cancer patients.

2. MYELOID GROWTH FACTORS

When it was recognized that the mature cells present in the peripheral blood were being continuously produced by a common pluripotent progenitor cell in the bone marrow, hematopoiesis became the most frequently used model for the study of cellular

From: *Cancer Drug Discovery and Development,*
Cytokines in the Genesis and Treatment of Cancer
Edited by: M. A. Caligiuri and M. T. Lotze © Humana Press Inc., Totowa, NJ

differentiation. It was shown that this process involved response to lineage commitment and proliferation signals mediated by glycoprotein ligands for receptors present on receptive progenitor cells. The first of these hematopoietic growth factors to be cloned and introduced into clinical trials in cancer patients, recombinant human granulocyte-macrophage colony-stimulating factor (GM-CSF) and recombinant human granulocyte colony-stimulating factor (G-CSF), were involved in regulating the production and functional activity of mature leukocytes.

A thorough review of the biology and early clinical development of these two proteins has been published *(1,2)*. The effects of GM-CSF and G-CSF on hematopoiesis, mature effector cell function and infection risk are quite distinct, with the result that these agents cannot be considered interchangeable in oncology practice. G-CSF is the regulator of basal and emergency neutrophil production, with endogenous levels rising in response to infection or neutropenia and mature neutrophils providing feedback inhibition of the hematopoietic effects of G-CSF mediated by the production of elastase *(3–5)*. G-CSF also regulates mature neutrophil function, activating and priming these cells to enhanced functional activity and response including, importantly, increased trans-endothelial migration to sites of inflammation *(6)*. GM-CSF is not essential to either basal or emergency neutrophil production, but plays a role in pulmonary homeostasis *(4,7)*, possibly by serving as an immune modulator produced and acting locally rather than as a systemic hematopoietic cytokine *(8)*. Although GM-CSF has some activating effects on mature neutrophils and macrophages, it enhances neutrophil adhesion, inhibiting trans-endothelial migration in inflamed or injured tissue *(6,9,10)*.

Worldwide, recombinant preparations of human G-CSF and GM-CSF expressed in either *E. coli* or yeast are available for clinical use. Because they are different proteins acting through different receptors and producing significantly different biologic effects, the clinical data for G-CSF and GM-CSF will be considered separately in this review. Because there are no studies demonstrating significant differences in the clinical effects of different preparations of each protein, clinical data for all recombinant human G-CSF preparations will be summarized as rhG-CSF data, and for recombinant human GM-CSF as rhGM-CSF data. Recently, a pegylated preparation of rhG-CSF has been introduced into clinical practice *(11)*. This preparation has a substantially prolonged half-life and, because it is cleared by mature neutrophils and their precursors, is self-regulating in terms of its pharmacokinetics and need be dosed only once per cycle. This preparation will be referred to as peg-rhuG-CSF.

2.1. Myeloid Growth Factors During Myelosuppressive Chemotherapy

Myeloid growth factors have been used during myelosuppressive chemotherapy to accomplish one of three goals: 1) to decrease the risk of infection, 2) to decrease the duration or severity of established febrile neutropenia, 3) to increase the efficacy of chemotherapy by permitting safe and meaningful increases in chemotherapy dose-intensity.

By far the best established application has been in the prevention of infection. The accepted outcome measure for the incidence of infection in good quality clinical trials has been the incidence of febrile neutropenia, a clinically meaningful entity that because it results in antibiotic use and known risks to patients, and often in hospitalization with obvious costs in terms of both health care resources and patient autonomy.

In several randomized, controlled clinical trials, rhuG-CSF, usually administered at a dose of 5 μg/kg/d commencing 1 d after chemotherapy and continuing until the neutrophil counts have recovered from their nadir, was consistently associated with a 40–60% reduction in the risk of febrile neutropenia, with a reduction in the duration of neutropenia and incidence of febrile neutropenia observed across all cycles of chemotherapy *(12–22)*. It is important to note that in these trials, the rates of febrile neutropenia observed in the control group were greater than 40%, leaving unanswered questions regarding the efficacy of rhuG-CSF in decreasing infection risk when baseline risk is lower.

Therapy with peg-rhG-CSF, with a single dose administered the day following chemotherapy has been shown in randomized controlled trials to be associated with a duration of neutropenia and rate of febrile neutropenia similar to that observed with daily rhuG-CSF therapy for patients receiving myelosuppressive chemotherapy *(23)*. A single, fixed dose of 6 mg has been shown to be comparable in efficacy to a weight-based dose of peg-huG-CSF, making appropriate, evidence-based therapy with this agent substantially simpler and more convenient for both providers and patients than daily rhuG-CSF *(24)*. Recently, the results of a very large, placebo controlled trial of peg-rhuG-CSF in women with breast cancer receiving docetaxel chemotherapy have been reported. Not unexpectedly, myeloid growth factor therapy was not only associated with a significant risk reduction when the control rate across all cycles was approx 20%, but the proportional reduction in risk was greater than 90%. Therapy with peg-rhuG-CSF is not only effective when used to abrogate lower risks of infection in patients receiving myelosuppressive chemotherapy, it is more effective than when peg-huG-CSF or rhG-CSF are used in high risk settings.

Randomized trials investigating the efficacy of therapy with rhuGM-CSF administered to decrease the incidence of infection during multi-cycle chemotherapy have yielded less consistent results *(25–31)*. In two trials, a decreased incidence of infection associated with rhGM-CSF therapy, one in an efficacy evaluable (as opposed to the more rigorous intent-to-treat analysis) subset of lymphoma patients treated with a daily dose of 400 µg/d for 7-d per cycle *(25)*, and the other in a very small trial involving 11 children *(28)*. Three studies observed a decreased incidence of infection limited to the first chemotherapy cycle despite continued rhGM-CSF therapy during subsequent cycles *(26,27,30)* and an equal number of trials have failed to detect a difference in infection risk associated with rhGM-CSF therapy, one in patients with breast cancer *(29)* and two in children *(31,32)*. One important question raised by these trials is the role, if any, of toxicity from rhuGM-CSF in decreasing or obscuring the observed benefit. Although four of these trials reported no increase in adverse events in the rhuGM-CSF arm *(25,29–31)* in the remaining trials an increased incidence of symptoms, including fever, myalgias, edema and rash *(26–28)* or thrombocytopenia *(26,28,32)* was reported in one of the trials, 14% of patients were withdrawn from study explicitly because of toxicity attributed to rhGM-CSF therapy *(27)*. Notwithstanding, the efficacy of rhGM-CSF for the prevention of infection during multi-cycle chemotherapy has not been established. Moreover, if it is effective, the dose and schedule yielding optimal results are not known. The dose finding study concluded that 10 µg/kg/d would be the appropriate dose for testing in a definitive randomized trial *(26)*, and the results of such a randomized trial have not been published. No pegylated preparation of rhuGM-CSF is available for clinical use.

Not surprisingly, the vast majority of cancer patients treated with the goal of reducing infection rates receive rhuG-CSF and increasingly peg rhuG-CSF. Several important questions remain. Because the impact of this therapy on health care costs depends upon: 1) the risk of febrile neutropenia without rhuG-CSF, 2) the proportional reduction in risk when rhuG-CSF is used, 3) the cost of caring for patients with febrile neutropenia and 4) the cost of rhuG-CSF therapy, several attempts have been made to use clinical trial data combined with assumptions and indirect estimates of hospital costs to determine the "breakeven point," defined as that risk of febrile neutropenia above which it becomes more expensive to the health care system to leave patients unprotected (33–35). Most analyses suggest that this breakeven point is a febrile neutropenia risk of approx 20%, although at lower risks there are some cost savings that partially offset drug acquisition costs. To date, theses analyses have made the assumption that rhuG-CSF or peg- rhuG-CSF therapy is always associated with approx a 50% reduction in febrile neutropenia risk; recent data suggesting that the magnitude of the reduction increases at lower baseline risk levels will likely result in a reassessment and further lowering of the estimated risk at which therapy becomes cost saving.

The utilization of rhuG-CSF or peg- rhuG-CSF in current oncologic practice is not always data-driven or rational or optimally convenient. In an effort to decrease the overall cost, many physicians wait until a patient's white count has reached its nadir and then administer rhuG-CSF for 4–6 d until neutrophil recovery. There has only been one randomized trial addressing the efficacy of rhuG-CSF when therapy is initiated at the onset of neutropenia, and this study failed to demonstrate any impact on infection risk, antibiotic use or febrile neuropenia (36). Some clinicians use rhuG-CSF therapy for a short period of time prechemotherapy in patients whose neutrophil counts, for whatever reason, are sufficiently low when the next cycle is due. There is no evidence that this approach lowers risk of infection during the next chemotherapy cycle; if it is believed that it is important that the chemotherapy be given, a more rationale approach would be to use rhuG-CSF or peg- rhuG-CSF in the fashion that has been shown to lower risk. Finally, as peg- rhuG-CSF becomes the most frequently used cytokine, the importance of the unstudied issues of safety of administration of this agent on the same day as chemotherapy (which would optimize patient convenience) and in conjunction with every-2-wk chemotherapy has increased. More studies will be needed.

The results of clinical trials investigating the impact of myeloid growth factor therapy initiated after the onset of febrile neutropenia during myelosuppressive chemotherapy have not conclusively demonstrated benefit in terms of complication rates, resource utilization or rapidity of recovery (37–42). Daily therapy initiated at the time of hospitalization was associated in some but not all studies with a decrease in the duration of neutropenia of approx 2 d, with a 1 or 2 d decrease in the duration of hospitalization (38,40). No study has demonstrated a statistically significant improvement is survival or health care costs, and in the one study in which quality of life was examined, this outcome was better in the placebo than growth factor group (39). Although the data do not support the routine initiation of myeloid growth factor therapy for patients with febrile neutropenia, this remains a reasonable option for cases in which the expected remaining period of neutropenia is several days or more, or in which the severity of the infection or the degree of co-morbidities are such that a 1 or 2 d decrease in the duration of neutropenia may make an important difference in outcome. No randomized trials of peg-rhuG-CSF in this setting have been published and, given that there is little benefit to hospitalized patients of once per cycle dosing and there are significant adverse economic effects to the hospital, it is unlikely that this preparation will find a role here.

Finally, myeloid growth factors are being used with increased frequency to facilitate the administration of full doses, on time, of relatively aggressive chemotherapy regimens aimed at improving survival in cancer patients. Randomized trials of higher dose intensities of chemotherapy facilitated by growth factor use have more often been negative *(43–51)* than positive *(52–56)*. Recently there have been two controlled trials of dose-intensified adjuvant chemotherapy for node positive breast cancer, one utilizing increased per-treatment dose intensity and the other decreased inter-treatment interval *(57)*, with each regimen compared to an accepted standard. Both approaches have shown some superiority in terms of relapse-free and overall survival and both have sufficient risk of febrile neutropenia to warrant the use of rhG-CSF or peg-rhG-CSF to decrease that risk. These are currently the best data documenting a benefit to patients of growth factor facilitated dose intensification.

Recent surveys of clinical practice in the United States have produced disturbing data that suggest that clinicians administering potentially curative chemotherapy, including both adjuvant treatment of breast cancer *(58)* and treatment for lymphoma *(59)* frequently administer lower doses or delay treatments as a strategy for dealing with neutropenia. Often, doses were reduced to levels which, based upon retrospective analyses, are suspected to be associated with inferior survival outcomes and myeloid growth factors were not employed as an alternative infection risk reduction strategy. In addition, the increasing emphasis in oncology upon providing optimal anticancer therapy to vulnerable populations, especially the elderly, is likely to result in a greater awareness of the importance of utilizing myeloid growth factors to maintain full dose on time while avoiding unnecessary toxicities. It is likely that the greatest growth in myeloid factor use in oncology in the next several years will be to establish and maintain chemotherapy dose intensity.

3. BONE MARROW AND PERIPHERAL BLOOD PROGENITOR CELL TRANSPLANTATION

3.1. Growth Factors and Bone Marrow / Progenitor Cell Transplantation

The introduction of myeloid growth factors has transformed the field of bone marrow transplantation. Years ago, when unprimed marrow was the only available source of hematopoietic support following myeloablative therapy, rhGM-CSF *(60,61)* or rhG-CSF *(62,63)* administered daily following marrow infusion was shown to decrease the duration of neutropenia, antibiotic use and hospitalization. In the allogeneic transplant setting, growth factor therapy was not associated with increases in graft-vs-host disease. Unfortunately, results of trials using rhG-CSF or rhGM-CSF to treat graft failure were been disappointing.

Major developments rapidly followed the recognition that hematopoietic progenitor cells circulate in increased numbers during myeloid growth factor therapy, followed by the discovery that it was feasible to harvest sufficient quantities with leukapheresis to provide an alternative and source of support. The infusion of peripheral blood progenitor cells (PBPC) harvested during therapy with rhG-CSF *(64–68)* or rhGM-CSF *(64,69–72)* following ablation were shown to be associated with significantly more rapid neutrophil and platelet engraftment compared to unprimed marrow. Similarly rapid engraftment profiles were observed when rhG-CSF primed marrow was used *(73)*. Comparative studies of the effects of PBPC harvested during rhuG-CSF vs during rhuGM-CSF therapy have suggested that the rhG-CSF mobilized cells may be superior in terms of efficacy and/or toxicity *(74,75)*.

Because the consistency of engraftment is related to the quantity of PBPC infused, substantial efforts have been made to optimize harvests. Improved yields have been obtained when myeloid growth factors are administered following chemotherapy, although chemotherapy is often not necessary for adequate graft acquisition (76,77) and this approach is obviously not feasible for donors in allogeneic transplantation. There has been significant interest in the optimal rhG-CSF dose for obtaining an adequate graft. For patients not receiving chemotherapy, rhG-CSF at 10 µg/kg/d may produce better yields than lower doses (78). Splitting the daily dose and administering rhG-CSF twice daily may (79) or may not (80) improve PBPC yields. Very high dose rhG-CSF, 12 µg/kg twice daily, may be superior to 10 µg/kg daily (81). For patients mobilized with chemotherapy plus rhG-CSF, 16 µg/kg/d is associated with greater cell yields that 8 µg/kg/d, although the increased cell dose may not translate into faster engraftment (82). Similar dose finding studies have not been reported for rhGM-CSF for PBPC harvesting. The combination of rhG-CSF and rhGM-CSF is an effective mobilizing regimen (83), however there are no studies demonstrating that this approach is superior to single factor mobilization. Preliminary data suggesting that peg-rhG-CSF is an excellent PBPC mobilizer, and may replace rhuG-CSF for this purpose.

Because neutrophil engraftment was so accelerated when PBPC were substituted for marrow, it was not clear that the administration of myeloid growth factors following PBPC infusion would provide any incremental benefit. In sufficiently-powered randomized clinical trials, rhG-CSF, given at a daily dose of 5 µg/kg or less until neutrophil recovery, has been associated with a reduction in the duration of neutropenia, and in some cases a decrease in days of hospitalization and overall costs (84–88). It may be possible to delay the initiation of growth factor therapy until day 6 post-transplant without compromising efficacy (89). Very little data exist for the efficacy of rhGM-CSF during recovery from PBPC transplant. There are no data available for peg-rhuG-CSF therapy following PBPC infusion.

The replacement of bone marrow with PBPC as the preferred source of cellular support has brought flexibility in terms of cell dose as well as the potential for promising graft engineering strategies including: tumor cell purging, "split grafts" for multiple cycles of high dose therapy, ex vivo expansion, selective removal of particular effector cells to reduce or manage graft-vs-host reactions, acquisition of dendritic cell precursors for anticancer vaccines, and gene therapy.

3.2. Myeloid Growth Factors for Patients With Myelodysplasia or Myeloid Malignancies

Patients with myelodysplastic syndrome (MDS) complicated by clinically significant neutropenia are at high risk for death from infection. Studies of short-term administration of either rhGM-CSF or rhG-CSF to patients with MDS and neutropenia have shown that neutrophil counts increase in the majority of patients, and baseline neutrophil dysfunction frequently improves, although these effects are usually lost within a few days to weeks. Moreover, MDS appears to be the one setting in which "lineage steal" occurs, and sustained therapy with myeloid growth factors can be complicated by worsening thrombocytopenia and bleeding. Hence, therapy with myeloid factors may be useful for short-term therapy of infected, neutropenic MDS patient in whom excess marrow blasts are not present. More recently, both rhG-CSF(90-92) and rhGM-CSF

(93,94) have been used in conjunction with recombinant erythropoietin to enhance the benefit of that agent in the management of MDS associated anemia.

Myeloid growth factors have been used in the treatment of patients with acute myelogenous leukemia undergoing induction or maintenance therapy with two distinct goals: to decrease the duration of neutropenia and its associated complications, especially in "elderly" patients at risk for toxic death, and to recruit malignant cells into a cell cycle phase in which they may be more sensitive to cell cycle specific chemotherapeutic agents. When the goal is prevention of infection alone, the factor has been started after the completion of chemotherapy in patients undergoing induction or consolidation therapy; when the goal is to increase chemosensitivity, the factor has been given during chemotherapy and most studies have been limited to patients with refractory leukemia.

Randomized clinical trials of rhGM-CSF given to elderly patients either following induction therapy *(95,96)* or during and after induction therapy *(97)* or to a general population of de-novo patients during and after induction therapy *(98)* have demonstrated that this therapy is safe and usually associated with a reduction in the duration of neutropenia following induction or consolidation chemotherapy. However, these trials have failed to consistently show a significant clinical benefit to patients. Although one trial that focused on the subset of patients in whom bone marrow was hypocellular on day 10 of standard leukemia therapy, suggested that growth factor therapy was associated with an improved median survival *(95)*, this finding was not reproduced in a larger study *(96)*. Therapy with rhGM-CSF is this setting has not been found to be cost effective *(99)*. Randomized clinical trials of rhG-CSF given to "elderly" patients following induction chemotherapy *(100,101)*, to younger patients during intensive induction chemotherapy *(102)* and to adults following induction or consolidation chemotherapy *(103,104)* have consistently observed a decrease in the duration of neutropenia, but have not consistently documented significant reductions in infections or hospital days nor a significant increase in survival. Two studies have observed a decreased duration of hospital stay *(102,103)* and in one study each a decrease in significant fungal infections *(103)* and an increase in complete response rates *(100)* were reported. In a randomized trial of rhG-CSF before and during chemotherapy for refractory leukemia, no change in response rate was observed *(104)*. No data are available for peg-rhG-CSF therapy in patients with leukemia.

Trials of rhGM-CSF of rhG-CSF for patients with acute myelogenous leukemia have demonstrated that this therapy is safe but failed to show a significant impact on survival or resource consumption. If a clinician chooses to use these agents in patients undergoing therapy for leukemia, daily doses of 5 µg/kg/d of either agent are reasonable choices.

3.3. Summary

It is difficult to overestimate the impact myeloid growth factors have had on the practice of oncology or on the lives or our patients. In addition to lowering infection and hospitalization risks for patients receiving chemotherapy, with the attendant decreases in lost productivity, disrupted personal lives and anxiety, they have dramatically reduced the duration of hospitalization in the transplant setting and facilitated the development of promising strategies for cellular therapy. More recently, we have learned that there is still substantial potential for these agents to further advance the care of cancer patients by allowing us to administer full, curative doses of chemotherapy on time for patients with early stage breast cancer or lymphoma, while protecting the safety and functional status of medically frail and vulnerable populations, particularly the elderly.

4. ERYTHROPOIETIC PROTEINS

The second significant hematopoietic growth factor to be introduced into clinical trials in cancer patients was recombinant human erythropoietin (rhuEPO). Erythropoietin is the humoral regulator of erythropoiesis; this molecule differs somewhat from the myeloid growth factors in that its anti-apoptotic effects predominate over mitogenic effects on precursor cells, with the practical result that it appears that this factor can be administered to patients on the same day that chemotherapy is given without enhancing the myelosuppressive effects of chemotherapy. Because rhuEPO is inactive unless the molecule is glycosylated, all preparations are expressed in mammalian cells. Most of the clinical data available relate to the two major rhuEPO preparations in use in the world today, epoetin alfa and epoetin beta. Although these two preparations differ slightly in their isoform composition and in whether albumin is used as a stabilizer (epoetin alfa used in the United States, but not the European preparation or epoetin beta) their half lives are very similar, and data for both molecules will be summarized under the term rhu-EPO, except for the brief discussion of pure red cell aplasia. Based upon the recognition that rhuEPO isoforms containing more carbohydrate moieties have greater in vivo potency, two additional glycosylation sites were introduced into the molecule through site-directed mutagenesis *(105)*. The product of this modified gene, darbepoetin alfa, has approx a threefold longer half-life than rhuEPO and a greater, protein-corrected in vivo potency. This molecule is now in clinical use in oncology practice throughout the world, and these data will also be summarized.

Patients with cancer are frequently anemic, due both to the underlying disease and to the effects of myelosuppressive chemotherapy. When it was recognized that cancer is a chronic illness characterized both by a cytokine mediated resistance of the marrow to the erythropoietic effects of erythropoietin and to a relative endogenous erythropoietin deficiency *(106)* it was logical to initiate clinical trials of erythropoietic proteins for the treatment of cancer-associated anemia. Initially, the focus of this therapy was a reduction in the frequency of red cell transfusion.

4.1. Cancer and Cancer Chemotherapy: Reducing Transfusions

Ten years ago, it was widely believed that cancer patients, because of their multiple morbidities and global functional impairments, did not suffer symptoms from anemia until hemoglobin levels fell to 8 g/dL or lower, and red cell transfusions became necessary. This assumption, coupled with the difficulties of using quality of life or symptom reduction as a primary endpoint in pivotal clinical trials, underlay the choice of transfusions reduction as the primary endpoint in the phase III clinical trials of rhuEPO in cancer patients. After several phase I and II trials demonstrated the potential for rhuEPO therapy to induce erythropoiesis in anemic cancer patients, randomized phase III trials using a starting dose of 150 U/kg thrice weekly for anemic patients receiving chemotherapy and 100 U/kg thrice weekly for anemic cancer patients not receiving chemotherapy were carried out *(107)*. Dose increases were incorporated for patients in whom an increase in hemoglobin level was not observed after the first 6 wk of therapy. These trials demonstrated that, for anemic cancer patients receiving chemotherapy,

12 wk of therapy with rhuEPO was associated with approx a 50% reduction in the proportion of patients requiring transfusion and the number of units transfused to the whole cohort compared to placebo. This finding was later confirmed in subsequent randomized trials *(108–110)*. Unfortunately, the trial in patients not receiving chemotherapy was only 8 wk in duration and, although treated patients responded in terms of hemoglobin increase as well or better than was observed in the chemotherapy trial, the difference between rhuEPO and placebo in terms of transfusion reduction was not statistically significant, presumably because of a significantly reduced power associated with the shorter duration of the trial. The results of this unfortunate outcome remain with us today; although it is obvious that anemic cancer patients not receiving chemotherapy respond as well or better to rhuEPO therapy *(111)* than patients receiving chemotherapy, no regulatory agency anywhere in the world has approved rhuEPO for this indication, and reimbursement policies and hence access to treatment vary widely within the United States as a result.

For several years, in the United States the dosing of rhuEPO in clinical practice has been flat dose rather than weight-based, and weekly rather than thrice weekly, with 40,000 U/wk being the usual starting dose, with dose increases for nonresponders after 4–6 wk. Recently, this dose and frequency was approved by the Food and Drug Administration.

Early clinical trials of darbepoetin alfa administered to anemic cancer patients receiving chemotherapy demonstrated that the drug was effective in increasing hemoglobin levels when administered weekly or every 2 or 3 wk *(112,113)*. In randomized, placebo controlled trials in anemic patients with lung cancer *(114)* or lymphoproliferative malignancies *(115)* undergoing chemotherapy, darbepoetin alfa dosed at 2.25 µg/kg/wk, with a dose increase permitted for patients not experiencing a substantial hemoglobin rise, were associated with significant reductions in transfusion requirements and decreases in fatigue. Studies of the efficacy of darbepoetin alfa in cancer patients not receiving chemotherapy have shown that these patients respond well, and can be treated as infrequently as every 4 wk *(116)*.

Fixed and weight-based dosing strategies for darbepoetin alfa appear to provide equivalent clinical results, regardless of patient weight *(117)*. In the United States, the most frequently used dose and schedule for darbepoetin alfa is a flat dose of 200 µg every 2 wk, with a dose increase to 300 µg every 2 wk for patients in whom the response is judged to be inadequate *(118)*. Clinical experience suggests that the results obtained with this approach are similar to those observed with currently used doses of rhuEPO *(119)*. Two large, randomized trials comparing rhuEPO, at a starting dose of 40,000 U/wk to darbepoetin, at a starting dose of 200 µg every 2 wk, with both drugs subject to dose increases for inadequate response, are in progress and near completion, and should determine whether the current dose of either agent is significantly better in terms of patient benefit.

Recently, we have carried out studies exploring the safety and efficacy of darbepoetin administered every 3 wk to anemic patients receiving every-3-week chemotherapy, with the darbepoetin given either on the same day as chemotherapy, or 1 wk earlier. Our data have shown that chemotherapy is associated with increased levels of endogenous erythropoietin, lasting approx 1 wk, as well as reduced clearance of darbepoetin, presumably owing to suppressed receptor-mediated clearance. Every-3-wk dosing is effective, and synchronous dosing is both safe and no less effective. In Europe, darbepoetin alfa is now approved for every-3-wk dosing in clinical practice, and one would expect similar developments in the United States in the future, given the obvious increase in patient convenience for patients receiving every-3-wk chemotherapy.

4.2. Cancer and Cancer Chemotherapy: Improving Quality of Life and functional Status

The year 1997 was a watershed in our understanding of the potential for erythropoietic therapy to enhance our supportive care of cancer patients. In that year, the results of a large survey of cancer patients was published, and revealed that fatigue rather than pain was the symptom most limiting to the function and quality of life of cancer patients *(120)*, a finding that was later confirmed in a second even larger survey *(121)*. Also in 1997, the results of a large, community-based study of anemic cancer chemotherapy patients receiving rhuEPO was published, with results demonstrating that treatment of anemia was associated with significant reductions in fatigue, and that the magnitude of the fatigue reduction was very strongly correlated with the magnitude of the hemoglobin increase *(122)*. These findings were confirmed and the fatigue reduction was shown to occur in all chemotherapy response categories in two subsequent community-based studies *(123,124)*. Finally, a randomized, double-blind placebo controlled trial demonstrated the improvement of quality of life enjoyed by patients treated for degrees of anemia that had until that time been thought to be asymptomatic and hence clinically insignificant in cancer patients *(108)*. Analyses of the pooled data from two of the large community based studies suggested that the greatest gains in energy, functional status and quality of life occurred when hemoglobin levels rose from 11 to 12g/dL, further challenging ingrained beliefs regarding the importance of mild anemia in the supportive care of cancer *(125)*.

Although these findings were astounding to oncologist, nephrologists had for years recognized that their patients felt best when hemoglobin levels were maintained in the 12 g/dL range and established standards of care for their field to insure that patients enjoyed the benefits of that insight. In a meta-analysis comparing observed quality of life gained for a given hemoglobin increase in studies of anemic dialysis patients to studies of anemic cancer chemotherapy patients, it was shown that the relationship between rising hemoglobin and increased quality of life was essentially the same for the two populations of patients *(126)*. Not only are cancer patients symptomatic from the pervasive mild and moderate degrees of anemia we have been trained to ignore, they are as symptomatic and likely to benefit from successful treatment as a group of patients for whom the value of treating anemia to levels that optimize function is widely accepted. These observations have resulted in a paradigm shift in our thinking about anemia management in the cancer patient and optimizing patient function and comfort is now the major goal of erythropoietic therapy in these patients. This more enlightened goal, which has taken more than 10 yr to evolve, suggests that earlier intervention, before patients have developed significant anemia-related fatigue or are at immediate risk of red cell transfusion, would be the logical next step in our efforts to optimally support our patients.

4.3. Cancer and Cancer Chemotherapy: Safety

Three issues have been raised regarding the safety of using erythropoietic agents in cancer patients. First, more than one hundred dialysis patients in Europe and Canada who had been receiving erythropoietic therapy, most frequently administered subcutaneously, recently developed severe, refractory, hypoplastic anemia *(127)*. This pure red cell aplasia (PRCA) has been found to be owing to the development of antibodies that are neutralizing to endogenous EPO, rHuEPO, and darbepoetin alfa. The epidemiologic data suggest that a significant increase in the incidence of PRCA followed the introduction into the market of a new preparation of epoetin alfa, produced in response to a European mandate aimed at minimizing the chances of transmission of prions by eliminating albumin from all pharmaceuticals. PRCA is uncommon even when this albumin-free epoetin alfa preparation is used, is very unlikely to occur when the drug is given intravenously as opposed to subcutaneously, has not occurred in cancer patients, and has not been observed with the epoetin alfa preparation that is marketed in the United States. Hence, PRCA is not currently a safety issue in this country.

The second issue regards the risk of thrombosis during therapy with erythopoietic proteins. It has been well documented that there is a slightly higher risk of thrombotic events, especially graft occlusions, in dialysis patients receiving rHuEPO. Until recently, it was less clear whether this was also an issue in cancer patients treated with these drugs, in part because the higher background rate of thrombosis in this population obscures the attribution of this adverse event. Based upon an examination of pooled data from all controlled trials in cancer patients, it is now clear that there is an increased risk of thrombotic events, especially, but not limited to, catheter-associated and deep venous thrombosis associated with both rhuEPO and darbepoetin therapy. The best estimates are that the overall risk across all tumor types is approx 3% in the control group and 5% in the treated group. It is not clear that these thromboses are mediated by the rheological effects of rising or high hemoglobin levels; in some reviews, thrombosis risk has been lower for patients with higher hemoglobin levels, but this may reflect more severe cancer and thrombotic diathesis in the more anemic patients. Several other mechanisms for thrombosis associated with erythropoietic therapy have been proposed including: activation of receptor bearing vascular endothelial cells *(128)*, activation of platelets by young erythrocytes *(129)* and synergy between erythropoietin and thrombopoietin in the activation of platelets *(130)*. Of course, more than one mechanism may be operative. The recent Cochrane meta-analysis of randomized controlled trials of rhuEPO during chemotherapy for anemic cancer patients found an increased risk of thrombotic events, with a calculated relative risk of 1.5 *(131)*. Not surprisingly, the risk of thrombosis is increased in patients with a history of thrombosis. It is now fairly clear that there is a real but small increase in thombosis risk when cancer patients receive erythropoietic proteins, and this should be factored into treatment decisions and discussed with patients. The role of prophylactic measures, such as low dose warfarin, in addressing this issue has not been explored.

The final safety issue arose recently when two randomized trials of the role of rhuEPO in enhancing survival in nonanemic patients with head and neck cancer undergoing radiotherapy without chemotherapy *(132)* or with metastatic breast cancer undergoing chemotherapy (paper not yet published if full) reported a decreased survival in the rHuEPO treated groups. It is not yet clear whether these observations are the result of baseline prognostic imbalances, methodologic flaws, or a real effect of the erythropoietic therapy. Until additional studies have been carried out, therapy with any erythropoietic protein for nonanemic cancer patients outside the setting of a clinical trial should not be contemplated.

These findings raised a concern that erythropoietin receptors (EPO-R) on cancer cells may be involved, and EPO may be a growth or anti-apoptotic factor for cancers. There are profound technical challenges to further exploring this hypothesis including: the difficulty in determining whether receptors identified are on tumor or stromal cells, the possibility that immuno-reagents are reacting with proteins other than EPO-R and giving false positive readings, the inability to determine whether receptors are functional even if present and on tumor cells, and the fact that functional EPO-R expression beneath current levels of detection would be sufficient to mediate an effect on tumor cells. These technical challenges notwithstanding, it seems doubtful that erythropoietic agent induced tumor progression will prove to be an issue for cancer patients for several reasons: 1) two randomized clinical trials in anemic cancer patients receiving chemotherapy have shown an trend toward improved survival with rhuEPO *(108)* and with darbepoetin *(114)* and no trial to date has reported an adverse effect on survival, 2) the Cochrane meta-analysis of randomized trials of rhuEPO treatment for anemic cancer patients reported a trend favoring improved survival in the rhuEPO treated patients *(131)* and 3) there is indirect evidence and strong theoretical support for the proposition that anemia decreases the survival of cancer patients *(133,134)*. To date, there is no evidence that treating anemic cancer patients with erythropoietic proteins is associated with any decrease in survival.

4.4. Cancer and Cancer Chemotherapy: Challenges for the Future

Although we now have an appreciation of the importance of anemia management in addressing the most important symptom experienced by cancer patients, we still have widely varying practice patterns and a significant proportion of patients who would benefit from treatment go untreated. It is likely that this is in part owing to the fact that 40 to 50% of treated patients do not "respond" if response is defined as a 2 g/dL increase in hemoglobin level that is clearly owing to the erythropoietic therapy. Parenthetically, it is important to note that it is not clear that a nonresponder is not benefiting from therapy; it is possible, for instance, that hemoglobin levels would have fallen further in the absence of therapy. Nevertheless, nonresponse is a critical issue and four strategies are available to address it: 1) initiate therapy early before the anemia is symptomatic and a significant increase in hemoglobin level is not needed, 2) add parenteral iron therapy, 3) administer cytokine blocking agents to decrease marrow resistance to the effects of EPO, and 4) change the dose and schedule of administration (frontloading). There are minimal data available for cytokine blockers, and frontloaded regimens have failed to solve this problem. As noted above, early initiation is consistent with the new goals of erythropoietic therapy.

The use of parenteral iron to support rhuEPO treatment in dialysis patients has become commonplace, and has shown both response enhancing and dose sparing impacts on erythropoietic therapy. Now that safer iron preparations are available, it is time to consider the potential of parenteral iron in oncology. It might be difficult for normal and iron replete individuals to mobilize iron from stores rapidly enough to prevent iron-restricted erythropoiesis in the face of pharmacologic levels of erythropoietic proteins. For cancer patients, who have the anemia of chronic disease impairing iron mobilization *(135)*, one might expect the problem of functional iron deficiency to be worse. Moreover, patients with the anemia of chronic disease also have decreased gastrointestinal absorption, making oral iron an even more unattractive prospect than it is in other settings. In a recent trial, anemic cancer chemotherapy patients receiving huEPO were randomized to receive no iron, oral iron, or two different schedules of parenteral iron dextran *(136)*. The mean increases in hemoglobin concentration were significantly

Table 1
Erythropoietic Therapy: Nephrology vs Hematology–Oncology

	Hematologic response	Transfusion risk reduction	QOL improvement	Mean weekly cost
Nephrology	>90%	>90%	Documented	$X
Oncology	50–60%	50–70%	Equally documented	$3X
MDS	20–40%	Observed but unquantified	Assumed	$4–6X

better in the parenteral iron groups than in the oral iron or no therapy groups, and in the oral iron group they were not significantly better than no iron therapy. This observation has recently been confirmed in a second randomized trial that enrolled more iron replete patients and use the safer parenteral iron salt preparation. The recognition that at least a part of the nonresponsiveness of cancer patients to erythropoietic proteins can be overcome with parenteral iron is the most important recent development in this field.

A second, related, less often discussed explanation for our failure to implement standards in oncology similar to nephrology's that insure that as many of our patients benefit as possible is the relatively high cost of treatment in the cancer patient. Because the doses of erythropoietic proteins are approx threefold higher in oncology, the per benefit (prevented transfusion, gained QOL unit) is much higher (see Table 1). Although it is hoped that early initiation and parenteral iron will help, it is likely that the disparities in terms of access will remain until novel drug pricing strategies are developed, or less expensive agents become available.

4.5. Myelodysplastic Syndrome

Anemia associated with MDS is a common, vexing problem in oncology practice. These patients are frequently elderly, tolerate anemia poorly, become transfusion dependent and inevitably develop complications of transfusion including allo-immunization and iron overload. Sufficient data have accumulated regarding the safety of rhEPO therapy in this setting to demonstrate that rhEPO therapy is safe, and not associated with either an increased risk of progression to acute leukemia (an interesting observation given the recent concerns about the effects of rhuEPO on cancer cells that have not been shown to have functional receptors) or with lineage steal. Unfortunately, rhEPO therapy is frequently ineffective, failing to increase hemoglobin levels in approx 60% of patients.

Recombinant human EPO doses of 200–3000 U/kg/wk intravenously, and 150–2000 U/kg subcutaneously have been studied, with hemoglobin increases noted mainly with doses of at least 60,000 U/wk and primarily in the subset of patients in the refractory anemia without excess blasts subset of the MDS syndrome (137–145). The addition of myeloid growth factor to rhEPO therapy may increase the erythropoietic response in patients with MDS.

For patients with symptomatic refractory anemia without excess blasts, it is very reasonable for the clinician to initiate an 8-wk trial of rhEPO therapy, with or without myeloid growth factor therapy, using the highest dose that is feasible in the particular reimbursement environment (146,147). For responding patients, therapy can be continued and doses adjusted to maintain an asymptomatic hemoglobin level. Recently, darbepoetin alfa has been shown to be effective in increasing hemoglobin levels in patients with MDS.

5. THROMBOPOIETIC AGENTS

Thrombopoietin is the physiologic regulator of platelet production in humans, with levels rising in response to thrombocytopenia owing to decreased clearance by megakaryocytes and platelets. Several cloned preparations of this hematopoietic cytokine have been introduced into clinical trials, however none of these have yet been approved by the Food and Drug Administration. Recombinant human interleukin-11 or oprelvekin, does stimulate platelet production, and this drug is available for clinical use *(148)*. It is not commonly used both because thrombocytopenia is not a frequent problem limiting our ability administer chemotherapy and its administration is associated with fluid shifts that complicate management. Currently, there are at least two promising small molecule thrombopoietin receptor agonists in clinical development, which may provide us with the ability to induce thrombopoiesis when necessary without complicating patient management.

REFERENCES

1. Lieschke GJ, Burgess AW. Granulocyte colony-stimulating factor and granulocyte-macrophage colony-stimulating factor (1). N Engl J Med 1992; 327(1): 28–35.
2. Lieschke GJ, Burgess AW. Granulocyte colony-stimulating factor and granulocyte-macrophage colony-stimulating factor (2). N Engl J Med 1992; 327(2):99–106.
3. Lieschke GJ, et al. Mice lacking granulocyte colony-stimulating factor have chronic neutropenia, granulocyte and macrophage progenitor cell deficiency, and impaired neutrophil mobilization. Blood 1994; 84(6): 1737–1746.
4. Dranoff G, et al. Involvement of granulocyte-macrophage colony-stimulating factor in pulmonary homeostasis. Science 1994; 264(5159):713–716.
5. El Ouriaghli F, et al. Neutrophil elastase enzymatically antagonizes the in vitro action of G-CSF: Implications for the regulation of granulopoiesis. Blood 2003; 101(5):1752–1758.
6. Yong KL. Granulocyte colony-stimulating factor (G-CSF) increases neutrophil migration across vascular endothelium independent of an effect on adhesion: Comparison with granulocyte-macrophage colony-stimulating factor (GM-CSF). Br J Haematol 1996; 94(1): 40–47.
7. Lieschke GJ, et al. Mice lacking both macrophage- and granulocyte-macrophage colony- stimulating factor have macrophages and coexistent osteopetrosis and severe lung disease. Blood 1994; 84(1):27–35.
8. Wang J, et al. Transgenic expression of granulocyte-macrophage colony-stimulating factor induces the differentiation and activation of a novel dendritic cell population in the lung. Blood 2000; 95(7): 2337–2345.
9. Peters WP, et al. Neutrophil migration is defective during recombinant human granulocyte-macrophage colony-stimulating factor infusion after autologous bone marrow transplantation in humans. Blood 1988; 72(4):1310–1315.
10. Yong KL, et al. Granulocyte-macrophage colony-stimulating factor induces neutrophil adhesion to pulmonary vascular endothelium in vivo: Role of beta 2 integrins. Blood 1992; 80(6):1565–1575.
11. Johnston E, et al. Randomized, dose-escalation study of SD/01 compared with daily filgrastim in patients receiving chemotherapy. J Clin Oncol 2000; 18(13):2522–2528.
12. Crawford J, et al. Reduction by granulocyte colony-stimulating factor of fever and neutropenia induced by chemotherapy in patients with small-cell lung cancer (see comments). N Engl J Med 1991; 325(3): 164–170.
13. Pettengell R et al. Granulocyte colony-stimulating factor to prevent dose-limiting neutropenia in non-Hodgkin's lymphoma: A randomized controlled trial. Blood 1992; 80(6): 1430–1436.
14. Trillet-Lenoir V, et al. Recombinant granulocyte colony stimulating factor reduces the infectious complications of cytotoxic chemotherapy. Eur J Cancer 1993; 29A(3): 319–324.
15. Ottmann OG, et al. Concomitant granulocyte colony-stimulating factor and induction chemoradiotherapy in adult acute lymphoblastic leukemia: A randomized phase III trial. Blood 1995; 86(2): 444–450.
16. Bui BN, et al. Efficacy of lenograstim on hematologic tolerance to MAID chemotherapy in patients with advanced soft tissue sarcoma and consequences on treatment dose-intensity. J Clin Oncol 1995; 13(10): 2629–2636.

17. Welte K, et al. A randomized phase-III study of the efficacy of granulocyte colony- stimulating factor in children with high-risk acute lymphoblastic leukemia. Berlin-Frankfurt-Munster Study Group. Blood 1996; 87(8): 3143–3150.
18. Zinzani PL, et al. Randomized trial with or without granulocyte colony-stimulating factor as adjunct to induction VNCOP-B treatment of elderly high- grade non-Hodgkin's lymphoma. Blood 1997; 89(11): 3974–3979.
19. Geissler K, et al. Granulocyte colony-stimulating factor as an adjunct to induction chemotherapy for adult acute lymphoblastic leukemia—a randomized phase-III study. Blood 1997; 90(2): 590–596.
20. Gisselbrecht C, et al. Placebo-controlled phase III study of lenograstim (glycosylated recombinant human granulocyte colony-stimulating factor) in aggressive non-Hodgkin's lymphoma: Factors influencing chemotherapy administration. Groupe d'Etude des Lymphomes de l'Adulte. Leuk Lymphoma, 1997;25(3,4): 289–300.
21. Larson RA, et al. A randomized controlled trial of filgrastim during remission induction and consolidation chemotherapy for adults with acute lymphoblastic leukemia: CALGB study 9111. Blood 1998;92(5): 1556–1564.
22. Ibrahim NK, et al. Phase I study of vinorelbine and paclitaxel by 3-hour simultaneous infusion with and without granulocyte colony-stimulating factor support in metastatic breast carcinoma. Cancer 2001; 91(4): 664–671.
23. Holmes FA, et al. Blinded, randomized, multicenter study to evaluate single administration pegfilgrastim once per cycle versus daily filgrastim as an adjunct to chemotherapy in patients with high-risk stage II or stage III/IV breast cancer. J Clin Oncol 2002; 20(3): 727–731.
24. Green MD, et al. A randomized double-blind multicenter phase III study of fixed-dose single-administration pegfilgrastim versus daily filgrastim in patients receiving myelosuppressive chemotherapy. Ann Oncol 2003; 14(1): 29–35.
25. Gerhartz HH, et al. Randomized, double-blind, placebo-controlled, phase III study of recombinant human granulocyte-macrophage colony-stimulating factor as adjunct to induction treatment of high-grade malignant non-Hodgkin's lymphomas (see comments). Blood 1993; 82(8): 2329–2339.
26. Hamm J, et al. Dose-ranging study of recombinant human granulocyte-macrophage colony-stimulating factor in small-cell lung carcinoma. J Clin Oncol 1994;12(12): 2667–2676.
27. Bajorin DF, et al. Recombinant human granulocyte-macrophage colony-stimulating factor as an adjunct to conventional-dose ifosfamide-based chemotherapy for patients with advanced or relapsed germ cell tumors: A randomized trial. J Clin Oncol 1995; 13(1): 79–86.
28. Burdach SE, et al. Granulocyte-macrophage-colony stimulating factor for prevention of neutropenia and infections in children and adolescents with solid tumors. Results of a prospective randomized study. Cancer 1995; 76(3): 510–516.
29. Jones SE, et al. Randomized double-blind prospective trial to evaluate the effects of sargramostim versus placebo in a moderate-dose fluorouracil, doxorubicin, and cyclophosphamide adjuvant chemotherapy program for stage II and III breast cancer. J Clin Oncol 1996; 14(11): 2976–2983.
30. Yau JC, et al. Randomized placebo-controlled trial of granulocyte-macrophage colony- stimulating-factor support for dose-intensive cyclophosphamide, etoposide, and cisplatin. Am J Hematol 1996; 51(4): 289–295.
31. van Pelt LJ, et al. Granulocyte-macrophage colony-stimulating factor (GM-CSF) ameliorates chemotherapy-induced neutropenia in children with solid tumors. Pediatr Hematol Oncol 1997; 14(6): 539–545.
32. Wexler LH, et al. Randomized trial of recombinant human granulocyte-macrophage colony- stimulating factor in pediatric patients receiving intensive myelosuppressive chemotherapy. J Clin Oncol 1996; 14(3): 901–910.
33. Glaspy JA, Economic outcomes associated with the use of hematopoietic growth factors. Oncology 1995; 9(11 Suppl): 93–105.
34. Silber JH, et al. Modeling the cost-effectiveness of granulocyte colony-stimulating factor use in early-stage breast cancer. J Clin Oncol 1998; 16(7): 2435–2444.
35. Lyman GH, Kuderer NM, Balducci L. Economic impact of granulopoiesis stimulating agents on the management of febrile neutropenia. Curr Opin Oncol 1998;10(4): 291–296.
36. Hartmann LC, et al. Granulocyte colony-stimulating factor in severe chemotherapy-induced afebrile neutropenia. N Engl J Med 1997; 336(25): 1776–1780.
37. Maher DW, et al. Filgrastim in patients with chemotherapy-induced febrile neutropenia. A double-blind, placebo-controlled trial. Ann Intern Med 1994; 121(7): 492–501.

38. Mayordomo JI, et al. Improving treatment of chemotherapy-induced neutropenic fever by adminis-
    tration of colony-stimulating factors. J Natl Cancer Inst 1995; 87(11): 803–808.
39. Vellenga E, et al. Randomized placebo-controlled trial of granulocyte-macrophage colony-stimulating
    factor in patients with chemotherapy-related febrile neutropenia. J Clin Oncol 1996; 14(2):
    619–627.
40. Mitchell PL, et al. Granulocyte colony-stimulating factor in established febrile neutropenia: A ran-
    domized study of pediatric patients. J Clin Oncol 1997; 15(3): 1163–1170.
41. Ravaud A, et al. Granulocyte-macrophage colony-stimulating factor in patients with neutropenic
    fever is potent after low-risk but not after high-risk neutropenic chemotherapy regimens: Results of a
    randomized phase III trial. J Clin Oncol 1998; 16(9): 2930–2936.
42. Arnberg H, et al. GM-CSF in chemotherapy-induced febrile neutropenia—a double-blind random-
    ized study. Anticancer Res 1998; 18(2B): 1255–1260.
43. Logothetis CJ, et al. Escalated MVAC with or without recombinant human granulocyte- macrophage
    colony-stimulating factor for the initial treatment of advanced malignant urothelial tumors: Results of
    a randomized trial. J Clin Oncol 1995; 13(9): 2272–2277.
44. Furuse K, et al. Phase III study of intensive weekly chemotherapy with recombinant human granulo-
    cyte colony-stimulating factor versus standard chemotherapy in extensive-disease small-cell lung
    cancer. The Japan Clinical Oncology Group. J Clin Oncol 1998; 16(6): 2126–2132.
45. Fossa SD, et al. Filgrastim during combination chemotherapy of patients with poor- prognosis
    metastatic germ cell malignancy. European Organization for Research and Treatment of Cancer,
    Genito-Urinary Group, and the Medical Research Council Testicular Cancer Working Party,
    Cambridge, United Kingdom. J Clin Oncol 1998; 16(2): 716–724.
46. Font A, et al. Increasing dose intensity of cisplatin-etoposide in advanced nonsmall cell lung carci-
    noma: A phase III randomized trial of the Spanish Lung Cancer Group. Cancer 1999; 85(4): 855–863.
47. Michel G, et al. Use of recombinant human granulocyte colony-stimulating factor to increase
    chemotherapy dose-intensity: A randomized trial in very high- risk childhood acute lymphoblastic
    leukemia. J Clin Oncol 2000; 18(7): 1517–1524.
48. Le Cesne A, et al. Randomized phase III study comparing conventional-dose doxorubicin plus ifos-
    famide versus high-dose doxorubicin plus ifosfamide plus recombinant human granulocyte-
    macrophage colony-stimulating factor in advanced soft tissue sarcomas: A trial of the European
    Organization for Research and Treatment of Cancer/Soft Tissue and Bone Sarcoma Group. J Clin
    Oncol 2000; 18(14): 2676–2684.
49. Pfreundschuh M, et al. Dose escalation of cytotoxic drugs using haematopoietic growth factors: A
    randomized trial to determine the magnitude of increase provided by GM-CSF. Ann Oncol 2001;
    12(4): 471–477.
50. Forastiere AA, et al. Phase III comparison of high-dose paclitaxel + cisplatin + granulocyte colony-
    stimulating factor versus low-dose paclitaxel + cisplatin in advanced head and neck cancer: Eastern
    Cooperative Oncology Group Study E1393. J Clin Oncol 2001; 19(4): 1088–1095.
51. Fumoleau P, et al. Intensification of adjuvant chemotherapy: 5-year results of a randomized trial com-
    paring conventional doxorubicin and cyclophosphamide with high-dose mitoxantrone and cyclophos-
    phamide with filgrastim in operable breast cancer with 10 or more involved axillary nodes. J Clin
    Oncol 2001; 19(3): 612–620.
52. Woll PJ, et al. Can cytotoxic dose-intensity be increased by using granulocyte colony- stimulating
    factor? A randomized controlled trial of lenograstim in small-cell lung cancer. J Clin Oncol 1995;
    13(3): 652–659.
53. Thatcher N, et al. Improving survival without reducing quality of life in small-cell lung cancer
    patients by increasing the dose-intensity of chemotherapy with granulocyte colony-stimulating factor
    support: Results of a British Medical Research Council Multicenter Randomized Trial. Medical
    Research Council Lung Cancer Working Party. J Clin Oncol 2000; 18(2): 395–404.
54. Sternberg CN, et al. Randomized phase III trial of high-dose-intensity methotrexate, vinblastine, dox-
    orubicin, and cisplatin (MVAC) chemotherapy and recombinant human granulocyte colony-stimulating
    factor versus classic MVAC in advanced urothelial tract tumors: European Organization for Research
    and Treatment of Cancer Protocol no. 30924. J Clin Oncol 2001; 19(10): 2638–2646.
55. Pfreundschuh M, et al. Two-weekly or 3-weekly CHOP chemotherapy with or without etoposide for
    the treatment of elderly patients with aggressive lymphomas: Results of the NHL-B2 trial of the
    DSHNHL. Blood 2004; 104(3): 634–641.

56. Pfreundschuh M, et al. Two-weekly or 3-weekly CHOP chemotherapy with or without etoposide for the treatment of young patients with good-prognosis (normal LDH) aggressive lymphomas: Results of the NHL-B1 trial of the DSHNHL. Blood 2004; 104(3): 626–633.

57. Citron ML, et al. Randomized trial of dose-dense versus conventionally scheduled and sequential versus concurrent combination chemotherapy as postoperative adjuvant treatment of node-positive primary breast cancer: First report of Intergroup Trial C9741/Cancer and Leukemia Group B Trial 9741. J Clin Oncol 2003; 21(8): 1431–1439.

58. Lyman GH, Dale DC, Crawford J, Incidence and predictors of low dose-intensity in adjuvant breast cancer chemotherapy: A nationwide study of community practices. J Clin Oncol 2003; 21(24): 4524–4531.

59. Lyman GH, et al. Incidence and predictors of low chemotherapy dose-intensity in aggressive non-Hodgkin's lymphoma: A nationwide study. J Clin Oncol 2004; 22(21): 4302–4311.

60. Brandt SJ, et al. Effect of recombinant human granulocyte-macrophage colony-stimulating factor on hematopoietic reconstitution after high-dose chemotherapy and autologous bone marrow transplantation. N Engl J Med 1988; 318(14): 869–876.

61. Nemunaitis J, et al. Recombinant granulocyte-macrophage colony-stimulating factor after autologous bone marrow transplantation for lymphoid cancer. N Engl J Med 1991; 324(25): 1773–1778.

62. Sheridan WP, et al. Granulocyte colony-stimulating factor and neutrophil recovery after high-dose chemotherapy and autologous bone marrow transplantation. Lancet 1989; 2(8668): 891–895.

63. Kennedy MJ, et al. Administration of human recombinant granulocyte colony-stimulating factor (filgrastim) accelerates granulocyte recovery following high- dose chemotherapy and autologous marrow transplantation with 4- hydroperoxycyclophosphamide-purged marrow in women with metastatic breast cancer. Cancer Res 1993; 53(22): 5424–5428.

64. Peters WP, et al. Comparative effects of granulocyte-macrophage colony-stimulating factor (GM-CSF) and granulocyte colony-stimulating factor (G-CSF) on priming peripheral blood progenitor cells for use with autologous bone marrow after high-dose chemotherapy. Blood 1993; 81(7): 1709–17019.

65. Chao NJ, et al. Granulocyte colony-stimulating factor "mobilized" peripheral blood progenitor cells accelerate granulocyte and platelet recovery after high-dose chemotherapy. Blood 1993; 81(8): 2031–2035.

66. Beyer J, et al. Hematopoietic rescue after high-dose chemotherapy using autologous peripheral-blood progenitor cells or bone marrow: A randomized comparison. J Clin Oncol 1995; 13(6): 1328–1335.

67. Schmitz N, et al. Randomised trial of filgrastim-mobilised peripheral blood progenitor cell transplantation versus autologous bone-marrow transplantation in lymphoma patients (see comments) (published erratum appears in Lancet 1996 Mar 30;347(9005):914). Lancet 1996; 347(8998): 353–357.

68. Kawano Y, et al. Efficacy of the mobilization of peripheral blood stem cells by granulocyte colony-stimulating factor in pediatric donors. Cancer Res 1999; 59(14): 3321–3324.

69. Gianni AM, et al. Granulocyte-macrophage colony-stimulating factor to harvest circulating haemopoietic stem cells for autotransplantation. Lancet 1989; 2(8663): 580–585.

70. Huan SD, et al. Influence of mobilized peripheral blood cells on the hematopoietic recovery by autologous marrow and recombinant human granulocyte- macrophage colony-stimulating factor after high-dose cyclophosphamide, etoposide, and cisplatin. Blood 1992; 79(12): 3388–3393.

71. Elias AD, et al. Mobilization of peripheral blood progenitor cells by chemotherapy and granulocyte-macrophage colony-stimulating factor for hematologic support after high-dose intensification for breast cancer. Blood 1992; 79(11): 3036–3044.

72. Kritz A, et al. Beneficial impact of peripheral blood progenitor cells in patients with metastatic breast cancer treated with high-dose chemotherapy plus granulocyte-macrophage colony-stimulating factor. A randomized trial. Cancer 1993; 71(8): 2515–2521.

73. Damiani D, et al. Randomized trial of autologous filgrastim-primed bone marrow transplantation versus filgrastim-mobilized peripheral blood stem cell transplantation in lymphoma patients. Blood 1997; 90(1): 36–42.

74. Demuynck H, et al. Comparative study of peripheral blood progenitor cell collection in patients with multiple myeloma after single-dose cyclophosphamide combined with rhGM-CSF or rhG-CSF (see comments). Br J Haematol 1995; 90(2): 384–292.

75. Weaver CH, et al. Randomized trial of filgrastim, sargramostim, or sequential sargramostim and filgrastim after myelosuppressive chemotherapy for the harvesting of peripheral-blood stem cells. J Clin Oncol 2000; 18(1): 43–53.

76. Kroger N, et al. Mobilizing peripheral blood stem cells with high-dose G-CSF alone is as effective as with Dexa-BEAM plus G-CSF in lymphoma patients. Br J Haematol 1998; 102(4): 1101–1106.

77. Narayanasami U, et al. Randomized trial of filgrastim versus chemotherapy and filgrastim mobilization of hematopoietic progenitor cells for rescue in autologous transplantation. Blood 2001; 98(7): 2059–2064.

78. Grigg AP, et al. Optimizing dose and scheduling of filgrastim (granulocyte colony- stimulating factor) for mobilization and collection of peripheral blood progenitor cells in normal volunteers (see comments). Blood 1995;86(12): 4437–4445.

79. Kroger N, et al. A randomized comparison of once versus twice daily recombinant human granulocyte colony-stimulating factor (filgrastim) for stem cell mobilization in healthy donors for allogeneic transplantation. Br J Haematol 2000; 111(3): 761–765.

80. Anderlini P, et al. A comparative study of once-daily versus twice-daily filgrastim administration for the mobilization and collection of CD34+ peripheral blood progenitor cells in normal donors. Br J Haematol 2000; 109(4): 770–772.

81. Engelhardt M, et al. High-versus standard-dose filgrastim (rhG-CSF) for mobilization of peripheral-blood progenitor cells from allogeneic donors and CD34(+) immunoselection. J Clin Oncol 1999; 17(7): 2160–2172.

82. Demirer T, et al. Mobilization of peripheral blood stem cells with chemotherapy and recombinant human granulocyte colony-stimulating factor (rhG-CSF): a randomized evaluation of different doses of rhG-CSF. Br J Haematol 2002; 116(2): 468–474.

83. Winter JN, et al. Phase I/II study of combined granulocyte colony-stimulating factor and granulocyte-macrophage colony-stimulating factor administration for the mobilization of hematopoietic progenitor cells. J Clin Oncol 1996; 14(1): 277–286.

84. Klumpp TR, et al. Granulocyte colony-stimulating factor accelerates neutrophil engraftment following peripheral-blood stem-cell transplantation: A prospective, randomized trial. J Clin Oncol 1995; 13(6): 1323–1327.

85. McQuaker IG, et al. Low-dose filgrastim significantly enhances neutrophil recovery following autologous peripheral-blood stem-cell transplantation in patients with lymphoproliferative disorders: Evidence for clinical and economic benefit. J Clin Oncol 1997; 15(2): 451–457.

86. Lee SM, et al. Recombinant human granulocyte colony-stimulating factor (filgrastim) following high-dose chemotherapy and peripheral blood progenitor cell rescue in high-grade non-Hodgkin's lymphoma: Clinical benefits at no extra cost. Br J Cancer 1998; 77(8): 1294–1299.

87. Linch DC, et al. G-CSF after peripheral blood stem cell transplantation in lymphoma patients significantly accelerated neutrophil recovery and shortened time in hospital: Results of a randomized BNLI trial. Br J Haematol 1997; 99(4): 933–938.

88. Bishop MR, et al. A randomized, double-blind trial of filgrastim (granulocyte colony- stimulating factor) versus placebo following allogeneic blood stem cell transplantation. Blood 2000; 96(1): 80–85.

89. Faucher C, et al. Administration of G-CSF can be delayed after transplantation of autologous G-CSF-primed blood stem cells: A randomized study. Bone Marrow Transplant 1996; 17(4): 533–536.

90. Negrin RS, et al. Maintenance treatment of the anemia of myelodysplastic syndromes with recombinant human granulocyte colony-stimulating factor and erythropoietin: Evidence for in vivo synergy. Blood 1996; 87(10): 4076–4081.

91. Hellstrom-Lindberg E, et al. Treatment of anemia in myelodysplastic syndromes with granulocyte colony-stimulating factor plus erythropoietin: Results from a randomized phase II study and long-term follow-up of 71 patients. Blood 1998; 92(1): 68–75.

92. Mantovani L, et al. Treatment of anaemia in myelodysplastic syndromes with prolonged administration of recombinant human granulocyte colony-stimulating factor and erythropoietin. Br J Haematol 2000; 109(2): 367–375.

93. Stasi R, et al. Recombinant human granulocyte-macrophage colony-stimulating factor plus erythropoietin for the treatment of cytopenias in patients with myelodysplastic syndromes. Br J Haematol 1999; 105(1): 141–148.

94. Thompson JA, et al. Effect of recombinant human erythropoietin combined with granulocyte/macrophage colony-stimulating factor in the treatment of patients with myelodysplastic syndrome. GM/EPO MDS Study Group. Blood 2000; 95(4): 1175–1179.

95. Rowe JM, et al. A randomized placebo-controlled phase III study of granulocyte- macrophage colony-stimulating factor in adult patients (> 55 to 70 years of age) with acute myelogenous leukemia: A study of the Eastern Cooperative Oncology Group (E1490). Blood 1995; 86(2): 457–462.

96. Stone RM, et al. Granulocyte-macrophage colony-stimulating factor after initial chemotherapy for elderly patients with primary acute myelogenous leukemia. Cancer and Leukemia Group B (see comments). N Engl J Med 1995; 332(25): 1671–1677.

97. Lowenberg B, et al. Use of recombinant GM-CSF during and after remission induction chemotherapy in patients aged 61 years and older with acute myeloid leukemia: Final report of AML-11, a phase III randomized study of the Leukemia Cooperative Group of European Organisation for the Research and Treatment of Cancer and the Dutch Belgian Hemato-Oncology Cooperative Group. Blood 1997; 90(8): 2952–2961.

98. Heil G, et al. GM-CSF in a double-blind randomized, placebo controlled trial in therapy of adult patients with de novo acute myeloid leukemia (AML). Leukemia 1995; 9(1): 3–9.

99. Uyl-de Groot CA, et al. Cost-effectiveness and quality-of-life assessment of GM-CSF as an adjunct to intensive remission induction chemotherapy in elderly patients with acute myeloid leukemia. Br J Haematol 1998; 100(4): 629–636.

100. Dombret H, et al. A controlled study of recombinant human granulocyte colony- stimulating factor in elderly patients after treatment for acute myelogenous leukemia. AML Cooperative Study Group (see comments). N Engl J Med 1995; 332(25): 1678–1683.

101. Godwin JE, et al. A double-blind placebo-controlled trial of granulocyte colony- stimulating factor in elderly patients with previously untreated acute myeloid leukemia: A Southwest oncology group study (9031). Blood 1998. 91(10): 3607–3615.

102. Moore JO, et al. Granulocyte-colony stimulating factor (filgrastim) accelerates granulocyte recovery after intensive postremission chemotherapy for acute myeloid leukemia with aziridinyl benzoquinone and mitoxantrone: Cancer and Leukemia Group B study 9022. Blood 1997;1989(3): 780–788.

103. Heil G, et al. A randomized, double-blind, placebo-controlled, phase III study of filgrastim in remission induction and consolidation therapy for adults with de novo acute myeloid leukemia. The International Acute Myeloid Leukemia Study Group. Blood 1997; 90(12): 4710–4718.

104. Usuki K, et al. Efficacy of granulocyte colony-stimulating factor in the treatment of acute myelogenous leukaemia: A multicentre randomized study. Br J Haematol 2002;116(1): 103–112.

105. Egrie JC, Browne JK, Development and characterization of novel erythropoiesis stimulating protein (NESP). Br J Cancer 2001; 84 Suppl 1: 3–10.

106. Miller CB, et al. Decreased erythropoietin response in patients with the anemia of cancer. N Engl J Med 1990; 322(24): 1689–1692.

107. Henry DH, Abels RI, Recombinant human erythropoietin in the treatment of cancer and chemotherapy-induced anemia: Results of double-blind and open-label follow-up studies. Semin Oncol 1994; 21(2 Suppl 3): 21–28.

108. Littlewood TJ, et al. Effects of epoetin alfa on hematologic parameters and quality of life in cancer patients receiving nonplatinum chemotherapy: Results of a randomized, double-blind, placebo-controlled trial. J Clin Oncol 2001; 19(11): 2865–2874.

109. Osterborg A, et al. Randomized, double-blind, placebo-controlled trial of recombinant human erythropoietin, epoetin Beta, in hematologic malignancies. J Clin Oncol 2002; 20(10): 2486–2494.

110. Cazzola M, et al. Once-weekly epoetin beta is highly effective in treating anaemic patients with lymphoproliferative malignancy and defective endogenous erythropoietin production. Br J Haematol 2003;122(3): 386–393.

111. Kasper C, et al. Recombinant human erythropoietin in the treatment of cancer-related anaemia. Eur J Haematol 1997; 58(4): 251–256.

112. Glaspy JA, et al. A randomized, active-control, pilot trial of front-loaded dosing regimens of darbepoetin-alfa for the treatment of patients with anemia during chemotherapy for malignant disease. Cancer 2003; 97(5): 1312–1320.

113. Kotasek D, et al. Darbepoetin alfa administered every 3 weeks alleviates anaemia in patients with solid tumours receiving chemotherapy; results of a double-blind, placebo-controlled, randomised study. Eur J Cancer 2003; 39(14): 2026–2034.

114. Vansteenkiste J, et al. Double-blind, placebo-controlled, randomized phase III trial of darbepoetin alfa in lung cancer patients receiving chemotherapy. J Natl Cancer Inst 2002;94(16): 1211–1220.

115. Hedenus M, et al. Randomized, dose-finding study of darbepoetin alfa in anaemic patients with lymphoproliferative malignancies. Br J Haematol 2002; 119(1): 79–86.

116. Smith RE, et al. A dose- and schedule-finding study of darbepoetin alpha for the treatment of chronic anaemia of cancer. Br J Cancer 2003; 88(12): 1851–1858.

117. Hesketh PJ, et al. A randomized controlled trial of darbepoetin alfa administered as a fixed or weight-based dose using a front-loading schedule in patients with anemia who have nonmyeloid malignancies. Cancer 2004; 100(4): 859–868.
118. Schwartzberg L, et al. A multicenter retrospective cohort study of practice patterns and clinical outcomes of the use of darbepoetin alfa and epoetin alfa for chemotherapy-induced anemia. Clin Ther 2003; 25(11): 2781–2796.
119. Schwartzberg LS, et al. A randomized comparison of every-2-week darbepoetin alfa and weekly epoetin alfa for the treatment of chemotherapy-induced anemia in patients with breast, lung, or gynecologic cancer. Oncologist 2004; 9(6): 696–707.
120. Vogelzang NJ, et al. Patient, caregiver, and oncologist perceptions of cancer-related fatigue: Results of a tripart assessment survey. The Fatigue Coalition. Semin Hematol 1997; 34(3 Suppl 2): 4–12.
121. Curt GA, et al. Impact of cancer-related fatigue on the lives of patients: New findings from the Fatigue Coalition. Oncologist 2000; 5(5): 353–360.
122. Glaspy J, et al. Impact of therapy with epoetin alfa on clinical outcomes in patients with nonmyeloid malignancies during cancer chemotherapy in community oncology practice. Procrit Study Group. J Clin Oncol 1997; 15(3): 1218–1234.
123. Demetri GD, et al. Quality-of-life benefit in chemotherapy patients treated with epoetin alfa is independent of disease response or tumor type: Results from a prospective community oncology study. Procrit Study Group. J Clin Oncol 1998; 16(10): 3412–3425.
124. Gabrilove JL, et al. Clinical evaluation of once-weekly dosing of epoetin alfa in chemotherapy patients: Improvements in hemoglobin and quality of life are similar to three-times-weekly dosing. J Clin Oncol 2001; 19(11): 2875–2882.
125. Crawford J, et al. Relationship between changes in hemoglobin level and quality of life during chemotherapy in anemic cancer patients receiving epoetin alfa therapy. Cancer 2002; 95(4): 888–895.
126. Ross SD, et al. The effect of anemia treatment on selected health-related quality-of- life domains: A systematic review. Clin Ther 2003; 25(6): 1786–1805.
127. Casadevall N, et al. Pure red-cell aplasia and antierythropoietin antibodies in patients treated with recombinant erythropoietin. N Engl J Med 2002; 346(7): 469–475.
128. Stohlawetz PJ, et al. Effects of erythropoietin on platelet reactivity and thrombopoiesis in humans. Blood 2000; 95(9): 2983–2989.
129. Valles J, et al. Platelet-erythrocyte interactions enhance alpha(IIb)beta(3) integrin receptor activation and P-selectin expression during platelet recruitment: Down-regulation by aspirin ex vivo. Blood 2002; 99(11): 3978–3984.
130. Wun T, et al. Thrombopoietin is synergistic with other hematopoietic growth factors and physiologic platelet agonists for platelet activation in vitro. Am J Hematol 1997; 54(3): 225–232.
131. Bohlius J, et al. Erythropoietin for patients with malignant disease. Cochrane Database Syst Rev 2004;3.
132. Henke M, et al. Erythropoietin to treat head and neck cancer patients with anaemia undergoing radiotherapy: Randomised, double-blind, placebo-controlled trial. Lancet 2003; 362(9392): 1255–1260.
133. Glaspy JA, The potential for anemia treatment to improve survival in cancer patients. Oncology (Huntingt) 2002; 16(9 Suppl 10): 35–40.
134. Glaspy J, Dunst J. Can erythropoietin therapy improve survival? Oncology 2004; 1: 5–11.
135. Glaspy J, Cavill I. Role of iron in optimizing responses of anemic cancer patients to erythropoietin. Oncology (Huntingt) 1999; 13(4): 461–473; discussion 477–478, 483–488.
136. Auerbach M, et al. Intravenous iron optimizes the response to recombinant human erythropoietin in cancer patients with chemotherapy-related anemia: A multicenter, open-label, randomized trial. J Clin Oncol 2004; 22(7): 1301–1307.
137. Stebler C, et al. High-dose recombinant human erythropoietin for treatment of anemia in myelodysplastic syndromes and paroxysmal nocturnal hemoglobinuria: A pilot study. Exp Hematol 1990; 18(11): 1204–1208.
138. Bowen D, Culligan D, Jacobs A, The treatment of anaemia in the myelodysplastic syndromes with recombinant human erythropoietin. Br J Haematol 1991; 77(3): 419–423.
139. Stein RS, Abels RI, Krantz SB. Pharmacologic doses of recombinant human erythropoietin in the treatment of myelodysplastic syndromes. Blood 1991; 78(7): 1658–1663.
140. Hellstrom E, et al. Treatment of myelodysplastic syndromes with recombinant human erythropoietin. Eur J Haematol 1991; 47(5): 355–360.

141. Rafanelli D, et al. Recombinant human erythropoietin for treatment of myelodysplastic syndromes. Leukemia 1992; 6(4): 323–327.
142. Casadevall N, et al. High-dose recombinant human erythropoietin administered intravenously for the treatment of anaemia in myelodysplastic syndromes. Acta Haematol 1992; 87 Suppl 1: 25–27.
143. Goy A, et al. High doses of intravenous recombinant erythropoietin for the treatment of anaemia in myelodysplastic syndrome. Br J Haematol 1993; 84(2): 232–237.
144. Stone RM, et al. Therapy with recombinant human erythropoietin in patients with myelodysplastic syndromes. Leuk Res 1994; 18(10): 769–776.
145. Stasi R, et al. Response to recombinant human erythropoietin in patients with myelodysplastic syndromes. Clin Cancer Res 1997; 3(5): 733–739.
146. Isnard F, et al. Efficacy of recombinant human erythropoietin in the treatment of refractory anemias without excess of blasts in myelodysplastic syndromes. Leuk Lymphoma 1994; 12(3-4): 307–314.
147. Di Raimondo F, et al. A good response rate to recombinant erythropoietin alone may be expected in selected myelodysplastic patients. A preliminary clinical study. Eur J Haematol 1996; 56(1-2): 7–11.
148. Sitaraman SV, Gewirtz AT. Oprelvekin. Genetics Institute. Curr Opin Investig Drugs 2001; 2(10): 1395–1400.

Index